Immunopharmacology of Neutrophils

THE HANDBOOK OF IMMUNOPHARMACOLOGY

Series Editor: Clive Page
King's College London, UK

Titles in this series

Cells and Mediators

Immunopharmacology of Eosinophils
(edited by H. Smith and R. Cook)

Immunopharmacology of Mast
Cells and Basophils
(edited by J.C. Foreman)

Lipid Mediators
(edited by F. Cunningham)

Immunopharmacology of
Neutrophils
(edited by P.G. Hellewell and
T.J. Williams)

Immunopharmacology of
Macrophages and Other
Antigen-Presenting Cells
(edited by C.A.F.M. Bruijnzeel-
Koomen and E.C.M. Hoefsmit)

Immunopharmacology of
Lymphocytes
(edited by M. Rola-Pleszczynski)

Adhesion Molecules
(edited by C.D. Wegner,
forthcoming)

Immunopharmacology of Platelets
(edited by M. Joseph, forthcoming)

Systems

Immunopharmacology of the
Gastrointestinal System
(edited by J.L. Wallace)

Immunopharmacology of Joints
and Connective Tissue
(edited by M.E. Davies and
J.T. Dingle)

Immunopharmacology of the Heart
(edited by M.J. Curtis)

Immunopharmacology of Epithelial
Barriers
(edited by R. Goldie)

Immunopharmacology of the
Renal System
(edited by C. Tetta)

Immunopharmacology of the
Microcirculation
(edited by S.D. Brain)

Drugs

Immunotherapy for Immune-
related Diseases
(edited by W.J. Metzger,
forthcoming)

Immunopharmacology of AIDS
(forthcoming)

Immunosuppressive Drugs
(forthcoming)

Glucocorticosteroids
(forthcoming)

Angiogenesis
(forthcoming)

Immunopharmacology of Free
Radical Species
(forthcoming)

Immunopharmacology
of
Neutrophils

edited by

Paul G. Hellewell
and Timothy J. Williams
National Heart and Lung Institute, London, UK

ACADEMIC PRESS
Harcourt Brace and Company, Publishers
London   San Diego   New York
Boston   Sydney   Tokyo   Toronto

ACADEMIC PRESS LIMITED
24/28 Oval Road
London NW1 7DX

United States Edition published by
ACADEMIC PRESS INC.
San Diego, CA 92101

A catalogue record for this book
is available from the British Library

ISBN 0-12-339250-0

Typeset by Mathematical Composition Setters Ltd, Salisbury, Wiltshire
Printed and bound in Great Britain by The Bath Press, Avon

Contents

1. The Neutrophil
P.G. Hellewell *and* T.J. Williams

2. Origin and Development of Neutrophils 5
M.Y. Gordon

6. Molecular Biology of Human Neutrophil Chemotactic Receptors 115

C. Gerard and N.P. Gerard

7. Neutrophil Adhesion Receptors 133

A.J. Wardlaw and G.M. Walsh

8. Receptor-mediated Signal Transduction Pathways in Neutrophils: Regulatory Mechanisms that Control Phospholipases C, D and A_2 159

S. Cockcroft

9. *Priming of Neutrophils* 195

M.J. Pabst

13. *Role of Neutrophils in Adult Respiratory Distress Syndrome and Cryptogenic Fibrosing Alveolitis* 275

S. Braude, T.W. Evans *and* R.M. du Bois

14. *Fate of Neutrophils* 295

J. Savill *and* C. Haslett

Contributors

S. Braude
Critical Care and Pulmonary Medicine
Manly Hospital
Sydney NSW 2095
Australia

C.M. Casimir
Department of Medicine
Rayne Institute
University College and Middlesex School of Medicine
University Street
London WC1E 6JJ, UK

S. Cockcroft
Department of Physiology
Rockefeller Building
University College London
University Street
London WC1E 6JJ, UK

N.S. Doherty
Central Research
Pfizer Inc
Eastern Point Road
Groton, CT 06340
USA

R.M. du Bois
Royal Brompton National Heart and Lung Institute
Emmanuel Kaye Building
Manresa Road
London SW3 6LR, UK

T.W. Evans
Department of Thoracic Medicine
Royal Brompton National Heart and Lung Institute
London, UK

C. Gerard
Department of Pediatrics
Ina Sue Perlmutter Laboratory
Childrens' Hospital
320 Longwood Avenue
Boston, MA 02115, USA

N.P. Gerard
Department of Pediatrics
Ina Sue Perlmutter Laboratory
Childrens' Hospital
320 Longwood Avenue
Boston, MA 02115, USA

M.Y. Gordon
Leukaemia Research Fund Centre
Chester Beatty Laboratories
Fulham Road
London SW3 6JB, UK

C. Haslett
Respiratory Medicine Unit
University of Edinburgh
City Hospital
Greenbank Drive
Edinburgh EH10 5SB, UK

P.G. Hellewell
Department of Applied Pharmacology
Royal Brompton National Heart and Lung Institute
Dovehouse Street
London SW3 6LY, UK

M.J. Janusz
Marion Merrell Dow Research Institute
2110 East Galbraith Road
Cincinnati, OH 45215,
USA

S.R. McColl
Le Centre de Recherche en Inflammation
Immunologie et Rheumatologie
Centre Hospitalier de l'Université Laval
Québec
Canada G1V 4G2

M.J. Pabst
Room 221 Nash Building
894 Union Avenue
Memphis, TN 38163
USA

A.J. Rees
Renal Unit
Department of Medicine
Hammersmith Hospital
Du Cane Road
London W12 0HS, UK

A.G. Rossi
Department of Applied Pharmacology
Royal Brompton National Heart and Lung Institute
Dovehouse Street
London SW3 6LY, UK

C.O.S. Savage
Vascular Immunobiology Group
Centre for Clinical Research in Immunology and
Signalling
The Medical School
University of Birmingham
Edgbaston
Birmingham B15 2TT, UK

J. Savill
Division of Renal and Inflammatory Disease
Department of Medicine
University Hospital
Nottingham NG7 2GH, UK

H.J. Showell
Department of Immunology and Infectious Diseases
Pfizer Central Research
Eastern Point Road
Groton, CT 06340
USA

C.G. Teahan
Department of Medicine
Rayne Institute
University College and Middlesex School of Medicine
University Street
London WC1E 6JJ, UK

G.M. Walsh
Department of Respiratory Medicine
Glenfield General Hospital
Groby Road
Leicester LE3 9QP, UK

A.J. Wardlaw
Department of Respiratory Medicine
Glenfield General Hospital
Groby Road
Leicester LE3 9QP, UK

F.M. Williams
Department of Applied Pharmacology
Royal Brompton National Heart and Lung Institute
Dovehouse Street
London SW3 6LY, UK

T.J. Williams
Department of Applied Pharmacology
Royal Brompton National Heart and Lung Institute
Dovehouse Street
London SW3 6LY, UK

Series Preface

The consequences of diseases involving the immune system such as AIDS, and chronic inflammatory diseases such as bronchial asthma, rheumatoid arthritis and atherosclerosis, now account for a considerable economic burden to governments worldwide. In response to this, there has been a massive research effort investigating the basic mechanisms underlying such diseases, and a tremendous drive to identify novel therapeutic applications for the prevention and treatment of such diseases. Despite this effort, however, much of it within the pharmaceutical industries, this area of medical research has not gained the prominence of cardiovascular pharmacology or neuropharmacology. Over the last decade there has been a plethora of research papers and publications on immunology, but comparatively little written about the implications of such research for drug development. There is also no focal information source for pharmacologists with an interest in diseases affecting the immune system or the inflammatory response to consult, whether as a teaching aid or as a research reference. The main impetus behind the creation of this series was to provide such a source by commissioning a comprehensive collection of volumes on all aspects of immunopharmacology. It has been a deliberate policy to seek editors for each volume who are not only active in their respective areas of expertise, but who also have a distinctly *pharmacological* bias to their research. My hope is that *The Handbook of Immunopharmacology* will become indispensable to researchers and teachers for many years to come, with volumes being regularly updated.

The series follows three main themes, each theme represented by volumes on individual component topics. The first covers each of the major cell types and classes of inflammatory mediators. The second covers each of the major organ systems and the diseases involving the immune and inflammatory responses that can affect them. The series will thus include clinical aspects along with basic science. The third covers different classes of drugs that are currently being used to treat inflammatory disease or diseases involving the immune system, as well as novel classes of drugs under development for the treatment of such diseases.

To enhance the usefulness of the series as a reference and teaching aid, a standardized artwork policy has been adopted. A particular cell type, for instance, is represented identically throughout the series. An appendix of these standard drawings is published in each volume. Likewise, a standardized system of abbreviations of terms has been implemented and will be developed by the editors involved in individual volumes as the series grows. A glossary of abbreviated terms is also published in each volume. This should facilitate cross-referencing between volumes. In time, it is hoped that the glossary will be regarded as a source of standard terms.

While the series has been developed to be an integrated whole, each volume is complete in itself and may be used as an authoritative review of its designated topic.

I am extremely grateful to the officers of Academic Press, and in particular to Dr Carey Chapman, for their vision in agreeing to collaborate on such a venture, and greatly hope that the series does indeed prove to be invaluable to the medical and scientific community.

C.P. Page

Preface

With the invention of the microscope came the first description of "globules" in the blood that differed from other blood cells in that they had the capacity to adhere to the walls of small blood vessels and migrate into the tissues. The predominant population of these cells was subsequently shown to have multilobed nuclei and a cytoplasm neutral to eosin staining. The discovery that these cells had the capacity to phagocytose and kill foreign organisms set the stage for a fascinating research field that continues to stimulate exciting new findings in laboratories throughout the world.

Approximately 10^{11} neutrophils, loaded with potentially destructive proteolytic and oxidative enzymes, set out from the bone marrow of the average man every day. Their life in the circulation is a matter of a few hours. The challenge, in terms of biological mechanisms, is to target these cells to sites of infection or injury with a rapid response time. Thus, neutrophils are equipped with sensors for soluble signals ("chemoattractants") generated in the tissue in response to tissue infection of injury, and sensors for molecules on surfaces. These receptors are important so that the cell can distinguish, for example, activated endothelium to stimulate adherence and emigration, or alternatively the bacterial surface to stimulate phagocytosis and killing. A deficiency in any of these mechanisms can result in life-threatening infection. An over-reaction can result in damage to the tissues that the neutrophil should be programmed to protect. This book addresses the key issues that face the neutrophil during its short but very important life.

We should like to thank all the authors for their scholarly contributions to this volume and hope that readers find what they are looking for amongst its pages.

Paul G. Hellewell
Timothy J. Williams

1. The Neutrophil

P.G. Hellewell and T.J. Williams

1. Introduction

The purpose of this chapter is to introduce the reader to the neutrophil, making reference as much as possible to other chapters in this handbook.

Neutrophils (polymorphonuclear neutrophil leucocytes) constitute approximately half the circulating white cell population in most species, and are characterized by a multilobed nucleus and distinctive cytoplasmic granules. These include primary (azurophilic), secondary (specific) and tertiary granules which contain an armoury of enzymes, proteins and glycosaminoglycans believed to participate in many of the functions of the cell. The primary function of neutrophils is in host defence, specifically the phagocytosis and killing of pathogens in tissues. To fulfil this role, the cell must respond to a chemical signal generated in the affected tissue, interact with and penetrate the vessel wall in the microcirculation, migrate to the site of infection, and recognize, phagocytose and kill foreign cells. These stages represent key elements of neutrophil function. The critical role of neutrophils in host defence is epitomized by patients who suffer from the disease LAD. Neutrophils from these individuals show a deficiency in the CD11/18 group of leucocyte cell adhesion molecules and are unable to accumulate at sites of inflammation, with the result that the patients suffer from life-threatening recurrent bacterial infections (see Chapter 7). Thus, the process of neutrophil accumulation in tissues for the purpose of host defence is essential for survival. Neutrophil accumulation is a controlled event such that inflammatory responses usually resolve acutely with the efficient removal (within days) of the inciting stimulus.

However, if the control mechanisms fail and there is an over-response or the response does not resolve, then neutrophil accumulation and activation can lead to tissue destruction and crippling inflammatory diseases. A detailed understanding of neutrophil functions will provide the potential to target therapeutically neutrophil-mediated disease processes.

The life span of the neutrophil from stem cell to its removal in tissues is approximately 12–14 days (discussed in detail in Chapter 2). A normal adult releases approximately 10^{11} neutrophils per day from the bone marrow into the circulation. The mature neutrophils then egress from the bone marrow into the circulation where they are distributed between the circulating pool and marginating pool (see Chapter 10). The rate of neutrophil egress is controlled by several known pathophysiological factors such as infection and stress, and also by several humoral factors (see Chapter 2). Whether the same factors control neutrophil marrow egress in healthy, uninfected and unstressed individuals is not known. However, mature neutrophils in the marrow constitute an important reserve pool of cells which can be stimulated to enter the blood (for example, by a fall in the neutrophil count in blood perfusing the marrow). This implies a sensitive feedback mechanism whereby neutropenia is sensed in some manner by the bone marrow and initiates the release. Presumably this involves some form of mediator but at this point the mechanism is not known.

Studies using radiolabelled neutrophils suggest that they have a half-life in the blood of approximately 4 h (Price and Dale, 1977). However, to determine the circulation time involves labelling a population of cells of different intrinsic ages and the actual life span of any one neutrophil in the blood is difficult to assess. It is thought that the circulating neutrophils are in dynamic equilibrium with a so-called marginating pool of the cells in the lungs. This marginated pool is a reflection of the different transit times of neutrophils as they pass through the capillary networks of the pulmonary circulation.

Once a neutrophil has migrated into the tissue, its primary purpose is to recognize, phagocytose and destroy pathogens. Phagocytosis comprises two steps; recognition and internalization of microorganisms or particulate matter into the phagosome. Killing or neutralization and subsequent digestion of the material then follows and involves a secretory response. For engulfment to occur, the particle must first be recognized by the neutrophil. In some cases the cell may be able to bind directly to materials such as LPS on the surface of the foreign organism. For the most part, however, the particle must be opsonized by binding of proteins from plasma. These may be either specific (immunoglobulin) or non-specific (e.g. complement, fibronectin, C-reactive protein). The neutrophil then recognizes the bound protein by means of specific receptors (i.e. Fc and complement receptors, CR1 and CR3, which are discussed in Chapter 7).

The intracellular killing of microorganisms generally involves initiation of the respiratory burst with the intraphagosomal release of toxic oxygen metabolites such as hypohalide (particularly hypochlorite, OCl^-), superoxide anion (O_2^-), hydroxyl radical ($^{\cdot}OH$) and hydrogen peroxide (H_2O_2). The importance of this process is seen in patients with CGD whose neutrophils cannot undergo an oxidative burst and are deficient in killing bacteria; these individuals frequently suffer life-threatening infection (discussed in Chapter 3). Oxygen metabolites may also be secreted to the outside of the cell under certain conditions (e.g. during phagocytosis) and a large body of evidence has accumulated for the participation of such metabolites in tissue damage (Henson and Johnston, 1987). Alternative or supplementary mechanisms also exist in the neutrophil for killing bacteria and include a number of unique bactericidal peptides secreted from granules into the phagosome (Chapters 4 and 5). However, some of these also may contribute to tissue injury if released to the outside of the cell.

Secretion of granule contents from neutrophils to the outside of the cell is usually referred to as degranulation and is generally thought to involve a process of exocytosis. However, the cell also actively releases a number of other materials to the outside, including lipid mediators of inflammation. It has become clear in recent years that neutrophils are also capable of gene transcription and synthesis of new proteins; they are therefore a rich source of cytokines including IL-8 but also the IL-1 receptor antagonist (Chapter 5). The mechanisms by which such molecules are released is largely unknown, although a transport process for LTB_4 has been described.

Phagocytosis is a good stimulus for secretion from the neutrophil but despite many observations, the mechanisms by which this occurs have not been fully established (see Henson *et al.* (1988) for full discussion). A role for secretion in the process of neutrophil migration has been proposed, where proteases such as elastase (Chapter 4) may degrade basement membrane and facilitate the movement of cells into tissue (Wright and Gallin, 1979; Huber and Weiss, 1989). Teleologically, a degree of secretion and digestion that was just enough to allow neutrophil migration but not so much as to produce major tissue damage would seem optimal.

As far as agents that induce degranulation are concerned, it should be noted that chemotactic agents (e.g. C5a and FMLP) are themselves poor secretagogues for the neutrophil, at least those cells that have been prepared from the blood in a non-activated state. This usually means that they have not been exposed to LPS which, as discussed in Chapter 9, is very effective at priming neutrophils. Priming is the phenomenon whereby a given mediator which does not induce a response in itself nevertheless alters the reactivity of the neutrophil to other stimuli to enhance their effects. Mediators which induce priming include molecules that can act as direct stimulants at higher concentrations. Priming for superoxide anion release from human neutrophils has been demonstrated (Chapter 9), but similar results are found when examining other neutrophil responses such as adherence, enzyme secretion and lipid mediator synthesis. Many of the studies in the literature use the enhancing agent cytochalasin B to investigate secretion, although its mechanism of action in this context is not fully understood.

The first step in activation of neutrophils is detection of the stimulus. Neutrophils possess receptors on their plasma membrane for a range of mediators, although receptors for all the mediators that activate neutrophils have not been identified. The molecular biology of these is discussed in Chapter 6. There are mediators that act on the neutrophil (Chapters 6 and 10), mediators produced by the neutrophil that may or may not act upon it (Chapter 5), and mediators which prime the neutrophil (Chapter 9).

The events occurring in the neutrophil following interaction of a mediator with its receptor (stimulus–receptor coupling), in particular the role of phospholipase enzymes in delivering intracellular signals which determine the final response of the cell are discussed in Chapter 8.

Neutrophil sequestration or retention in the microvasculature initiates the interaction between the leucocyte and the endothelial cells that is required for migration into the tissue. Direct visualization of the microvasculature (e.g. mesentery and ear chambers) has shown that in the peripheral circulation, the site of neutrophil sequestration and migration is the post-capillary venule where cells have been observed to roll slowly along the walls of vessels (Chapter 10). This rolling process is now known to be mediated by the selectin family of cell adhesion molecules, in particular L-selectin on the leucocyte and E- and P-selectin on the endothelial cell. The pulmonary circulation, however, appears to be an exception and there is accumulating evidence to suggest that neutrophils are sequestered primarily in the capillaries (Chapter 10). Part of this may relate to geometric constraints on the neutrophil as it passes through a pulmonary capillary of smaller diameter causing physical retention at these sites rather than active adhesive processes.

The rolling process does not necessarily lead to neutrophil emigration. The adherence of neutrophils to endothelium needs to become strengthened if emigration is to follow. This is mediated by chemoattractant molecules stimulating neutrophils to change their CD11/CD18 molecules from a non-adhesive conformation to an adhesive one. Firm adhesion to ligands (ICAM-1, ICAM-2) on the endothelial cells then occurs (Chapters 7 and 10).

The passage of neutrophils through the vessel wall was studied in detail by Clark and Clark (1935) who observed the emigration of neutrophils through the endothelium into tissue. This process was rapid, taking only a few minutes. In subsequent ultrastructural studies, Marchesi and Florey (1960) suggested that from an adherent neutrophil, a pseudopodium emerged which penetrated the endothelial cell layer followed by the rest of the neutrophil. A common finding was a neutrophil located between the endothelium and basement membrane, which suggests the latter to be an additional barrier to migration. The neutrophils were thought to emigrate between the endothelial cells, i.e. through the cell junctions. This route is still considered the most likely but definitive proof of such a process is lacking, largely because of the static nature of ultrastructural studies.

The mechanisms by which neutrophils sense a chemotactic gradient and respond by directed locomotion are still relatively poorly understood. The process of chemotaxis has been extensively studied *in vitro*, however, the mechanisms of emigration *in vivo* may be significantly different or at least more complex. For example, the endothelial cell itself is known to contribute significantly to the process of emigration by expressing ICAM–1 (Chapter 10). Moreover, recent observations question the relevance of chemotaxis (along a transendothelial gradient of soluble mediator) to neutrophil accumulation *in vivo* and suggest that haptotaxis (i.e. a surface-bound gradient) is the predominant mechanism. This idea (which was first proposed in the early 1980s (Henson *et al.*, 1981)) has been put forward as a result of experiments which indicate that endothelial cells can bind chemotactic factors and present them to the neutrophil (Rot, 1992; Tanaka *et al.*, 1993).

As discussed above, the primary function of the neutrophil is the phagocytosis and killing of microorganisms. To achieve this, neutrophils adhere to endothelium and migrate into the tissue in response to a stimulus. This

Table 1.1 Diseases in which neutrophils may damage tissues

Organ	Disease
Lung	Adult Respiratory Distress Syndrome
	Asthma
	Asbestosis
	Emphysema
	Idiopathic pulmonary fibrosis
Kidney	Glomerulonephritis
	Interstitial nephritis
Heart	Myocardial reperfusion injury
	Ischaemic heart disease
Joint	Rheumatoid arthritis
	Gout
Gut	Inflammatory bowel disease
Systemic	Scleroderma
	Vasculitis
Others	Burns
	Frostbite
	Dermatitis
	Malignant neoplasms at sites of chronic inflammation

process of inflammation is a protective response of the host and, in general, does not lead to tissue injury (i.e. actual tissue damage and ultimately, cell death). Thus, within a period of days following the initial influx of neutrophils into the tissue, the inflammatory lesion may be completely resolved (see Chapter 14).

In other situations, injury to tissue is more severe and neutrophil accumulation is accompanied by significant changes in the endothelium and morphological evidence of injury (cell destruction). Some of these diseases are listed in Table 1.1, but specific examples are discussed fully in Chapters 11, 12 and 13.

There is a long history of major scientific findings concerned with the neutrophil. There continues to be a considerable international multidisciplinary research effort dedicated to understanding the mysteries surrounding this evanescent cell. We have been fortunate to assemble work from experts who have specialized in different aspects of neutrophil function and are confident that you as the reader will find their contributions comprehensive, informative and interesting.

2. References

Clark, E.R. and Clark E.L. (1935). Observations on changes in blood vascular endothelium in the living animal. Am. J. Anat. 57, 385–438.

Henson, P.M., Webster, R.O. and Henson, J.E. (1981). In Cellular Interactions (eds J.C. Dingle and J.L. Gordon), pp 43–56. Elsevier/North Holland Biomedical Press, Amsterdam.

Henson, P.M., Henson, J.E., Fittschen, C., Kimani, G., Bratton, D.L. and Riches, D.W.H. (1988). In "Inflammation: Basic Principles and Clinical Correlates" (eds J.I. Gallin, I.M. Goldstein and R. Snyderman) pp 363–381. Raven Press, New York.

Henson, P.M. and Johnston, R.B. Jr (1987). Tissue injury in inflammation. Oxidants, proteinases and cationic proteins. J. Clin. Invest. 79, 669–674.

Huber, A.R. and Weiss, S.J. (1989). Disruption of the sub-endothelial basement membrane during neutrophil diapedesis in an in vitro construct of a blood vessel wall. J. Clin. Invest. 83, 1122–1136.

Marchesi, V. and Florey, H.W. (1960). Electron microscope observations on the emigration of leukocytes. Q. J. Exp. Physiol. 45, 343–374.

Price, T.H. and Dale, D.C. (1977). Neutrophil preservation: the effect of short-term storage on in vivo kinetics. J. Clin. Invest. 59, 475–485.

Rot, A. (1992). Endothelial cell binding of NAP-1/IL-8: role in neutrophil emigration. Immunol. Today 13, 291–294.

Tanaka, Y., Adams, D.H. and Shaw, S. (1993). Proteoglycans on endothelial cells present adhesion-inducing cytokines to leukocytes. Immunol. Today 14, 111–115.

Wright, D.G. and Gallin, J.I. (1979). Secretory responses of human neutrophils: exocytosis of specific (secondary) granules by human neutrophils during adherence in vitro and during exudation in vivo. J. Immunol. 123, 285–294.

2. Origin and Development of Neutrophils

M.Y. Gordon

1. Introduction

Neutrophils are complex mature haemopoietic cells that provide a major body defence against infection by microorganisms. They are short-lived cells (their half-life in the circulation is only 6–7 h) and therefore they need to be replaced at a great rate in order to maintain a stable circulating neutrophil count. A person weighing 70 kg will produce about 1×10^{11} neutrophils during each day of adult life and the total weight of neutrophils produced in a lifetime exceeds the adult body weight. Production on this scale is not possible unless there is a precursor pool, from which the mature neutrophils are derived, with a vast capacity for proliferation. These precursor cells are the haemopoietic stem cells and, in fact, are the origin of all mature white cells, red cells and platelets that circulate in the bloodstream (i.e. the stem cells are pluripotent). The development of mature neutrophils

Immunopharmacology of Neutrophils
ISBN 0–12–339250–0

from stem cells involves the processes of differentiation, amplification of cell numbers and cellular maturation. These processes are strictly regulated in order to maintain the neutrophil count within normal limits and this regulation is imposed by soluble haemopoietic growth factors and the microenvironment in which haemopoiesis occurs. The neutrophils must be able to leave the bloodstream and enter the tissues when necessary and this involves the development of mechanisms for migration and cell adhesion (see Chapter 10) and the secretion of matrix-degrading enzymes (Chapter 4). Finally, the acquisition of the apparatus for killing microorganisms completes the requirements for a neutrophil's existence.

In this chapter, I shall address the origin and development of neutrophils in terms of their phylogeny, ontogeny and adult haemopoiesis.

2. Phylogeny of Neutrophil Production

The phylogeny of haemopoiesis has been reviewed by Tavassoli and Yoffey (1983). White blood cells can be related to cells found at a very early stage in the evolution of multicellular organisms. In metazoan sponges, motile phagocytic cells derived from mesenchymal cells are involved in digestion, excretion and clotting. The circulatory system starts to develop in invertebrates and in its simplest form consists of a tube with occasional branches. In some species, there is a pulsatile region that may function as a primitive heart. The localization of blood cells occurs in different sites in different species and in molluscs, for example, the haemopoietic tissue ("white bodies") is found behind the eyes. In piscean evolution, blood islands condense to form a spleen which, in cartilagenous fishes, is the major site of haemopoiesis. In the bony fishes, the kidney is the predominant haemopoietic organ, although granulocytes are also produced in the spleen, intestinal submucosa and periportal pancreatic tissue.

Haemopoietic bone marrow first appears in the frog. However, in frogs, haemopoiesis only occurs transiently in the marrow, immediately after metamorphosis and hibernation. Otherwise, erythropoiesis takes place in the spleen and granulocytes are produced in the kidney and intestinal submucosa. The bone marrow becomes increasingly prominent as a site for haemopoiesis in reptiles, and a sequence of development can be discerned in toads, turtles and lizards. In toads, the spleen is dominant, in turtles the spleen and bone marrow are of equal importance, and in lizards the marrow is dominant. Haemopoiesis becomes restricted to the bone marrow in birds and the marrow:blood barrier imposed by sinusoidal endothelium is a characteristic of mammalian bone marrow. The spleen of lower mammals retains some haemopoietic function but, in adult primates, haemopoiesis occurs exclusively in the bone marrow and extramedullary haemopoiesis is abnormal.

This brief account shows that phylogenetically, as ontogenetically (see below), haemopoiesis does not originate in the bone marrow and that in amphibians and reptiles haemopoiesis is not dependent on the microenvironment provided by the bone marrow.

3. Mammalian Neutrophil Production

The haemopoietic stem cells that are the ultimate source of all mature blood cells cannot be recognized microscopically because of their low incidence in haemopoietic tissue and their undistinguished morphology. Candidate stem cells have been identified morphologically in bone marrow cell populations. They are generally thought to have the appearance of small lymphocytes and have been referred to in the past as small transitional cells (see Tavassoli and Yoffey (1983) for review). These are 7–8 μm in diameter with a high nuclear:cytoplasmic ratio, basophilic cytoplasm and leptochromatic nuclei with one or two nucleoli. Others have referred to candidate haemopoietic stem cells by the operational term "cells meeting our morphological criteria" or CMOMC (Dicke et al., 1973). In humans, they are amongst the population of progenitor cells defined by expression of the CD34 antigen (Greaves et al., 1992). These cells can be purified by flow cytometry or using immunomagnetic beads (Figure 2.1). Experimentally, the presence of stem cells is detected indirectly by placing single cell suspensions of haemopoietic tissue in conditions that will stimulate stem cell proliferation and the maturation of their offspring. Thus, in 1961, Till and McCulloch found that injecting murine bone marrow cells into lethally irradiated syngeneic recipient mice resulted in the formation of colonies of haemopoietic cells on the

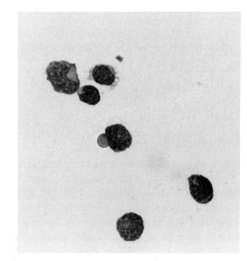

Figure 2.1 Morphology of CD34⁺ human bone marrow cells isolated using immunomagnetic beads (courtesy P.G. Grimsley).

recipients' spleens. Since the lethal irradiation had destroyed the haemopoietic system of the recipient, the colonies must have been produced by some of the injected cells. Some of the colonies consisted of more than one lineage of haemopoietic cell differentiation and the spleen colony assay, or CFU-S assay, became a widely accepted measure of haemopoietic stem cells in mice. Although the principle of ablating haemopoiesis and reconstituting it by injecting viable haemopoietic stem cells is the basis of clinical bone marrow transplantation, this approach is obviously not applicable to studies of haemopoiesis in humans. In man, the existence of equivalent pluripotent stem cells was established by analysing karyotypic or enzyme markers in patients with CML which is a clonal haematological neoplasm derived from a transformed haemopoietic stem cell. In these patients, the Philadelphia (Ph) chromosome abnormality (t9;22) is virtually pathognomic for the disease and is found in the erythroid, granulocytic and megakaryocytic lineages (Fialkow, 1982). Thus, these three lineages arise from a common precursor. Similarly, in CML patients who are G6PD heterozygotes, all haemopoietic lineages express the same type of enzyme showing that they are clones derived from the same original cell. If they were not, the cell populations would express approximately the same amounts of the two possible types of enzyme.

In the mid-1960s, methods were developed for growing colonies of haemopoietic cells from mouse bone marrow cells in semi-solid culture systems. These assays were initiated by suspending bone marrow cells in agar medium supplemented with a conditioned medium that contained CSF. About one per 1000 bone marrow cells

was a target for the CSF and proliferated in response to it. The progeny of the original target cells were unable to migrate far, because of the viscosity of the agar, and formed a colony (Figure 2.2). By 1970, similar colony assays were available for human bone marrow cells. At first, these assays detected the proliferative activity of the precursors for granulocytes and monocytes (colony-forming unit for granulocytes and macrophages (CFU-GM)) but it was not long before assays for the progenitors of the other lineages of haemopoiesis were developed. Alongside this progress, it became apparent that more than one CSF existed and that they stimulated target cells of particular lineages and at particular stages of development (Table 2.1). These CSFs have now been molecularly cloned and those that influence the production of neutrophils are discussed in more detail below. The use of the colony assay systems has been instrumental in building up a hierarchical impression of haemopoietic cell development and it is now possible to envisage the processes involved in neutrophil production in the context of haemopoiesis as a whole (Figure 2.3).

Haemopoiesis in semi-solid cultures is stimulated by the action of haemopoietic growth factors and these systems give no idea about the influence of the haemopoietic microenvironment. Studies of this aspect were facilitated when Dexter et al. (1977) developed the long-term bone marrow culture system which permitted the maintenance of murine haemopoiesis in the presence of cultured stromal cells (Figure 2.4). It is assumed that the stromal cells are the in vitro equivalent of the haemopoietic microenvironment and that their ability to sustain haemopoiesis for a long period of time reflects their importance for haemopoietic regulation in vivo. Similar

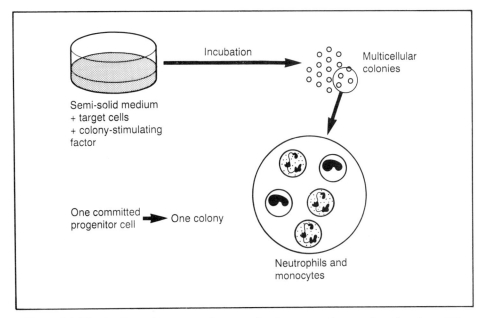

Figure 2.2 The *in vitro* colony assay for granulocyte–macrophage colony-forming cells.

Table 2.1 Haemopoietic growth factors influencing the production of neutrophils

Factor	Abbreviation	Target cells[a]
Granulocyte–macrophage colony-stimulating factor	GM-CSF	**CFU-GEMM, GM and M** CFU-M, Eo and Mk
Granulocyte colony-stimulating factor	G-CSF	**CFU-G**; CFU-M
Macrophage colony-stimulating factor	M-CSF	**GFU-G**; CFU-M
Interleukin-3	IL-3	**Stem cells; GEMM, G and GM**; CFU-M, CFU-Eo; CFU-Mk; mast cells
Interleukin-6	IL-6	**Stem cells**; CFU-Mk; B cells; T cells

[a] Target cells on the neutrophil lineage are indicated in bold print.
Abbreviations are as follows:

CFU-GEMM, colony-forming unit for granulocytes, erythrocytes, monocytes and megakaryocytes; -GM, granulocytes and monocytes; -G, granulocytes; -M, monocytes; -Eo, eosinophils; -Mk, megakaryocytes.

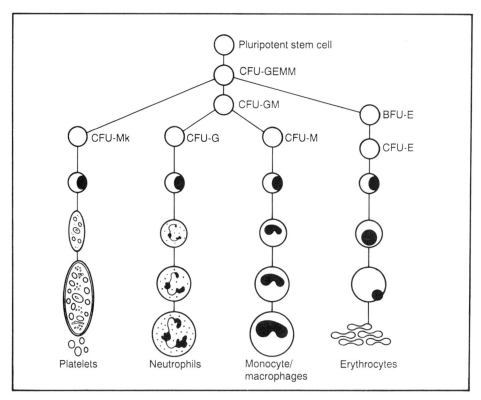

Figure 2.3 Hierarchical scheme for the development of mature blood cells from pluripotent stem cells.

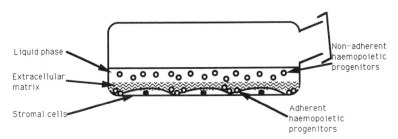

Figure 2.4 The long-term bone marrow culture system.

methods have been developed for the long-term culture of human haemopoietic cells and, although human cultures are not as durable as murine cultures, they have provided valuable information about the interrelationships between stromal cells and haemopoietic cells in haemopoietic tissue.

4. Ontogeny of Human Neutrophil Production

Keleman *et al.* (1979) performed an extensive study of 190 human embryos and fetuses, ranging in gestational age from 3 to 28 weeks. This work was a valuable contribution to understanding the chronology of haemopoiesis during intrauterine human development.

Stem cell migration and seeding in suitable microenvironments is an important principle for the development of the haemopoietic system. In the embryo, haemopoiesis is first established in the mesenchyme of the yolk sac as a consequence of the differentiation of the mesenchymal cells into endothelial cells on the one hand and haemopoietic stem cells on the other. Once the circulation is established, haemopoietic stem cells can be delivered to the embryo and this starts at the beginning of the fourth week of gestation. Thereafter, the stem cells sequentially seed the liver, spleen and bone marrow.

In the yolk sac, haemopoiesis can first be detected on the 18th–19th day of gestation and consists of blood islands, partially or completely surrounded by endothelial cells. At this stage, the haemopoietic cells consist predominantly of primitive primordial cells (haemocytoblasts) in the yolk sac and predominantly more differentiated erythroblastoid cells in the umbilical, chorionic and amniotic vessels. Primitive erythropoiesis persists as the major visible haemopoietic activity in the fetal blood vessels, liver and spleen. However, haemopoiesis also occurs in connective tissue, outside the organs, for most of intrauterine life and large numbers of granulocytes can be found in these sites.

Relatively few granulopoietic cells are produced in the liver and spleen during the early stages of embryonic development and these cells are not produced in large numbers until haemopoiesis is established in the bone marrow. At 7–8 weeks of gestation, neutrophilic promyelocytes and myelocytes account for about 0.2% of all nucleated cells in umbilical cord blood and at 21 weeks for 3% in cardiac blood. Band and segmented neutrophils appear in the blood at 9–10 weeks and increase in number to account for some 16% of total nucleated cells at 21 weeks. In the liver, granulocytes are present in only small numbers for the first 15 weeks but increase in number beyond the 21st week. The granulocytic cells, of both the neutrophilic and eosinophilic series at varying stages of maturation, are found almost exclusively in the connective tissue of the portal spaces. Neutrophilic granulocytes are present in the spleen from the 11th week of gestation and in the bone marrow from the 10th–13th week, where they account for 30–40% of the total nucleated cellularity. Bone marrow haemopoiesis becomes established at different times in different bones. It coincides with the process of ossification which is spread over a long period during fetal development.

The migration of haemopoietic stem cells from the yolk sac to the bone marrow probably involves specific interactions between these cells and cells of the microenvironment. These interactions should govern both the entry and exit of the transit stem cell populations but little is known of how this might be achieved. The microenvironments provided by fetal liver and fetal bone marrow have certain special structural features. First, macrophages are a prominent component of non-hepatic elements in the early stages of human fetal liver development; second, the fat cells that are typical of adult human bone marrow are not found in fetal human bone marrow (Keleman *et al.*, 1979; Keleman and Janossa, 1983). To a large extent, these differences are reproduced in culture since fetal liver cells generate populations of macrophages and fetal marrow cells generate fibroblasts but do not form fat cells (Riley and Gordon, 1987).

An influence of the microenvironment is indicated also by the capacity of fetal liver, spleen and cord blood cells to produce multilineage and granulocytic colonies, as well as erythroid colonies, in semi-solid culture systems (Moore and Williams, 1973; Rowley *et al.*, 1978; Hassan *et al.*, 1979; Barak *et al.*, 1980; Peschle *et al.*, 1981; Hann *et al.*, 1983). This also is consistent with data obtained from *in vitro* cultures which shows that macrophages encourage erythropoiesis whereas fibroblasts encourage granulopoiesis (Westen and Bainton, 1979; Gordon, 1981; Gordon *et al.*, 1983). Also, when human fetal liver is cultured in the long-term culture system, there is a dramatic shift from erythroid to granulocytic cell production. Moreover, granulopoiesis could be sustained for up to a year when fetal liver cells were cultured on preformed adult bone marrow-derived stromal layers (Capellini *et al.*, 1985).

At birth, haemopoietic activity is distributed throughout the human skeleton. During early childhood, significant numbers of granulopoietic colony-forming cells can be detected in the long bones but, in adult life they are found almost exclusively in the sternum and pelvis (Gordon *et al.*, 1976).

5. Neutrophil Production in the Adult

5.1 REGULATION OF NEUTROPHIL DEVELOPMENT BY CYTOKINES

Neutrophil development is regulated by three major haemopoietic growth factors that originally were defined by their biological activities in semi-solid bone marrow culture systems. They are G-CSF, GM-CSF and IL-3 and are necessary for the survival, proliferation and differentiation of their corresponding target cells. In addition to these positive influences on granulopoiesis, negative-feedback regulators that restrain production have been proposed.

Initially, conditioned culture medium, serum from endotoxin-treated animals or tissue extracts were used as sources of the CSFs. These crude preparations turned out, on further investigation, to contain more than one activity attributable to different proteins. It was very difficult to purify the individual CSFs in the various biological sources and it was not possible to define the biological properties of the individual factors until expression cloning and the production of recombinant proteins was achieved.

5.1.1 Granulocyte Colony-stimulating Factor

Murine G-CSF was purified by Nicola et al. (1983) who described a hydrophobic glycoprotein (Mr 24–25 kD) with a neuraminidase-sensitive component and internal disulphide bond(s) which were necessary for biological activity. The purified human G-CSF had similar properties (Nicola et al., 1985) and, in fact, G-CSF differs from GM-CSF and IL-3 in being active on human and murine target cells; the activities of GM-CSF and IL-3 are species-specific.

Souza et al. (1986) cloned a cDNA encoding human G-CSF from the 5637 bladder carcinoma cell line and Nagata et al. (1986a) cloned G-CSF cDNA from a squamous carcinoma cell line. The cDNAs encoded proteins of 174 and 177 amino acids, respectively, and the smaller protein, which had properties very similar to those of native murine G-CSF, was significantly more active than the larger protein. There is a single gene locus of 2.3 kb for human G-CSF (Nagata et al., 1986a,b) located on chromosome 17q11–22 (Le Beau et al., 1987; Simmers et al., 1987). Thus, the localization of the human G-CSF gene is separated from that of haemopoietic growth factors such as GM-CSF, IL-3, IL-4 and IL-5 which are clustered together on the long arm of chromosome 5 (Nicola, 1989).

G-CSF can be produced by many types of cells and production can be induced or amplified by a wide spectrum of stimuli. Monocytes and macrophages are a major source of G-CSF but it can also be produced by normal mesodermal cells such as vascular endothelial cells, fibroblasts and mesothelial cells (Demetri et al., 1989; Zsebo et al. 1988; Koeffler et al., 1987). These cells can be induced to produce G-CSF in vitro by treatment with LPS. TNF, GM-CSF and other cytokines (Herrmann et al., 1986; Koeffler et al., 1987, 1988; Fibbe et al., 1988; Vellenga et al., 1988; Zsebo et al., 1988; Demetri et al., 1989; Ernst et al., 1989; Oster et al., 1989; Wieser et al., 1989). Production of G-CSF in all of these normal cell types is not constitutive but is highly regulated. In contrast, malignant cells may produce

G-CSF constitutively (Gabrilove et al., 1985; Welte et al., 1985; Lilly et al., 1987) and produce haematological changes in solid tumour patients. Transcriptional and post-transcriptional mechanisms (Taniguchi, 1988) have been implicated in the regulation of G-CSF gene expression. Transcriptional regulation is indicated by the identification of regulatory elements upstream of the G-CSF gene (Tsuchiya et al., 1987; Muller et al., 1988; Nishizawa and Nagata, 1990; Nishizawa et al., 1990) whilst post-transcriptional mechanisms are indicated by increases in the half-life of G-CSF mRNA following exposure to inducing agents (Ernst et al., 1989). G-CSF may be regulated coordinately with other cytokine genes, as it is in fibroblasts and mesothelial cells (Koeffler et al., 1988; Demetri et al. 1989, 1990), or independently, as it can be in human blood monocytes (Vellenga et al., 1988; Ernst et al., 1989).

In vitro, the effects of G-CSF on normal haemopoietic cells are primarily restricted to the neutrophil lineage where it stimulates the development of neutrophil colonies and enhances the functions of mature neutrophils (Metcalf and Nicola, 1983). In addition, there is some evidence that G-CSF can affect the proliferation of primitive haemopoietic stem cells if it is added in combination with cytokines such as IL-3 or IL-6 (Ikebuchi et al., 1988; Kateyama et al., 1990). These synergistic effects of combinations of growth factors have been demonstrated in culture systems designed for the formation of colonies by primitive cells that are not in the cell cycle whilst they remain undisturbed in vivo. The in vitro data suggest that the combined actions of G-CSF plus IL-3 or IL-6 shorten the time taken for the resting cells to enter the cell cycle and commence colony formation.

Exposure of human neutrophils to G-CSF in vitro "primes" the neutrophils so that, following exposure to the chemotactic peptide FMLP, superoxide production is increased (Nathan, 1989; Yuo et al., 1990). G-CSF treatment also increases the adherence properties of neutrophils and increases the affinity of the neutrophil cell adhesion molecule, L-selectin (Chapter 7), for its ligand that is involved in binding neutrophils to endothelial cells (Yuo et al., 1989; Spertini et al., 1991). It does not, however, alter the level of L-selectin expression at the cell surface.

In vivo, it is uncertain whether G-CSF plays a role in maintaining normal steady-state haemopoiesis or is important only in states of granulopoietic stress. Normally, the serum levels of G-CSF in humans are below the limit of detection of the most sensitive assay systems available (Watari et al., 1989; Kawakami et al., 1990), suggesting that it may not be important for base rate granulocyte production However, some normal dogs treated with human G-CSF developed neutralizing antibodies. In these dogs, the antibodies cross-reacted with the endogenous canine G-CSF and neutralized it also. The dogs became profoundly neutropenic and this is the strongest piece of evidence that G-CSF is necessary for the maintenance of normal neutrophil numbers (Hammond *et al.*, 1991).

The involvement of G-CSF in stressed granulopoiesis is easier to support. The levels of G-CSF are greatly elevated in infected individuals or patients treated with myelo-toxic chemotherapy and bone marrow transplantation (Watari *et al.*, 1989). Moreover, several situations are associated with reciprocity between G-CSF levels and the neutrophil count, such as recovery from chemotherapy and cyclic neutropenia (Watari *et al.*, 1989), suggesting that G-CSF regulates the circulating neutrophil count during recovery from neutropenia. Very high levels have been contrived by retroviral expression of G-CSF trans-genic mice (Chang *et al.*, 1989a) which, although they develop very high granulocyte counts, do not suffer the toxicity experienced by GM-CSF transgenic mice (see below).

5.1.2 Granulocyte–Macrophage Colony-Stimulating Factor

GM-CSF was first purified from medium conditioned by mouse lung tissue (Burgess *et al.*, 1977) and was found to be a glycoprotein (MW 23–29 kD). Human GM-CSF is also a glycoprotein with an apparent molecular weight of 22 kD (Wong *et al.*, 1985). Initially, the low yield of GM-CSF protein from biological sources delayed cloning of this haemopoietic growth factor but, as a result of reducing the charge heterogeneity by treatment with neuraminidase, sufficient sequence information was obtained (Gough *et al.*, 1984) and human GM-CSF was cloned from the Mo cell line (Golde *et al.*, 1978; Gasson *et al.*, 1984). The human GM-CSF cDNA encodes a polypeptide of 144 amino acids which is glycosylated and which has two intrachain disulphide bonds. Removal of the carbohydrate by mutagenesis or synthesis in bacteria has been shown to increase the biological activity of GM-CSF, but the disulphide bonds are necessary for full activity (De Lamarter *et al.*, 1985; Miyajama *et al.*, 1986; Burgess *et al.*, 1987; Moonen *et al.*, 1987). The gene for human GM-CSF has been mapped to the long arm of chromosome 5 (5q21–q32) (Huebner *et al.*, 1985; Le Beau *et al.*, 1986) and this is particularly interesting because it is the location of several other growth factor and growth factor receptor genes (IL-3, IL-4, IL-5, and M-CSF and its receptor, *c-fms*) (Yang *et al.*, 1988; van Leeuwen *et al.*, 1989). Also, deletion of the long arm of chromosome 5 characterizes the 5q- syndrome which is one of a group of myelodysplastic or "preleukaemic" disorders (Le Beau *et al.*, 1986; Nimer and Golde, 1987).

Activated cells of a variety of types synthesize and secrete GM-CSF. They include T cells and macrophages activated by immunological or inflammatory stimulation (Golde and Cline, 1972; Cline and Golde, 1974; Thorens *et al.*, 1987), and fibroblasts and endothelial cells activated by the monokines IL-1 and TNF (Bagby *et al.*, 1986; Munker *et al.*, 1986; Broudy *et al.*, 1987; Yamato

et al., 1989). These interactions fit in well with the physiological role of GM-CSF in enhancing host defence. Abnormal or increased production of GM-CSF has been reported in certain pathological circumstances. It is expressed by some myeloid leukaemias where it may act as an autocrine stimulator of cell proliferation (Young and Griffin, 1986; Young *et al.*, 1987; Young *et al.*, 1988; Delwel *et al.*, 1989; Salem *et al.*, 1990); it is produced by some solid tumours and may be associated with granulocytosis *in vivo* (Mano *et al.*, 1987; Hocking *et al.*, 1983) and it has been found in the synovial fluid of patients with inflammatory arthropathies where it may be involved in tissue damage associated with inflam-mation (Williamson *et al.*, 1988; Xu *et al.*, 1989). It is relevant that the very high levels of GM-CSF in mice expressing GM-CSF as a transgene or in mice trans-planted with GM-CSF-producing cells cause a lethal syndrome involving macrophage production and accumulation (Lang *et al.*, 1987; Johnson *et al.*, 1989) and that autocrine expression of GM-CSF has been impli-cated as one of a series of stages in the pathogenesis of acute myeloid leukaemia (Laker *et al.*, 1987).

GM-CSF does not circulate in the bloodstream at levels that can be detected and probably is produced and acts locally. Indeed, GM-CSF has been shown to bind to glycosaminoglycans in the extracellular matrix produced by cultured bone marrow stromal cells (Gordon *et al.*, 1987; Roberts *et al.*, 1988). This may represent one mechanism whereby GM-CSF can be localized in the vicinity of its production site and presented to the appropriate target cells.

Expression of GM-CSF is regulated by transcriptional and post-transcriptional controls. The GM-CSF gene is constitutively transcribed in monocytes, endothelial cells and fibroblasts but GM-CSF is not produced because mRNA does not accumulate (Thorens *et al.*, 1987; Koeffler *et al.*, 1988) However, mRNA does accumulate, as a result of increased transcription and stabilization of the mRNA (Seelentag *et al.*, 1987; Kaushansky, 1989; Slack *et al.*, 1990), in cells that have been activated. Thus, abnormalities of mRNA stability could explain the apparent autocrine expression of GM-CSF in some malignant cells (Schuler and Cole, 1988). There have been many approaches to the identification of the regu-latory sequences in the GM-CSF gene. They include comparison of sequences to identify important conserved sequences (Miyatake *et al.*, 1985; Stanley *et al.* 1985), identification of promotor regions and searches for transcription factors (James and Kazenwadel, 1989; Schreck and Baeuerle, 1990; Shannon *et al.*, 1990).

In vitro, GM-CSF operates as a multilineage haemo-poietic growth factor, and stimulates the proliferation and maturation of neutrophil, eosinophil and monocyte precursors (Metcalf *et al.*, 1986; Begley *et al.*, 1988; Emerson *et al.*, 1988; Sonoda *et al.*, 1988). It also stimu-lates proliferation during the early stages of erythroid burst formation and it is now known that the factor formerly called "burst promoting activity" is in fact the same as GM-CSF (Sonoda *et al.*, 1988; Donahue *et al.*, 1985; Emerson *et al.*, 1989). It enhances the functions of neutrophils, eosinophils (Lopez *et al.*, 1986; Silberstein *et al.*, 1986), basophils (Haak-Frendscho *et al.*, 1988; Hirai *et al.*, 1988), macrophages (Handman and Burgess, 1979; Cannistra *et al.*, 1988; Falk *et al.*, 1988), Langerhans cells (Witmer-Pack *et al.*, 1987; Heufler *et al.*, 1988) and possibly lymphocytes (Santoli *et al.*, 1988; Haas *et al.*, 1989). The direct effects of GM-CSF on neutrophils include degranulation, inhibition of migration, effects on the cytoskeleton, changes in cell shape and changes in receptor expression (Gasson *et al.*, 1984; Wiesbart *et al.*, 1985, 1986; Arnaout *et al.*, 1986; Lopez *et al.*, 1986; Richter *et al.*, 1989). Neutrophils "primed" by GM-CSF are more responsive to FMLP (English *et al.*, 1988; Fletcher and Gasson, 1988) and produce greater amounts of inflammatory mediators (Dahinden *et al.*, 1988; DiPersio *et al.*, 1988; Naccache, *et al.*, 1988).

In vivo, the physiological role of GM-CSF appears to be enhancement of host defence mechanisms and its role in homoeostatic neutrophil production is unclear. However, the ability of GM-CSF to improve neutrophil production in neutropenic patients (Donahue *et al.*, 1986; Mayer *et al.*, 1987; Monroy *et al.*, 1987) is central to its therapeutic applications.

5.1.3 Interleukin-3

IL-3 is the factor responsible for most of the haemopoietic growth factor activity in medium conditioned by WEHI-3B myelomonocytic leukaemia cells and by T-lymphocyte-related cells. A cDNA encoding the multi-lineage growth factor IL-3 was isolated from the gibbon T-cell line MLA-144 to obtain the 90% homologous sequence from a human genomic library (Yang *et al.*, 1986). In a separate study, Dorssers *et al.* (1987) exploited a non-coding murine sequence that is highly conserved to obtain a human cDNA clone by hybridization with murine IL-3 cDNA. This strategy was successful despite the fact that the predicted amino-acid sequence of human IL-3 is only 29% homologous with that of murine IL-3. More recently, cDNA clones encoding IL-3 have been isolated from a human T-cell library (Otsuka *et al.* 1988).

In vitro, IL-3 acts as a multilineage haemopoietic growth factor but appears to act on earlier stages of haemopoiesis than the other colony-stimulating factors (Bot *et al.*, 1988). *In vivo* in mice, high levels of IL-3 cause a myeloproliferative syndrome but this is not a malignant condition (Chang *et al.*, 1989b).

Murine IL-3 is a monomeric glycoprotein of MW 23 000–32 000 D of which about 40% is carbohydrate. There are four potential glycosylation sites and variable glycosylation probably accounts for the range of molecular weights that have been reported. Although glycosylation is not necessary for biological activity

in vitro, it may modify the kinetics of IL-3 *in vivo*. Divergence of the IL-3 gene during evolution has resulted in less homology between species than is found for the other haemopoietic growth factors. Comparison of the sequences for different species indicates that a conserved disulphide bridge found in murine and primate IL-3 is important for protein structure and function. There are two potential sites for N-linked glycosylation in human IL-3 and up to 50% of the recombinant molecule is carbohydrate (see Stocking and Ostertag (1990) for references.). Along with several other haemopoietic growth factors (see above), the gene for IL-3 has been mapped to human chromosome 5q.

In spite of the evidence obtained from *in vitro* studies, little is known of the production site(s) or role(s) of IL-3 *in vivo*. Evidence for its cellular production rests almost exclusively on studies using activated T cells and normal cells that constitutively express low levels of IL-3 have not been detected.

5.1.4 Negative Feedback Regulation of Granulopoiesis

The regulation of many biological systems involves mechanisms for negative feedback so that the final end-product inhibits excessive production by its progenitor or precursor. Such activities have been sought in relation to neutrophil production and a granulocyte chalone (i.e. a tissue-specific inhibitor) produced by mature neutrophils has been described (Foa *et al.*, 1982). In addition, neutrophil-derived lactoferrin and acidic isoferritins have been implicated (Broxmeyer, 1982), but their precise role is unclear.

5.2 CYTOKINE RECEPTORS ON NEUTROPHILS AND THEIR PRECURSORS

Each haemopoietic growth factor interacts with a specific, saturable, high-affinity receptor at the target cell surface. The molecular characterization of the growth factor receptors has shown that they can be grouped into families. Receptors for GM-CSF and IL-3 belong to the large "haematopoietin receptor superfamily" (Cosman *et al.*, 1990). The major region of homology resides in a stretch of 210 amino acids in the extracellular binding domain which, in all members, contains four cysteine residues and a sequence of five amino acids (WSXWS) just outside of the membrane spanning region. The G-CSF receptor has the 210 amino-acid sequence characteristic of the haematopoietin receptor superfamily but there is also an N-terminal immunoglobulin domain. By these criteria, the G-CSF receptor has features of the immunoglobulin superfamily as well as features of the haematopoietin receptor superfamily (Figure 2.5).

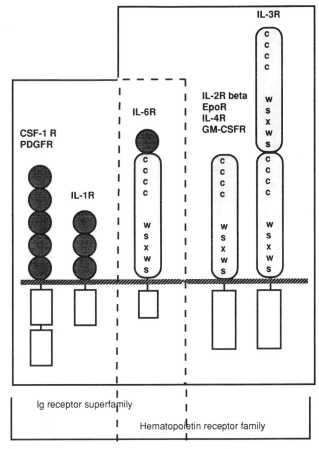

Figure 2.5 Relationships between the haemopoietic growth factor receptor gene families.

5.2.1 Granulocyte Colony-stimulating Factor Receptor

Receptors for G-CSF were first studied on murine cells by Nicola and Metcalf (1984, 1985) and similar receptors are found on human cells (Nicola *et al.*, 1986). The receptors are present on all stages of neutrophil development from the colony-forming cell to the mature neutrophil and on some monocytes. These receptors are not expressed by cells of the erythroid or megakaryocytic lineages. Mature neutrophils have the highest number of G-CSF receptors per cell and there is a general correlation between G-CSF receptor numbers and cellular maturation. The G-CSF binding site on human neutrophils, using murine G-CSF as a ligand, has an apparent K_d of 900 pmol/l and there are between 700 and 1500 receptors per cell. Two cDNAs encoding the human G-CSF receptor have been cloned from cDNA libraries obtained from human placenta (Larsen *et al.*, 1990). One predicted a protein of 759 amino acids whilst the other, which had a greater homology with the murine G-CSF receptor, predicted a protein of 812 amino acids. These two proteins appear to result from alternative processing of the same gene product. The extracellular domain contains several

sequences that are reminiscent of other, otherwise unrelated, proteins and this type of composite structure is characteristic of several cytokine receptor molecules. In particular, the G-CSF receptor has the characteristic properties of the "haematopoietin receptor superfamily" (four conserved cysteines and a WSXWS sequence near to the cell membrane). Also, there are sequences that are similar to sequences found in fibronectin type III, the prolactin receptor and N-CAM, and there is an N-terminal immunoglobulin-like domain. The human G-CSF receptor gene has been mapped to chromosome 1p32–34 where it is telomeric to the CSF-1 (M-CSF), jun and TCL-5 loci (Tweady *et al.* 1992).

5.2.2 Granulocyte–macrophage Colony-stimulating Factor Receptor

Walker and Burgess (1985) first characterized the GM-CSF receptor on murine myelomonocytic cells and their results of ^{125}I-labelled GM-CSF suggested that the cells expressed two classes of receptor of high and lower affinity respectively. Neutrophil GM-CSF receptors, on the other hand, are represented by a single high affinity class of binding sites (K_d 50 pmol/l). The numbers of receptors per cell are quite low (800–1000) but the highest numbers are expressed on the most mature polymorphonuclear neutrophils (Gasson *et al.*, 1986). Recombinant human GM-CSF-binding protein, encoded by cDNA obtained from a placental cDNA library (Gearing *et al.*, 1989), is a protein with a large open reading frame of 400 amino acids (Mr 85 kD) and is a member of the "haematopoietin receptor superfamily". Transfection of the cDNA into COS cells and ^{125}I-GM-CSF binding studies showed that the binding protein was of the lower affinity. This, plus the fact that GM-CSF and IL-3 can apparently compete for the same receptor to a certain extent (see below), has led to the suggestion that the GM-CSF receptor, like the IL-2 and IL-6 receptors, consist of multiple subunits. Further, it is suggested that the competition between GM-CSF and IL-3 results from competition for a shared subunit.

5.2.3   Interleukin-3 Receptors

An IL-3-binding component of the murine IL-3 receptor has been cloned and is a member of the haematopoietin receptor superfamily in which the characteristic extra-cellular domain is duplicated (Itoh *et al.*, 1990). The protein expressed in COS cells or fibroblasts showed specific low-affinity binding of IL-3 with no ligand-dependent receptor internalization and no tyrosine phosphorylation in IL-3-stimulated transfected cells. The cytoplasmic domain lacks a consensus sequence for tyrosine kinase activity and this finding, plus the low binding affinity of IL-3, suggests that additional components are necessary for the functional high-affinity IL-3 receptor. These have been identified as β components and appear to be shared between the GM-CSF and IL-3 receptors in human cells whereas murine cells express two distinct β subunits (Kitamura *et al.*, 1991a,b).

5.3   SIGNAL TRANSDUCTION IN NEUTROPHIL DEVELOPMENT

The process of signal transduction involves complex bio-chemical pathways that link the binding of growth factors to their cell surface receptors with their effects on gene expression in the nucleus. In spite of recent progress, the sequence of signals that links these two events is poorly understood although two important pathways, the phosphoinositide pathway and the pathway initiated by tyrosine kinase activity, have been identified. Signal transduction mechanisms in neutrophils are discussed in detail in Chapter 8.

The sequence of the G-CSF receptor does not suggest that it can function as a kinase and the mechanisms responsible for signal transduction via this receptor are unknown (Larsen *et al.*, 1990). It is possible that, like the IL-6 receptor (Kishimoto, 1989), the G-CSF receptor associates with another unknown component in the cell membrane in order to be able to transduce a signal.

Human neutrophils exposed to G-CSF do not display any signs of the several indicators of signal transduction such as an increase in the concentration of intracellular calcium ions, the electrical potential across the membrane or intracellular pH. However, exposure to G-CSF does seem to induce the release of arachidonic acid from membrane phospholipids, possibly as a consequence of rapid activation of a phospholipase. Neutrophils exposed to G-CSF do not translocate protein kinase C from the cytoplasm to the cell membrane. There is, however, a transient increase in the intracellular levels of cAMP (Sullivan *et al.*, 1987; Matsuda *et al.*, 1989).

Serine and tyrosine phosphorylation stimulated by GM-CSF binding to its receptor (Morla *et al.*, 1988; Sorensen *et al.*, 1989) must be an indirect effect because the GM-CSF-binding protein does not have kinase activity. Other signal transduction pathways that have been implicated in responses to GM-CSF involve guanine nucleotide-binding proteins (Coffey *et al.*, 1988; McColl *et al.*, 1989) but the role of these mediators is not well understood.

5.4   THE MICROENVIRONMENTS FOR NEUTROPHIL DEVELOPMENT

The various stages in the lifetime of a neutrophil are distributed between three environments. Neutrophil production to the stage of terminal maturation occurs in the bone marrow; cells are released from the storage pool in the marrow into the peripheral blood where they circulate for some hours and, finally, they enter the tissues where they probably live for 1–2 days (see Chapter 14 for a discussion on the fate of neutrophils). The controlled movement of the stages in neutrophil production from one compartment to another implies that the cells interact differently with their surrounding microenvironment at different stages in their development. At least part of this migratory process can be explained by adhesive interactions with microenvironmental cells and there is a growing body of evidence to support the proposal that the adhesive properties of haemopoietic progenitor cells alter as the cells mature.

In the bone marrow, the earliest haemopoietic stem cells are found close to the subendothelial layer of the marrow cavity. These early cells appear to be the most adhesive of the progenitor cells and bind to plastic *in vitro* (Gordon, 1988; Kiefer *et al.*, 1991). These primitive cells can also be shown to bind to cultured bone marrow-derived stromal cells (Gordon, 1988; Ploemacher *et al.*, 1991) but there is also a distinct population that binds only to stroma and not to plastic.

The physiological significance of binding to plastic is unclear but it is reasonable to suggest that binding to stromal cells is relevant to the localization of haemo-poietic cell development in the marrow cavity and the fact that transplanted (i.e. intravenously infused) stem cells can "home" to the bone marrow and reconstitute depleted haemopoietic tissue (Gordon and Greaves, 1989). These associations led to experimental investigation of binding interactions between haemopoietic progenitors and cultured stromal cells *in vitro*. A particular class of haemopoietic progenitor, the blast colony-forming cell or Bl-CFC, binds avidly to cultured stroma and forms colonies. This system, therefore, provides a suitable experimental model for investigating cellular interactions (Gordon and Greaves, 1989).

The mechanism for binding Bl-CFCs to stroma seems to involve a combination of receptors (cell adhesion molecules) and their respective ligands. It requires the formation of a specific HS-PG in the extracellular matrix of the stromal cells that is induced by growing the stromal cells in the presence of methylprednisolone (Siczkowski *et al.*, 1992). The Bl-CFCs bind to the HS-PG via a PI-anchored cell adhesion molecule whose expression is regulated by treatment with haemopoietic growth factors (Gordon *et al.*, 1991). The engagement of the PI-achored adhesion molecule with the HS-PG is thought to be a specific recognition event that occurs early in the binding interaction and is of sufficiently high affinity to overcome mutually repulsive negative charges at the cell surfaces. This facilitates the engagement of further, uncharacterized, cell adhesion molecules with their cognate ligands and strengthening of the bond between the cells (Siczkowski *et al.*, 1992). Other requirements for binding of Bl-CFCs do not include the presence of divalent cations or serum (Gordon *et al.*, 1990).

The majority of committed haemopoietic progenitor cells, including the CFU-GM, do not bind to either plastic or to cultured stroma and can be considered "non-adherent" according to this functional classification (Gordon, 1988). However, these haemopoietic progenitor cells are retained in the marrow *in vivo* and are found amongst stromal cells in long-term marrow cultures *in vitro*. Thus, whilst they do not adhere to plastic or to cultured stromal layers, they are obviously capable of some interaction with their microenvironment (Gordon, 1988). Also, haemopoietic progenitors express the integrin molecule, VLA-4, and other cell adhesion molecules which give them further potential for adhesive interactions (see Long (1992) for review). It seems likely that granulopoietic cells retain some capacity for interaction with the marrow microenvironment until they mature to the polymorphonuclear stage and are released into the bloodstream.

There is a large storage pool of neutrophils in the bone marrow that is equivalent in size to some 30 times the circulating leucocyte mass. The egress of neutrophils from the bone marrow spaces into the venous sinuses is related to the capacity of the mature cells to move in an amoeboid fashion between the endothelial cells by a process known as diapedesis. In the blood, neutrophils circulate for a relatively short period of time and are lost in a random fashion from the vascular compartment. This compartment can be divided into a circulating pool and the so-called marginated pool of cells (see Chapter 10).

5.5 MORPHOLOGICAL AND CYTOCHEMICAL DEVELOPMENT OF NEUTROPHILS

The granulocyte progenitor cells (CFU-GM) in the bone marrow produce myeloblasts which in turn differentiate via several recognizable morphological stages into mature non-dividing polymorphonuclear neutrophils. These morphological changes partly occur because of the acquisition of granules which serve to isolate enzymes required for the destruction of microorganisms and other functions. These enzymes, if free in the cytoplasm, would be damaging to the cell. The granules and their contents confer characteristic staining properties on the neutrophils and changes in morphology and cytochemistry are therefore considered together. The stages in neutrophil development are represented by the myeloblasts, promyelocytes, myelocytes, band cells and polymorphonuclear neutrophils.

Myeloblasts are undifferentiated cells with a high nuclear:cytoplasmic ratio. The nucleus is large and oval, and nucleoli are prominent. The reaction product for peroxidase is present in the cytoplasm in the RER, in the Golgi apparatus and in the occasional precocious azurophilic (primary) granule. These granules contain myeloperoxidase and are formed mainly in the promyelocytes but are not found after the myelocyte stage. The contents of the azurophilic granules are listed in Table 2.2.

Promyelocytes produce and accumulate large numbers of mainly spherical peroxidase-positive azurophilic granules and peroxidase-positive material is present also throughout the RER and the Golgi. At the onset of myelocyte differentiation, peroxidase-staining disappears from the RER and the Golgi, and the production of azurophilic granules ceases. The myelocyte stage begins with the formation of peroxidase-negative specific (secondary) granules which are formed by the Golgi complex and are typically spherical or rod shaped. Their contents are also listed in Table 2.2. The myelocyte can undergo about three cell divisions and the granules are fairly equally divided amongst the daughter cells.

The myelocyte stage is the final mitotic stage in neutrophil development. The identifying features of the non-dividing metamyelocytes, band cells and polymorphs are their characteristic nuclear morphology, their mixed primary and secondary granule population, and small Golgi region. The peroxidase-positive azurophilic granules and peroxidase-negative specific granules are distinct entities. Specific granules are twice as numerous as azurophilic granules in mature polymorphs because

Table 2.2 Contents of azurophilic and specific granules from human neutrophils

		Azurophilic granules	Specific granules
Microbicidal enzymes		Myeloperoxidase	Lysozyme
		Lysozyme	
Neutral proteinases		Elastase	Collagenase
		Cathepsin G	
		Proteinase 3	
Acid hydrolases		β-Glycerophosphatase	
		β-Glucuronidase	
		N-acetyl-β-glucosaminidase	
		α-Mannosidase	
		Cathepsins B and D	
Miscellaneous		Cationic proteins	Lactoferrin
		Defensins	Vitamin B12 binding proteins
		Bacterial permeability increasing protein	Plasminogen activator
		Azurophil-derived bacterial factors	Histaminase
			FMLP, C3bi, and laminin receptors
			Cytochrome *b*

azurophilic granule production ceases after the promyelocyte stage and are diluted by cell division and because production of specific granules continues in the daughter myelocytes.

The specific granules are small and cannot be resolved by light microscopy. They are responsible for the pink coloration of the neutrophil cytoplasm in Romanowsky-stained blood smears. The violet-coloured granules in mature neutrophils are, in fact, azurophilic primary granules whose staining properties have been altered during cellular maturation.

5.6 FUNCTIONAL DEVELOPMENT OF NEUTROPHILS

The ability of the neutrophil to kill microorganisms depends on a complicated series of events (see Chapter 3) involving phagocytosis and the generation of toxic oxygen derivatives produced by the respiratory burst (Holmes *et al.*, 1967; Boxer *et al.*, 1974). They undergo liquefaction and form pus in the process. These functions are not expressed by myeloblasts but are acquired as the cells mature. Their development appears to be associated with the development of specific granules (Segel *et al.*, 1987). Indeed, there is a correlation between respiratory burst activity and content of cytochrome *b* which has been shown to be located in the membrane of specific granules (Borregaard and Herlin, 1982). The capacity to phagocytose complement-opsonized particles also correlates with the development of specific granules and may be associated with the location of C3bi receptors in the membranes of the specific granules (Todd *et al.*, 1984; Segel *et al.*, 1987).

5.7 KINETICS OF NEUTROPHIL PRODUCTION

The lifetime of a neutrophil is spent sequentially in the bone marrow, peripheral blood and the tissues, and this distribution provides a spatial framework for discussing the kinetics of neutrophil development. Also, stages in neutrophil development can be divided into the mitotic or proliferating compartment, the maturation compartment and the storage compartment (Figure 2.6). Neutrophil kinetics have been studied using a range of techniques. Labelling with radioisotopes is the most widely applicable method for studying the production, distribution and fate of neutrophils, and commonly uses ^{3}HTdR, diisopropyl fluorophosphate DF^{32}P and radioactive chromium (^{51}Cr). These different reagents all have advantages and disadvantages. Tritiated thymidine is selectively incorporated into the DNA of dividing cells and is ideal for autoradiography but cannot be used for *in vivo* studies of human granulopoiesis. Labelled DF^{32}P binds to granulocytes and monocytes, but not appreciably to other white cells, and can be used as an *in vivo* or *in vitro* label. Similarly, ^{51}Cr is used as a leucocyte label and allows surface monitoring of its γ emission. However, ^{51}Cr labels cells indiscriminately and elutes easily from the cells. The information about neutrophil kinetics has been thoroughly reviewed (Dancey *et al.*, 1976; Vincent, 1977; Cronkite, 1979). Other, less widely applicable, methods include depletion or destruction of granulocytes to measure the size and mobilization kinetics of reserves; determination of the mitotic index of myeloid precursor cells and the induction of inflammatory

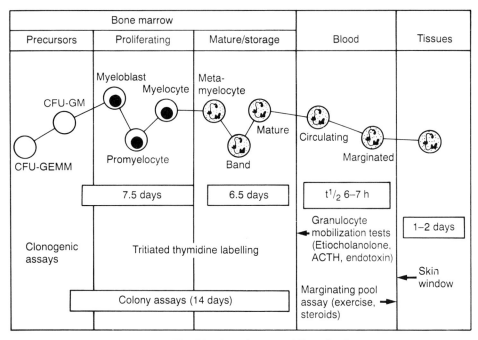

Figure 2.6 The kinetics of neutrophil production.

lesions to evaluate the rate of migration into damaged tissues.

In the bone marrow, stem cell and CFU-GM kinetics are largely undefined and it is not yet possible to assess accurately the size of the stem-cell pool in humans. Although attempts to analyse the detailed kinetic parameters of the stem-cell pool have led to discordant information (see Cronkite, 1979), some features have been established. The majority of stem cells in the stem-cell compartment are normally quiescent. When they do divide, they are capable of producing, overall, equal numbers of stem-cell progeny and progeny destined to differentiate. As a result of the equal balance between self-replication and differentiation at the stem cell level, the size of the stem-cell pool is normally static. The idea that the pluripotent stem-cell compartment is capable of perpetual self-renewal has largely given way to the impression that there is an age structure in the stem-cell compartment such that stem cells that have a history of mitosis have a relatively reduced life-span compared with stem cells that have not divided as many times or have not divided at all. This is compatible with the concept that the stem cells with a mitotic history are preferentially directed to enter one or another of the differentiation pathways and are replaced by cells that are, mitotically, one step behind them. In essence, this means that haemopoiesis is sustained by clonal succession at the stem cell level. The later progenitors of neutrophils, the CFU-GM, are in more active cell cycle as judged by the [3]HTdR suicide technique. These cells still have the potential to differentiate into neutrophils or monocytes but rapidly become committed to one or the other of these lineages.

Identifiable marrow neutrophils belong to the proliferating, maturing and storage compartments. The morphologically recognizable proliferating granulocytes include the myeloblasts, promyelocytes and myelocytes, all of which are capable of cell division. The metamyelocytes and mature polymorphonuclear neutrophils do not divide. About 4–5 cell divisions occur between the myeloblast and the metamyelocyte in the proliferating compartment, and three of them may occur at the myelocyte stage, although this number may not be fixed.

The myelocyte pool is at least four times the size of the promyelocyte pool which indicates that the major increase in neutrophil number occurs at the myelocyte level. It is difficult to provide a precise dynamic model of the kinetics of the human proliferating granulocyte pool but some estimates of the marrow neutrophil compartments, transit times and proliferation kinetics have been made (see Cronkite, 1979; Table 2.3).

6. Abnormalities of Neutrophil Development

Neutrophil disorders can be very variable but can be broadly divided into conditions that are quantitative (i.e. the neutrophil count is decreased or increased) and those that are qualitative (i.e. dysfunction of some aspect of neutrophil behaviour). Clearly, the complexity of the neutrophil provides the background, for example, for defects in adhesion, locomotion, phagocytosis and

Table 2.3 Kinetic parameters of marrow neutrophil production

	Mitotic index (%)	Cells in S phase (%)	Transit time (h)	Total cells/kg × 10^{-9}
Mitotic cells				
Myeloblasts	2.5	85	23	0.14
Promyelocytes	1.5	65	26–78	0.51
Myelocytes	1.1	33	17–126	1.95
Maturing/ stored cells				
Metamyelocytes	0	0	8–108	2.7
Bands	0	0	12–96	3.6
Polymorphs	0	0	0–120	2.5

microbial killing. It is not possible here to cover all of the disorders involving abnormalities in neutrophil development, only to give selected examples.

6.1 NEUTROPENIA

Neutropenia due to decreased granulocyte production can occur either as an isolated deficiency or in combination with other cytopenias. The most severe and striking example of the latter conditions is aplastic anaemia in which production of red cells, white cells and platelets is dangerously reduced. The major clinical manifestation of neutropenia is a marked increase in susceptibility to infection. Neutropenia can be predicted when patients are treated with cytotoxic therapy or it may be congenital, constitutional or idiopathic. Some examples are summarized below.

6.1.1 Congenital Neutropenia

The congenital neutropenias are a heterogeneous group of disorders that may be benign or aggressive, stable or cycling. The haematological manifestations are variable and they may be associated with other phenotypic abnormalities.

Kostmann's syndrome is a congenital neutropenia involving agranulocytosis, monocytosis and maturation arrest at the promyelocyte–myelocyte stage in the marrow. However, the numbers and affinities of the G-CSF receptors appear normal (Kyas *et al.*, 1992) and the cells in granulocyte colonies mature normally despite the maturation arrest that occurs *in vivo* (Falk *et al.*, 1977). Normal granulocytic colony formation *in vitro* in the absence of any demonstrable inhibitors of granulopoiesis provides indirect evidence for a microenvironmental defect (Wreidt *et al.*, 1970; Amato *et al.*, 1976). However, Kostmann's syndrome has been successfully treated by bone marrow transplantation (Rappeport *et al.*, 1980) which suggests that the microenvironment in the marrow of these patients is normal.

Schwachmann Diamond syndrome is a congenital trilineage cytopenia that is accompanied by exocrine pancreatic insufficiency and skeletal abnormalities. Cartilage–Hair syndrome and Chediak–Higashi syndrome are associated with mild to moderate neutropenia and, on the one hand, impaired T-cell formation, dwarfism and very fine hair, and on the other hand, partial occulo-cutaneous albinism and neuropathies.

Family studies have demonstrated that granulopoiesis is abnormal in some parents of children with congenital neutropenia. In one family, only the mother was affected. In another family, cells from both parents differentiated abnormally *in vitro* whilst, in a third, marrow from both parents contained reduced numbers of CFU-GM (Rich *et al.*, 1977; Chusid *et al.*, 1980).

6.1.2 Cyclic Neutropenia

Cyclic neutropenia is characterized by fluctuations in the reticulocyte and platelet counts, as well as fluctuations in the neutrophil count, with a remarkably constant periodicity of about 3 weeks (reviewed by Lange, 1983). Susceptibility to infections is increased during the periods of neutropenia. The probable origin of the condition from a defect in haemopoietic stem cells was indicated when a patient was given a bone marrow transplant from a donor with cyclic neutropenia and subsequently developed the disorder (Krance *et al.*, 1982) and it is thought to reflect a regulatory abnormality at the stem cell level. No abnormalities of G-CSF receptors, in terms of numbers or affinities, have been demonstrated (Kyas *et al.*, 1992) and cyclic neutropenia has been effectively treated with recombinant G-CSF (Hammond *et al.*, 1989).

6.1.3 Constitutional Neutropenia

Yemenite Jews and people of African origin have a stable genetic neutropenia associated with a normal myeloid: erythroid ratio in the marrow and no relative increase in immature cells ("shift to the left"). The incidence of colony-forming cells (CFU-GM) in the marrow is about twice the normal and the cells do not display any morphological abnormalities (Mintz and Sachs, 1973). Neutropenia in these individuals could be due to the defective release of neutrophils from the bone marrow, to destruction of neutrophils at the periphery or to subnormal corticosteroid production (Schoenfield *et al.*, 1983).

A second cause of peripheral neutropenia is accelerated neutrophil destruction. This occurs in a group of auto-immune neutropenias which may be idiopathic or drug induced and characterizes disorders such as Felty's syndrome and SLE. Felty's syndrome is a triad of symptoms, described by Felty (1924). Neutropenia may be caused by excessive margination in some patients (Vincent *et al.*, 1974) and reduced production in others.

Third, a condition referred to as "pseudoneutropenia" is caused by abnormalities in the distribution of neutrophils.

6.2 LEUCOCYTE ADHESION DEFICIENCY

This inherited disorder involves defective cell adhesion and has now been well characterized. The affected individuals are deficient in the leucocyte adhesion molecules LFA-1, Mac-1 and P150,95. This is caused by a mutation in the common β chain of these hetero-dimeric $\alpha\beta$ integrin molecules which consists of a single amino-acid substitution in the ligand-binding domain. The patients suffer life-threatening bacterial and fungal infections, and severely affected individuals rarely survive beyond childhood. Their neutrophils do not orient and migrate in response to chemotactic stimuli or emigrate to skin windows, and cannot cross vascular endothelium. They are, therefore, unable to manufacture pus and this has been confirmed by examining surgical biopsies from sites of bacterial infection in LAD patients. The existence of LAD is the most dramatic demonstration of the importance of neutrophil adhesion via integrin molecules. Interestingly, other cell adhesion mechanisms on neutro-phils appear to be intact in LAD patients and intra-alveolar accumulations have been found, post mortem, in the lung of a severely affected LAD patient but not in extravascular sites of infection in the skin or gut. It is thought that a different mechanism is responsible for neutrophil emigration into the lungs (see Chapter 10).

6.3 INFLAMMATORY DISORDERS

Trafficking of phagocytic cells across vessel walls is essen-tial for defence against microbial infection and tissue repair but can, in certain circumstances, cause tissue injury (see Chapter 10). Aggregation of cells in the vessel lumen is suggested to result in ischaemia and potentially injurious products, such as oxidants, enzymes, phospho-lipase products and cytokines are released during the processes of cell activation, binding to endothelium and transendothelial migration. Mechanisms of this type have been implicated in a variety of clinical disorders. It is

possible that some conditions might be counteracted by "anti-adhesion" therapy using monoclonal antibodies to prevent adhesion and, since cells that do not bind to endothelium cannot enter the tissues, thus prevent tissue damage (see Chapter 10).

6.4 CHRONIC GRANULOMATOUS DISEASE

There are X-linked and rarer autosomal recessive forms of CGD, both of which affect components of the NADPH oxidase system which results in failure of microbicidal activity following phagocytosis (see Chapter 3). Diagnosis is made by the failure of neutrophils to reduce NBT following stimulation of the intracellular oxidase system by PMA The autosomal recessive forms may have a tendency to be less severe clinically, but serious morbidity and mortality can occur in all forms of CGD.

Bone marrow transplantation has been used success-fully to treat CGD (Rappeport *et al.*, 1982). Anti-microbial prophylaxis remarkably improves the outlook for these patients and γ-interferon may further reduce their susceptibility to infection (International Chronic Granulomatous Disease Study Group, 1991).

6.5 GRANULE ABNORMALITIES

6.5.1 Congenital Dysgranulopoietic Neutropenia

The condition involves defective synthesis or degenera-tion of azurophilic/primary granules, absence or marked deficiency of specific/secondary granules and autophagia (Parmley *et al.*, 1980). There are normal numbers of granulocytic colony-forming cells in the peripheral blood and bone marrow,and the levels of colony-stimulating activity also are normal, although the morphological abnormalities seen *in vivo* also occur in the cultured cells. There are no demonstrable antibodies or inhibitors of granulopoiesis and the condition is best described as an intrinsic progenitor cell defect.

6.5.2 Hereditary Myeloperoxidase Deficiency

The azurophilic granules of the neutrophils and mono-cytes lack MPO (Kitahara *et al.*, 1981). This deficiency occurs in 1/2000–1/5000 people and is not usually associated with any clinical abnormalities. The carrier state, or partial MPO deficiency, is inherited in an autosomal dominant fashion. Total MPO deficiency impairs the bacteriocidal functions of the neutrophils.

6.5.3 Auer Bodies

These are found in some blast cells in AML. They are abnormally large, elongated azurophilic granules con-taining peroxidase, lysosomal enzymes and crystalline inclusions (Bainton *et al.*, 1971).

6.5.4 Chediak–Higashi Syndrome

This is a rare autosomal recessive disorder characterized by oculocutaneous albinism, increased susceptibility to infection and abnormally large granules in most granular cells (Rausch *et al.*, 1978).

6.6 NUCLEAR ABNORMALITIES

Abnormalities of the nucleus occur in the Pelger–Huet anomaly (failure of nuclear lobe formation), in folate and vitamin B12 deficiency (hypersegmentation) and in severe alcoholism (formation of ring nuclei).

7. *References*

Amato, D., Freedman, M.H. and Saunders, E.F. (1976). Granulopoiesis in severe congenital neutropenia. Blood 47, 531–538.

Arnaout, M.A., Wang, E.A., Clark, S.C. and Sieff, C.A. (1986). Human recombinant granulocyte–macrophage colony-stimulating factor increases cell-to-cell adhesion and surface expression of adhesion-promoting surface glycoproteins on mature granulocytes. J. Clin. Invest. 78, 597–601.

Bagby, G.C., Dinarello, D., Wallace, P., Warner, C., Hefeneider, S. and McCall, E. (1986). Interleukin 1 stimulates granulocyte macrophage colony-stimulating activity release by vascular endothelial cells. J. Clin. Invest. 78, 1316–1323.

Bainton, D.F., Ullyot, J.L. and Farquar, M.G. (1971). The development of neutrophil polymorphonuclear leukocytes in human bone marrow. Origin and composition of azurophil and specific granules. J. Exp. Med. 134, 907–934.

Barak, Y., Levin, S., Soroker, N., Barash, A., Lancet, M. and Nir, E. (1980) Granulocyte–macrophage colonies in cultures of human fetal liver cells: morphological and ultrastructural analysis of proliferation and differentiation. Exp. Hematol. 8, 837–842.

Begley, C.G., Nicola, N.A. and Metcalf, D. (1988). Proliferation of normal human promyelocytes and myelocytes after single pulse stimulation by purified GM-CSF or G-CSF. Blood 71, 640–645.

Borregaard, N. and Herlin, T. (1982). Energy metabolism of human neutrophils during phagocytosis. J. Clin. Invest. 70, 550–557.

Bot, F.J., Dorssers, L., Wagemaker, G. and Lowenberg, B. (1988). Stimulating spectrum of human recombinant multi-CSF (IL-3) on human marrow precursors: importance in accessory cells. Blood 71, 1600–1614.

Boxer, I.A., Hedley-Whyte, E.T. and Stossel, T.P. (1974). Neutrophil actin dysfunction and abnormal neutrophil behaviour. N. Engl. J. Med. 291, 1093–1099.

Broudy, V.C., Kaushansky, K., Harlan, J.M. and Adamson, J.W. (1987). Interleukin-1 stimulates human endothelial cells to produce granulocyte–macrophage colony-stimulating factor and granulocyte colony-stimulating factor. J. Immunol. 139, 464–468.

Broxmeyer, H.E. (1982). In "The Human Bone Marrow: Anatomy, Physiology and Pathophysiology", Vol. 1 (eds S. Trubowitz and S. Davis), pp 77–91. CRC Press, Boca Raton, Florida.

Burgess, A.W., Camakaris, J. and Metcalf, D. (1977). Purification and properties of colony-stimulating factor from mouse lung-conditioned medium. J. Biol. Chem. 252, 1998–2003.

Burgess, A.W., Begley, C.G., Johnson, G.R., Lopez, A.F., Williamson, D.J., Mermod, J-J., Simpson, R.J., Schmitz, A. and Delamarter, J.F. (1987). Purification and properties of bacterially synthesized human granulocyte–macrophage colony stimulating factor. Blood 69, 43–51.

Cannistra, S.A., Vellenga, E., Groshek, P., Rambaldi, A. and Griffin, J.D. (1988). Human granulocyte–monocyte colony-stimulating factor and interleukin 3 stimulate monocyte cytotoxicity through a tumor necrosis factor-dependent mechanism. Blood 71, 672–676.

Capellini, M.D., Potter, C.G. and Wood, W.G. (1985). In "Fetal Liver Transplantation" (eds R.P. Gale, J.-P. Touraine and G. Lucarelli) pp 113–118. Alan R. Liss, Inc., New York.

Chang, J.M, Metcalf, D., Gonda, T.J. and Johnson, G.R. (1989a). Long-term exposure to retrovirally expressed granulocyte colony-stimulating factor induces a nonneoplastic granulocyte and progenitor cell hyperplasia without tissue damage in mice. J. Clin. Invest. 84, 1488–1496.

Chang, J.M., Metcalf, D., Lang, R.A., Gonda, T.J. and Johnson, G.R. (1989b). Nonneoplastic hematopoietic myeloproliferative syndrome induced by dysregulated multi-CSF (IL-3) expression. Blood 73, 1487–1497.

Chusid, M.J., Pisciotta, A.V., Duquesnoy, R.J., Cammitta, B.M. and Tomasulo, P.A. (1980). Congenital neutropenia: studies of pathogenesis. Am. J. Hemat. 8, 315–324.

Cline, M.J. and Golde, D.W. (1974). Production of colony-stimulating activity by human lymphocytes. Nature 248, 703–704.

Coffey, R.G., Davis, J.S. and Djeu, J.Y. (1988). Stimulation of guanylate cyclase activity and reduction of adenylate cyclase activity by granulocyte–macrophage colony-stimulating factor in human blood neutrophils. J. Immunol. 140, 2695–2701.

Cosman D., Lyman, S.D., Idzerda, R.L., Beckmann, M.P., Park, L.S., Goodwin, R.G. and March, C.J. (1990). A new cytokine receptor superfamily. Trends Biochem. Sci. 15, 265–270.

Cronkite, E.P. (1979). Kinetics of granulopoiesis. Clin. Haematol. 8, 351–370.

Dahinden, C.A., Zingg, J., Maly, F.E. and de Weck, A.L. (1988). Leukotriene production in human neutrophils primed by recombinant human granulocyte/macrophage colony-stimulating factor and stimulated with the complement component C5a and FMLP as second signals. J. Exp. Med. 167, 1281–1295.

Dancey, J.T., Deubelbeisse, K.A., Harker, L.A.and Finch, C.A. (1976). Neutrophil kinetics in man. J. Clin. Invest. 58, 705–715.

De Lamarter, J.F., Mermod, J.J., Liang, C-M., Eliason, J.F. and Thatcher, D.R. (1985). Recombinant murine GM-CSF from *E. coli* has biological activity and is neutralised by a specific antiserum. EMBO J. 4, 2575–2581.

Delwel, R., van Buitenen, C., Salem, M., Bot, F., Gillis, S., Kaushansky, K., Altrock, B. and Lowenberg, B. (1989). Interleukin-1 stimulates proliferation of acute myeloblastic leukemia cells by induction of granulocyte–macrophage colony-stimulating factor release. Blood 74, 586–593.

Demetri, G., Ernst, T., Pratt, E., Zenzie, B., Rheinwald, J. and Griffin, J. (1990). Expression of ras oncogenes in cultured human cells alters the transcriptional and posttranscriptional regulation of cytokine genes. J. Clin. Invest. 86, 1261–1269.

Demetri, G., Zenzie, B., Rheinwald, J. and Griffin, J. (1989). Expression of colony-stimulating factor genes by normal mesothelial cells and human malignant mesothelioma cell lines in vitro. Blood 74, 940–946.

Dexter, T.M., Allen, T.D. and Lajtha, L.G. (1977). Conditions controlling the proliferation of haemopoietic stem cells in vitro. J. Cell. Physiol. 91, 335–344.

Dicke, K.A., van Noord, M.J., Moat, B., Schaeffer, B. and van Bekkum, D.W. (1973). Identification of cells in primate bone marrow resembling the haemophoietic stem cell of the mouse. Blood 42, 195–208.

Donahue, R.E., Emerson, S.G., Wang, E.A., Wong, G.G., Clark, S.C. and Nathan, D.G. (1985). Demonstration of burst-promoting activity of recombinant human GM-CSF on circulating erythroid progenitors using an assay involving the delayed addition of erythropoietin. Blood 66, 1479–1481.

Donahue, R.E., Wang, E.A., Stone, D.K., Kamen, R., Wong, G.G., Sehgal, P.K., Nathan, D.G. and Clark, S.C. (1986), Stimulation of haematopoiesis in primates by continuous infusion of recombinant human GM-CSF. Nature 321, 878–875.

Dorssers, L., Burger, H., Bot, F., Delwel, R., Guerts van Kessel, A.H.M., Lowenberg, B. and Wagemaker, G. (1987). Characterization of a human multilineage-colony-stimulating factor cDNA identified by a conserved non coding sequence in mouse interkeukin-3. Gene 55, 115–124.

DiPersio, J.F., Billing, P., Williams, R. and Gasson, J.C. (1988). Human granulocyte–macrophage colony-stimulating factor (GM-CSF) and other cytokines prime neutrophils for enhanced arachidonic acid release and leukotriene B_4 synthesis. J. Immunol. 140, 4315–4322.

Emerson, S.G., Yang, Y.-C., Clark, S.C. and Long, M.W. (1988). Human recombinant granulocyte–macrophage colony stimulating factor and interleukin 3 have overlapping but distinct hematopoietic activities. J. Clin. Invest. 82, 1282–1287.

Emerson, S.G., Thomas, S., Ferrara, J.L. and Greenstein, J.L. (1989). Developmental regulation of erythropoiesis by hematopoietic growth factors: analysis on populations of BFU-E from bone marrow, peripheral blood and fetal liver. Blood 74, 49–55.

English, D., Broxmeyer, H.E., Gabig, T.G., Akard, L.P., Williams, D.E. and Hoffman, D. (1988). Temporal adaptation of neutrophil oxidative responsiveness to n-formyl-methionyl-leucyl-phenylalanine. Acceleration by granulocyte–macrophage colony-stimulating factor. J. Immunol. 141, 2400–2406.

Ernst, T.J., Ritchie, A.R., Demetri, G.D. and Griffin, J.D. (1989). Regulation of granulocyte- and monocyte-colony stimulating factor mRNA levels in human blood monocytes is mediated primarily at a post-transcriptional level. J. Biol. Chem. 264, 5700–5703.

Falk, P.M., Rich, K., Feig, S. Stiehm, R., Golde, D.W. and Cline, M.J. (1977). Evaluation of congenital neutropenic disorders by in vitro bone marrow culture. Pediatrics 59, 739–748.

Falk, L.A., Wahl, L.M. and Vogel, S.N. (1988). Analysis of Ia antigen expression in macrophages derived from bone marrow cells cultured in granulocyte–macrophage colony-stimulating factor or macrophage colony-stimulating factor. J. Immunol. 140, 2652–2660.

Felty, A.R. (1924). Chronic arthritis in the adult associated with splenomegaly and leukopenia: a report of five cases of an unusual clinical syndrome. Bull. Johns Hopkins Hosp. 35, 16–20.

Fialkow, P.J. (1982). Cell lineages in hematopoietic neoplasia studies using glucose-6-phosphate dehydrogenase. J. Cell. Physiol. (Suppl. 1), 37–43.

Fibbe, W.E., van Damme, J., Billiau, A., Goselink, H.M., Voogt, P.J., van E.G., Ralph, P., Altrock, B.W. and Falkenberg, J.H. (1988). Interleukin 1 induces human marrow stromal cells in long term culture to produce granulocyte colony-stimulating factor and macrophage colony-stimulating factor. Blood 71, 430–435.

Fletcher, M.P. and Gasson, J.C. (1988). Enhancement of neutrophil function by granulocyte–macrophage colony-stimulating factor involves recruitment of a less responsive subpopulation. Blood 71, 652–658.

Foa, P., Maiolo, A.T., Lombardi, L., Rytomaa, T. and Polli, E.E. (1982). Effect of granulocytic chalone on the growth rate of continuous cell lines propagated in vitro. Scand. J. Haematol. 29, 257–264.

Gabrilove, J., Welte, K., Lu, L., Castr-Malaspina, H. and Moore, M. (1985). Constitutive production of leukemia differentiation, colony-stimulating, erythroid burst-promoting and pluripoietic factors by a human hepatoma cell line. Characterization of the leukemia differentiation factor. Blood 66, 407–415.

Gasson, J.C., Weisbart, R.H., Kaufman, S.E., Clark, S.C., Hewick, R.M., Wong, G.G. and Golde, D.W. (1984). Purified human granulocyte–macrophage colony-stimulating factor: direct action on neutrophils. Science 226, 1339–1342.

Gasson, J.C., Kaufman, S.E., Weisbart, R.H., Tomonaga, M. and Golde, D.W. (1986). High affinity binding of granulocyte–macrophage colony-stimulating factor to normal and leukemic human myeloid cells. Proc. Natl Acad. Sci. USA 83, 669–673.

Gearing, D.P., King, J.A., Gough, N.M. and Nicola, N.A. (1989). Expression cloning of a receptor for human granulocyte–macrophage colony-stimulating factor. EMBO J. 8, 3667–3676.

Golde, D.W. and Cline, M.J. (1972). Identification of the colony-stimulating cell in human peripheral blood. J. Clin. Invest. 51, 2981–2983.

Golde, D.W., Quan, S.G. and Cline, M.J. (1978). Human T lymphocyte cell line producing colony-stimulating activity. Blood 52, 1068–1072.

Gordon, M.Y. (1981). Granulopoietic effects of factors produced by cultured human bone marrow fibroblastoid cells. Stem Cells 1, 180–192.

Gordon, M.Y. (1988). Annotation: adhesive properties of haemopoietic stem cells. Br. J. Haematol. 68, 149–151.

Gordon, M.Y. and Greaves, M.F. (1989. Physiological mechanisms of stem cell regulation in bone marrow transplantation and haemopoiesis. Bone Marrow Transplant. 4, 335–338.

Gordon, M.Y., Douglas, I.D.C., Clink, H.M. and Pickering, B.M.J. (1976). Distribution of granulopoietic activity in the human skeleton, studied by colony growth in agar diffusion chambers. Br. J. Haematol. 32, 537–542.

Gordon, M.Y., Kearney, L.U. and Hibbin, J.A. (1983). Effects of human marrow stromal cells on proliferation by human granulocytic (GM-CFC), erythroid (BFU-E) and mixed (Mix-CFC) colony-forming cells. Br. J. Haematol. 53, 317–325.

Gordon, M.Y., Riley, G.P., Watt, S.M. and Greaves, M.F. (1987). Compartmentalization of a haemopoietic growth factor (GM-CSF) by glycosaminoglycans in the bone marrow microenvironment. Nature 326, 403–405.

Gordon, M.Y., Clarke, D., Atkinson, J. and Greaves, M.F. (1990). Hemopoietic progenitor cell binding to the stromal microenvironment in vitro. Exp. Hematol. 18, 837–842.

Gordon, M.Y., Atkinson, J., Clarke, D., Goldman, J.M., Grimsley, P.G., Siczkowski, M. and Greaves, M.F. (1991). Deficiency of a phosphatidylinositol-anchored cell adhesion molecule influences haemopoietic progenitor binding to marrow stroma in chronic myeloid leukaemia. Leukemia 5, 693–698.

Gough, N.M., Gough, J., Metcalf, D., Kelso, A., Grail, D., Nicola, N.A., Burgess, A.W. and Dunn, A.R. (1984). Molecular cloning of cDNA encoding a murine haematopoietic growth regulator, granulocyte–macrophage colony stimulating factor. Nature 309, 763–767.

Greaves, M.F., Brown, J., Molgaard, H.V., Spurr, N.K., Robertson, D., Delia, D. and Sutherland, D.R. (1992). Molecular features of CD34: a hemopoietic cell-associated molecule. Leukemia 6 (Suppl.), 31–36.

Haak-Frendscho, M., Arai, N., Arai K-I., Baeza, M.L., Finn, A. and Kaplan, A.P. (1988). Human recombinant granulocyte–macrophage colony-stimulating factor and interleukin 3 cause basophil histamine release. J. Clin. Invest. 82, 17–20.

Haas, R., Hohaus, S., Kiesel, S., Ogniben, E. and Hunstein, W. (1989). Effect of recombinant human granulocyte–macrophage colony-stimulating factor (rhuGM-CSF) on normal peripheral B lymphocytes and B lymphoblastoid cell lines. Immunol. Lett. 20, 133–138.

Hammond, W.P., Price, T.H., Souza, L.M. and Dale, D.C. (1989). Treatment of cyclic neutropenia with granulocyte colony-stimulating factor. N. Engl. J. Med. 320, 1306–1311.

Hammond, W., Csiba, E., Canin, A., Hockman, H., Souza, L., Layton, J. and Dale, D. (1991). Chronic neutropenia: a new canine model induced by human granulocyte colony-stimulating factor. J. Clin. Invest. 87, 704–710.

Handman, E. and Burgess, A.W. (1979). Stimulation by granulocyte–macrophage colony-stimulating factor of Leishmania tropica killing by macrophages. J. Immunol. 122, 1134–1137.

Hann, I.M., Bodger, M.P. and Hoffbrand, A.V. (1983). Development of pluripotent hemopoietic progenitor cells in the human fetus. Blood 62, 118–123.

Hassan, M.W., Lutton, J.D., Levere, R.D., Reider, R.F. and Cederqvist, L.L. (1979). In vitro culture of erythroid colonies from human fetal liver and umbilical cord blood. Br. J. Haematol. 41, 477–484.

Herrmann, F., Cannistra, S. and Griffin, J. (1986). T-cell/monocyte interactions in the production of humoral factors regulating human granulopoiesis in vitro. J. Immunol. 136, 2856–2861.

Heufler, C., Koch, F. and Schuler, G. (1988). Granulocyte/macrophage colony-stimulating factor and interleukin 1 mediate the maturation of murine epidermal Langerhans cells into potent immunostimulatory dendritic cells. J. Exp. Med. 167, 700–705.

Hirai, K., Morita, Y., Misaki, Y., Ohta, K., Takaishi, T., Suzuki, S., Motoyoshi, K. and Miyamoto, T. (1988). Modulation of human basophil histamine release by hemopoietic growth factors. J. Immunol. 141, 3958–3964.

Hocking, W., Goodman, J. and Golde, D (1983). Granulocytosis associated with production of colony-stimulating activity. Blood 61, 600–603.

Holmes, B., Page, A.R. and Good, R.A. (1967). Studies on the metabolic activity of leukocytes from patients with a genetic abnormality of phagocyte function. J. Clin. Invest. 46, 1422–1432.

Huebner, K., Isobe, M., Croce, C.M., Golde, D.W., Kaufman, S.E. and Gasson, J.C. (1985). The human gene encoding GM-CSF is at 5q21–q32, the chromosome region deleted in the 5q- anomaly. Science 230, 1282–1285.

Ikebuchi, K., Clarke S.C., Ihle, J.N., Souza, L.M. and Ogawa, M. (1988). Granulocyte colony-stimulating factor enhances interleukin-3-dependent proliferation of multipotential hemopoietic progenitors. Proc. Natl Acad. Sci. USA 85, 3445–3449.

International Chronic Granulomatous Disease Cooperative Study Group (1991). A controlled trial of interferon gamma to prevent infection in chronic granulomatous disease. N. Engl. J. Med. 324, 509–517.

Itoh, N., Yonehara, S., Schreurs, J., Gorman, G.M., Maruyama, K., Ishii, A., Yahara, I., Akai, K-I. and Miyajima, A. (1990). Cloning of an interleukin-3 receptor gene: a member of a distinct receptor gene family. Science 247, 324–327.

James, R. and Kazenwadel, J. (1989). T-cell nuclei contain a protein that binds upstream of the murine granulocyte–macrophage colony-stimulating factor gene. Proc. Natl Acad. Sci. USA 86, 7392–7396.

Johnson, G.R., Gonda, T.J., Metcalf, D., Hariharan, I.K. and Cory, S. (1989). A lethal myeloproliferative syndrome in mice transplanted with bone marrow cells infected with a retrovirus expressing granulocyte–macrophage colony stimulating factor. EMBO J. 8, 441–448.

Katayama, K., Koizumi, S., Ueno, Y., Ohno, I., Ichihara, T., Horita, S., Miyawaki, T. and Taniguchi, N. (1990). Antagonistic effects of interleukin 6 and G-CSF at the later stage of human granulopoiesis in vitro. Exp. Hematol. 18, 390–394.

Kaushansky, K. (1989). Control of granulocyte–macrophage colony-stimulating factor production in normal endothelial cells by positive and negative regulatory elements. J. Immunol. 143, 2525–2529.

Kawakami, M., Tsusumi, H., Kumakawa, T., Abe, H., Hirai, M., Kurosawa, S., Mori, M. and Fukushima, M. (1990). Levels of serum granulocyte colony-stimulating factor in patients with infections. Blood 76, 1962–1964.

Keleman, E. and Janossa, M. (1983). Macrophages are the first differentiated blood cells formed in human embryonic liver. Exp. Hematol. 8, 996–1001.

Keleman, E., Calvo, W. and Fliedner, T.M. (1979). "Atlas of Human Hemopoietic Development". Springer-Verlag, Berlin, Heidelberg.

Kiefer, F., Wagner, E.F., and Keller, G. (1991) Fractionation of mouse bone marrow by adherence separates primitive hematopoietic stem cells from in vitro colony-forming cells and spleen colony-forming cells. Blood 78, 2577–2582.

Kishimoto, T. (1989). The biology of interleukin-6. Blood 74, 1–10.

Kitahara, M., Eyre, H.J., Simonian, Y., Atkin, C.L. and Hasstedt, S.J. (1981). Hereditary myeloperoxidase deficiency. Blood 57, 888–893.

Kitamura, T., Hayashida, K., Sakamaki, K., Yokota, T., Arai, K.-I. and Miyajima, A. (1991a). Reconstitution of functional receptors for human granulocyte/macrophage colony-stimulating factor (GM-CSF): evidence that the protein encoded by the AIC2B cDNA is a subunit of the murine GM-CSF receptor. Proc. Natl Acad. Sci. USA 88, 5082–5086.

Kitamura, T., Sato, N., Arai, K.-I. and Miyajima, A. (1991b). Expression cloning of the human IL-3 receptor cDNA reveals a shared β subunit for the human IL-3 and GM-CSF receptors. Cell 66, 1165–1174.

Koeffler, H.P., Gasson, J., Ranyard, J., Souza, L., Shepard, M. and Munker, R. (1987). Recombinant human TNF alpha stimulates production of granulocyte colony-stimulating factor. Blood 70, 55–59.

Koeffler, H.P., Gasson, J. and Tobler, A. (1988). Transcriptional and posttranscriptional modulation of myeloid colony-stimulating factor expression by tumor necrosis factor and other agents. Mol. Cell. Biol. 8, 3432–3438.

Krance, R.A., Spruce, W.E., Forman, S.J., Rosen, R.B., Hecht, T., Hammond, W.P. and Blum, K.G. (1982). Human cyclic neutropenia transferred by allogeneic marrow grafting. Blood 60, 1263–1266.

Kyas, U., Pietsch, T. and Welte, K. (1992). Expression of receptors for granulocyte colony-stimulating factor on neutrophils from patients with severe congenital neutropenia and cyclic neutropenia. Blood 79, 1144–1147.

Laker, C., Stocking, C., Bergholz, U., Hess, N., De Lamarter, J.F. and Ostertag, W. (1987). Autocrine stimulation after transfer of the granulocyte/macrophage colony-stimulating factor gene and autonomous growth are distinct but interdependent steps in the oncogenic pathway. Proc. Natl Acad. Sci. USA 84, 8458–8462.

Lang, R.A., Metcalf, D., Cuthbertson, R.A., Lyons, J., Stanley, E., Kelso, E., Kannourakis, G., Williamson, D.J., Klintworth, G.K., Gonda, T.J. and Dunn, A.R. (1987). Transgenic mice expressing a hemopoietic growth factor gene (GM-CSF) develop accumulations of macrophages, blindness and a fatal syndrome of tissue damage. Cell 51, 675–686.

Lange, R.D. (1983). Cyclic hematopoiesis: human cyclic neutropenia. Exp. Hematol. 11, 435–438.

Larsen, A., Davis, T., Curtis, B., Gimpel, S., Sims, J., Cosman, D., Park, L., Sorensen, E., March, C.J. and Smith, C. (1990). Expression cloning of a human granulocyte colony-stimulating factor receptor: a structural mosaic of hemopoietin receptor, immunoglobulin and fibronectin domains. J. Exp. Med. 172, 1559–1564.

Le Beau, M., Lemons, R., Carrino, J., Pettenati, M., Souza, L., Diaz, M. and Rowley, J. (1987). Chromosomal localization of the human G-CSF gene to 17q11 proximal to the breakpoint of the t(15;17) in acute promyelocytic leukemia. Leukemia 1, 795–799.

Le Beau, M.M., Westbrook, C.A., Diaz, M.O., Larson, R.A., Rowley, J.D., Gasson, J.C., Golde, D.W. and Scherr, C.J. (1986). Evidence for the involvement of GM-CSF and FMS in the deletion (5q) in myeloid disorders. Science 231, 984–987.

Lilly, M.B., Devlin, P.E., Devlin, J.J. and Rado, T.A. (1987). Production of granulocyte colony-stimulating factor by a human melanoma cell line. Exp. Hematol. 15, 966–971.

Long, M.W. (1992). Review: Blood cell cytoadhesion molecules. Exp. Hematol. 20, 288–301.

Lopez, A.F., Williamson, J, Gamble, J.R., Begley, C.G., Harlan, J.M., Klebanoff, S.J., Waltersdorph, A., Wong, G., Clark, S.C. and Vadas, M.A. (1986). Recombinant human granulocyte–macrophage colony-stimulating factor stimulates in vitro mature neutrophil and eosinophil functions, surface receptor expression and survival. J. Clin. Invest. 78, 1220–1228.

Mano, H., Nishida, J., Usuki, K., Maru, Y., Kobayashi, Y., Hirai, H., Ukabe, T., Ukabe, A. and Takaku, F. (1987). Constitutive expression of the granulocyte–macrophage colony-stimulating factor gene in human solid tumors. Jpn. J. Cancer Res. 78, 1041–1043.

Matsuda, S., Shirafuji, N. and Asano, S. (1989). Human granulocyte colony-stimulating factor specifically binds to murine myeloblastic NFS-60 cells and activates their guanosine triphosphate binding proteins/adenylate cyclase system. Blood 74, 2343–2348.

Mayer, P., Lam, C., Obenaus, H., Liehl, E. and Bessemer, J. (1987). Recombinant human GM-CSF induces leukocytosis and activates peripheral blood polymorphonuclear neutrophils in nonhuman primates. Blood 70, 206–213.

McColl, S.R., Kreis, C., DiPersio, J.F., Borgeat, P. and Nacchache, P.H. (1989). Involvement of guanine nucleotide binding proteins in neutrophil activation and priming by granulocyte–macrophage colony-stimulating factor. Blood 73, 588–591.

Metcalf, D. and Nicola, N.A (1983). Proliferative effects of purified granulocyte colony-stimulating factor (G-CSF) on normal mouse hemopoietic cells. J. Cell. Physiol. 116, 198–206.

Metcalf, D., Begley, C.G., Johnson, G.R., Nicola, N.A., Vadas, M.A., Lopez, A.F., Williamson, D.J., Wong, G.G., Clarke, S.C. and Wang, E.A. (1986). Biological properties in vitro of a recombinant human granulocyte–macrophage colony-stimulating factor. Blood, 67, 37–45.

Mintz, U. and Sachs, L. (1973). Normal granulocyte colony-forming cells in the bone marrow of Yemenite Jews with genetic neutropenia. Blood 41, 745–751.

Miyajima, A., Otsu, K, Schreurs, J., Bond, M.W., Abrams, J.S. and Arai, K. (1986). Expression of murine and human granulocyte–macrophage colony-stimulating factors in S. cerevisiae: Mutagenesis of the potential glycosylation sites. EMBO J. 5, 1193–1197.

Miyatake, S., Otsuka, T., Yokota, T., Lee, F. and Arai, K. (1985). Structure of the chromosomal gene for granulocyte macrophage colony stimulating factor: comparison of the mouse and human genes. EMBO J. 4, 2561–2568.

Monroy, R.L., Skelly, R.R., MacVittie, T.J., Davis, T.A., Sauber, J.J., Clark, S.C. and Donahue, R.E. (1987). The effect of recombinant GM-CSF on the recovery of monkeys transplanted with autologous bone marrow. Blood 70, 1696–1699.

Moonen, P., Mermod, J-J., Ernst, J.F., Hirschi, M. and Delamarter, J.F. (1987). Increased biological activity of deglycosylated recombinant human granulocyte/macrophage colony-stimulating factor produced by yeast or animal cells. Proc. Natl Acad. Sci. USA 84, 4428–4431.

Moore, M.A.S. and Williams, N. (1973). Analysis of proliferation and differentiation of fetal granulocyte–macrophage progenitor cells in hemopoietic tissues. Cell Tissue Kinet. 6, 461–476.

Morla, A.O., Schreurs, J., Miyajima, A. and Wang, J.Y.J. (1988). Hematopoietic growth factors activate the tyrosine phosphorylation of distinct sets of proteins in interleukin-3-dependent murine cell lines. Mol. Cell. Biol. 8, 2214–2218.

Muller, M., Ruppert, S., Schaffner, W. and Mattias, P. (1988). A cloned octamer transcription factor stimulates transcription from lymphoid-specific promoters in non-B cells. Nature 336, 544–551.

Munker, R., Gasson, J., Ogawa, M. and Koeffler, H.P. (1986). Recombinant human TNF induces production of granulocyte–monocyte colony-stimulating factor. Nature 323, 79–82.

Naccache, P.H., Faucher, N., Borgeat, P., Gasson, J.C. and DiPersio, J.F. (1988). Granulocyte–macrophage colony-stimulating factor modulates the excitation–response coupling sequence in human neutrophils. J. Immunol. 140, 3541–3546.

Nagata, S., Tsuchiya, M., Asano, S., Kaziro, Y., Yamazaki, T., Yamamoto, O., Hirata, Y., Kubota, N., Oheda, M., Nomura, H. and Ono, M. (1986a). Molecular cloning and expression of cDNA for human granulocyte colony-stimulating factor. Nature 319, 415–418.

Nagata, S., Tsuchiya, M., Asano, S., Yamamoto, O., Hirata, Y., Kubota, N., Oheda, M., Nomura, H. and Yamazaki, T. (1986b). The chromosomal gene structure and two mRNAs for human granulocyte colony-stimulating factor. EMBO J. 5, 575–579.

Nathan, C.F. (1989). Respiratory burst in adherent human neutrophils: triggering by colony-stimulating factors CSF-GM and CSF-G. Blood, 73, 301–306.

Nicola, N. (1989). Hemopoietic cell growth factors and their receptors. Annu. Rev. Biochem. 58, 45–77.

Nicola N.A. and Metcalf, D. (1984). Binding of the differentiation-inducer, granulocyte-colony-stimulating factor, to responsive but not unresponsive leukemia cell lines. Proc. Natl Acad. Sci. USA 81, 3765–3769.

Nicola, N.A. and Metcalf, D. (1985). Binding of [125]-Labelled granulocyte colony-stimulating factor to normal murine hemopoietic cells. J. Cell. Physiol. 124, 313–321.

Nicola, N.A., Metcalf, D., Matsumoto, M. and Johnson, G.R. (1983). Purification of a factor inducing differentiation in murine myelomonocytic leukemia cells. Identification as granulocyte colony-stimulating factor. J. Biol. Chem. 258, 9017–9023.

Nicola, N.A., Begley, C.G. and Metcalf, D. (1985). Identification of the human analogue of a regulator that induces differentiation in murine leukaemic cells. Nature 314, 625–628.

Nicola, N.A., Vadas, M.A. and Lopez, A.F. (1986). Down-modulation of receptors for granulocyte colony-stimulating factor on human neutrophils by granulocyte-activating agents. J. Cell. Physiol. 128, 501–509.

Nimer, S.D. and Golde, D.W. (1987). The 5q- abnormality. Blood 70, 1705–1712.

Nishizawa, M. and Nagata, S. (1990). Regulatory elements responsible for inducible expression of the granulocyte colony-stimulating factor gene in macrophages. Mol. Cell. Biol. 10, 2002–2011.

Nishizawa, M., Tsuchiya, M., Watanabe, F.R. and Nagata, S. (1990). Multiple elements in the promotor of granulocyte colony-stimulating factor gene regulate its constitutive expression in human carcinoma cells. J. Biol. Chem. 265, 5897–5902.

Oster, W., Lindemann, A., Mertelsmann, R. and Herrmann, F. (1989). Granulocyte–macrophage colony-stimulating factor (CSF) and multilineage CSF recruit human monocytes to express granulocyte CSF. Blood 73, 64–67.

Otsuka, T., Miyajima, A., Brown, N., Otsu, K., Abrams, J., Saeland, S., Caux, C., de Waal Malefijt, R., de Vries, J., Meyerson, P., Yokota, K., Gemmel, L., Rennick, D., Lee, F., Arai, K. and Yokota, T. (1988). Isolation and characterization of an expressible cDNA clone encoding human interleukin-3: induction of IL-3 mRNA in human T cell clones. J Immunol. 140, 2288–2295.

Parmley, R.T., Crist, W.M., Ragab, A.H., Boxer, L.A., Malluh, A., Lui, V.K. and Darby, C.P. (1980). Congenital dysgranulopoietic neutropenia: Clinical, serologic, ultrastructural and in vitro proliferative characteristics. Blood 56, 465–475.

Peschle, C., Migliaccio, A.R., Migliaccio, G., Ciccariello, R., Lettieri, F., Quattrin, S., Russo, G. and Mastroberardino, G. (1981). Identification and characterisation of three classes of erythroid progenitors in human fetal liver. Blood 58, 565–572.

Ploemacher, R.E., van der Sluijs, J.P., van Beurden, C.A.J., Baert, M.R.M. and Chan, P.L. (1991). Use of limiting-dilution type long-term marrow cultures in frequency analysis of marrow-repopulating and spleen colony-forming hematopoietic stem cells in the mouse. Blood 78, 2527–2533.

Rappeport, J.M., Smith, Parkman, R., Newburger, P., Camitta, B.M. and Chusid, M.J. (1980). Correction of infantile agranulocytosis (Kostmann's syndrome) by allogeneic bone marrow transplantation. Am. J. Med. 68, 605–609.

Rappeport, J.M., Newburger, P.E., Goldblum, R.M., Goldman, A.S., Nathan, D.G. and Parkman, R. (1982). Allogeneic bone marrow transplantation for chronic granulomatous disease. J. Pediatr. 101, 952–955.

Rausch, P.G., Pryzwansky, K.B. and Spitznagel, J.K. (1978). Immunocytochemical identification of azurophilic and specific granule markers in the giant granules of Chediak–Higashi neutrophils. N. Engl. J. Med. 298, 693–698.

Rich, D., Falk, P.M., Stiehm, E.R., Feig, S., Golde, D.W. and Cline, M.J. (1977). Abnormal in vitro granulopoiesis in phenotypically normal parents of some children with congenital neutropenia. Pediatrics 59, 396–401.

Richter, J., Andersson, T. and Olsson, I. (1989). Effect of tumor necrosis factor and granulocyte/macrophage colony-stimulating factor on neutrophil degranulation. J. Immunol. 142, 3199–3205.

Riley, G.P. and Gordon, M.Y. (1987). Characterization of cultured stromal layers derived from fetal and adult hemopoietic tissues. Exp. Hematol. 15, 78–84.

Roberts, R., Gallagher, J., Spooncer, E., Allen, T.D., Bloomfield, F, and Dexter, T.M. (1988). Heparan sulphate bound growth factors: a mechanism for stromal cell mediated haemopoiesis. Nature 332, 376–378.

Rowley, P.T., Ohlsson-Wilhelm, W.B.M. and Farley, B.A. (1978). Erythroid colony formation from human fetal liver. Proc. Natl Acad. Sci. USA 75, 984–988.

Salem, M., Delwel, R., Touw, I., Mahmoud, L.A., Elbasousy, E.M. and Lowenberg, B. (1990). Modulation of colony stimulating factor-(CSF) dependent growth of acute myeloid leukemia by tumor necrosis factor. Leukemia 4, 37–43.

Santoli, D., Clarke, S.C., Krieder, B.L., Maslin, P.A. and Rovera, G. (1988). Amplification of IL-2 driven T cell proliferation by recombinant human IL-3 and granulocyte–macrophage colony-stimulating factor. J. Immunol. 141, 519–526.

Schoenfield, Y., Shindel, D., Neri, A., Berliner, S., Lusky, A., Kaufman, C. and Pinkhas, J. (1983). Pregnancy induced leukocytosis in Yemenite Jews. Acta Haemat. 70, 170–177.

Schreck, R. and Baeuerle, P.A. (1990). NF-ϰB as inducible transcriptional activator of the granulocyte–macrophage colony-stimulating factor gene. Mol. Cell. Biol. 10, 1281–1286.

Schuler, G.D. and Cole, M.D. (1988). GM-CSF and oncogene mRNA stabilities are independently regulated in trans in a mouse monocytic tumor. Cell 55, 1115–1122.

Seelentag, W.K., Mermod, J.-J., Montesano, R. and Vassilli, P. (1987). Additive effects of interleukin 1 and tumor necrosis factor α on the accumulation of the three granulocyte and macrophage colony stimulating factor mRNAs in human endothelial cells. EMBO J. 6, 2261–2265.

Segel, E.K., Ellegaard, J. and Borregaard, N. (1987). Development of the phagocytic and cidal capacity during maturation of myeloid cells: studies on cells from patients with chronic myelogenous leukaemia. Br. J. Haematol. 67, 3–10.

Shannon, M.F., Pell, L.M., Lenardo, M.J., Kuczek, E.S., Occhiodoro, F.S., Dunn, S.M. and Vadas, M.A. (1990). A novel tumor necrosis factor-responsive transcription factor which recognizes a regulatory element in hemopoietic growth factor genes. Mol. Cell. Biol. 10, 2950–2959.

Siczkowski, M., Clarke, D. and Gordon, M.Y. (1992). Binding of primitive haemopoietic progenitor cells to marrow stromal cells involves heparan sulphate. Blood 80, 912–919.

Silberstein, D.S., Owen, W.F., Gasson, J.C., DiPersio, J.F., Golde, D.W., Bina, J.C., Soberman, R., Austen, K.F. and David, J.R. (1986). Enhancement of human eosinophil cytotoxicity and leukotriene synthesis by biosynthetic (recombinant) granulocyte–macrophage colony-stimulating factor. J. Immunol. 137, 3290–3294.

Simmers, R.N., Webber, L.M., Shannon, M.F., Garson, O.M., Wong, G., Vadas, M.A. and Sutherland, G.R. (1987). Localization of the G-CSF gene on chromosome 17 proximal to the breakpoint in the t(15;17) in acute promyelocytic leukemia. Blood 70, 330–332.

Slack, J.L., Nemunaitis, J., Andrews, D.F. and Singer, J.W. (1990). Regulation of cytokine and growth factor gene expression in human bone marrow stromal cells transformed with simian virus 40. Blood 75, 2319–2327.

Sonoda, Y., Yang, Y-C., Wang, G.G., Clark, S.C. and Ogawa, M. (1988). Analysis in serum-free culture of the targets of recombinant human hemopoietic growth factors: interleukin 3 and granulocyte/macrophage colony-stimulating factor are specific for early developmental stages. Proc. Natl Acad. Sci. USA 85, 4360–4364.

Sorenson, P.H.B., Mui, A.L.-F., Murthy, S.C. and Krystal, G. (1989). Interleukin-3, GM-CSF and TPA induce distinct phosphorylation events in an interleukin 3-dependent multipotential cell line. Blood 73, 406–418.

Souza, L.M, Boone, T.C., Gabrilove, J., Lai, P.H., Zsebo, K.M., Murdock, D.C., Chazin, V.R., Bruszewski, J., Lu, H., Chen, K.K., Barendt, J., Platzer, E., Moore, M.A.S., Mertelsmann, R. and Welte, K. (1986). Recombinant human granulocyte colony-stimulating factor: effects on normal and leukemic myeloid cells. Science 232, 61–65.

Spertini, O., Kansas, G., Munro, J., Griffin, J. and Tedder, T. (1991). Regulation of leukocyte migration by activation of the leukocyte adhesion molecule-1 (LAM-1) selectin. Nature 349, 691–694.

Stanley, E.R., Metcalf, D., Sobieszczuk, P., Gough, N.M. and Dunn, A.R. (1985). The structure and expression of the murine gene encoding granulocyte–macrophage colony-stimulating factor: evidence for the utilization of two alternative promotors. EMBO J. 4, 2569–2573.

Stocking, C. and Ostertag, W. (1990). In "Growth Factors, Differentiation Factors and Cytokines" (ed. A. Habenicht) pp 115–128. Springer Verlag, Berlin, Heidelberg.

Sullivan, R., Griffin, J.D., Simons, E.R., Schafer, A.I., Meshulam, T., Fredette, J.P., Maas, A.K., Gadenne, A.S., Leavitt, J.L. and Melnick, D.A. (1987). Effects of recombinant human granulocyte and macrophage colony-stimulating factors on signal transduction pathways in human granulocytes. J. Immunol. 139, 3422–3430.

Taniguchi, T. (1988). Regulation of cytokine gene expression. Annu. Rev. Immunol. 6, 439–464.

Tavassoli, M. and Yoffey, J.M. (1983). "Bone Marrow: Structure and Function". Alan R. Liss, Inc., New York.

Thorens, B., Mermod, J.J. and Vassilli, P. (1987). Phagocytosis and inflammatory stimuli induce GM-CSF mRNA in macrophages through posttranscriptional regulation. Cell 48, 671–679.

Till, J.E. and McCulloch, E.A. (1961). A direct measurement of the radiation sensitivity of normal mouse bone marrow cells. Radiat. Res. 14, 213–222.

Todd, R.F., Arnaout, M.A., Rosin, R.E., Crowley, C.A., Peters, W.A. and Babior, B.M. (1984). Subcellular localization of the large subunit of Mo1 ($Mo1_x$; formerly gp110) a surface glycoprotein associated with neutrophil adhesion. J. Clin. Invest. 74, 1280–1290.

Tsuchiya, M., Kaziro, Y. and Nagata, S. (1987). The chromosomal gene structure for murine granulocyte colony-stimulating factor. Eur. J. Biochem. 165, 7–12.

Tweady, D. J., Anderson, K., Cannizaro, L.A., Steinman, R.A., Croce, C.M. and Huebner, K. (1992). Molecular cloning of cDNAs for the human granulocyte colony-stimulating factor from HL-60 and mapping of the gene to chromosome region 1p32–34. Blood 79, 1148–1164.

Van Leeuwen, B.H., Martinson, M.E., Webb, G.C. and Young, I.G. (1989). Molecular organization of the cytokine gene cluster involving the human IL-3, IL-4, IL-5 and GM-CSF genes, on human chromosome 5. Blood 73, 1142–1148.

Vellenga, E., Rambaldi, A., Ernst, T.J., Ostapovicz, D. and Griffin, J.D. (1988). Independent regulation of M-CSF and G-CSF gene expression in human monocytes. Blood 71, 1529–1532.

Vincent, P.C. (1977). Granulocyte kinetics in health and disease. Clin. Haematol. 6, 695–717.

Vincent, P.C., Levi, J.A. and Macqueen, A. (1974). The mechanism of neutropenia in Felty's syndrome. Brit. J. Haematol. 27, 46.

Walker, F. and Burgess, A.W. (1985). Specific binding of radioiodinated granulocyte–macrophage colony-stimulating factor to hemopoietic cells. EMBO J. 4, 933–939.

Watari, K., Asano, S., Shirafuji, N., Kodo, H., Ozawa, K., Takaku, F. and Kamachi, S. (1989). Serum granulocyte colony-stimulating factor levels in healthy volunteers and patients with various disorders as estimated by enzyme immunoassay. Blood 73, 117–122.

Welte, K., Platzer, E., Lu, L., Gabrilove, J., Levi, E., Mertels-mann, R. and Moore, M. (1985). Purification and biological characterization of human pluripotent hematopoietic colony-stimulating factor. Proc. Natl Acad. Sci. USA 82, 1526–1530.

Westen, H. and Bainton, D.F. (1979). Association of alkaline phosphatase-positive reticulum cells in bone marrow with granulocytic precursors. J. Exp. Med. 150, 919–937.

Weisbart, R.H., Golde, D.W., Clark, S.C., Wong, G.G. and Gasson, J.C. (1985). Human granulocyte–macrophage colony-stimulating factor is a neutrophil activator. Nature 314, 361–363.

Weisbart, R.H., Golde, D.W. and Gasson, J.C. (1986). Bio-synthetic GM-CSF modulates the number and affinity of neutrophil f-met-leu-phe receptors. J. Immunol. 137, 3584–3587.

Wieser, M., Bonifer, R., Oster, W., Lindemann, A., Mertelsmann, R. and Herrmann, F. (1989). Interleukin-4 induces secretion of CSF for granulocytes and CSF for macro-phages by peripheral blood monocytes. Blood 73, 1105–1108.

Williamson, D.J., Begley, C.G., Vadas, M.A. and Metcalf, D. (1988). The detection and initial characterization of colony-stimulating factors in synovial fluid. Clin. Exp. Immunol. 72, 67–73.

Witmer-Pack, M.D., Olivier, W., Valinsky, J., Schuler, G. and Steinman, R.M. (1987). Granulocyte/macrophage colony-stimulating factor is essential for the viability and function of cultured murine epidermal Langerhans cells. J. Exp. Med. 166, 1484–1498.

Wong, G.G., Witek, J.S., Temple, P.A., Wilkens, K.M., Leary, A.C., Luxenberg, D.P., Jones, S.S., Brown, E.L., Kay, R.M., Orr, E.C., Shoemaker, C., Golde, D.W., Kaufman, R.J., Hewick, R.M. and Clarke, S.C. (1985). Human GM-CSF: molecular cloning of the complementary DNA and purification of the natural and recombinant proteins. Science 228, 810–815.

Wriedt, K., Kauder, E. and Mauer, A.M. (1970). Defective myelopoiesis in congenital neutropenia. N. Engl. J. Med. 283, 1072–1077.

Xu, W.D., Firestein, G.S., Taetle, R., Kaushansky, K. and Zvaifler, N.J. (1989). Cytokines in chronic inflammatory arthritis. II. Granulocyte–macrophage colony-stimulating factor in rheumatoid synovial effusions. J. Clin. Invest. 83, 876–882.

Yamato, K., El-Hajjaoui, Z., Kuo, J.F. and Koeffler, H.P. (1989). Granulocyte–macrophage colony-stimulating factor: signals for its mRNA accumulation. Blood 74, 1314–1320.

Yang, Y.C., Ciarletta, A.B., Temple, P.A., Chung, M., Kovacic, S., Witek-Giannotti, J.S., Leary, A.C., Kriz, R., Donahue, R.E., Wong, G.G. and Clarke, S.C. (1986). Human interleukin-3 (multi-CSF): identification by expres-sion cloning of a novel haematopoietic growth factor related to murine IL-3. Cell 47, 3–10.

Yang, Y.-C., Kovacic, S., Kriz, R., Wolf, S., Clark, S.C., Wellems, T.E., Nienhuis, A. and Epstein, N. (1988). The human genes for GM-CSF and IL-3 are closely linked in tandem on chromosome 5. Blood 71, 958–961.

Young, D.C. and Griffin, J.D. (1986). Autocrine secretion of GM-CSF in acute myeloblastic leukemia. Blood 68, 1178–1181.

Young, D.C., Wagner, K. and Griffin, J.D. (1987). Constitutive expression of the granulocyte–macrophage colony-stimulating factor gene in acute myeloblastic leukemia. J. Clin. Invest. 79, 100–106.

Young, D.C., Demetri, G.D., Ernst, T.J., Cannistra, S.A. and Griffin, J.D. (1988). In vitro expression of colony-stimulating factor genes by human acute myeloblastic leukemia cells. Exp. Hematol. 16, 378–382.

Yuo, A., Kitagawa, S., Ohsaka, A., Ohta, M., Miyazono, K., Okabe, T., Urabe, A., Saito, M. and Takaku, F. (1989). Recombinant human granulocyte colony-stimulating factor as an activator of human granulocytes: potentiation of responses triggered by receptor mediated agonists and stimulation of C3bi receptor expression and adherence. Blood 74, 2144–2149.

Yuo, A., Kitagawa, S., Ohsaka, A., Saito, M. and Takaku, F. (1990). Stimulation and priming of human neutrophils by granulocyte colony-stimulating factor and granulocyte–macrophage colony-stimulating factor: qualitative and quan-titative differences. Biochem. Biophys. Res. Comm. 171, 491–497.

Zsebo, K., Yuschenkoff, V., Schiffer, S., Chang, D., McCall, E., Dinarello, C., Brown, M., Altrock, B. and Bagby, G. (1988). Vascular endothelial cells and granulopoiesis: interleukin-1 stimulates release of G-CSF and GM-CSF. Blood 71, 99–103.

3. The Respiratory Burst of Neutrophils and Its Deficiency

C.M. Casimir and C.G. Teahan

1. The NADPH Oxidase of Phagocytes

1.1 INTRODUCTION

The first cells to accumulate at sites of inflammation are the neutrophils, whose function is to engulf (phagocytose) and kill invading microorganisms. Phagocytosis is accompanied by a burst of oxygen consumption referred to as "the respiratory burst", first observed in 1932 (Baldridge and Gerard, 1933). In fact this increased oxygen consumption is unconnected with respiration (neutrophils contain few mitochondria and derive most of their energy from glycolysis) but is due to activation of

Immunopharmacology of Neutrophils
ISBN 0-12-339250-0

an oxidase located in the plasma membrane that reduces molecular oxygen to the superoxide anion, O_2^- (Sbarra and Karnovsky, 1959). Since it has been shown that NADPH is the physiological electron donor for this system it is known as the NADPH oxidase (Rossi, 1986). It is found in all the phagocytic blood cells: neutrophils, monocytes, macrophages and eosinophils. It is also found, at very low levels, in a small proportion of immature B lymphocytes (Maly et al., 1988). The ability of neutrophils to kill microbes (but not their capacity for phagocytosis) is impaired under anaerobic conditions. Neutrophils from patients with a disease known as CGD (see Section 2) can phagocytose bacteria but cannot generate superoxide (Holmes et al., 1966, 1967). These patients suffer severe, often fatal, infections due to failure of the neutrophils to kill invading microorganisms. The respiratory burst is therefore an essential component of the neutrophil's microbicidal machinery.

1.2   PRODUCTION OF SUPEROXIDE

The NADPH oxidase catalyses the following reaction

$$NADPH + H^+ + 2O_2 \rightarrow NADP^+ + 2H^+ + 2O_2^-$$

whereby NADPH, produced in the cytosol by the hexose monophosphate shunt, donates two electrons, to effect a one electron reduction of each of two atoms of molecular oxygen (Babior et al., 1973). The K_M of the oxidase is 30–50 μM. The pK of the dissociation

$$O_2H \rightarrow O_2^- + H^+$$

is 4.7 indicating that the superoxide anion is the predominant species present at physiological pH. The superoxide thus formed then spontaneously dismutates to form hydrogen peroxide (H_2O_2).

$$2O_2^- + 2H^+ \rightarrow O_2 + H_2O_2$$

Other more reactive oxygen products may also arise via further reactions, e.g. the $OH^\bullet$ radical and oxygen singlet $^1O_2$.

The respiratory burst can be activated by a variety of stimuli. Physiological stimuli include opsonized micro-organisms and FMLP, a chemotactic peptide released by bacteria. Oxidase activity can be estimated by measuring any one of several different parameters: the increase in oxygen consumption using an oxygen electrode, production of superoxide as the superoxide dismutase-inhibitable reduction of cytochrome c at 550 nm, as the production of formazan by the reduction of nitroblue tetrazolium, fluorimetric or enzymatic measurement of hydrogen peroxide production, and by chemiluminescence. The most widely used method is that of cytochrome c reduction.

1.3   THE RESPIRATORY BURST AND ITS ROLE IN BACTERIAL KILLING

Early studies with pH-sensitive dyes coupled to phagocytosed particles suggested that the phagocytic vacuoles were an acidic environment (Mandell, 1970; Jacques and Bainton, 1978). However, it became apparent that the very earliest events were not being detected. Subsequent work demonstrated that the vacuolar pH initially rises to approximately pH 7.8–8.0 before falling slowly to pH 6.0 (Segal et al., 1981; Cech and Lehrer, 1984). The rise in pH is accompanied by the pumping of electrons by the oxidase into the vacuole (Henderson et al., 1987). This process has been shown to be electrogenic. The reduced oxygen products, superoxide and peroxide, then consume protons as they disproportionate to the protonated form with a concomitant rise in pH. Reduced oxygen products are not microbicidal in themselves. Cytoplasts (neutrophils from which the granules and nuclei are removed) are able to phagocytose bacteria and generate a respiratory burst but fail to kill Staphylococci in the normal way, suggesting that the granule contents, including many proteases, which would normally be dispensed into the vacuole, are required for killing (Odell and Segal, 1988; see Chapter 4). It is possible that the initial rise in intravacuolar pH which occurs concomitantly with the respiratory burst serves to create an environment in which the granular proteases are active and can destroy the microorganism.

Myeloperoxidase, released from azurophil granules during degranulation, catalyses the reaction of hydrogen peroxide with chloride ions to yield hypochlorous acid, a potent anti-microbial agent. In addition, the introduction of pure myeloperoxidase into the phagocytic vacuole of cytoplasts has been shown to reconstitute microbicidal activity (Odell and Segal, 1988). Clearly, however, this enzyme is not essential for the killing process, since myeloperoxidase-deficient individuals do not suffer from a higher incidence of infection than normal (Klebanoff and Clark, 1978).

1.4   CHARACTERIZATION OF THE OXIDASE

Two approaches have been central to the dissection of the NADPH oxidase into its individual components. One has been the study of cells from patients with CGD, a disease characterized by failure of the neutrophil to generate superoxide. This syndrome will be discussed in greater detail later (Section 2). The other has been the use of "cell free" systems of superoxide production in which the recombining of membranes and cytosol prepared from non-activated cells, in the presence of an amphiphile such as sodium dodecyl sulphate or arachidonic acid and the electron donor NADPH, results in the production of superoxide.

The application of these technologies during the last 15 years, together with some exceptional classical biochemistry and innovative molecular biology, has now provided us with a fairly complete picture of the structure of the active oxidase complex. A schematic is depicted in Figure 3.1. Precise understanding of the interactions between components and their three-dimensional structures remain, though, as problems for the future.

1.4.1 The Cell-Free System

The cell-free system was first described independently, by two groups in 1984 (Bromberg and Pick, 1984; Heyneman and Vercauteren, 1984) and has since been developed and widely used by many workers in the field (Bromberg and Pick, 1985; Curnutte, 1985; McPhail et al., 1985; Gabig et al., 1987; Ligeti et al., 1988; Tanaka et al., 1988). The rationale behind the approach is depicted in Figure 3.2. It has allowed investigators to identify and isolate components of the oxidase, since for the first time it provided an assay capable of assessing the involvement of individual components in superoxide production. A critical parameter in determining the levels of superoxide generated by the cell-free system is the ratio

of membrane and cytosolic protein to that of amphiphile (Pilloud et al., 1989). The addition of GTP or its non-hydrolysable analogue, GTP-γ-S, augments the activity of the cell-free system quite markedly when intact membranes are used in the assay (Seifert et al., 1986; Gabig et al., 1987; Ligeti et al., 1988; Aharoni and Pick, 1990; Eklund et al., 1991). These findings suggested that a G protein was involved in the system. A small G protein, rap 1 (see Section 1.7.2; Chapter 8), has been shown to be physically associated with cytochrome b_{-245} (Quinn et al., 1989). There is as yet, however, no direct evidence for its involvement in the oxidase. Interestingly, workers using solubilized membranes in the cell-free system have obtained maximal activity without a requirement for nucleotide (Pick et al., 1989; Shpungin et al., 1989; Abo and Pick, 1991; Abo et al., 1991).

1.5 MEMBRANE COMPONENTS OF THE OXIDASE

The dormant oxidase has components residing in the plasma membrane, specific granule membrane and cytosol.

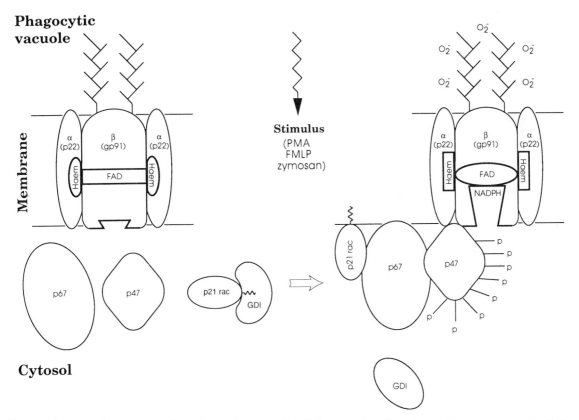

Figure 3.1 Schematic representation of complex formation between cytosolic and membrane components of the NADPH oxidase upon neutrophil activation. Oxidase components are identified using standard nomenclature. —p, phosphorylation. The changes in shape of the binding sites for haem and the nucleotide cofactors are used to represent speculated conformational changes in the protein structure.

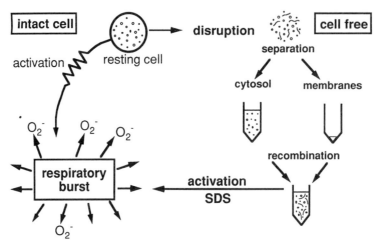

Figure 3.2 Schematic representation of cell-free oxidase assay system.

Upon stimulation the active enzyme is found in the plasma membrane where it appears as a complex of proteins from both membrane and cytosolic pools (Figure 3.1). There is now compelling evidence that the first component of the oxidase to be identified, the membrane-bound cytochrome b_{-245}, is the only true membrane component and the only redox molecule involved in electron transport (Rotrosen *et al.*, 1992; Segal *et al.*, 1992).

1.5.1 Discovery and Identification of Cytochrome b_{-245}

Cytochrome b_{-245} was first detected by spectroscopic analysis in equine neutrophils in 1961 and it was later suggested that it might be involved in the respiratory burst because of its cytochrome oxidase-like properties, namely an ability to bind carbon monoxide and to autoxidize (Hattori, 1961; Ohta *et al.*, 1966; Shinagawa *et al.*, 1966).

This earlier work was largely ignored until Segal and Jones in 1978 reported the presence of cytochrome b_{-245} in human neutrophils (Segal and Jones, 1978). The unusually low midpoint oxidation–reduction potential of this cytochrome (-245 mV) makes it distinguishable from b-cytochromes present in the mitochondria and microsomes and indicated that it was capable of reducing molecular oxygen (Wood, 1987). It is also known as cytochrome $b558$, the 558 referring to the wavelength of its alpha band of light absorption in reduced minus oxidized spectra. It is present in neutrophils and monocytes at a concentration of approximately 100 pmol/mg protein (Segal *et al.*, 1983). Using spectral analysis the association of the cytochrome with the phagocytic vacuole and its absence from, or gross abnormality in, cells from patients with CGD, was suggestive of a role in the oxidase (Segal and Jones, 1978, 1980; Segal *et al.*, 1978). Further work demonstrated a complete lack of this molecule in a large subset of CGD

patients (those with the X-linked form of the disease), strongly implicating it as one of the redox components of the oxidase (Segal *et al.*, 1983). Complementation studies using monocytes from cytochrome b_{-245} positive and negative forms of CGD further supported the involvement of this molecule in the respiratory burst (Hamers *et al.*, 1984).

Purification of the cytochrome proved difficult. The four initial purification schemes described isolated polypeptides ranging from 11 to 127 kD (Harper *et al.*, 1984; Pember *et al.*, 1984; Serra *et al.*, 1984; Lutter *et al.*, 1985). Proteolysis was a major problem in this work since neutrophils are a rich source of proteolytic enzymes. In addition the cytochrome was found to be composed of two subunits, one of which is heavily glycosylated and migrates as a diffuse band on polyacrylamide gels making reporting of molecular weight estimations confused (Harper *et al.*, 1984).

The cytochrome was shown to comprise two subunits, a small (22 kD) alpha subunit and a large (76–92 kD), heavily glycosylated, beta subunit (Segal, 1987; Parkos *et al.*, 1987). The beta subunit comprises approximately 21% carbohydrate, predominantly of the N-linked high-lactosamine complex type (Harper *et al.*, 1985). That of the guinea-pig macrophage has a lower molecular weight of 54–60 kD due to the fact that it is less heavily glycosylated than its human neutrophil counterpart (Knoller *et al.*, 1991). The significance of the degree of glycosylation is not known. Both polypeptides are missing from patients with X-linked CGD (Segal, 1987; Parkos *et al.*, 1987, 1988a) (see Section 2.2.1). In non-activated neutrophils the cytochrome is located in the plasma membrane and the specific granules (Segal and Jones, 1979a; Garcia and Segal, 1984; Morel *et al.*, 1985; Parkos *et al.*, 1985; Clark *et al.*, 1987; Ambruso *et al.*, 1990). Upon stimulation, the specific granules fuse with the phagocytic vacuoles, increasing the level of cytochrome present in the vacuolar membrane.

The gene responsible for most cases of X-linked CGD was identified in 1986 by one of the first applications of reverse genetics (Royer-Pokora *et al.*, 1986) (Section 2.2.1). Although some confusion occurred initially over the identity of the protein encoded by this gene, amino-acid sequence data obtained from the purified beta subunit of the cytochrome unequivocally identified this polypeptide as the defective molecule responsible for X-linked CGD (Teahan *et al.*, 1987). Studies using antibodies raised to the gene product also established the identity of the β-subunit and the X-CGD gene product (Dinauer *et al.*, 1987).

1.5.2 Biochemical and Structural Properties of Cytochrome b_{-245}

The alkaline pyridine spectrum of cytochrome b_{-245} is that of a protohaem pyridine haemochrome, characteristic of *b*-type cytochromes (Segal and Jones, 1979a). It has several unusual properties. Its low midpoint potential of -245 mV, the lowest potential of any mammalian *b* cytochrome, confers on it the capability of directly reducing molecular oxygen to superoxide (the midpoint potential of the O_2/O_2^- couple is -160 mV) (Cross *et al.*, 1984; Wood, 1987). It is capable of binding cytochrome oxidase, a property which it shares with bacterial cytochromes *o* (Cross *et al.*, 1981, 1982a). The oxidation of the reduced cytochrome is very rapid with a half-time of 4.7 ms (Cross *et al.*, 1982a). The recombination time after flash dissociation of the complex is approximately 6 ms indicating that it probably binds oxygen. Recent work has shown that reduction of the cytochrome b_{-245} by p450 reductase results in the production of superoxide, further evidence that it is the terminal component of the oxidase (Isogai *et al.*, 1991).

The smaller (22 kD, "alpha") subunit of cytochrome b_{-245} is thought to be the haem binding component of the complex. Evidence for this has come from two directions. Firstly, when the cytochrome subunits are separated by equilibrium centrifugation in the presence of octyl glucoside, the haem appears to be associated with the α-subunit. Secondly, radiation inactivation analysis indicated a molecular weight for the the haem-binding moiety of approximately 21 kD (Nugent *et al.*, 1989). In addition, purification studies from different cell types indicate a close correlation between the amount of haem and that of the small, but not the large, subunit (Capeillere-Blandin *et al.*, 1991). Raman spectroscopy indicates that the haem is bound to two histidine residues. The small subunit contains two histidines, one of which (His-93) is in a region having homology to the haem-binding subunit of cytochrome *c* oxidase (Parkos *et al.*, 1988b). The second histidine though, is the site of a naturally occurring polymorphism which does not affect haem binding or cytochrome function (Dinauer *et al.*, 1990). It would seem that the haem must be coordinated in a somewhat atypical fashion, either within a single alpha subunit, or perhaps bound *between* two small subunits, or *between* an α- and a β-subunit.

Cytochrome b_{-245} is a one-electron acceptor while NADPH is a two-electron donor. Flavoproteins are capable of accepting two electrons from NADPH and transferring them one at a time to the cytochrome which could then effect the single electron reduction of molecular oxygen to superoxide. In fact, it has been observed almost universally in electron transport chains that a flavoprotein intermediate is used to couple a reduced nicotinamide to a haem or iron–sulphur protein (Massey and Hemmerich, 1980). The involvement of a flavoprotein in the NADPH oxidase was postulated by Cagan and Karnovsky (1964). Evidence in support of this idea was obtained when it was found that FAD was able to restore lost activity to oxidase preparations obtained by detergent extraction of membranes (Klebanoff, 1971; Babior and Kipnes, 1977; Wakeyama *et al.*, 1982; Rossi, 1986; Bellavite, 1988). Furthermore, superoxide activity is inhibited by some flavin analogues and correlates with the redox potential of others (Light *et al.*, 1981; Parkinson and Gabig, 1988). FAD in membranes and membrane extracts can be reduced by NADPH under anaerobic conditions (Cross *et al.*, 1984; Gabig and Lefker, 1984a) and diphenylene iodonium, a flavoprotein inhibitor and an inhibitor of the oxidase, prevents the anaerobic reduction of both FAD and the cytochrome (Cross and Jones, 1986). An electron spin resonance spectrum characteristic of a flavin semiquinone has also been observed in membranes prepared from activated neutrophils in the presence of NADPH, but not using membranes from non-activated cells (Kakinuma *et al.*, 1986). This spectrum indicated a midpoint potential of -280 mV, intermediate between that of the $NADP^+/NADPH$ couple (-320 mV) and that of the oxidized/reduced cytochrome *b* (-245 mV). Analysis of the flavin content of these membranes revealed that it was almost exclusively FAD. This was released by denaturation with little covalently bound flavin evident. Since there was strong evidence implicating a flavoprotein in the NADPH oxidase, several groups have attempted to identify the flavoprotein involved. This body of work has been extensively reviewed elsewhere (Morel *et al.*, 1991).

There is now compelling evidence that cytochrome b_{-245} is in fact also the flavoprotein of the NADPH oxidase. This possibility was first conjectured in 1982 (Cross *et al.*, 1982b). The FAD content in the membranes of cells from CGD patients lacking cytochrome b_{-245} was found to be variable but was generally less than that of normal or autosomal recessive CGD (Cross *et al.*, 1982; Gabig and Lefker, 1984b; Bohler *et al.*, 1986; Ohno *et al.*, 1986) suggesting an association between the haem and flavin containing proteins, possibly within a flavocytochrome. Some partially purified preparations of the solubilized oxidase contained both FAD and haem (Bellavite *et al.*, 1983) which were reduced upon addition of NADPH (Bellavite *et al.*, 1984). However, others reported preparations containing only FAD (Markert *et al.*, 1985; Kakinuma *et al.*, 1987) or completely lacking cofactors (Doussiere and Vignais, 1985). The two known cytosolic components of the oxidase, p47-*phox* and p67-*phox* (see Section 1.6), did not bind flavin (Chiba *et al.*, 1990). Furthermore, Pick and co-workers have shown that, at least in the cell-free system, the cytochrome is the only membrane component required for activity (Knoller *et al.*, 1991).

Recently published reports appear to have solved the identity of the FAD binding component, providing strong evidence that the flavoprotein is a membrane component and is in fact cytochrome b_{-245} itself (Rotrosen *et al.*, 1992; Segal *et al.*, 1992). Using a very sensitive assay for FAD (the reconstitution of activity to apo D-amino acid oxidase by FAD) it was shown that membranes from X-linked CGD patients (who generally lack the cytochrome) contained less than 30% of the FAD present in normal neutrophil membranes (Segal *et al.*, 1992). In addition, normal levels of FAD were found in membranes from p47-*phox*-deficient autosomal recessive CGD cells which contain a normal amount of cytochrome b_{-245}. The low levels of FAD present in X-linked CGD membranes were considered to be unrelated to the oxidase, given that similar results were obtained with membranes from uninduced HL60 cells (a human promyelocytic cell line that can be induced to differentiate into mature neutrophil or macrophage-like cells with NADPH oxidase activity). By subtracting this fraction of membrane-associated FAD from the total, a 1:2 ratio of FAD to haem was found in both stimulated and unstimulated membranes. A very similar FAD:haem ratio was found by Bellavite *et al.* (1983) in peak fractions

of partially purified oxidase preparations. The purified cytochrome could be reflavinated to about 20% of maximum in the presence of lipid (Segal *et al.*, 1992).

When the sequence of the β-subunit of the cytochrome was determined in 1986/1987 there was no evidence, based on sequence homology, that the protein could bind nucleotides. More recently, the sequence of the β-subunit of the cytochrome was compared against libraries of common nucleotide-binding sites (Bork and Grunwald, 1990) and general motifs, but again without much success (Segal *et al.*, 1992). Studies demonstrating strong homologies in flavin and NADPH-binding domains in the nitric reductase family of proteins (Bredt *et al.*, 1991; Karplus *et al.*, 1991; Porter, 1991) provided the answer. A search employing the conserved glycine-rich region in the proposed NADPH-binding site of the FNR flavoenzyme family (Bredt *et al.*, 1991) demonstrated close homology between the β-subunit of the cytochrome and other members of this family (Rotrosen *et al.*, 1992; Segal *et al.*, 1992) (Figure 3.3). Homology was also detected in the region of the FAD–isoalloxazine binding site approximately 90 amino acids upstream of the NADPH–ribose binding site (Segal *et al.*, 1992). Although amino-acid identity was weak, those in the proposed nucleotide binding region corresponded closely to those in the FNR family in charge, size and function.

Attempts to label the NADPH binding component using NADPH dialdehyde have given contradictory results due to its lack of specificity as an affinity labelling agent. A 66 kD membrane protein was initially reported to be the NADPH-binding protein of the oxidase (Umei *et al.*, 1986). However, another group reported a 66 kD cytosolic protein as the NADPH binder (Smith *et al.*, 1989), and a 32 kD component has recently been proposed (Umei *et al.*, 1991).

	FAD	NADPH	NADPH
(1)	712 R A Y T P S S	783 L A M I A G - G T G I T P V Y Q V M	880 L A A C G P
(2)	66 R P Y T P I S	149 V G M I A G - G T G I T P M L Q V I	245 V L M C G P
(3)	337 H P F T L T S	402 V V M L V G A G I G V T P F A S I L	533 V F L C G P
(4)	386 R L Y S I A S	453 V I M I - G P G T G I A P F R S F M	549 I Y V C G D
(5)	93 R L Y S I A S	166 I I M L - G T G T G I A P F R S F L	269 V Y M C G L
(6)	367 R Y Y S I S S	436 L I M V - G P G T G V A P F R G F V	536 F Y I C G D
(7)	454 R Y Y S I A S	526 V I M V - G P G T G I A P F M G F I	627 I Y V C G D
(8)	1173 R Y Y S I S S	1242 C I L V - G P G T G I A P F R S F W	1345 I Y V C G D

Figure 3.3 Homologies between β-chain of cytochrome b and the FNR family of reductases. 1, NADH nitrate reductase; 2, NADH cytochrome b5 reductase; 3, NADPH cytochrome b_{-245} β-chain; 4, NADPH sulphite reductase; 5, ferredoxin NADP reductase; 6, NADPH cytochrome P450 reductase; 7, NADPH cytochrome P450 reductase; 8, NADPH nitric oxide synthase.

A CGD patient (Dinauer *et al.*, 1989) has been described, however, in whom the pattern of inheritance was clearly X-linked but had apparently normal cytochrome (Hurst *et al.*, 1991). Normal levels of FAD were found in the membranes. Sequencing of the cytochrome b_{-245} cDNA from this patient revealed a point mutation in the β-subunit leading to the substitution of a histidine for a proline at residue 415 (Dinauer *et al.*, 1989). This substitution is located in the glycine-rich region of the predicted NADPH-binding site. It was therefore likely that failure of the cytochrome to bind NADPH was the cause of CGD in this patient. To test this possibility, NADPH-binding studies, using the photoaffinity probe ^{32}P-labelled 2-azido-NADP, were performed on membranes from normal subjects, a patient with classical X-linked cytochrome *b*-negative CGD and this unusual X-linked cytochrome *b*-positive individual. Preparations from both X-linked patients failed to show NADP binding in the region of the β-subunit of the cytochrome (Segal *et al.*, 1992).

1.6 CYTOSOLIC COMPONENTS OF THE OXIDASE

1.6.1 p47-*phox*

Because the neutrophil membranes of X-linked CGD patients lacked cytochrome b_{-245}, attention focused on the abnormality responsible for the common autosomal recessive form of CGD (AR-CGD), which is cytochrome positive. In neutrophils from these patients it was discovered that the cytochrome failed to become reduced upon stimulation of the cells (Segal and Jones, 1980). A defect in the signalling pathway responsible for oxidase activation was a plausible mechanism, and to this end several groups studied patterns of phosphorylated proteins obtained when normal and AR-CGD cells were stimulated, in the hope of detecting differences. Segal *et al.* (1985) identified a newly phosphorylated band of approximately 47 kD (originally referred to as 44 kD) in cytosol from activated neutrophils that was absent from AR-CGD neutrophil cytosol. It was also shown that, in normal cells, this phosphoprotein translocated from the cytosol to the membrane upon stimulation of the cell (Heyworth *et al.*, 1989). Further evidence that the 47 kD phosphoprotein was involved in the oxidase came from the observation that this translocation did not occur in cells from patients with X-linked CGD, which lack the cytochrome (Heyworth *et al.*, 1989); this implied there was an association between the two molecules. It was also observed that phosphorylation of the 47 kD protein in the cytosol preceded the appearance of phosphorylated 47 kD protein in the membrane, suggesting a causal role for phosphorylation in this relocation (Heyworth *et al.*, 1989). More recently, it has been shown that this phosphorylation occurs in two successive stages, one set of phosphorylation events occurring in the cytosol and a second occurring subsequent to the protein's translocation to the membrane (Okamura *et al.*, 1988a, 1988b).

The breakthrough in the isolation of this molecule came from a rather unexpected direction. It had previously been reported that GTP-γ-S potentiated the cell-free system implicating the involvement of a G protein in the oxidase (Gabig *et al.*, 1987; Seifert and Schultz, 1987; Ligeti *et al.*, 1988). For this reason Clark and his colleagues analysed neutrophil cytosol for proteins that could bind to GTP agarose (Volpp *et al.*, 1988). Proteins that bound to the column and eluted in the presence of GTP were used to generate an antiserum referred to as B1 (Volpp *et al.*, 1988). Despite the fact that the protein fraction used to raise this antiserum contained quite a sizeable number of proteins, the B1 antiserum reacted basically against three proteins in neutrophil cytosol that were specific for cells of myeloid origin. Fractionation of the cytosol by gel filtration was used to test fractions for their ability to replace cytosol in the cell-free system. Comparing this assay with Western blot results, two proteins of molecular weight 47 kD and 67 kD were found to coelute with oxidase activity (Volpp *et al.*, 1988).

A broadly similar approach using the same antibody preparation was followed by Malech and his co-workers (Nunoi *et al.*, 1988). Anion exchange fractionation of normal cytosol was able to resolve three peaks (NCF-1, NCF-2, NCF-3) that were able to act synergistically with suboptimal amounts of cytosol in the cell-free system. The effect of adding some of these fractions to cytosols from patients with two different forms of autosomal recessive CGD was then investigated. NCF-1 and NCF-2 were able to correct the cytosolic defect in both forms of AR-CGD, each peak having the ability to correct only one of the two forms. Immunoblotting of NCF-1 and NCF-2 using the B1 antiserum revealed that NCF-1 contained the 47 kD protein and NCF-2 contained the 67 kD protein. These proteins are now referred to as p47-*phox* and p67-*phox* to indicate their involvement in the *pha*gocytic *ox*idase; this nomenclature has now become standard for all the NADPH oxidase components (see Table 3.1). The B1 antiserum was subsequently used by both groups to obtain cDNA clones encoding these proteins. The cDNA sequence of p47-*phox* was reported independently by Lomax *et al.* (1989b) and Volpp *et al.* (1989a), although owing to the high G-C content of the mRNA both groups made errors in the sequencing (Lomax *et al.*, 1989a; Volpp *et al.*, 1989b). The correct sequence was also reported by Rodaway *et al.* (1990) who identified the gene as one whose transcription increased dramatically upon induction of differentiation in HL60 cells.

The p47-*phox* cDNA encodes a protein of 390 amino acids, of predicted molecular weight, 44.7 kD, containing several potential phosphorylation sites [PKC, mitogen-activated protein (MAP) kinase, casein kinase,

Table 3.1   Specific components of the NADPH oxidase

	gp91-phox	p22-phox	p47-phox	p67-phox
Component	Cytochrome b_{-245} β-subunit	Cytochrome b_{-245} α-subunit	47 kD phosphoprotein	
Localization in resting cell	Membrane	Membrane	Cytoplasm	Cytoplasm
Locus	CYBB	CYBA	NCF-1	NCF-2
Chromosomal localization	Xp21.1	16q24	7q11.23	1q25
Gene size	30 kb	8.5 kb	17–20 kb	37 kb
Exons	13	5	9	16
mRNA size	4.8 kb	0.7 kb	1.4 kb	2.4 kb
Protein predicted mol.wt	65 kD	21 kD	44.6 kD	60.9 kD
(SDS PAGE)	(90 kD)	(22 kD)	(47 kD)	(67 kD)

calmodulin-dependent kinase]. Upon activation of neutrophils, eight distinct phosphorylated species have been detected (Rotrosen and Leto, 1990). Recombinant protein reconstituted oxidase activity to cytosol from p47-*phox*-deficient neutrophils (Lomax *et al.*, 1989b; Volpp *et al.*, 1989a). The net charge of the protein is +9, consistent with the basic isoelectric point of 10 reported by Curnutte *et al.* (1989).

The sequence shows little homology with other proteins and gives few clues as to its possible role in the oxidase. It does, however, contain regions of homology to SH3 domains (src homology 3), motifs of about 50 residues, first described in the regulatory region of pp60^{v-src}. A diverse group of proteins has been shown to contain SH3 domains (Rodaway *et al.*, 1990; Leto *et al.*, 1990), including phospholipase C gamma, ras-GAP and alpha fodrin. The function of these domains is not known, although in some proteins they are thought to mediate interaction with the cytoskeleton (Drubin *et al.*, 1990; Musacchio *et al.*, 1992). Both p47-*phox* and p67-*phox* contain two such domains, which has led to a deal of speculation on the role of the cytoskeleton in activation of the NADPH oxidase (Nauseef *et al.*, 1991; Woodman *et al.*, 1991). It seems that p67-*phox* may bind to actin (Woodman *et al.*, 1991) but this area generally is in need of clarification. The fact that both the cytosolic components of the oxidase are "bivalent" with respect to the SH3 domains suggests they may be involved in subunit–subunit interactions. Certainly, the translocation of p67-*phox* to the membrane has been shown to be dependent on the presence of p47-*phox*; translocation of p67-*phox* is not observed in p47-*phox*-deficient patients (Heyworth *et al.*, 1991). The converse seems not to be true but this would appear to support the notion that the two cytosolic factors normally interact in some way. Evidence that this may not be mediated through the SH3 domains though has come from study of recombinant p67-*phox* protein. In these studies, an *in vitro* mutant lacking both SH3 domains was found to function equivalently to the wild-type protein, when tested by its ability to stimulate superoxide generation in the cell-free system (Leto and Garrett, 1992).

That p47-*phox* and the 47 kD phosphoprotein missing in AR-CGD were one and the same was established by isolation of the phosphoprotein and determination of its N-terminal amino acid sequence. Its sequence was shown to correspond to that predicted from the cloned gene (Teahan *et al.*, 1990). A peptide antiserum raised to the C-terminus of the protein also demonstrated its absence from AR-CGD cells. The level of p47-*phox* in neutrophil cytosol has been estimated at 150 ng/10^6 cells (Leto *et al.*, 1991).

Although the role of p47-*phox* in the activation of the oxidase remains unknown, evidence has accumulated for its close interaction with other components of the system, namely p67-*phox* and the β-subunit of cytochrome b_{-245}. From its initial identification it was known that p47-*phox* translocates from the cytosol to the membrane on cell activation (Heyworth *et al.*, 1989; Clark *et al.*, 1990). That its membrane target was cytochrome b_{-245} was strongly suggested by its failure to translocate in cytochrome-deficient X-linked CGD cells (Heyworth *et al.*, 1989); a finding confirmed in later studies using antibodies to recombinant p47-*phox* protein (Rotrosen *et al.*, 1990). Further evidence for this interaction was obtained when it was shown that a C-terminal heptapeptide of the β-subunit of the cytochrome blocked both the cell-free generation of superoxide and that produced by cells which had been permeabilized and treated with the peptide prior to stimulation with FMLP (Rotrosen *et al.*, 1990).

1.6.2   p67-*phox*

As alluded to above, the B1 antiserum also identified a 67 kD protein, which was missing in a small minority of the AR-CGD cases not deficient in p47-*phox* (Clark *et al.*, 1989; Leto *et al.*, 1990; Casimir *et al.*, 1992). The antiserum was also used to isolate cDNA clones encoding this protein. Addition of recombinant p67-*phox* protein was able partially to restore NADPH oxidase activity to a cell-free system using cytosol from p67-*phox*-deficient neutrophils (Leto *et al.*, 1990). The nucleotide sequence predicts a protein of 526 amino acids with a calculated size of 60.9 kD. The sequence of p67-*phox* bears no obvious homology with any other proteins, apart from possessing two SH3 domains, as does p47-*phox*.

p67-*phox* has additionally been isolated as a 63 kD band from porcine and bovine neutrophils (Tanaka *et al.*, 1990; Pilloud-Dagher and Vignais, 1991). The porcine protein appears to exist as a trimer while the bovine molecule elutes from gel filtration columns as a dimer. It is present at a concentration of approximately 75 ng/10^6 human neutrophils (Leto *et al.*, 1991).

As described above, p67-*phox* has also been shown to translocate from the cytosol to the membranes upon activation of the cell (Clark *et al.*, 1990), although its translocation appears to be dependent on p47-*phox*. Since p47-*phox* does not translocate in cytochrome-negative X-linked CGD cells, p67-*phox* would be expected to behave similarly. In three out of four X-linked CGD patients this was indeed the case (Heyworth *et al.*, 1991). In the fourth patient, however, low levels of membrane-associated p67-*phox* were observed despite there being no evidence of p47-*phox* translocation. This anomaly remains unexplained.

A mixture of recombinant p47-*phox* and p67-*phox* failed to substitute for whole cytosol in the cell free system (Leto *et al.*, 1991). This was consistent with work from several groups which indicated that there were at least four cytosolic components involved in activation of the oxidase (Fujita *et al.*, 1987; Nunoi *et al.*, 1988; Curnutte *et al.*, 1989; Bolscher *et al.*, 1990).

1.7 SMALL G PROTEINS

The low molecular weight (20–30 kD) GTP-binding proteins comprise a family of proteins distinct from the heterotrimeric G proteins (see Chapter 8). The proteins cycle between an active GTP-bound form and an inactive GDP-bound form generated by hydrolysis of the GTP. They possess an intrinsic GTPase activity which may be modulated by other proteins such as the GTPase-activating factor, GDP dissociation inhibitor and the GDP dissociation stimulator. It is thought that the nature of the nucleotide bound affects the conformation of the G protein thus facilitating signal transduction.

1.7.1 p21 rac1 and 2

GTP-γ-S was first shown to augment the cell-free oxidase activity in 1987 (Gabig *et al.*, 1987; Seifert and Schültz, 1987) and from that time attempts were made to identify the G protein involved. Studies by Gabig and colleagues indicated that a pertussis toxin-insensitive cytosolic G protein was involved in activation of the oxidase (Gabig *et al.*, 1987, 1990). Pick and co-workers, using guinea-pig macrophages, found that the cytosol can be separated into two fractions, sigma 1 and sigma 2, which, when combined, can substitute for whole cytosol in the cell-free system (Pick *et al.*, 1989; Sha'ag and Pick, 1990). Sigma 2 contained both p47-*phox* and p67-*phox* and attention was focused on the identification and

characterization of the active component(s) present in sigma 1. Interestingly, the active component in sigma 1 was also found to be present in cytosol from non-phagocytic cells. This activity was purified to reveal a complex composed of 22 kD and 26 kD polypeptides which eluted as a molecular mass of 46 kD on gel filtration (Abo and Pick, 1991). Amino-acid sequencing of the mixture identified the 22kD as the small GTP-binding protein, p21 rac1, and the 26 kD as rho GDI (Abo *et al.*, 1991). There was no requirement for GTP when the purified complex was used to reconstitute sigma 1-depleted cytosol in the cell-free system. When recombinant p21 rac1 was added to the system in the absence of rho GDI, however, it was necessary to preload the recombinant protein with GTP. The nature of the guanine nucleotide in the complex has yet to be determined.

Other workers have identified the small G protein involved in the oxidase to be p21 rac2 rather than rac1 (Knaus *et al.*, 1992; Mizuno *et al.*, 1992). Antibody specific for p21 rac2 strongly inhibited the cell-free oxidase while that specific for rac1 had little effect (Knaus *et al.*, 1992). The sequences of the two proteins exhibit 92% identity and it is possible that the small G protein involved in the oxidase is a novel rac molecule. Contrary to the work of Abo and co-workers, Mizuno reported that recombinant p21 rac1 is *not* active in the cell-free system (Abo *et al.*, 1991; Mizuno *et al.*, 1992). These inconsistencies remain to be resolved.

The fact that a small G protein has been shown to be essential for a very specific and highly regulated enzyme system opens up a new field in the study of regulation of the oxidase in particular and signal transduction mediated by small G proteins in general.

1.7.2 p21 rap1

The small G protein, p21 rap1, has been reported to co-purify and cross-immunoprecipitate with cytochrome b_{-245} (Quinn *et al.*, 1989). The relevance of this to oxidase activity has not been established and, at least in a cell-free system (using recombinant p47-*phox*, p67-*phox*, GTP-loaded recombinant p21 rac1 and relipidated purified cytochrome b_{-245}), it is not required for superoxide production (Abo *et al.*, 1992).

1.8 ACTIVATION OF THE OXIDASE

Neutrophils can respond in many ways to different stimuli and in different ways to varying concentrations of a given stimulus. The mechanisms by which these responses are regulated and coordinated is a complex and as yet poorly understood area.

1.8.1 Oxidase Activators

Neutrophils respond to particular stimuli present near or at sites of inflammation. Among the most effective of these are opsonized microorganisms, the complement fragment C5a which is formed upon complement activation following interaction of microorganisms with antibodies, N-formyl-methionyl-peptides that are secreted by bacteria or released by the lysis of dead micro-organisms, PAF, LTB₄, neutrophil activating factors NAP-1 and NAP-2. All of these stimuli act via distinct surface receptors (see Chapter 6) coupled to hetero-trimeric G proteins not only to activate the respiratory burst but also, at an earlier stage in the sequence of events, to facilitate migration of neutrophils along an increasing concentration gradient of the stimulus to the site of infection. FMLP at concentrations of less than 10 nM does not activate the oxidase but does induce the migration of neutrophils to the inflamed area where, at concentrations of FMLP greater than 100 nM, the respiratory burst is triggered.

Artificial stimuli can also activate the oxidase. These include fluoride, PMA and other phorbol esters, the calcium ionophore A23187 and opsonized latex beads.

1.8.2 Priming of the Burst

Neutrophils may exist in a state between resting and acti-vated, termed "primed", whereby subsequent exposure of the cells to a stimulus results in an amplified respiratory burst with a much reduced lag phase (Johnston and Kitagawa, 1985; Haslett *et al.*, 1989; Walker *et al.*, 1991; see Chapter 9). Cytokines (IL-1, IL-2, IL-4, TNFα, G-CSF, GM-CSF and IFNγ), phorbol esters, chemo-attractants, bacterial lipopolysaccharide, ionomycin and DAG are some of the agents capable of priming neutro-phils (Bender *et al.*, 1983; Haslett *et al.*, 1989; Yuo *et al.*, 1990). The precise mechanisms involved in priming remain unknown. An increase in the concentration of cytosolic calcium appears to be a step common to many priming agents (Ingraham *et al.*, 1982; Finkel *et al.*, 1987; Forehand *et al.*, 1989). PKC has been shown to translocate to the membrane in primed neutrophils consistent with an increase in the levels of cytosolic calcium in these cells. Levels of diacylglycerol are also increased in the membranes of primed cells as are the number and affinity of various receptors.

1.8.3 Generation of Second Messengers

The involvement of phospholipase C in activation of the neutrophil has been recognized for almost a decade (Cockcroft *et al.*, 1984; Cockcroft and Gomperts, 1985; Ohta *et al.*, 1985; Smith *et al.*, 1985). Upon activation by a receptor-coupled stimulus PLC hydrolyses a membrane phospholipid, PIP₂, generating two second messengers, DAG and IP₃. DAG is a cofactor required for the activation of PKC. It is rapidly converted to phosphatidic acid by phosphorylation by DAG kinase. IP₃ effects the release of calcium from intracellular stores. These increased levels of intracellular calcium may activate several independent pathways including those involving PKC. This is discussed in detail in Chapter 8.

There is now growing evidence that phospholipases D and A₂ are also involved in neutrophil activation (also discussed in Chapter 8). Phospholipase D generates phosphatidic acid by the hydrolysis of the membrane lipid, phosphatidylcholine (Agwu *et al.*, 1989; Billah *et al.*, 1989). The phosphatidic acid formed is slowly converted into DAG by phosphatidate phosphohydro-lase (Billah *et al.*, 1989). Release of arachidonic acid from phosphatidylcholine by PLA₂ has also been shown to correlate with oxidase activity (Maridonneau-Parini and Tauber, 1986). Inhibitors of PLA₂ inhibit PMA acti-vation of the oxidase suggesting that arachidonic acid is involved in at least one of the signalling pathways (Henderson *et al.*, 1989). PLC is activated via a pertussis toxin-sensitive G protein and there is increasing evidence that PLD and PLA₂ are also activated by G proteins. PLD and PLA₂ may also be activated downstream of PLC activation via increases in levels of intracellular calcium.

1.8.4 The Role of Phosphorylation in Regulation of the Oxidase

The absolute requirement for p47-*phox* in superoxide production makes its role as a substrate for serine phos-phorylation of interest with regard to its regulation. The correlation of p47-*phox* phosphorylation in response to a wide range of stimuli, its subsequent translocation to the membrane and oxidase activity suggested a central role for protein kinase activity in the regulation of the burst.

PMA has been known as a potent activator of the oxidase since 1974 (Repine *et al.*, 1974). Up until the early 1980s, however, little was known regarding the intermediary steps involved in this activation. It was then found that treatment of neutrophils with PMA or FMLP resulted in enhanced protein phosphorylation within the cell (Schneider *et al.*, 1981). Of particular note were two proteins at 47 and 49 kD which underwent intense phosphorylation, the kinetics of which was compatible with their involvement in superoxide pro-duction. A year later it was reported that phorbol esters bind to and activate PKC and the connection was made between activation of protein phosphorylation by PKC and activation of the NADPH oxidase (Castagna *et al.*, 1982). Activation of PKC *in vivo* is thought to occur via the interaction of a stimulus, e.g. FMLP, with its receptor, which activates a pertussis-toxin-sensitive G protein which in turn activates PLC. PKC has been shown to translocate from the cytosol to the membrane within seconds of stimulation and prior to superoxide production (Wolfson *et al.*, 1985; Christiansen, 1988). At the membrane DAG, in conjunction with another phospholipid, PS, activates the kinase. Phorbol esters act by mimicking DAG. Synthetic DAGs and phorbol esters have been shown to activate the oxidase to an extent similar to that of physiological stimuli, supporting the argument that PKC is involved in at least one of the acti-vation pathways (Curnutte *et al.*, 1984; Robinson *et al.*, 1985; Badwey and Karnovsky, 1986; Pilloud *et al.*, 1989). It has been shown that in human neutrophils there are two PKC isotypes present, β-PKC, a calcium-dependent isotype, which translocates to the membrane upon stimulation, and a calcium-independent non-translocating PKC, termed n-PKC (Majumdar *et al.*, 1991). β-PKC was shown to phosphorylate a major 47 kD cytosolic protein (most likely p47-*phox*), while n-PKC did not. Of note is the fact that FMLP stimulates a rapid but transient increase in long-chain fatty acylCoA which was found to inhibit n-PKC (Majumdar *et al.*, 1991). It has been reported previously that PKC can act as negative signal and can down-regulate ligand-induced signalling (Della Bianca *et al.*, 1986) so it is possible that the presence of different PKC isotypes in the neutrophil could account for both positive and negative effects.

Studies with various inhibitors of PKC have led to contradictory reports as to the role of this kinase in the respiratory burst. The PKC inhibitor H7, an isoquinoline sulphonamide, does not inhibit FMLP-induced activation of the oxidase (Wright and Hoffman, 1987; Seifert and Schachtele, 1988). However, the lack of specificity of many of the inhibitors used in the study of PKC has raised doubts as to the reliability of results obtained with their use (Seifert and Schachtele, 1988). Moreover, the observation that PKC inhibitors do not inhibit all activators of the respiratory burst suggests that other kinases are also involved in activation (Cooke and Hallett, 1985; Gerard *et al.*, 1986; Pontremoli *et al.*, 1986; Berkow *et al.*, 1987; Grinstein and Furuya, 1988; Berkow and Dodson, 1990). Activation of neutrophils with PMA, PAF, FMLP, LTB4 and A23187 results in the tyrosine phosphorylation of a relatively small number of proteins over a time course similar to that of activation of the respiratory burst (Berkow *et al.*, 1987; Huang *et al.*, 1990). The tyrosine kinase inhibitor ST638 inhibited superoxide production in response to FMLP but not to PMA or A23187 (Berkow *et al.*, 1989; Gomez-Cambronero *et al.*, 1989). Tyrosine phosphorylation is also seen in electropermeabilized neutrophils stimulated with guanine nucleotides (Nasmith *et al.*, 1989). Since GTP-γ-S also activates the oxidase, there may be a link between activation and tyrosine phosphorylation. Pretreatment of electropermeabilized cells with PMA inhibited this phosphorylation indicating some interlinking of the two systems.

2. *Chronic Granulomatous Disease*

2.1 INTRODUCTION

Our knowledge of the NADPH oxidase and the discovery of CGD are intimately linked. Undoubtedly, were it not for CGD our understanding of the NADPH oxidase would be significantly diminished. CGD was first recognized as a hereditary condition affecting neutrophil function as long ago as 1957 (Berendes *et al.*, 1957) and is characterized by severe and recurrent infections. The condition affects between 1 in 1 000 000 and 1 in 250 000. Clinically, a very narrow spectrum of organisms

are responsible for the complications of CGD. Most commonly these are *Staphylococcus aureus* infections, or Gram-negative enteric bacteria, though often hardest to treat is *Aspergillus* pneumonia. Patients are routinely maintained on antibiotic prophylaxis, but the condition may still be fatal. Current actuarial data indicate a 50% mortality by age 20 in a patient population studied over the last 15 years (Finn *et al.*, 1990).

Despite its recognition some 35 years ago, it has taken until very recently to unravel the relationship between the genetics of CGD and the biochemistry of the NADPH oxidase completely. The problems have been that, far from being a single disorder, CGD has now been shown to derive from mutations in four distinct genes, each of which encodes a specific component of the NADPH oxidase. The individual properties of these components have been extensively discussed in Section 1 and are detailed in Table 3.1.

Historically, the classic presentation of CGD was in small boys which led to the supposition that the gene responsible was X-linked (Hohn and Lehrer, 1975). Pedigree analysis soon confirmed this to be the case. This classic presentation was associated with an absence of cytochrome b_{-245} (see Section 1.5) from the neutrophil membranes of these patients (Segal and Jones, 1979b; Segal *et al.*, 1983; Bohler *et al.*, 1986; Riccardi *et al.*, 1986; Segal, 1987; Minegishi *et al.*, 1988). It fairly soon became clear, however, that another significant patient group existed. These were CGD patients, in that they completely lacked a respiratory burst (see Section 1.3) but were cytochrome b_{-245}-positive individuals whose CGD displayed an autosomal inheritance pattern, affecting boys and girls equally (Holmes *et al.*, 1970; Segal and Jones, 1980; Segal *et al.*, 1983; D'Amelio *et al.*, 1984; Weening *et al.*, 1985a; Bohler *et al.*, 1986; Segal, 1988). The existence of these patients was a major stimulus in the search for a cytosolic component to the NADPH oxidase (Sections 1.6 and 2.2.3). The observation that has caused the most confusion between the genetics of CGD and the biochemistry of the NADPH oxidase was the discovery of rare CGD patients who lacked cytochrome b_{-245} but showed an autosomal inheritance pattern (Weening *et al.*, 1985b; Ohno *et al.*, 1986; Okamura *et al.*, 1988b). These patients have subsequently been demonstrated to have defects in the smaller, α-subunit of cytochrome b_{-245} (Dinauer *et al.*, 1990; Parkos *et al.*, 1987, 1988b).

2.2 ISOLATION OF DNA SEQUENCES ENCODING GENES AFFECTED IN CGD

2.2.1 X-Linked CGD

As described above, the classical "CGD gene" was known to be located on the X chromosome. More detailed mapping of the locus using X-chromosome deletions was able to map the position of this gene to Xp21.1 (Franke et al., 1985; Baehner et al., 1986). This information led to the "CGD gene" becoming the first human gene to be cloned based purely on a knowledge of its chromosomal location (Royer Pokora et al., 1986). Orkin and Kunkel took a revolutionary approach to the problem but were presented with the possibility of doing so by the existence of an exceptional patient having an X chromosome deletion causing no fewer than four different genetic disorders; these were Duchenne muscular dystrophy, retinitis pigmentosa, CGD and the MacCloud phenotype (Franke et al., 1985; Monaco et al., 1985; Royer Pokora et al., 1986). In order to isolate DNA sequences residing in the region covered by the deletion, an excess of DNA from the patient's cells was hybridized with Hae-III-digested DNA isolated from a cell line containing three X chromosomes. To achieve the necessarily fast hybridization kinetics a technique of hybridizing in a phenol emulsion was developed known as PERT (phenol-enhanced reassociation technique). The DNA fragments deriving from the region deleted in the patient's DNA will have no homologous hybridization partners and will not therefore form hybrids. The single-stranded DNA was separated from the duplexed DNA using hydroxyapatite, self-annealed and cloned into a plasmid DNA vector, to produce a library of sequences specific for the region deleted in the patient (Kunkel et al., 1985). In addition, it was reasoned that the X-CGD specific gene transcript would be expressed at high level in differentiated myeloid cells. DNA sequences fulfilling this criterion were isolated from the HL60 cell line. This is a promyelocytic leukaemia line, that can be induced to undergo myeloid differentiation on treatment with a number of chemical agents (Collins et al., 1978). RNA sequences that were expressed at high level in induced HL60 cells were isolated from a whole cell cDNA by hybridization to a large excess of RNA from uninduced cells. As before, sequences specific for the differentiated cells will have no hybridization partners and will therefore remain single stranded. The single-stranded cDNA was separated from RNA–DNA hybrids on hydroxyapatite and then used as a hybridization probe on the PERT library. Using this strategy Kunkel and Orkin were able to isolate a DNA fragment that mapped to the deleted region in the CGD patient and also was expressed as a myeloid cell-specific mRNA. One of the clones so identified was found to hybridize to an mRNA of 4.3 kb which in a particular CGD patient was found to be altered in size. This patient was found to have a genomic DNA deletion that ended within the RNA transcript and caused a chain-terminating mutation. The sequence of the normal transcript was obtained from the cDNA clone. The predicted protein was completely unlike any previously identified sequence. Certainly, the sequence looked quite unlike any known cytochrome. This led the authors to doubt whether cytochrome b_{-245} was in fact implicated in CGD. Subsequently, however, this controversy was resolved when the N-terminal sequence of

cytochrome b_{-245} was determined by Teahan et al. (1987). This was found to match with DNA sequence from the cDNA clone which had originally been thought to be part of the 5' untranslated region of the mRNA (Dinauer et al., 1987; Teahan et al., 1987), owing to an error in the original sequence (Royer Pokora et al., 1986).

2.2.2 The α-Subunit of Cytochrome b_{-245}

An element of the confusion over the identity of the protein encoded by the "CGD locus" was caused by amino-acid compositional analysis of purified cytochrome b_{-245} which did not correlate with that deduced from the cDNA sequence of the PERT clone. The reason for this became clear when cytochrome b_{-245} was found to consist of two subunits (Dinauer et al., 1987; Teahan et al., 1987). The previously unrecognized subunit is a molecule of approximately 23 kD (Parkos et al., 1987) having a small amount of homology to other cytochromes b (Parkos et al., 1988b). It is now thought to be the haem-binding moiety of the cytochrome (Nugent et al., 1989), though its precise stoichiometry with regard to gp91-phox remains unclear. The smaller subunit was cloned from an HL60 cell cDNA library using an antibody to the purified protein (Parkos et al., 1988) and the gene has been localized to chromosome 16 (Bu-Ghanim et al., 1990; Dinauer et al., 1990). Interestingly, on Northern blot analysis, the mRNA of approximately 650 nt was found to be expressed virtually ubiquitously. Unusually, however, the 22 kD subunit protein is only found to be present in phagocytic cells. In fact it appears that the 90 kD and 23 kD proteins are only stable in each other's presence, where interactions between the subunits stabilize the complex. This almost certainly accounts for the fact that in both X-linked and autosomal forms of CGD which are cytochrome deficient, both subunits of the cytochrome are found to be missing (Segal 1987, 1988; Parkos et al., 1988; Clark et al., 1989; Curnutte and Smith, 1991).

2.2.3 Cytosolic Factors

In addition to the cytochrome, two cytosolic components have been identified which are specific to the NADPH oxidase and therefore affected in CGD. The first of these is p47-phox, a 47 kD protein whose existence was first implicated from studies by Heyworth and Segal on neutrophil phosphoproteins (Segal et al., 1985; Heyworth and Segal, 1986) (see Section 1.6.1). Some contention existed originally over whether these patients actually lacked p47-phox, or simply failed to phosphorylate this molecule (Kramer et al., 1988). It has subsequently become clear that AR-CGD patients fail to synthesize p47-phox (Nunoi et al., 1988; Volpp et al., 1988; Teahan et al., 1990).

The isolation of cDNA encoding this molecule was greatly facilitated by the availability of an antiserum (B1) raised to GTP-binding proteins from neutrophil cytosol (see Section 1.6). Analysis with this serum on fractionated cytosol highlighted two proteins that were recognized by the antiserum and which were present in fractions that were able to stimulate oxidase production in cell-free oxidase systems (Nunoi *et al.*, 1988; Volpp *et al.*, 1988). Moreover, these fractions contained a 47 kD protein that reacted with the B1 serum and which was missing from the cytosol of AR-CGD patients. The real surprise for both these groups was the unexpected finding of a second protein with similar characteristics to p47-*phox*, present in slightly different column fractions and, crucially, missing from the cytosol of an AR-CGD patient who did not lack p47-*phox* (Nunoi *et al.*, 1988; Volpp *et al.*, 1988). This protein had a molecular weight of 67 kD and is now referred to as p67-*phox*. That this CGD patient had a disease distinct from p47-*phox*-deficient AR-CGD was demonstrated by complementation analysis using cytosol extracts in a cell-free oxidase system.

The cDNAs encoding both these molecules were cloned using the B1 antiserum to screen HL60 cell expression libraries (Lomax *et al.*, 1989b; Volpp *et al.*, 1989a; Leto *et al.*, 1990). In addition, the 47 kD phosphoprotein was demonstrated to be the same protein as p47-*phox* when it was similarly cloned using an antibody raised against the purified phosphoprotein (Rodaway *et al.*, 1990; Teahan *et al.*, 1990). The primary amino-acid sequences of these proteins have thus far shed little light on their supposed functions other than the identification of SH3 domains in both proteins (see Section 1.6). A number of potential phosphorylation sites have been identified in p47-*phox* molecule, but it remains to be established which of these are the true *in vivo* targets. Neither protein appears to have the ability to bind FAD (Chiba *et al.*, 1990) and are therefore unlikely to take part in electron-transfer functions.

2.3 GENE STRUCTURE AND REGULATION

2.3.1 gp91-*phox*

As was indicated above, the primary sequence data on the gp91-*phox* gene did not originally indicate any homology to other known proteins. More recently, however, homology to a ferric reductase of yeast (Dancis *et al.*, 1992) and to bacterial flavocytochromes (Porter, 1991) has been identified. This led Segal to identify some highly conserved regions of gp91-*phox* which were consistent with their being the binding sites for the nucleotides FAD and NADPH (Segal *et al.*, 1992) (see Figure 3.3). Evidence from flavin measurement of CGD cell membranes and binding studies using NADPH analogues (Segal *et al.*, 1992) have confirmed that gp91-*phox* is indeed the protein that binds both these cofactors and therefore that the complete cytochrome b_{-245} is responsible for all the electron-transfer functions of the NADPH oxidase. Cell-free reconstitution experiments using pure or recombinant components have now also

unequivocally demonstrated this fact (Abo *et al.*, 1992). Similar conclusions have also been drawn by others (Rotrosen *et al.*, 1992).

Molecular modelling, based on the deduced amino-acid sequence, has suggested a conjectural structure for this molecule (Segal *et al.*, 1992). There are six potential membrane-spanning helices, two binding clefts and a large cytoplasmic domain. The C-terminal region has been suggested to interact with p47-*phox* based on experiments with permeabilized PMNs. Firstly, immuno-precipitation of p47-*phox* from activated cells was able to co-precipitate gp91-*phox* and vice versa. Moreover, a peptide antibody to the six amino acids at amino-acid positions 559–565 (11 residues from the C-terminus), or the peptide itself, were shown to block activation of the oxidase in the cell-free system or permeabilized cells, respectively (Rotrosen *et al.*, 1990).

The structure of the gp91-*phox* gene has now been elucidated (Skalnik *et al.*, 1991) and has been shown to comprise 13 exons spanning some 30 kb in the genome. Expression of the mRNA has been found to be highly tissue specific, transcripts being observed only in myeloid cells and in EBV-transformed B lymphocytes (which express all the components of the NADPH oxidase to varying degrees, see also Section 2.4.1). Analysis of the promoter region of this gene has revealed the presence of a number of recognized regulatory elements (Skalnik *et al.*, 1991). The first of these is a classical TATA box motif at position -30 common to most genes and probably responsible for directing the precise initiation site for transcription. In addition, a repeated CAAT box motif was found at positions -110 and -124. These were observed to bind CP1 transcription factor when incubated with nuclear extracts from myeloid cells. This binding was inhibited in nuclear extracts from non-myeloid cells by a protein known as CAAT displacement factor, first observed in sea-urchin histone gene regulation. The binding site specificities of these two proteins overlap in the gp91-*phox* promoter and this led the authors to suggest that myeloid specificity is achieved by a repressor activity of the CAAT displacement factor. This was tested by functional analysis using growth hormone cDNA as a "reporter" for gene activity directed by the gp91-*phox* promoter region. Myeloid cell specificity is therefore achieved by repressing transcription in non-myeloid cells, owning the greater stability of binding of CAAT displacement factor over CP1. Experiments with transgenic mice have further corroborated this picture, but strangely the gp91-*phox* promoter region was able to direct expression of its associated growth hormone reporter gene only in the monocyte–macrophage lineage and not in neutrophils (Skalnik *et al.*, 1991). Other sequences not yet identified must be necessary to direct expression in this cell type.

2.3.2 p22-*phox*

The gene for the smaller subunit of cytochrome b_{-245}

has been isolated (Dinauer *et al.*, 1990). It consists of five exons and spans some 8.5 kb in the genome.

The regulation of this gene stands in marked contrast to gp91-*phox* in that p22-*phox* appears to be regulated as a housekeeping gene. The mRNA is found ubiquitously, but with the exception of recombinant protein expression in COS cells (Parkos *et al.*, 1988), p22-*phox* protein is only observed in cells that also express gp91-*phox*. Modelling of the three-dimensional structure based on the primary amino-acid data has suggested the existence of two membrane-spanning helices, but its precise relationship to gp91-*phox* is not resolved. On energetic grounds it would be expected that there would be two small subunits per single large subunit in the whole cytochrome b_{-245}. This is because a single FAD can transfer two electrons but a haem is only capable of transferring one (see Section 1.5.2). Precisely where the haem is bound on p22-*phox* is similarly not established, and a recent report has presented some evidence for the haem being bound between both subunits (Quinn *et al.*, 1992).

2.3.3 p47-*phox*

The p47-*phox* gene maps to chromosome 7 (Franke *et al.*, 1990) and has also recently been cloned, having nine exons and spanning about 18 kb (Chanock *et al.*, 1991). Details of its regulation are still somewhat sketchy at present, but the basis of the tissue specificity of this gene would appear to be fundamentally different from gp91-*phox* with which it interestingly shares a similar tissue specific distribution. The 1.4 kb p47-*phox* mRNA essentially is found exclusively in PMNs and myeloid cell lines (HL60, U937), but it is also transcribed at similar levels in EBV-transformed B lymphocytes (Casimir *et al.*, 1991), which is not so true of the X-CGD gene. The p47-*phox* gene is strongly induced during myeloid cell differentiation, the steady-state level of mRNA in HL60 cells increases around 50 fold on differentiation (Rodaway *et al.*, 1990; Casimir *et al.*, 1991). Some evidence for regulation by retinoic acid has been obtained; "run-off" transcription analysis of retinoid enhanced transcription was shown to be insensitive to cycloheximide and therefore attributable to a direct transcriptional effect (Rodaway *et al.*, 1990). Undoubtedly more data on the regulation of this gene will be forthcoming in the near future.

2.3.4 p67-*phox*

The gene for p67-*phox* has been localized to the long arm of chromosome 1 (Franke *et al.*, 1990), and there has been a recent report identifying the gene size and total number of exons. There is little information on specificity of expression, save a putative IFNγ regulatory site (Kenney *et al.*, 1992).

2.4 GENETIC LESIONS

2.4.1 gp91-*phox*

Being the first of the genes encoding an NADPH oxidase component to be cloned, more mutations have been found in the gene for gp91-*phox* than for any of the other components. As might be expected, a wide variety of different types of lesion have been found in this gene. Originally, it was thought that large deletions of the type seen in the earliest cases of X-CGD analysed would

Table 3.2 Deletion and insertion mutations in the β-subunit of cytochrome b_{-245}

CGD class[a]	Mutation	Size	Nucleotide position	Amino-acid change
X91[0]	Deletion	3.5 kb[b]	?	Deletion of exons 6 + 7 (aa 162–225)
X91[0]	Deletion	3 kb[b]	?	Deletion of exon 5 (aa 113–161) and frameshift
X91[0]	Deletion	1 kb[b]	?	Deletion of exons 4–9 (aa 85–384)
X91[0]	Deletion	120 bp[c]	?	Delete of aa 530–570
X91[0]	Insertion	40 bp[b]	Between G(702) and C(703)	13 additional aa at Gly-230 and frameshift

[a] See Table 3.6.
[b] Data from Roos (1992).
[c] Data from Royer Pokora *et al.* (1986).
aa, amino acids.

predominate over other types of defect but this has not proven to be the case. A number of the point mutations that have been found have also helped to shed new light on structure/function relationships in this molecule.

2.4.1.1 Deletions and Insertions

The X chromosome is seemingly somewhat prone to deletion and this is perhaps reflected in the fact that a number of X-CGD mutations are caused by large deletions, sometimes affecting other genetic loci in addition to gp91-*phox* (Franke *et al.*, 1985; Royer Pokora *et al.*, 1986; Pelham *et al.*, 1990). In addition, a few small deletions between 1 and 3.5 kb have been documented (Roos, 1992) (see Table 3.2), although the precise breakpoints are not yet always elucidated.

2.4.1.2 Splicing Defects

A group of mutations affecting splicing of the gp91-*phox* mRNA have recently been identified by Roos and his co-workers (de Boer *et al.*, 1992a) suggesting this may be a relatively common mechanism (Table 3.3). These are most commonly point mutations in the DNA affecting the highly conserved nucleotides adjacent to the intron–exon boundary. This gives rise to mRNA molecules with the precise deletion of a single exon, so-called "exon-skipping" mutations. These patients can be identified by deletions in the mRNA, sometimes visible on Northern blot analysis but, more commonly, revealed by PCR amplification of selected regions of the transcript. Five such patients have been identified. Three of these affect splice donor sites leading to the loss of exons 7, 5 and 3, respectively. One affected a splice acceptor causing deletion of exon 2. The last of these was a mutation in exon 6 which activates a cryptic splice site. This is unusually

preferred over the natural splice donor and resulted in a frameshift in the mRNA generating a premature stop codon. Some speculation has occurred as to why these mutations appear to reduce the level of mRNA expression as observed on Northern blots (de Boer *et al.*, 1992a). One possible explanation for this is that a number of alternatively spliced molecules are produced but the only type seen in the patients are the one stable configuration, which is only a proportion of the total output from the gene. This could explain why splice donor-site mutations often lead to deletion of the intron proximal to the site of the lesion rather than distally, as might be expected. The distally deleted mRNA may well not be stable.

One further splicing-related mutation has been observed in an extremely unusual case described by Dinauer and colleagues (Schapiro *et al.*, 1991) of a man who remained asymptomatic until the age of 69. This patient had a single nucleotide substitution at the acceptor site of intron 11. This resulted in the activation of a cryptic splice site within exon 12, leading to the deletion of amino acids 488–497. Interestingly, this creates a significantly milder phenotype than is common, implying that this region of gp91-*phox* is less critical for function than some other regions of the protein.

2.4.1.3 Point Mutations

Some ten patients with point mutations have been identified (Table 3.4), all of whom have different lesions (excepting families with more than one affected individual). These consist primarily of non-conservative amino-acid substitutions. One of these cases is female with extreme lyonization, such that despite being heterozygous for the His (101) → Arg mutation, 95–98% of

Table 3.3 Splicing mutations in the β-subunit of cytochrome b_{-245}

CGD class[a]	Nucleotide position	Mutation	Nucleotides changed	Amino acids changed
X91^0	Intron 7 donor site (+2)	T → A[b]	Exon 7 deleted and frameshift	225 onwards
X91^0	Intron 5 donor site (+3)	A → T[b]	Exon 5 deleted and frameshift	113 onwards
X91^0	Intron 3 donor site (+5)	G → A[b]	Exon 3 deleted	48–85
X91^0	Intron 1 acceptor site (−1)	G → A[b]	Exon 2 deleted	16–47
X91$^+$	Intron 11 acceptor site (−1)	A → G[c]	nts 1471–1501 in exon 12 deleted	aa 488–497 deleted
X91^0	nt633	C → A[b]	New splice donor	Trp-206 → stop

[a] See Table 3.6.
[b] Data from de Boer *et al.* (1992a).
[c] Data from Schapiro *et al.* (1991).
nt(s), nucleotide(s); aa, amino acids.

Table 3.4 Point mutations in the β-subunit of cytochrome b_{-245}

CGD class[a]	Mutation	Nucleotide position	Nucleotide change	Amino acid position	Amino acid change
X91^0	Missense	637	C → T[b]	209	His → Tyr
X91^0	Missense	229	C → T[b]	73	Arg → stop
X91^0	Missense	314	A → G[b]	101	His → Arg
X91$^-$	Missense	1178	G → C[b]	389	Gly →Ala
X91$^-$	Missense	734	G → C[b]	244	Cys → Ser
X91$^-$	Missense		?[b]	309	Glu → Lys
X91$^+$	Missense	1256	C → A[c]	415	Pro → His
X91^0	Deletion	134	ΔT[d]	42	Frameshift
X91^0	Deletion	59	ΔT[d]	17	Frameshift

[a] See Table 3.6.
[b] Data from Bolscher et al. (1991).
[c] Data from Dinauer et al. (1989).
[d] Data from Roos (1992).

her neutrophils are expressing the X chromosome carrying the mutant gene (Bolscher et al., 1991). One chain-terminating mutation has been documented at Arg 73 (Bolscher et al., 1991).

By far the most illuminating point mutation is that of a Pro → His mutation at residue 415 (Dinauer et al., 1989). This patient is of a very rare phenotype in that a completely normal amount of a totally non-functional cytochrome b_{-245} is present in the patient's cells. Clearly this mutation does not affect the interaction of the two cytochrome subunits. The Pro 415 is, however, located in the region of the molecule identified as the NADPH binding site and binding studies with an NADPH analogue have suggested that this mutation destroys the ability of the molecule to bind NADPH. Comparison with amino-acid sequences of other NADPH-binding proteins also indicated that this proline residue was invariant, within the binding cleft (Segal et al., 1992).

Two single nucleotide deletions causing frameshift mutations have also been observed (Roos, 1992).

2.4.2 p22-phox

Mutations in the smaller subunit of cytochrome b_{-245} are much rarer than for the large, notwithstanding the fact that it is autosomally encoded. Seven patients have now been characterized and all but one carry different lesions (see Table 3.5). Six of these cases have arisen due to consanguinity and are therefore homozygous defects. The remaining case is a compound heterozygote carrying two distinct mutant alleles (Dinauer et al., 1990). As for the large subunit, mutations of heterogeneous origin underlay defective p22-phox synthesis. Most are amino-acid substitutions, the two independent cases with the same defect are Arg(90) → Gln substitutions (Dinauer et al., 1990; de Boer et al., 1992b). One large deletion (>10 kb) (Dinauer et al., 1990), one single nucleotide

Table 3.5 Mutations in the α-subunit of cytochrome b_{-245}

CGD class[a]	Mutation	Nucleotide position	Nucleotides changed	Amino-acid position	Amino acids changed
A22^0	Deletion	?	>10 kb[b]	—	—
A22^0	Deletion	272	ΔC[b]	81	Frameshift
A22^0	Splice donor intron 4 (+1)	Exon 4 deleted (232–315)	G → A[c]	68–97	Deleted
A22^0	Missense	297	G → A[c]	90	Arg → Gln
A22^0	Missense	382	C → A[b]	118	Ser → Arg
A22$^+$	Missense	495	C → A[d]	156	Pro → Gln
A22^0	Missense	297	G → A[b]	90	Arg → Gln
A22^0	Missense	309	A → G[c]	94	His → Arg

[a] See Table 3.6.
[b] Data from Dinauer et al. (1990).
[c] Data from de Boer et al. (1992b).
[d] Data from Dinauer et al. (1991).

deletion and one "exon skipping" mutation (de Boer *et al.*, 1992b) have been found. As for gp91-*phox*, most of the mutations result in the absence of p22-*phox* protein. One patient, however, has normal levels of non-functional cytochrome *b*₋₂₄₅ and this results from Pro156, which is mutated to Gln, by a C to A transversion (Dinauer *et al.*, 1991). The biochemical basis for the lack of function of this molecule is not yet understood.

2.4.3 p47-*phox* and p67-*phox*

Lesions in p47-*phox* are the second most common cause of CGD accounting for between 23% and 30% of all cases. Because it is autosomally inherited, this indicates a very high incidence of mutant alleles, some 200 times more frequent than mutant gp91-*phox* alleles at around 1 in 2000 of the population (Casimir *et al.*, 1991). In rather stark contrast to the cytochrome *b*₋₂₄₅ mutations, a single lesion in p47-*phox* predominates, accounting for about 90% of all mutant alleles. This mutation is a deletion of a GT dinucleotide found at GTGT repeat located at the border of the first intron and second exon (Casimir *et al.*, 1991). The deletion is frameshifting and produces a chain terminator at amino-acid residue 51 (Figure 3.4). It is not known if the patients produce the predicted truncated product of around 6 kD. Duplication of the GT base pair accounts for the fact that p47-*phox*-deficient patients have normal amounts of a normal-sized mRNA (Lomax *et al.*, 1989b; Casimir *et al.*, 1991). The GT

deletion is homozygous in all but two documented cases, which are compound heterozygotes having the GT deletion balanced against missense mutations, resulting in Lys → Glu or Thr → Ala substitutions (Chanock *et al.*, 1991). Both of these mutations presumably produce proteins that are unstable as no immunoreactive material is present in these individuals.

In this laboratory (unpublished observations) we have also now identified two patients not carrying the GT deletion but these are incompletely characterized. One of these patients is a compound heterozygote who has inherited a single T deletion from her mother. Interestingly, this is located at a triple GT repeat sequence.

The reason for the prevalence of the GT dinucleotide deletion is not completely clear. All the studied cases are independent occurrences and none involve consanguinity. The question then arises as to whether these are newly originating mutations, or represent the spread of a single mutant allele throughout the population. No association with any particular ethnic group has been found, but no haplotype analysis is currently available. Perhaps the recent discovery of silent polymorphisms in the p47-*phox* coding sequence will make this possible. One salient fact, however, is our own observation that PCR amplification of normal genomic DNA across this region leads to the generation of the GT deletion in many of the amplification products *in vitro*. Some 50% of the PCR products are found to have the deletion following 30 amplification

```
                  1                      25
  +/CGD    GAGCACTGGAGGCCACCCAGTC ATG GGG GAC ACC TTC
                                  met gly asp thr phe   5


                        50                   XmnI
  +/CGD    ATC CGT CAC ATC GCC GTG CTG GGC TTT GAG AAG CGC

           ile arg his ile ala leu leu gly phe glu lys arg  17


           75                       **  100
  +/CGD    TTC GTA CCC AGC CAG CAC TAT GTG TAC ATG TTC CTG
           phe val pro ser gln his tyr val tyr met phe leu  29

  CGD                                GTA CAT GTT CCT GGT
                                     val his val pro gly  29


                         125                Acc I
  +        GTG AAA TGG CAG GAC CTG TCG GAG AAG GTG GTC TAC
           val lys trp gln asp leu ser glu lys val val tyr  41

  CGD      GAA ATG GCA GGA CCT GTC GGA GAA GGT GGT CTA CCG
           glu met ala gly pro val gly glu gly gly leu pro  41


                150         Bgl II          175
  +        CGG CGC TTC ACC GAG ATC TAC GAG TTC CAT AAA ACC
           arg arg phe thr glu ile tyr glu phe his lys thr  53


  CGD      GCG CTT CAC CGA GAT CTA CGA GTT CCA TAA AAC CTT
           ala leu his arg asp leu arg val pro ***          50
```

Figure 3.4 Prevalent deletion mutation in p47-*phox* causing autosomal recessive CGD. Nucleotide numbers are depicted above the cDNA sequence. Amino-acid numbers are shown in italics at the end of each line. +, normal sequence; CGD, patient's sequence.

cycles. Thus, this appears to mimic the situation found *in vivo*. We take this to imply that there is some feature of the DNA milieu around the GTGT repeat that creates significant problems for copying by DNA polymerases. Clearly, more work will be required to resolve these questions.

Only one preliminary report of a defect in p67-*phox* exists, which identifies an insertion of about 100 bases between codons 212 and 324 (Kenney *et al.*, 1990).

2.5   MOLECULAR GENETICS AND CLASSIFICATION

The four genetic loci that encode components of the NADPH oxidase have all been mapped to specific chromosomal locations (Bu-Ghanim *et al.*, 1990; Dinauer *et al.*, 1990; Franke *et al.*, 1985, 1990). All four reside on different chromosomes (see Table 3.1).

The major cytochrome subunit gp91-*phox* is encoded on the X chromosome and is therefore the most prevalent cause of CGD; the three remaining components are autosomal. Genetically, therefore, CGD can be divided into X-linked and autosomal recessive forms. Biochemically, CGD has often been divided into cytochrome b_{-245}-negative and cytochrome b_{-245}-positive types. Classically, the X-linked form is cytochrome negative and the autosomal recessive form cytochrome positive. However, the discovery of cytochrome-negative autosomal recessive individuals was able to presage the discovery of p22-*phox*, the small subunit of cytochrome b_{-245}. To further complicate matters a small number of X-linked cytochrome-positive individuals have been identified (Borregaard *et al.*, 1983; Newburger *et al.*, 1986; Dinauer *et al.*, 1989). Some of these are the classic "variants" who have reduced amounts of cytochrome but usually retain partial activity. An important observation here is that the superoxide-generating ability of variant neutrophils overlaps with values obtained for the carriers of X-linked cytochrome-deficient CGD. This demonstrates that a reduced number of fully active cells is more effective than a circulation composed entirely of partially active cells.

To clarify this situation, a new classification of CGD based on the recent discovery of all the components has been agreed (Table 3.6). It seems unlikely, after two major surveys (Clark *et al.*, 1989; Casimir *et al.*, 1992) that any more specific components of the NADPH oxidase, that is ones whose deficiency causes CGD, remain to be discovered. All known cases can be accounted for by mutations in one of the four recognized components. As the involvement of p21rac has demonstrated (see Section 1.7.1), however, there may well be extra factors with more general cellular functions that have involvement in the oxidase. Mutations in these types of factors would most likely give rise to a lethal phenotype in homozygous form.

The new classification uses the known molecular weights of the oxidase components to distinguish the different genes and the identifier X or A for the inheritance pattern. As for other genetic conditions, superscripts are used to distinguish different types of mutations in the same gene. At present, this mainly applies to gp91-*phox*, so that mutations leading to deficiency carry a superscript "0", those with detectable but reduced protein carry a "−" and those with a normal amount of protein a "+".

2.6   DIAGNOSIS AND TREATMENT

2.6.1   Diagnosis

The classic diagnostic tool for CGD has been the NBT slide test (Segal 1974; Levinsky *et al.*, 1983), which is a microscopical test performed on blood smears. In this test, individual neutrophils that are able to produce superoxide reduce NBT giving rise to an insoluble formazan that produces an intense blue colour. The cells of a CGD patient are unable to do this and a negative NBT test is still a good indicator of a CGD diagnosis. It is still the best diagnostic tool for identifying carrier mothers of X-CGD as the X linkage produces a mosaic of positively staining and negative cells. This is due to the stochastic nature of X-inactivation so that only one of the two X chromosomes is active in any individual cell. Cases

Table 3.6   New classification of CGD

Classification	Oxidase activity	Affected oxidase component	Level of protein expression	Prevalence
X-91^0	<1%	Cytochrome β-subunit	None	60%
X-91$^-$	5–40%	Cytochrome β-subunit	Reduced	3%
X-91$^+$	<1%	Cytochrome β-subunit	Normal	<1%
A22^0	<1%	Cytochrome α-subunit	None	5%
A22$^+$	<1%	Cytochrome α-subunit	Normal	<1%
A47	<1%	p47-*phox*	None	25%
A67	<1%	p67-*phox*	None	5%

of extreme lyonization and variable levels of background staining have produced problems of interpretation in the past, so it is good also to have newer alternative strategies.

A negative NBT test can be corroborated by direct estimate of superoxide generation, for which a number of assays exist. The most commonly used is the reduction of cytochrome *c*, measured by analysis of differential spectrum at 540 nm. This assay is genuinely quantitative but less sensitive than chemiluminescent assay. Chemiluminescent detection is most reliably performed in its luminol enhanced form where H_2O_2 generated by the NADPH oxidase is used by added peroxidase to activate luminol (Wymann *et al.*, 1987; Porter *et al.*, 1992). This assay has the advantage of extreme sensitivity but is difficult to quantify.

At present, the most complete diagnosis can be provided by a combination of NBT test and analysis of neutrophil proteins by Western blot. In this latter technique, total neutrophil proteins are separated by SDS–PAGE and transferred on to a nitrocellulose membrane. The membrane is then incubated in the presence of a specific antiserum directed against one (or more) of the oxidase components. Binding of antibody to proteins in the mixture can be visualized using an alkaline phosphatase-conjugated second antibody, or with [125]-I-labelled protein A. Absence of any particular band can identify the affected component of the NADPH oxidase. This has worked particularly well for the cytoplasmic components as good antibodies have been available for some time (Nunoi *et al.*, 1988; Volpp *et al.*, 1988; Clark *et al.*, 1989; Rodaway *et al.*, 1990; Teahan *et al.*, 1990; Casimir *et al.*, 1992) and both proteins are relatively abundant. Antibodies to p22-*phox* have also been produced and used with good effect (Nakamura *et al.*, 1987; Parkos *et al.*, 1988b; Casimir *et al.*, 1992). The problem up to now has been in obtaining a good reactivity against gp91-*phox*. The heavy glycosylation of the human protein probably is a hindrance both to its immunogenicity and causes it to run very diffusely on SDS–PAGE (Harper *et al.*, 1985; Segal *et al.*, 1986). Antiserum to a C-terminal peptide sequence has worked adequately, but a fairly recent monoclonal antibody (Verhoven *et al.*, 1989) seems to be the most sensitive reagent currently available. Antibody-based diagnosis has been used in two major patient studies in America (Clark *et al.*, 1989) and in Europe (Casimir *et al.*, 1992). These studies have been used to evaluate the relative frequencies of defects in the four different components of the NADPH oxidase (Table 3.1).

The problem with antibody-based methods derives from the observation that both subunits of cytochrome b_{-245} are missing, regardless of the site of the lesion (Segal *et al.*, 1978, 1983; Segal, 1987; Parkos *et al.*, 1989). In this context an NBT test on the mother's blood can substantiate the X-chromosome linkage. In male patients with no family history and a normal maternal NBT test it is still very difficult to assign the site of the lesion to gp91-*phox* or p22-*phox* gene. The patient may have acquired a new X91 mutation or have inherited two A22 mutations. Most often the former seems to be the case, but although small, the number of A22 female patients (whose A22 diagnosis is unequivocal) we have identified in our own studies (Casimir *et al.*, 1992) makes it likely that a few male patients are still incorrectly diagnosed.

2.6.2 Antenatal Diagnosis

Antenatal diagnosis can be made at present by an NBT test on cord blood at about 14–16 weeks gestation but this is complicated by the possibility of contamination with maternally derived cells and necessitates late-stage termination should the fetus be affected. An anti-p22-*phox* monoclonal has been reported to identify positive macrophages successfully from chorionic villus sampling (Nakamura *et al.*, 1990) but false negatives are a concern for this method of antenatal diagnosis.

This situation could be improved by the availability of nucleic acid-based tests, which should be applicable to antenatal diagnosis. Linkage of X-CGD to two different RFLP markers has been described (Battat and Franke, 1989; Muhlebach *et al.*, 1990; Pelham *et al.*, 1990) and together these should be informative in up to 50% of cases. Sufficient DNA can be obtained from CVS to enable this to be used antenatally (A. Pelham and C. Kinnon, personal communication). Tests based on PCR should ideally be the most flexible and reliable. Exon skipping mutations could be reliably identified this way, but this again requires an RNA analysis. The elucidation of the intron junction sequences means that multiplex PCR can be used to identify individuals with major X91 deletions but these are less common than previously anticipated. Knowledge of a specific familial lesion does allow the design of a customized molecular analysis where diagnosis may be obtained by direct sequence analysis. It may eventually be possible to use pools of primer pairs to identify all the known lesions using PCR, but with so much heterogeneity in X-CGD mutations it seems unlikely that previously unencountered lesions will not continue to appear. For A47 CGD the situation is better as a single mutation seems to dominate. Diagnosis for this GT deletion by restriction enzyme digestion of PCR-amplified material has been described (Rodaway *et al.*, 1990), but again this can only be applied to RNA. A DNA-based competitive PCR diagnostic assay for this mutation has now been developed in our laboratory, which should be applicable to all diagnostic situations. It remains to be seen whether the other lesions that occur in this molecule are found at a limited number of sites, or if they have the heterogeneity seen for the other genes involved in CGD.

2.6.3 Treatment

Management of CGD patients has improved significantly

over the last 15 years, but still carries a risk of fatality. The most usual form of treatment is antibiotic prophylaxis, for which sulphamethoxazole–trimethoprim has been found valuable. Patients are very variable in age of first presentation, ranging in the extreme from within the first year of life to the 69th year of life (Finn *et al.*, 1990; Schapiro *et al.*, 1991). Age of first presentation, however, is quite a good indicator of the severity of disease. What determines its severity still seems extremely arcane. Some researchers have indicated that patients lacking cytochrome b_{-245} have more severe disease than those with cytosolic defects (Weening *et al.*, 1985), but there is little solid evidence to support this notion. From our own experience, we have treated cousins who share the same genetic lesion, yet whose clinical course has been strikingly different.

The most recent development in treatment of CGD has been the use of rhIFN-γ. A number of early reports documented enhanced superoxide generation on treatment of neutrophils or monocytes both *in vitro* (Berton *et al.*, 1986; Cassatella *et al.*, 1988; Ezekowitz *et al.*, 1988; Sechler *et al.*, 1988) and *in vivo* (Ezekowitz *et al.*, 1988; Sechler *et al.*, 1988). Increased levels of mRNA for various of the oxidase components (Cassatella *et al.*, 1989, 1990, 1991) and increased rate of transcription of gp91-*phox* (Newburger *et al.*, 1988) were also described in response to IFN-γ treatment. On the basis of these findings a multicentre placebo-controlled double-blind trial was initiated to test their validity and potential therapeutic benefit (Gallin *et al.*, 1991). This study demonstrated that IFN-γ given at a subcutaneous dose of 0.05 mg/m^2 three times weekly, can reduce the number of serious infectious episodes. This was true regardless of the nature of the genetic lesion giving rise to CGD. This study failed, however, to find any conclusive changes in any measurable NADPH oxidase parameter, either in terms of O_2^- production or microbial killing activity. The only conclusion must be that increased immunity is provided by mechanisms independent of NADPH oxidase function.

One treatment available now that could be described as a cure for CGD is bone marrow transplantation. The use has been sparing and the record of success for allogeneic grafts in CGD has been poor and sporadic (Westminster Hospital Transplant Team, 1977; Rappeport *et al.*, 1982; Kamani *et al.*, 1988). For the future, a real cure for the majority of CGD patients will most probably come from somatic gene therapy (Gallin and Malech, 1990; Karlsson, 1991). CGD rates as a good candidate disorder, having well-defined molecular genetics, an accessible target organ (the marrow) and in essence is a single gene defect. This treatment aims to introduce a functional copy of the defective NADPH oxidase gene into pluripotent stem cells from the patient's marrow and repopulate the patient's peripheral blood using this autologous graft.

Introduction of a suitable vehicle into a true stem cell, one capable of self renewal, has yet to be demonstrated

in any context. Recently, however, correction of the CGD phenotype in A47⁰-derived EBV-immortalized B lymphocytes was described by Thrasher *et al.* (1992). B lymphocytes transformed by EBV express all the known components of the NADPH oxidase and are capable of generating small amounts of superoxide (Maly *et al.*, 1988, 1990). B cell lines established from CGD patients lack the same oxidase component as their neutrophils and similarly fail to generate O_2^- in response to stimuli, such as PMA. Cells from a B cell line established from a p47-*phox*-deficient patient were used as recipients for transfer of retroviral vector containing a functional p47-*phox* cDNA. Following transfer, blotting experiments were used to demonstrate the presence of a single copy of the viral genome in the transduced cells, a virally encoded p47-*phox* mRNA of the expected size and p47-*phox* protein at a level equivalent to about half that of a normal neutrophil. Chemiluminescent and cytochrome *c* assay of superoxide generation by the transduced cells showed restoration of function to a level approximately 35% of normal.

These data have clearly underlined the feasibility of the gene therapy approach. Although not yet duplicated in cells of myeloid origin, the restoration of NADPH oxidase function to CGD cells by retroviral transfer marks a significant first step on the road to development of gene therapy as the definitive treatment for CGD.

3.   Acknowledgements

We would like to thank Drs D. Roos and M. de Boer for making available some of their unpublished data, and the Wellcome Trust, The Birth Defects Foundation and the MRC for their support.

4.   References

Abo, A. and Pick, E. (1991). Purification and characterization of a third cytosolic component of the superoxide-generating NADPH oxidase of macrophages. J. Biol. Chem. 266, 23577–23585.

Abo, A., Pick, E., Hall, A., Totty, N., Teahan, C.G. and Segal, A.W. (1991). The small GTP-binding protein, p21rac 1, is involved in activation of the NADPH oxidase. Nature 353, 668–670.

Abo, A., Boyhan, A., West, I., Thrasher, A.J. and Segal, A.W. (1992). Reconstitution of neutrophil NADPH oxidase activity in the cell-free system by four components: p67-phox, p47-phox, p21rac1, and cytochrome b-245. J. Biol. Chem. 267, 16767–16770.

Agwu, D.E., McPhail, L.C., Chabot, M.C., Daniel, L.W., Wykle, R.L. and McCall, C.E. (1989). Choline-linked phosphoglycerides. J. Biol. Chem. 264, 1405–1413.

Aharoni, I. and Pick, E. (1990). Activation of the superoxide-generating NADPH oxidase of macrophages by sodium dodecyl sulfate in a soluble cell-free system: evidence for involvement of a G protein. J. Leuk. Biol. 48, 107–115.

Ambruso, D.R., Bolscher, B.G.J.M., Stokman, P.M., Verhoeven, A.J. and Roos, D. (1990). Assembly and activation of the NADPH:O₂ oxidoreductase in human neutrophils after stimulation with phorbol myristate acetate. J. Biol. Chem. 265, 924–930.

Babior, B.M. and Kipnes, R.S. (1977). Superoxide forming enzyme from human neutrophils: evidence for a flavin requirement. Blood 50, 517–524.

Babior, B.M., Kipnes, R.S. and Curnutte, J.T. (1973). Biological defence mechanisms: the production by leukocytes of superoxide, a potential bactericidal agent. J. Clin. Invest. 52, 741–744.

Badwey, J.A. and Karnovsky, M.L. (1986). Production of superoxide by phagocytic leukocytes: a paradigm for stimulus–response phenomena. Curr. Top. Cell Regul. 28, 183–208.

Baehner, R.L., Kunkel, L.M., Monaco, A.P., Haines, P.M., Palmer, C., Heerema, N. and Orkin, S.H. (1986). DNA linkage analysis of X-linked chronic granulomatous disease. Proc. Natl Acad. Sci. USA 83, 3398–3401.

Baldridge, C.W. and Gerard, R.W. (1933). The extra respiration of phagocytosis. Am. J. Physiol. 103, 235–236.

Battat, L. and Franke, U. (1989). Nsi I RFLP at the X-linked chronic granulomatous disease locus (CYBB). Nucleic Acids Res. 17, 3619.

Bellavite, P. (1988). The superoxide-forming enzyme system of phagocytes. J. Free Rad. Biol. Med. 4, 225–261.

Bellavite, P., Cross, A.R., Serra, M.C., Davoli, A., Jones, O.T. and Rossi, F. (1983). The cytochrome b and flavin content and properties of the O₂⁻-forming NADPH oxidase solubilized from activated neutrophils. Biochim. Biophys. Acta 746, 40–47.

Bellavite, P., Jones, O.T., Cross, A.R., Papini, E. and Rossi, F. (1984). Composition of partially purified NADPH oxidase from pig neutrophils. Biochem. J. 223, 639–648.

Bender, J.G., McPhail, L.C. and Van Epps, D.E. (1983). Exposure of human neutrophils to chemotactic factors potentiates activation of the respiratory burst enzyme. J. Immunol. 130, 2316–2323.

Berendes, H., Bridges, R.A. and Good, R.A. (1957). A fatal granulomatosus of childhood. Minn. Med. 40, 309.

Berkow, R.L. and Dodson, R.W. (1990). Tyrosine-specific protein phosphorylation during activation of human neutrophils. Blood 75, 2445–2452.

Berkow, R.L., Dodson, R.W. and Kraft, A.S. (1987). The effect of a protein kinase C inhibitor, H-7, on human neutrophil oxidative burst and degranulation. J. Leuk. Biol. 41, 441–446.

Berkow, R.L., Dodson, R.W. and Kraft, A.S. (1989). Human neutrophils contain distinct cytosolic and particulate tyrosine kinase activities: possible role in neutrophil activation. Biochim. Biophys. Acta 997, 292–301.

Berton, G., Zani, L., Cassatella, M.A. and Rossi, F. (1986). Gamma interferon is able to enhance the oxidative metabolism of human neutrophils. Biochem. Biophys. Res. Commun. 138, 1276–1282.

Billah, M.M., Eckel, S., Mullmann, T.J., Egan, R.W. and Siegel, M.I. (1989). Phosphatidylcholine hydrolysis by phospholipase D determines phosphatidate and diglyceride levels in chemotactic peptide-stimulated human neutrophils. J. Biol. Chem. 264, 17069–17077.

Bohler, M.C., Seger, R.A., Mouy, R., Vilmer, E., Fischer, A. and Griscelli, C. (1986). A study of 25 patients with chronic granulomatous disease: a new classification by correlating respiratory burst, cytochrome b, and flavoprotein. J. Clin Immunol. 6, 136–145.

Bolscher, B.G.J.M., Denis, S.W., Verhoeven, A.J. and Roos, D. (1990). The activity of one soluble component of the cell-free NADPH:O₂ oxidoreductase of human neutrophils depends on guanosine 5′-o-(3-thio)triphosphate. J. Biol. Chem. 265, 15782–15787.

Bolscher, B.G.J.M., de Boer, M., De Klein, A., Weening, R.S. and Roos, D. (1991). Point mutations in the β-subunit of cytochrome b558 leading to X-linked chronic granulomatous disease. Blood 77, 2482–2487.

Bork, P. and Grunwald, C. (1990). Recognition of different nucleotide-binding sites in primary structures using a property-pattern approach. Eur. J. Biochem. 191, 347–358.

Borregaard, N., Cross, A.R., Herlin, T., Jones, O.T. and Segal, A.W. (1983). A variant form of X-linked chronic granulomatous disease with normal nitroblue tetrazolium slide test and cytochrome b. Eur. J. Clin. Invest. 13, 243–248.

Bredt, D.S., Hwang, P.M., Glatt, C.E., Lowenstein, C., Reed, R.R. and Snyder, S.H. (1991). Cloned and expressed nitric oxide synthase structurally resembles cytochrome P-450 reductase. Nature 351, 714–718.

Bromberg, Y. and Pick, E. (1984). Unsaturated fatty acids stimulate NADPH-dependent superoxide production by cell-free system derived from macrophages. Cell Immunol. 88, 213–221.

Bromberg, Y. and Pick, E. (1985). Activation of NADPH-dependent superoxide production in a cell-free system by sodium dodecyl sulfate. J. Biol. Chem. 260, 13539–13545.

Bu-Ghanim, H.N., Casimir, C.M., Povey, S. and Segal, A.W. (1990). The α subunit of cytochrome b-245 mapped to human chromosome 16. Genomics 8, 568–570.

Cagan, R.H. and Karnovsky, M.L. (1964). Enzymic basis of the respiratory stimulation during phagocytosis. Nature 204, 255–257.

Capeillere-Blandin, C., Masson, A. and Descamps-Latscha, B. (1991). Molecular characteristics of cytochrome b558 isolated from human granulocytes, monocytes and HL60 and U937 cells differentiated into monocyte/macrophages. Biochim. Biophys. Acta 1094, 55–65.

Casimir, C.M., Bu-Ghanim, H.N., Rodaway, A.R.F., Bentley, D.L., Rowe, P. and Segal, A.W. (1991). Autosomal recessive chronic granulomatous disease caused by deletion at a dinucleotide repeat. Proc. Natl Acad. Sci. USA 88, 2753–2757.

Casimir, C.M., Chetty, M., Bohler, M.-C., Garcia, R., Fischer, A., Griscelli, C., Johnson, B. and Segal, A.W. (1992). Identification of the defective NADPH-oxidase component in chronic granulomatous disease: a study of 57 European families. Eur. J. Clin. Invest. 22, 403–406.

Cassatella, M.A., Cappelli, R., Della Bianca, V., Grzeskowiak, M., Dusi, S. and Berton, G. (1988). Interferon-gamma activates human neutrophil oxygen metabolism and exocytosis. Immunology 63, 499–506.

Cassatella, M.A., Hartman, L., Perussia, B. and Trinchieri, G. (1989). Tumor necrosis factor and immune interferon synergistically induce cytochrome b-245 heavy chain gene expression and NADPH oxidase in human leukemic myeloid cells. J. Clin. Invest. 83, 1570–1579.

Cassatella, M.A., Bazzoni F., Flynn, R.M., Dusi, S., Trinchieri, G. and Rossi, P. (1990). Molecular basis of interferon-gamma and liposaccharide enhancement of phagocyte respiratory burst capability-studies on the gene expression of several NADPH oxidase components. J. Biol. Chem. 265, 20241–20246.

Cassatella, M.A., Bazzoni, F., Calzetti, F., Guasparri, I., Rossi, F. and Trinchieri, G. (1991). Interferon-gamma transcriptionally modulates the expression of the genes for the high affinity IgG-Fc receptor and the 47-kDa cytosolic component of NADPH oxidase in human polymorphonuclear leukocytes. J. Biol. Chem. 266, 22079–22082.

Castagna, M., Takai, Y., Kaibuchi, K., Sano, K., Kikkawa, U. and Nishizuka, Y. (1982). Direct activation of calcium-activated phospholipid-dependent protein kinase by tumor-promoting phorbol esters. J. Biol. Chem. 257, 7847–7851.

Cech, P. and Lehrer, R.I. (1984). Phagolysosomal pH of human neutrophils. Blood 63, 88–95.

Chanock, S.J., Barrett, D.M., Curnutte, J.T. and Orkin, S.H. (1991). Gene structure of the cytosolic component, p47-phox and mutations in autosomal recessive chronic granulomatous disease. Blood 78, 165a.

Chiba, T., Kaneda, M., Fujii, H., Clark, R.A. and Nauseef, W.M. (1990). Two cytosolic components of the neutrophil NADPH oxidase, P47-phox and P67-phox, are not flavoproteins. Biochem. Biophys. Res. Comm. 173, 376–381.

Christiansen, N.O. (1988). A time-course study on superoxide generation and protein kinase C activation in human neutrophils. FEBS Lett. 239, 195–198.

Clark, R.A., Leidal, K.G., Pearson, D.W. and Nauseef, W.M. (1987). NADPH oxidase of human neutrophils. Subcellular localization and characterization of an arachidonate-activatable superoxide-generating system. J. Biol. Chem. 262, 4065–4074.

Clark, R.A., Malech, H.L., Gallin, J.I., Nunoi, H., Volpp, B.D., Pearson, D.W., Nauseef, W.M. and Curnutte, J.T. (1989). Genetic variants of chronic granulomatous disease: prevalence of deficiencies of two cytosolic components of the NADPH oxidase system. N. Engl. J. Med. 321, 647–652.

Clark, R.A., Volpp, B.D., Leidal, K.G. and Nauseef, W.M. (1990). Two cytosolic components of the human neutrophil respiratory burst oxidase translocate to the plasma membrane during cell activation. J. Clin. Invest. 85, 714–721.

Cockcroft, S. and Gomperts, B.D. (1985). Role of guanine nucleotide binding protein in the activation of polyphosphoinositide phosphodiesterase. Nature 314, 534–536.

Cockcroft, S., Baldwin, J.M. and Allan, D. (1984). The Ca^+-activated polyphosphoinositide phosphodiesterase of human and rabbit neutrophil membranes. Biochem. J. 221, 477–482.

Collins, S.J., Ruscetti, E.W., Gallagher, R.E. and Gallo, R.C. (1978). Terminal differentiation of human promyelocytic leukemia cells induced by dimethyl sulphoxide and other polar compounds. Proc. Natl Acad. Sci. USA 75, 2458–2463.

Cooke, E. and Hallett, M.B. (1985). The role of C-kinase in the physiological activation of the neutrophil oxidase. Biochem. J. 232, 323–327.

Cross, A.R. and Jones, O.T. (1986). The effect of the inhibitor diphenylene iodonium on the superoxide-generating system of neutrophils. Specific labelling of a component polypeptide of the oxidase. Biochem. J. 237, 111–116.

Cross, A.R., Jones, O.T., Harper, A.M. and Segal, A.W. (1981). Oxidation–reduction properties of the cytochrome b found in the plasma-membrane fraction of human neutrophils. A possible oxidase in the respiratory burst. Biochem. J. 194, 599–606.

Cross, A.R., Higson, F.K., Jones, O.T., Harper, A.M. and Segal, A.W. (1982a). The enzymic reduction and kinetics of oxidation of cytochrome b-245 of neutrophils. Biochem. J. 204, 479–485.

Cross, A.R., Jones, O.T., Garcia, R. and Segal, A.W. (1982b). The association of FAD with the cytochrome b- 245 of human neutrophils. Biochem. J. 208, 759–763.

Cross, A.R., Parkinson, J.F. and Jones, O.T. (1984). The superoxide-generating oxidase of leucocytes. NADPH-dependent reduction of flavin and cytochrome b in solubilized preparations. Biochem. J. 223, 337–344.

Curnutte, J.T. (1985). Activation of human neutrophil nicotinamide adenine dinucleotide phosphate, reduced (triphosphopyridine nucleotide, reduced) oxidase by arachidonic acid in a cell-free system. J. Clin. Invest. 75, 1740–1743.

Curnutte, J.T. and Smith, R.M. (1991). Molecular basis of chronic granulomatous disease. Blood 77, 673–686.

Curnutte, J.T., Badwey, J.A., Robinson, J.M., Karnovsky, M.J. and Karnovsky, M.L. (1984). Studies on the mechanism of superoxide release from human neutrophils stimulated with arachidonate. J. Biol. chem. 259, 11851–11857.

Curnutte, J.T, Scott, P.J. and Mayo, L.A. (1989). Cytosolic components of the respiratory burst oxidase: Resolution of four components, two of which are missing in complementing types of chronic granulomatous disease. Proc. Natl Acad. Sci. USA 86, 825–829.

D'Amelio, R., Bellavite, P., Bianco, P., de Sole, P., Le Moli, S., Lippa, S., Seminara, R., Vercelli, B., Rossi, F., Rocchi, G. and Ainti, F. (1984). Chronic granulomatous disease in two sisters. J. Clin. Immunol. 4, 220–227.

Dancis, A., Roman, D.G., Anderson, G.J., Hinnebusch, A.G. and Klausner, R.D. (1992). Ferric reductase of Saccharomyces cerevisiae: molecular characterization, role in iron uptake and transcriptional control by iron. Prod. Natl Acad. Sci. USA 89, 3869–3873.

de Boer, M., Bolscher, B.G.J.M., Dinauer, M.C., Orkin, S.H., Smith, C.I.E., Ahlin, A., Weening, R.S. and Roos, D. (1992a). Splice site mutations are a common cause of X-linked chronic granulomatous disease. Blood 80, 1553–1558.

de Boer, M., De Klein, A., Hossle, J, P., Seger, R., Corbeel, L., Weening, R.S. and Roos, D. (1992b). Cytochrome b558-negative, autosomal recessive-chronic granulomatous disease; two new mutations in the cytochrome b558 light chain of the NADPH oxidase (p22-phox). Am. J. Hum. Genet. 51, 1127–1135.

Della Bianca, V., Grzeskowiak, M., Cassatella, M.A., Zeni, L. and Rossi, F. (1986). Phorbol 12-myristate 13-acetate potentiates the respiratory burst while inhibits phosphoinositide hydrolysis and calcium mobilization by formyl-methionyl-leucyl-phenylalanine in human neutrophils. Biochem. Biophys. Res. Comm. 135, 556–565.

Dinauer, M.C., Orkin, S.H., Brown, R., Jesaitis, A.J. and Parkos, C.A. (1987). The glycoprotein encoded by the X-linked chronic granulomatous disease locus is a component of the neutrophil cytochrome b complex. Nature 327, 717–720.

Dinauer, M.C., Curnutte, J.T., Rosen, H. and Orkin, S.H. (1989). A missense mutation in the neutrophil cytochrome b heavy chain in cytochrome-positive X-linked chronic granulomatous disease. J. Clin. Invest. 84, 2012–2016.

Dinauer, M.C., Pierce, E.A., Bruns, G.A.P., Curnutte, J.T. and Orkin, S.H. (1990). Human neutrophil cytochrome b light chain (p22-phox): gene structure, chromosomal location and mutations in cytochrome-negative autosomal recessive chronic granulomatous disease. J. Clin. Invest. 86, 1729–1737.

Dinauer, M.C., Pierce, E.A., Erickson, R.W., Muhlebach, T.J., Messner, H., Orkin, S.H., Seger, R.A. and Curnutte, J.T. (1991). Point mutation in the cytoplasmic domain of the neutrophil p22-phox cytochrome b subunit is associated with a nonfunctional NADPH oxidase and chronic granulomatous disease. Proc. Natl Acad Sci. USA 88, 11231–11235.

Doussiere, J. and Vignais, P.V. (1985). Purification and properties of an O_2^--generating oxidase from bovine polymorphonuclear neutrophils. Biochemistry 24, 7231–7239.

Drubin, D.G., Mulholland, J., Zhu, Z. and Botstein, D. (1990). Homology of a yeast actin-binding protein to signal transduction proteins and myosin-1. Nature 343, 288–290.

Eklund, E.A., Marshall, M., Gibbs, J.B., Crean, C.D. and Gabig, T.G. (1991). Resolution of a low molecular weight G protein in neutrophil cytosol required for NADPH oxidase activation and reconstitution by recombinant Krev-1 protein. J. Biol. Chem. 266, 13964–13970.

Ezekowitz, R.A.B., Dinauer, M.C., Jaffe, H.S., Orkin, S.H. and Newburger, P.E. (1988). Partial correction of the phagocyte defect in patients with X-linked chronic granulomatous disease by subcutaneous interferon gamma. N. Engl. J. Med. 319, 146–151.

Finkel, T.H., Pabst, M.J., Suzuki, H., Guthrie, L.A., Forehand, J.R., Phillips, W.A. and Johnston, R.B. (1987). Priming of neutrophils and macrophages for enhanced release of superoxide anion by the calcium ionophore ionomycin. J. Biol. Chem. 262, 12589–12596.

Finn, A., Hadzic, N., Morgan, G., Strobel, S. and Levinsky, R.J. (1990). Prognosis of chronic granulomatous disease. Arch. Dis. Child. 65, 942–945.

Forehand, J.R., Pabst, M.J., Phillips, W.A. and Johnston, R.B. (1989). Lipopolysaccharide priming of human neutrophils for an enhanced respiratory burst. J. Clin. Invest. 83, 74–93.

Franke, U., Ochs, H.D., deMartinville, B., Giacolone, J., Lindren, V., Disteche, C., Pagon, R.A., Hofker, M.H., van Ommen, G.-J., Pearson, P.L. and Wedgewood, R.J. (1985). Minor Xp21 chromosome deletion in a male associated with expression of Duchenne muscular dystrophy, chronic granulomatous disease, retinitis pigmentosa and McLeod syndrome. Am. J. Hum. Genet. 37, 250–267.

Franke, U., Hseih, C.-L., Foellmer, B.E., Lomax, K.J., Malech, H.L. and Leto, T.L. (1990). Genes for two autosomal recessive forms of chronic granulomatous disease assigned to 1q25 (NCF2) and 7q11.23 (NCF1). Am. J. Hum. Genet. 47, 483–492.

Fujita, I., Takeshige, K. and Minakami, S. (1987). Characterization of the NADPH-dependent superoxide production activated by sodium dodecyl sulfate in a cell-free system of pig neutrophils. Biochim. Biophys. Acta 931, 41–48.

Gabig, T.G. and Lefker, B.A. (1984a). Catalytic properties of the resolved flavoprotein and cytochrome B components of the NADPH dependent O_2^--generating oxidase from human neutrophils. Biochem. Biophys. Res Commun. 118, 430–436.

Gabig, T.G. and Lefker, B.A. (1984b). Deficient flavoprotein component of the NADPH-dependent O_2^--generating oxidase in the neutrophils from three male patients with chronic granulomatous disease. J. Clin. Invest. 73, 701–705.

Gabig, T.G., English, D., Akard, L.P. and Schell, M.J. (1987). Regulation of neutrophil NADPH oxidase activation in a cell-free system by guanine nucleotides and fluoride. Evidence for participation of a pertussis and cholera toxin-insensitive G protein. J. Biol. Chem. 262, 1685–1690.

Gabig, T.G., Eklund, E.A., Bruce Potter, G. and Dykes, J.R. (1990). A neutrophil GTP-binding protein that regulates cellfree NADPH oxidase activation is located in the cytosolic fraction. J. Immunol. 145, 945–951.

Gallin, J.I. and Malech, H.L. (1990). Update on chronic granulomatous diseases of childhood. Immunotherapy and potential for gene therapy. JAMA 263, 1533–1537.

Gallin, J.I. Malech, H.L., Weening, R.S., Curnutte, J.T., Quie, P.G., Jaffe, H.S. and Esekowitz, R.A.B. (1991). A controlled trial of interferon gamma to prevent infection in chronic granulomatous disease. N. Engl. J. Med. 324, 509–516.

Garcia, R.C. and Segal, A.W. (1984). Changes in the subcellular distribution of the cytochrome b-245 on stimulation of human neutrophils. Biochem. J. 219, 233–242.

Gerard, C., McPhail, L.C., Marfat, A., Bass, D.A. and McCall, C.E. (1986). Role of protein kinases in stimulation of human polymorphonuclear leukocyte oxidative metabolism by various agonists. J. Clin. Invest. 77, 61–65.

Gomez-Cambronero, J., Huang, C.-K., Bonak, V.A., Wang, E., Casnellie, J.E., Shiraishi, T. and Sha'aft, R.I. (1989). Tyrosine phosphorylation in human neutrophil. Biochem. Biophys. Res. Comm. 162, 1478–1485.

Grinstein, S. and Furuya, W. (1988). Receptor-mediated activation of electropermiablized neutrophils. Evidence for a Ca^{2+}- and protein kinase C-independent signaling pathway. J. Biol. Chem. 263, 1779–1783.

Hamers, M.N., de Boer, M., Meerhof, L.J., Weening, R.S. and Roos, D. (1984). Complementation in monocyte hybrids revealing genetic heterogeneity in chronic granulomatous disease. Nature 307, 553–555.

Harper, A.M., Dunne, M.J. and Segal, A.W. (1984). Purification of cytochrome b-245 from human neutrophils. Biochem. J. 219, 519–527.

Harper, A.M., Chaplin, M.F. and Segal, A.W. (1985). Cytochrome b-245 from human neutrophils is a glycoprotein. Biochem. J. 227, 783–788.

Haslett, C., Savill, J.S. and Meagher, L. (1989). The neutrophil. Curr. Opin. Immunol. Curr. Sci. 2, 10–18.

Hattori, H. (1961). Studies on the labile, stable NADI oxidase and peroxidase staining reactions in the isolated particles of horse granulocyte. Nagoya J. Med. Sci. 23, 362–378.

Henderson, L.M., Chappell, J.B. and Jones, O.T. (1987). The superoxide-generating NADPH oxidase of human neutrophils is electrogenic and associated with an H^+ channel. Biochem. J. 246, 325–329.

Henderson, L.M., Chappell, J.B. and Jones, O.T.G. (1989). Superoxide generation is inhibited by phospholipase A2 inhibitors. Biochem. J. 264, 249–255.

Heyneman, R.A. and Vercauteren, R.E. (1984). Activation of a NADPH oxidase from horse polymorphonuclear leukocytes in a cell-free system. J. Leuk. Biol. 36, 751–759.

Heyworth, P.G. and Segal, A.W. (1986). Further evidence for the involvement of a phosphoprotein in the respiratory burst oxidase of human neutrophils. Biochem. J. 239, 723–731.

Heyworth, P.G., Shrimpton, C.F. and Segal, A.W. (1989). Localisation of the 47 kDa phosphoprotein involved in the respiratory burst NADPH oxidase of phagocytic cells. Evidence for its translocation from the cytosol to plasma membrane. Biochem. J. 260, 243–248.

Heyworth, P.G., Curnutte, J.T., Nauseef, W.M., Volpp, B.D., Pearson, D.W., Rosen, H. and Clark, R.A. (1991). Neutrophil nicotinamide adenine dinucleotide phosphate oxidase assembly. Translocation of p47-phox and p67-phox requires interaction between p47-phox and cytochrome b558. J. Clin. Invest. 87, 352–356.

Hohn, D.C. and Lehrer, R.I. (1975). NADPH oxidase deficiency in X-linked chronic granulomatous disease. J. Clin. Invest. 55, 707–713.

Holmes, B., Quie, P.G., Windhorst, D.B. and Good, R.A. (1966). Fatal granulomatous disease of childhood. An inborn abnormality of phagocytic function. Lancet 1, 1225–1228.

Holmes, B., Page, A.R. and Good, R.A. (1967). Studies of the metabolic activity of leukocytes from patients with a genetic abnormality of phagocyte function. J. Clin. Invest. 46, 1422–1432.

Holmes, B., Park, B.H., Malawista, S.E., Quie, P.G., Nelson, D.L. and Good, R.A. (1970). Chronic granulomatous disease in females. N. Engl. J. Med. 283, 217–221.

Huang, C.K., Bonak, V., Laramee, G.R. and Casnellie, J.E. (1990). Protein phosphorylation in rabbit peritoneal neutrophils. Biochem. J. 269, 431–436.

Hurst, J.K., Loehr, T.M., Curnutte, J.T. and Rosen, H. (1991). Resonance Raman and electron paramagnetic resonance structural investigations of neutrophil cytochrome b558. J. Biol. Chem. 266, 1627–1634.

Ingraham, L.M., Coates, T.D., Allen, J.M., Higgins, C.P., Baehner, R.L. and Boxer, L.A. (1982). Metabolic, membrane and functional responses of human polymorphonuclear leukocytes to platelet-activating factor. Blood 59, 1259–1266.

Isogai, Y., Shiro, Y., Nasuda-Kouyama, A. and Iizuka, T. (1991). Superoxide production by cytochrome b558 purified from neutrophils in a reconstituted system with an exogenous reductase. J. Biol. Chem. 266, 13481–13484.

Jacques, Y.V. and Bainton, D.F. (1978). Changes in pH within the phagocytic vacuoles of human neutrophils and monocytes. Lab. Invest. 39, 179–185.

Johnston, R.B. and Kitagawa, S. (1985). Molecular basis for the enhanced respiratory burst of activated macrophages. Fed. Proc. 44, 2927–2932.

Kakinuma, K., Kaneda, M., Chiba, T. and Ohnishi, T. (1986). Electron spin resonance studies on a flavoprotein in neutrophil plasma membranes. Redox potentials of the flavin and its participation in NADPH oxidase. J. Biol. Chem. 261, 9426–9432.

Kakinuma, K., Fukuhara, Y. and Kaneda, M. (1987). The respiratory burst oxidase of neutrophils. Separation of an FAD enzyme and its characterization. J. Biol. Chem. 262, 12316–12322.

Kamani, N., August, C.S., Campbell, D.E., Nassan, N.F. and Douglas, S.D. (1988). Marrow transplantation in chronic granulomatous disease: an update with 6-year follow-up. J. Pediatr. 113, 697–700.

Karlsson, S. (1991). Treatment of genetic defects in hematopoietic cell function by gene transfer. Blood 78, 2481–2492.

Karplus, P.A., Daniels, M.J. and Herriott, J.R. (1991). Atomic structure of ferredoxin-NADP$^+$ reductase: prototype for a structurally novel flavoenzyme family. Science 251, 60–66.

Kenney, R.T., Malech, H.L., Gallin, J.I. and Leto, T.L. (1990). Amplification mapping of p67-phox deficient chronic granulomatous disease. Clin. Res. 38, 434A.

Kenney, R.T., Malech, H.L. and Leto, T.L. (1992). Structural characterization of the p67-phox gene. Clin. Res. 40, 261A.

Klebanoff, S.J. (1971). Intraleukocytic microbicidal defects. Annu. Rev. Med. 22, 39–62.

Klebanoff, S.J. and Clark, R.A. (1978). "The Neutrophil Function and Clinical Disorders". North-Holland, New York.

Knaus, U.G., Heyworth, P.G., Evans, T., Curnutte, J.T. and Bokoch, G.M. (1992). Regulation of phagocyte oxygen radical production by the GTP-binding protein rac2. Science 254, 1512–1515.

Knoller, S., Shpungin, S. and Pick, E. (1991). The membrane-associated component of the amphiphile-activated, cytosol-dependent superoxide-forming NADPH oxidase of macrophages is identical to cytochrome b 559. J. Biol. Chem. 266, 2795–2804.

Kramer, I.M., Verhoeven, A.J., van der Bend, R.L., Weening, R.S. and Roos, D. (1988). Purified protein kinase C phosphorylates a 47-kDa protein in control neutrophil cytoplasts but not in neutrophil cytoplasts from patients with the autosomal form of chronic granulomatous disease. J. Biol. Chem. 263, 2352–2357.

Kunkel, L.M., Monaco, A.P., Middlesworth, W., Ochs, H.D. and Latt, S.A. (1985). Specific cloning of DNA fragments absent from the DNA of a male patient with an X chromosome deletion. Proc. Natl Acad. Sci. USA 82, 4778–4782.

Leto, T.L. and Garrett, M.C. (1992). SRC-like (SH3) domains of p67-phox are not essential for cell-free reconstitution of NADPH oxidase activity. Clin. Res. 40, 175A.

Leto, T.L., Lomax, K.J., Volpp, B.D., Nunoi, H., Sechler, J.M.G., Nauseef, W.M., Clark, R.A., Gallin, J.I. and Malech, H.L. (1990). Cloning of a 67-kD neutrophil oxidase factor with similarity to a noncatalytic region of p60^{c-src}. Science 248, 727–730.

Leto, T.L., Garrett, M.C., Fujii, H. and Nunoi, H. (1991). Characterization of neutrophil NADPH oxidase factors p47-phox and p67-phox from recombinant baculoviruses. J. Biol. Chem. 266, 19812–19818.

Levinsky, R.J., Harvey, B.A.M., Rodeck, C.H. and Soothill, J.F. (1983). Phorbol-myristate acetate stimulated NBT test; a simple method suitable for antenatal diagnosis of chronic granulomatous disease. Clin. Exp. Immunol. 54, 595–598.

Ligeti, E., Doussiere, J. and Vignais, P.V. (1988). Activation of the $O_2^{\cdot-}$-generating oxidase in plasma membrane from bovine polymorphonuclear neutrophils by arachidonic acid, a cytosolic factor of protein nature, and nonhydrolyzable analogues of GTP. Biochemistry 27, 193–200.

Light, D.R., Walsh, C., O'Callaghan, A.M., Goetzl, E.J. and Tauber, A.I. (1981). Characteristics of the cofactor requirements for the superoxide-generating NADPH oxidase of human polymorphonuclear leukocytes. Biochemistry 20, 1468–1476.

Lomax, K.J., Leto, T.L., Nunoi, H., Gallin, J.I. and Malech, H.J. (1989a). Recombinant 47-kilodalton cytosol factor restores NADPH oxidase in chronic granulomatous disease (Author's correction). Science 245, 987.

Lomax, K.J., Leto, T.L., Nunoi, H., Gallin, J.I. and Malech, H.L. (1989b). Recombinant 47-kilodalton cytosol factor restores NADPH oxidase in chronic granulomatous disease. Science 245, 409–412.

Lutter, R., van Schaik, M.L., van Zwieten, R., Wever, R., Roos, D. and Hamers, M.N. (1985). Purification and partial characterization of the b-type cytochrome from human polymorphonuclear leukocytes. J. Biol. Chem. 260, 2237–2244.

Majumdar, S., Rossi, M.W., Fujiki, T., Phillips, W.A., Disa, S., Queen, C.F., Johnston, R.B., Jr, Rosen, O.M., Corkey, B.E. and Korchak, H.M. (1991). Protein kinase C isotopes and signaling in neutrophils. J. Biol. Chem. 266, 9285–9294.

Maly, F.E., Cross, A.R., Jones, O.T., Wolf Vorbeck, G., Walker, C. and De Weck, A.L. (1988). The superoxide generating system of B cell lines. Structural homology with the phagocytic oxidase and triggering via surface Ig. J. Immunol. 140, 2334–2339.

Maly, F.E., Nakamura, M., Gauchat, A., Urwyler, C., Walker, C., Dahinden, C.A., Cross, A.R., Jones, O.T. and DeWeck, A.L. (1990). Superoxide dependent nitroblue tetrazolium reduction and expression of cytochrome b245 components by human B-lymphocytes and B-cell lines. J. Immunol. 142, 1260–1267.

Mandell, G.L. (1970). Intraphagosomal pH of human polymorphonuclear neutrophils. Proc. Soc. Exp. Biol. Med. 134, 447–449.

Maridonneau-Parini, I. and Tauber, A.I. (1986). Activation of NADPH-oxidase by arachidonate acid involves phospholipase A2 in human neutrophils but not in the cell free system. Biochem. Biophys. Res. Comm. 138, 1099–1105.

Markert, M., Glass, G.A. and Babior, B.M. (1985). Respiratory burst oxidase from human neutrophils: purification and some properties. Proc. Natl Acad. Sci. USA 82, 3144–3148.

Massey, V. and Hemmerich, P. (1980). Active-site probes of flavoproteins. Biochem. Soc. Trans. 8, 246–257.

McPhail, L.C., Shirley, P.S., Clayton, C.C. and Snyderman, R. (1985). Activation of the respiratory burst enzyme from human neutrophils in a cell-free system. J. Clin. Invest. 75, 1735–1739.

Minegishi, N., Nakamura, M., Suzaki, K., Terasawa, M., Minegishi, M. and Konno, T. (1988). Chronic granulomatous disease with neutrophil membrane cytochrome b deficiency: demonstration by immunochemical staining with monoclonal antibody. Tohoku. J. Exp. Med. 154, 143–148.

Mizuno, T., Kaibuchi, K., Ando, S., Musha, T., Hiraoka, K., Takaishi, K., Asada, M., Nunio, H., Matsuda, I. and Takai, Y. (1992). Regulation of the superoxide-generating NADPH oxidase by a small GTP-binding protein and its stimulatory and inhibitory GDP/GTP exchange proteins. J. Biol. Chem. 267, 10215–10218.

Monaco, A.P., Bertelson, C.J., Middlesworth, W., Colletti, C.A., Aldridge, J., Fischbeck, K.H., Bartlett, R., Pericak Vance, M.A., Roses, A.D. and Kunkel, L.M. (1985). Detection of deletions spanning the Duchenne muscular dystrophy locus using a tightly linked DNA segment. Nature 316, 842–845.

Morel, F., Doussiere, J., Stasia, M.J. and Vignais, P.V. (1985).

The respiratory burst of bovine neutrophils. Role of a b type cytochrome and coenzyme specificity. Eur. J. Biochem. 152, 669–679.

Morel, F., Doussiere, J. and Vignais, P.V. (1991). The superoxide-generating oxidase of phagocytic cells. Physiological, molecular and pathological aspects. Eur. J. Biochem. 201, 523–546.

Muhlebach, T.J., Robinson, W., Seger, R.A. and Machler, M. (1990). A second NSI1 RFLP at the CYBB locus. Nucleic Acids Res. 18, 4966.

Musacchio, A., Gibson, T., Lehto, V-P. and Saraste, M. (1992). SH3-an abundant protein domain in search of a function. FEBS 307, 55–61.

Nakamura, M., Imajoh-Ohmi, S., Kanegesaki, S., Kurozumi, H., Sato, K., Kato, S. and Miyazaki, Y. (1990). Prenatal diagnosis of cytochrome-deficient chronic granulomatous disease. Lancet 336, 118–119.

Nakamura, M., Murakami, M., Koga, T., Tanaka, Y. and Minakami, S. (1987). Monoclonal antibody 7D5 raised to cytochrome b558 of human neutrophils: immunocytochemical detection of the antigen in peripheral phagocytes of normal subjects, patients with chronic granulomatous disease, and their carrier mothers. Blood 69, 1404–1408.

Nasmith, P.E., Mills, G.B. and Grinstein, S. (1989). Guanine nucleotides induce tyrosine phosphorylation and activation of the respiratory burst in neutrophils. Biochem. J. 257, 893–897.

Nauseef, W.M., Volpp, B.D., McCormick, S., Leidal, K.G. and Clark, R.A. (1991). Assembly of the neutrophil respiratory burst oxidase. J. Biol. Chem. 266, 5911–5917.

Newburger, P.E., Luscinskas, F.W., Ryan, T., Beard, C.J., Wright, J., Simons, E.R. and Tauber, A.I. (1986). Variant chronic granulomatous disease: modulation of the neutrophil defect by severe infection. Blood 68, 914–919.

Newburger, P.E., Ezekowitz, R.A.B., Whitney, C., Wright, J. and Orkin, S.H. (1988). Induction of phagocyte cytochrome b heavy chain gene expression by interferon γ Proc. Natl Acad. Sci. USA 85, 5215–5219.

Nugent, J.H.A., Gratzer, W. and Segal, A.W. (1989). Identification of the haem binding subunit of cytochrome b-245. Biochem. J. 264, 921–924.

Nunoi, H., Rotrosen, D., Gallin, J.I. and Malech, H.L. (1988). Two forms of autosomal chronic granulomatous disease lack distinct neutrophil cytosol factors. Science 242, 1298–1301.

Odell, E.W. and Segal, A.W. (1988). The bactericidal effects of the respiratory burst and the myeloperoxidase system isolated in neutrophil cytoplasts. Biochim. Biophys. Acta 971, 266–274.

Ohno, Y., Buescher, E.S., Roberts, R., Metcalf, J.A. and Gallin, J.I. (1986). Reevaluation of cytochrome b and flavin adenine dinucleotide in neutrophils from patients with chronic granulomatous disease and description of a family with probable autosomal recessive inheritance of cytochrome b deficiency. Blood 67, 1132–1138.

Ohta, H., Takahashi, H., Hattori, H., Yamada, H. and Takikawa, K. (1966). Some oxidative enzymes and cytochrome in the specific granules of neutrophil leukocytes. Acta Haematol. Jap. 29, 799–808.

Ohta, H., Okajima, F. and Ui, M. (1985). Inhibition by islet-activating protein of a chemotactic peptide-induced early breakdown of inositol phospholipids and Ca^{2+} mobilization in guinea pig neutrophils. J. Biol. Chem. 260, 15771–5780.

Okamura, N., Curnutte, J.T., Roberts, R.L. and Babior, B.M. (1988a). Relationship of protein phosphorylation to the activation of the respiratory burst in human neutrophils. Defects in the phosphorylation of a group of closely related 48-kDa proteins in two forms of chronic granulomatous disease. J. Biol. Chem. 263, 6777–6782.

Okamura, N., Malawista, S.E., Roberts, R.L., Rosen, H., Ochs, H.D., Babior, B.M. and Curnutte, J.T. (1988b). Phosphorylation of the oxidase-related 48K phosphoprotein family in the unusual autosomal cytochrome-negative and X-linked cytochrome-positive types of chronic granulomatous disease. Blood 72, 811–816.

Parkinson, J.F. and Gabig, T.G. (1988). Phagocyte NADPH-oxidase. Studies with flavin analogues as active site probes in triton X-100-solubilized preparations. J. Biol. Chem. 263, 8859–8863.

Parkos, C.A., Cochrane, C.G., Schmitt, M. and Jesaitis, A.J. (1985). Regulation of the oxidative response of human granulocytes to chemoattractants. J. Biol. Chem. 260, 6541–6547.

Parkos, C.A., Allen, R.A., Cochrane, C.G. and Jesaitis, A.J. (1987). Purified cytochrome b from human granulocyte plasma membrane is comprised of two polypeptides with relative molecular weights of 91,000 and 22,000. J. Clin. Invest. 80, 732–742.

Parkos, C.A., Allen, R.A., Cochrane, C.G. and Jesaitis, A.J. (1988a) The quaternary structure of the plasma membrane b-type cytochrome of human granulocytes. Biochim. Biophys. Acta 932, 71–83.

Parkos, C.A., Dinauer, M.C., Walker, L.E., Allen, R.A., Jesaitis, A.J. and Orkin, S.H. (1988b). Primary structure and unique expression of the 22-kilodalton light chain of human neutrophil cytochrome b. Proc. Natl Acad. Sci. USA 85, 3319–3323.

Parkos, C.A., Dinauer, M.C., Jesaitis, A.J., Orkin, S.H. and Curnutte, J.T. (1989). Absence of both the 91kD and 22kD subunits of human neutrophil cytochrome b in two genetic forms of chronic granulomatous disease. Blood 73, 1416–1420.

Pelham, A., O'Reilly, M.-A.J., Malcolm, S., Levinsky, R.J. and Kinnon, C. (1990). RFLP and deletion analysis for X-linked chronic granulomatous disease using the cDNA probe: potential for improved prenatal diagnosis and carrier demonstration. Blood 76, 820–824.

Pember, S.O., Heyl, B.L., Kinkade, J.M., Jr and Lambeth, J.D. (1984). Cytochrome b558 from (bovine) granulocytes. Partial purification from Triton X-114 extracts and properties of the isolated cytochrome. J. Biol. Chem. 259, 10590–10595.

Pick, E., Kroizman, T. and Abo, A. (1989). Activation of the superoxide-forming NADPH oxidase of macrophages requires two cytosolic components – one of them is also present in certain nonphagocytic cells. J. Immunol. 143, 4180–4187.

Pilloud, M.C., Doussiere, J. and Vignais, P.V. (1989). Parameters of activation of the membrane-bound O_2^--generating oxidase from bovine neutrophils in a cell-free system. Biochem. Biophys. Res. Comm. 159, 783–790.

Pilloud-Dagher, M.-C. and Vignais, P.V. (1991). Purification and characterization of an oxidase activating factor of 63 kilodaltons from bovine neutrophils. Biochemistry 30, 2753–2760.

Pontremoli, S., Melloni, E., Michetti, M., Sacco, O., Sparatore, B., Damiani, G. and Horecker, B.L. (1986). Cytolytic effects of neutrophils: role for a membrane-bound neutral proteinase. Proc. Natl Acad. Sci. USA 83, 1685-1689.

Porter, C.D., Parkar, M.H., Collins, M.K.L., Levinsky, R.J. and Kinnon, C. (1992). Superoxide production by normal and chronic granulomatous disease (CGD) patient-derived EBV-transformed B cell lines. Measured by chemiluminescence-based assays. J. Immunol. Meth. 155, 151–157.

Porter, T.D. (1991). An unusual yet strongly conserved flavoprotein reductase in bacteria and mammals. Trends Biochem. Sci. 16, 154–158.

Quinn, M.T., Parkos, C.A., Walker, L., Orkin, S.H., Dinauer, M.C. and Jesaitis, A.J. (1989). Association of a ras-related protein with cytochrome b of human neutrophils. Nature 342, 198–200.

Quinn, M.T., Mullen, L.M. and Jesaitis, A.J. (1992). Human neutrophil cytochrome b contains multiple hemes. J. Biol. Chem. 267, 7303–7309.

Rappeport, J.M., Newburger, P.E. and Goldblum, R.M. (1982). Allogeneic bone marrow transplantation for chronic granulomatous disease. J. Pediatr. 101, 952–955.

Repine, J.E., White, J.G., Clawson, C.C. and Holmes, B.M. (1974). Effects of phorbol myristate acetate on the metabolism and ultrastructure of neutrophils in chronic granulomatous disease. J. Clin. Invest. 54, 83–90.

Riccardi, S., Giordano, D., Schettini, F., De Mattia, D., Lovecchio, T., Santoro, N. and Fumarulo, R. (1986). Cytochrome b and FAD content in polymorphonuclear leucocytes in a family with X-linked chronic granulomatous disease. Scand. J. Haematol. 37, 333–336.

Robinson, J.M., Badwey, J.A., Karnovsky, M.L. and Karnovsky, M.J. (1985). Release of superoxide and change in morphology by neutrophils in response to phorbol esters: antagonism by inhibitors of calcium-binding proteins. J. Cell. Biol. 101, 1052–1058.

Rodaway, A.R.F., Teahan, C.G., Casimir, C.M., Segal, A.W. and Bentley, D.L. (1990). Characterisation of the 47 kD autosomal chronic granulomatous disease protein; tissue specific expression and transcriptional control by retinoic acid. Mol. Cell. Biol. 10, 5388–5396.

Roos, D. (1992). In "New Concepts in Immunodeficiency Diseases" (eds C. Griscelli and S. Gupta). John Wiley and Sons, Chichester.

Rossi, F. (1986). The O_2^--forming NADPH oxidase of the phagocytes: nature, mechanisms of activation and function. Biochim. Biophys. Acta 853, 65–89.

Rotrosen, D. and Leto, T.L. (1990). Phosphorylation of neutrophil 47-kDa cytosolic factor. Translocation to membrane is associated with distinct phosphorylation events. J. Biol. Chem. 265, 19910–19915.

Rotrosen, D., Kleinberg, M.E., Nunoi, H., Leto, T.L., Gallin, J.I. and Malech, H.L. (1990). Evidence for a functional cytoplasmic domain of phagocyte oxidase cytochrome b558. J. Biol. Chem. 265, 8745–8750.

Rotrosen, D., Yeung, C.L., Leto, T.L., Malech, H.L. and Kwong, C.H. (1992). Cytochrome b558: the flavin-binding component of the phagocyte NADPH oxidase. Science 256, 1459–1462.

Royer Pokora, B., Kunkel, L.M., Monaco, A.P., Goff, S.C., Newburger, P.E., Baehner, R.L., Cole, F.S., Curnutte, J.T.

and Orkin, S.H. (1986). Cloning the gene for an inherited human disorder – chronic granulomatous disease – on the basis of its chromosomal location. Nature 322, 32–38.

Sbarra, A.J. and Karnovsky, M.L. (1959). The biochemical basis of phagocytosis. 1. Metabolic changes during the ingestion of particles by polymorphonuclear leukocytes. J. Biol. Chem. 234, 1355–1362.

Schapiro, B.L., Newburger, P.E., Klempner, M.S. and Dinauer, M.C. (1991). Chronic granulomatous disease presenting in a 69-year-old man. N. Engl. J. Med. 325, 1786–1790.

Schneider, C., Zanetti M. and Romeo, D. (1981). Surface-active stimuli selectively increase protein phosphorylation in human neutrophils. FEBS Lett. 127, 4–8.

Sechler, J.M.G., Malech, H.L., White, C.J. and Gallin, J.I. (1988). Recombinant human interferon-γ reconstitutes defective phagocyte function in patients with chronic granulomatous disease of childhood. Proc. Natl Acad. Sci. USA 85, 4874–4878.

Segal, A.W. (1974). Nitroblue-tetrazolium tests. Lancet 2, 1248–1252.

Segal, A.W. (1987). Absence of both cytochrome b-245 subunits from neutrophils in X-linked chronic granulomatous disease. Nature 326, 88–91.

Segal, A.W. (1988). Cytochrome b-245 and its involvement in the molecular pathology of chronic granulomatous disease. Hematol. Oncol. Clin. North. Am. 2, 213–223.

Segal, A.W. and Jones, O.T.G. (1978). Novel cytochrome b system in phagocytic vacuoles from human granulocytes. Nature 276, 515–517.

Segal, A.W. and Jones, O.T. (1979a). The subcellular distribution and some properties of the cytochrome b component of the microbicidal oxidase system of human neutrophils. Biochem. J. 182, 181–188.

Segal, A.W. and Jones, O.T. (1979b). Neutrophil cytochrome b in chronic granulomatous disease (letter). Lancet 1, 1036–1037.

Segal, A.W. and Jones, O.T.G. (1980). Absence of cytochrome b reduction in stimulated neutrophils from both female and male patients with chronic granulomatous disease. FEBS Lett. 110, 111–114.

Segal, A.W., Jones, O.T., Webster, D. and Allison, A.C. (1978). Absence of a newly described cytochrome b from neutrophils of patients with chronic granulomatous disease. Lancet 2, 446–449.

Segal, A.W., Geisow, M., Garcia, R., Harper, A. and Miller, R. (1981). The respiratory burst of phagocytic cells is associated with a rise in vacuolar pH. Nature 290, 406–409.

Segal, A.W., Cross, A.R., Garcia, R.C., Borregaard, N., Valerius, N.H., Soothill, J.F. and Jones, O.T. (1983). Absence of cytochrome b-245 in chronic granulomatous disease. A multicenter European evaluation of its incidence and relevance. N. Engl. J. Med. 308, 245–251.

Segal, A.W., Heyworth, P.G., Cockcroft, S. and Barrowman, M.M. (1985). Stimulated neutrophils from patients with autosomal recessive chronic granulomatous disease fail to phosphorylate a Mr- 44,000 protein. Nature 316, 547–549.

Segal, A.W., Harper, A.M., Cross, A.R. and Jones, O.T. (1986). Cytochrome b-245. Meth. Enzymol. 132, 378–394.

Segal, A.W., West, I., Wientjes, F., Nugent, J.H.A., Chavan, A.J., Haley, B., Garcia, R.C., Rosen, H. and Scrace, G.

(1992). Cytochrome b-245 is a flavocytochrome containing FAD and the NADPH-binding site of the microbicidal oxidase of phagocytes. Biochem. J. 284, 781–788.

Seifert, R. and Schachtele, C. (1988). Studies with protein kinase C inhibitors presently available cannot elucidate the role of protein kinase C in the activation of NADPH oxidase. Biochem. Biophys Res. Comm. 152, 585–592.

Seifert, R. and Schultz, G. (1987). Fatty-acid-induced activation of NADPH oxidase in plasma membranes of human neutrophils depends on neutrophil cytosol and is potentiated by stable guanine nucleotides. Eur. J. Biochem. 162, 563–569.

Seifert, R., Rosenthal, W. and Schultz, G. (1986). Guanine nucleotides stimulate NADPH oxidase in membranes of human neutrophils. FEBS Lett. 205, 161–165.

Serra, M.C., Bellavite, P., Davoli, A., Bannister, J.V. and Rossi, F. (1984). Isolation from neutrophil membranes of a complex containing active NADPH oxidase and cytochrome b-245. Biochim. Biophys. Acta 788, 138–146.

Sha'ag, D. and Pick, E. (1990). Nucleotide binding properties of cytosolic components required for expression of activity of the superoxide generating NADPH oxidase. Biochim. Biophys. Acta 1037, 405–412.

Shinagawa, Y., Tanaka, C. and Teraoka, A. (1966). A new cytochrome in neutrophilic granules of rabbit leucocyte. J. Biochem. (Tokyo) 59, 622–624.

Shpungin, S., Dotan, I., Abo, A. and Pick, E. (1989). Activation of the superoxide forming NADPH oxidase in a cell free system by sodium dodecyl sulfate. Absolute lipid dependence of the solubilized enzyme. J. Biol. Chem. 264, 9195–9203.

Skalnik, D.G., Dorfman, D.M., Perkins, A.S., Jenkins, N.A., Copeland, N.G. and Orkin, S.H. (1991a). Targeting of transgene expression to monocyte/macrophages by the gp91-phox promoter and consequent histiocytic malignancies. Proc. Natl Acad. Sci. USA 88, 8505–8509.

Skalnik, D.G., Strauss, E.C. and Orkin, S.H. (1991b). CCAAT displacement protein as a repressor of the myelomonocytic-specific gp91-phox gene promoter. J. Biol. Chem. 266, 16736–16744.

Smith, C.D., Lane, B.C., Kusaka, I., Verghese, M.W. and Snyderman, R. (1985). Chemoattractant receptor induced hydrolysis of phosphatidylinositol 4,5-bisphosphate in human polymorphonuclear leukocyte membranes. Requirement for a guanine nucleotide regulatory protein. J. Biol. Chem. 260, 5875–5878.

Smith, R.M., Curnutte, J.T. and Babior, B.M. (1989). Affinity labeling of the cytosolic membrane components of the respiratory burst oxidase by the 2′,3′-dialdehyde derivative of NADPH. J. Biol. Chem. 264, 1958–1962.

Tanaka, A., Makino, R., Iisuka, T., Ishimura, Y. and Kanegasaki, S. (1988). Activation by saturated and monosaturated fatty acids of the O_2^--generating system in a cell-free preparation from neutrophils. J. Biol. Chem. 263, 13670–13676.

Tanaka, T., Imajoh-Ohmi, S., Kanegasaki, S., Takagi, Y., Makino, R. and Ishimura, Y. (1990). A 63-kilodalton cytosolic polypeptide involved in superoxide generation in porcine neutrophils. J. Biol. Chem. 265, 18717–18720.

Teahan, C., Rowe, P., Parker, P., Totty, N. and Segal, A.W. (1987). The X-linked chronic granulomatous disease gene codes for the beta-chain of cytochrome b-245. Nature 327, 720–721.

Teahan, C.G., Totty, N., Casimir, C.M. and Segal, A.W. (1990). Purification of the 47 kDa phosphoprotein associated with the NADPH oxidase of human neutrophils. Biochem. J. 267, 485–489.

Thrasher, A.J., Chetty, M., Casimir, C.M. and Segal, A.W. (1992). Restoration of superoxide generation to a chronic ganulomatous disease derived B cell line by retrovirus mediated gene transfer. Blood 80, 1125–1129.

Umei, T., Babior, B.M., Curnutte, J.T. and Smith, R.M. (1991). Identification of the NADPH-binding subunit of the respiratory burst oxidase. J. Biol, Chem. 266, 6019–6022.

Umei, T., Takeshige, K. and Minakami, S. (1986). NADPH binding component of neutrophil superoxide-generating oxidase. J. Biol. Chem. 261, 5229–5232.

Verhoven, A.J., Bolscher, B.G.J.M., Meerhof, L.F., van Zwieten, R., Keijer, J., Weening, R.S. and Roos, D. (1989). Characterisation of two monoclonal antibodies against cytochrome b558 of human neutrophils. Blood 73, 1686–1694.

Volpp, B.D., Nauseef, W.M. and Clark, R.A. (1988). Two cytosolic neutrophil oxidase components absent in autosomal chronic granulomatous disease. Science 242, 1295–1297.

Volpp, B.D., Nauseef, W.M., Donelson, J.E., Moser, D.R. and Clark, R.A. (1989a). Cloning of the cDNA and functional expression of the 47-kilodalton cytosolic component of human neutrophil respiratory burst oxidase. Proc. Natl Acad. Sci. USA 86, 7195–7199.

Volpp, B.D., Nauseef, W.M., Donelson, J.E., Moser, D.R. and Clark, R.A. (1989b). Cloning of the cDNA and functional expression of the 47 kilodalton cytosolic component of human neutrophil respiratory burst oxidase (Author's correction). Proc. Natl Acad. Sci. USA 86, 9563.

Wakeyama, H., Takeshige, K., Takayanagi, R. and Minakami, S. (1982). Superoxide-forming NADPH oxidase preparation of pig polymorphonuclear leucocyte. Biochem. J. 205, 593–601.

Walker, B.A.M., Hagenlocker, B.E. and Ward, P.A. (1991). Superoxide responses to formyl-methionyl-leucyl-phenylalanine in primed neutrophils. J. Immunol. 146, 3124–3131.

Weening, R.S., Adriaansz, L.H., Weemaes, C.M., Lutter, R. and Roos, D. (1985a) Clinical differences in chronic granulomatous disease in patients with cytochrome b-negative or cytochrome b-positive neutrophils. J. Pediatr. 107, 102–104.

Weening, R.S., Corbeel, L., de Boer, M., Lutter, R., van Zwieten, R. and Roos, D. (1985b). Cytochrome b deficiency in an autosomal form of chronic granulomatous disease. A third form of chronic granulomatous disease recognized by monocyte hybridization. J. Clin. Invest. 75, 915–920.

Westminster Hospital Transplant Team (1977). Bone marrow transplant from an unrelated donor for chronic granulomatous disease. Lancet 263, 210–213.

Wolfson, M., McPhail, L.C., Nasrallah, V.N. and Snyderman, R. (1985). Phorbol myristate acetate mediates redistribution of protein kinase C in human neutrophils: potential role in the activation of the respiratory burst enzyme. J. Immunol. 135, 2057–2062.

Wood, P.M. (1987). The two redox potentials for oxygen reduction to superoxide. Trends Biochem. Sci. 12, 250–251.

Woodman, R.C., Ruedi, J.M., Jesaitis, A.J., Okamura, N., Quinn, M.T., Smith, R.M., Curnutte, J.T. and Babior, B.M. (1991). Respiratory burst oxidase and three of four oxidase-related polypeptides are associated with the cytoskeleton of human neutrophils. J. Clin Invest. 87, 1345–1351.

Wright, C.D. and Hoffman, M.D. (1987). Comparison of the roles of calmodulin and protein kinase C in activation of the human neutrophil respiratory burst. Biochem. Biophys. Res. Comm. 142, 53–62.

Wymann, M.P., von Tscharner, V., Deranleau, D.A. and Baggiolini, M. (1987). Chemiluminescence detection of H_2O_2 produced by human neutrophils during the respiratory burst. Anal. Biochem. 165, 371–378.

Yuo, A., Kitagawa, S., Ohsaka, A., Saito, M. and Takaku, F. (1990). Stimulation and priming of human neutrophils by granulocyte colony-stimulating factor and granulocyte–macrophage colony-stimulating factor: qualitative and quantitative differences. Biochem. Biophys. Res. Commun. 171, 491–497.

4. Neutrophil Proteases:[1] Their Physiological and Pathological Roles

Niall S. Doherty and Michael J. Janusz

1. Introduction

Neutrophils play a vital role in host defence. They are usually the first cells to arrive at the site of an infection or injury and frequently are the most numerous cells present in a lesion. Their efficacy in host defence depends on their ability to kill a wide range of microorganisms. This lethal activity is provided by a broad range of weapons which includes proteases and other hydrolases, cationic proteins, low pH, and generation of reactive oxygen and nitrogen species. However, it is clearly not sufficient to just kill the invading microorganisms; the remains must be cleared from the battlefield and irreparably damaged tissue components must be removed to allow repair and remodelling to take place. The neutrophil is equipped with a powerful destructive potential of enormously broad specificity which enables it to fulfil these roles in host defence. Much of this destructive potential is provided by hydrolases located in the intracellular granules. As proteins comprise a major component of all organisms, it is only natural that proteases should account for a very high proportion of the destructive enzymes in neutrophil granules.

In addition to the granule proteases, neutrophils contain proteases in nearly all other subcellular locations. Many of these proteases are involved in housekeeping roles and are common to many cell types; others have a limited cellular distribution and fulfil cell- or tissue-specific roles. This discussion will emphasize those proteases which are unique to neutrophils or have been shown to play a role in their specialized functional properties. Discussion of neutrophil proteases will be

---

[1] The terms protease and proteinase will be used interchangeably.

Immunopharmacology of Neutrophils
ISBN 0–12–339250–0

Table 4.1 The subcellular location of the neutrophil proteases

Subcellular compartment	Proteases present	Functional characteristics
Granules		
Primary (Azurophilic)	Elastase Cathepsins B, D, G Proteinase 3	Proteases discharged into endocytic vesicles or the extracellular space
Secondary/tertiary	Collagenase Gelatinase	
Plasma membrane	Plasminogen activator Neutral endopeptidase Aminopeptidase M	Proteases anchored in the plasma membrane with the catalytic site facing the extracellular space
Cytosol	Calpain IL-1 converting enzyme	Proteases located in the cytosol. Some have a variable, but regulated, degree of binding to subcellular organelles or the interior of the plasma membrane

organized on the basis of their subcellular location, since this to a large extent also groups them by function. A list of the subcellular compartments to be discussed and a summary of their important characteristics is shown in Table 4.1.

Although the powerful destructive potential of neutrophil proteases is essential for the normal physiological function of these cells, it is also a liability to the host. It is easy to imagine how unregulated action of these enzymes could wreak havoc on normal healthy tissue. In fact, neutrophil proteases are implicated as important contributors to the pathology of many inflammatory diseases, particularly with reference to tissue damage. However, the evidence for their involvement is usually circumstantial and controversial. As will be discussed, it has proved impossible so far to assess the contribution made by any particular neutrophil protease in any disease unambiguously. The difficulties encountered are partly because a complex array of regulatory mechanisms and a screen of anti-proteases normally limits the action of neutrophil proteases. In order to understand the physiological and pathological roles of these enzymes, the control of, and possible escape from, these protective mechanisms will be described.

Because of their presumed role in inflammatory tissue damage, the neutrophil proteases are prime targets for therapeutic intervention and drug discovery. Since synthetic protease inhibitors not only have therapeutic potential but are also valuable tools for probing the biology of neutrophil proteases, data obtained using such agents will be presented. Many studies have relied on the use of "specific" synthetic inhibitors to identify roles for proteases in neutrophil function. Unfortunately the specificity of inhibitors cannot be assumed simply because they are described as, for example, serine protease inhibitors or elastase inhibitors. Many of these inhibitors have multiple activities and are, at best, imperfect tools. Unequivocal identification of a functional role for a particular protease is best achieved by identification

of its normal substrate and correlation of cleavage of substrate with functional effects in the presence of a range of inhibitors of different structural classes (natural and synthetic) and antibodies.

2. The Granules

Neutrophils are distinguished from other members of the family of leucocytes known as PMNs by differences in granule composition. The granules are such a marked characteristic of the appearance of PMNs when stained with standard haematological (Romanowsky) stains, e.g. Giemsa, that these cells are also collectively known as granulocytes. Since the granules contain important proteases and play a major role in the physiological and pathological functions of neutrophils, it is necessary to clarify some of the confusing terminology and claims for the existence of novel granule types (Table 4.2), prior to discussing the enzymes themselves.

Bainton (1988) has reviewed the information available up to 1988 concerning morphology and nomenclature of neutrophil granules. In conventionally prepared smears of whole blood, neutrophils show neither the large, blue (azurophilic, basophilic) granules of basophils nor the large red/orange (eosinophilic, acidophilic) granules of eosinophils; hence the name neutrophil. However, numerous small blue/lilac (azurophilic) granules can be seen. The faint pinkish colour which is often seen in the cytoplasm is due to the presence of a large number of smaller eosinophilic granules which cannot be resolved at the light microscope level. The azurophilic granules appear earlier in the bone marrow differentiation of neutrophils and are therefore also known as primary granules (Smolen, 1989), to distinguish them from the smaller eosinophilic granules which appear later and are known as secondary granules. Since the primary granules appear to be analogous to lysosomes, in that they contain the characteristic acid hydrolases found in the lysosomes

Table 4.2 The granules of human neutrophils

	Granules[a]				
	Primary	Secondary	Tertiary[b]	Phosphasomes	Calciosomes
Synonyms	Azurophilic, non-specific, basophilic	Specific, eosinophilic, acidophilic, adhesomes[1]	C-Particles[2] Secretory vesicles[3]	Secretory vesicles[4]	
Size/shape	Mostly spheres, some elipsoid, approx. 500 nm diameter[5]	Spherical (approx. 200 nm diameter) or rod-shaped (130 × 1000 nm)[5]			Variable shape, (sperical to pleiomorphic) 50–200 nm diameter[6]
Lysosomal acid hydrolases	β-Glucuronidase, acid-phosphatase, cathepsin B, cathepsin D, etc.				
Neutral serine proteases	Elastase, Cathepsin G, Proteinase 3, etc.	Plasminogen activator			
Neutral metalloproteases		Collagenase	Gelatinase		
Microbicidal factors	Myeloperoxidase, lysozyme, defensins, cationic proteins	Lysozyme, Cytochrome b_{558}[7]		NADPH oxidase[8]	
Adhesion molecules/ chemotactic factor receptors		Receptors for laminin, fibrinogen, vitronectin,[9] fMet-Leu-Phe receptor, C3 (Mac-1),[10] p150,95[10]		FcRIII (speculative)[11]	
Miscellaneous		Vitamin B12-binding protein, lactoferrin		Alkaline phosphatase,[11,12] plasma proteins,[13] decay accelerating factor (speculative)[11]	Calsequestrin[6]

[a] Unless otherwise indicated the data are taken from Baggiolini (1980).
[b] The existence of tertiary granules as a distinct population is disputed (see text).
References: [1]Singer et al. (1989); [2]Dewald et al. (1982); [3]Lew et al. (1986); [4]Borregaard et al. (1990); [5]Bainton (1988); [6]Volpe et al. (1988); [7]Borregaard et al. (1983); [8]Sengelov et al. (1992); [9]Singer et al. (1989); [10]Bainton et al. (1987); [11]Kobayashi and Robinson (1991); [12]Smith et al. (1985); [13]Borregaard et al. (1992).

of other cell types (in addition to some components unique to the neutrophil), the term non-specific granules has also been used. The secondary granules do not appear to have obvious counterparts in other cell types and have been termed specific granules.

This pattern of development is not accepted by all authors. Brederoo et al. (1983) have shown in morphological studies with the electron microscope that, during the development of human neutrophils, granules containing crystalloid or fibrillar inclusions are formed prior to the formation of azurophilic granules. If the nomenclature is to be based on the sequence in which the granules appear during neutrophil differentiation in the bone marrow, Brederoo et al. indicate that the azurophilic granule should be regarded as the secondary granule and the specific granule as the tertiary granule. This suggestion has not found general acceptance, perhaps because a biochemical correlate of the crystalloid/fibril-containing "primary" granule of Brederoo et al. has not been identified. Singer et al. (1989) have suggested that, because they contain a large complement of CAMs, the azurophilic/secondary granules could be referred to as

"adhesomes". To avoid confusion, the widely accepted terms, primary and secondary granules, will be used in this review and a summary of their properties is given in Table 4.2.

The existence of another type of granule, characterized by the presence of gelatinase, cytochrome b_{588} and ubiquinone but not myeloperoxidase or lactoferrin (Table 4.2), has been proposed on the basis of fractionation studies and evidence of selective release of gelatinase in the absence of release of azurophilic or specific granule components (Bretz and Bagiolini, 1982; Dewald et al., 1982; Mollinedo and Schneider, 1984). These putative granules have been widely referred to as tertiary granules even though it is not known whether they appear later in the differentiation of neutrophils than the other two granule populations (Rice et al., 1986). They have also been referred to as C-particles (Bretz and Baggiolini, 1982) and occasionally as secretory vesicles (Lew et al., 1986). The latter term, unfortunately, is also used to describe distinct organelles also known as phosphasomes (see Table 4.2). However, ultrastructural studies have failed to confirm the existence of "tertiary granules"

(Hibbs and Bainton, 1989) and, although the issue is not resolved, it is possible that the tertiary granule does not exist as a separate population and many of the data which suggested its existence could be interpreted on the basis of the existence of only two distinct populations, i.e. primary and secondary granules. Within each population, heterogeneity of composition and sensitivity to agents which induce release of granule contents have been widely reported (Rice *et al.*, 1986; Perez *et al.*, 1987; Damiano *et al.*, 1988; Hibbs and Bainton, 1989; Schettler *et al.*, 1991). The primary and secondary populations appear to contain granules with a continuous range of composition and one extreme of the specific granule spectrum may have the composition attributed to tertiary granules. The sources of such heterogeneity may be: (a) the existence of sub-populations of neutrophils; (b) the presence of granules at different stages of maturity; and/or (c) the intracellular trafficking/fusion events associated with neutrophil function (Rice *et al.*, 1986). Thus, the issue of whether tertiary granules exist in human neutrophils may be more a question of semantics than of substance. However, through the use of an immunoassay for gelatinase, instead of the usual enzyme assay, data have been obtained which strengthen the argument in favour of a distinct granule population (Kjeldson *et al.*, 1992). Clearly, the question is still open. Recent reports describe two other distinctly different granule populations, calciosomes and phosphasomes (Table 4.2). Although neither of these organelles have been shown to contain proteases, it may only be a matter of time before proteases are located there.

In unstimulated neutrophils the granules act as storage containers: they isolate the proteases and other potentially destructive granule components in a manner which prevents their destructive properties from being fully expressed and causing damage either to the neutrophil itself or surrounding normal tissue. Apart from this physical separation from potential substrates. a number of additional mechanisms are utilized to enable the proteases to be stored safely, i.e. storage as inactive proenzymes, storage at non-optimal pH and storage of enzyme/inhibitor complexes. The metalloproteases (gelatinase, collagenase) can be considered binary chemical weapons since generation of enzyme activity requires delivery to the site of action of both the inactive proenzyme and an activating agent. However, in all cases the generation of catalytically active granule proteases requires fusion of the granule membrane with either the plasma membrane (exocytosis) or with endocytic vesicles such as phagosomes, pinosomes or coated vesicles, resulting in a change in location and environment of the granule contents. Therefore, although the following proteases are classified as granule enzymes by most authors they can be found in other cellular compartments or extracellularly under appropriate conditions.

3. *Primary Granules*

Neutrophil primary granules contain an abundance of proteinases which play an important role in host defence. One important function of primary granule proteinases is the degradation of microbial proteins in the phagolysosomes, although a range of additional physiological and pathological roles is now recognized. Primary granules contain proteases with pH optima varying from neutrality (elastase, CatG) to pH 3.5–4.0 (cathepsin B, cathepsin D). It is uncertain whether conditions exist under which they are all functional simultaneously or whether they are selectively activated under different conditions. The development of specific cell-penetrating substrates that generate fluorescent products, combined with the use of microscopy and flow cytometry (Rothe *et al.*, 1992), should help clarify these questions. The properties of primary granule proteinases are summarized in Table 4.3.

3.1 HUMAN NEUTROPHIL ELASTASE

HNE (EC 3.4.21.37) is an abundant primary granule serine proteinase with the ability to degrade a wide variety of connective tissue macromolecules. In addition to elasin (Baugh and Travis, 1976), HNE can degrade fibronectin (McDonald and Kelley, 1980), proteoglycan (Malemud and Janoff, 1975; Janoff *et al.*, 1976; Kaiser *et al.*, 1976), collagen telopeptides (Starkey *et al.*, 1977; Mainardi *et al.*, 1980) and laminin (Heck *et al.*, 1990) (Table 4.3). HNE consists of 218 amino acids, four disulphide bonds and two asparagine-linked carbohydrate side chains (Sinha *et al.*, 1987). The gene for HNE consists of five exons and four introns, and codes for a translation product of 267 residues including an N-terminal extension of 29 residues and a C-terminal extension of 20 residues (Farley *et al.*, 1988; Takahashi *et al.*, 1988b). A 238 amino-acid serine protease isolated from bone marrow and named medullasin (Aoki *et al.*, 1975; Aoki, 1978) was subsequently found to be identical to a form of HNE which retained the 20 amino-acid carboxy terminal extension (Nakamura *et al.*, 1987; Okano *et al.*, 1987; Farley *et al.*, 1988; Takahashi *et al.*, 1988b). Retention of this additional sequence changes the catalytic activity of HNE and confers significant differences in its biological properties (reviewed in Aoki, 1992). It is uncertain whether this form of HNE has a distinct physiological/pathological role or is an intermediate form, which can be found in immature neutrophils, on the way to the mature 218 amino-acid form of HNE. The mature HNE protein has an *Mr* of approximately 30 000, an isoelectric point of 10.8 and a preference for cleaving peptide bonds at the carboxyl side of valine, methionine and leucine residues (Travis, 1988). The cationic nature of HNE is due to the presence of

Table 4.3 The enzymes of the primary granules

Enzyme	Molecular weight (kD)	Protease class	Biological substrates	Synthetic substrates	Endogenous inhibitors	Selected synthetic inhibitors
Elastase	25–30[1-4]	Serine	Elastin[4] Fibronectin[5] Proteoglycan[6-8] Collagen[9,10] Laminin[26]	MeO-Suc-Ala-Ala-Pro-Val-nitroanilide[11,12]	α_1-PI[3,13] SLPI[3,13,14,15] α_2-M[3,13] Elafin[16]	Boronic acids[17] Triflouromethyl ketones[18] Aldehydes[19] α-Ketoesters[20] Chloromethylketones[21,22] Cephalosporins[23,24]
Cathepsin G	26–30[25,26]	Serine	Elastin (weak)[3] Proteoglycan[3] Fibronectin[28] Laminin[27]	MeO-Suc-Ala-Ala-Pro-Phe-nitroanilide[12]	α_1-ACT[3,13] SLPI[3,14,15] α_2-M[3,13]	Diketones[19,20] Ketoesters[29,30] Chloromethylketones[21,23]
Proteinase 3	27–29[31,32]	Serine	Elastin[32] Fibronectin[33] Laminin[33] Vitronectin[33] Collagen[33]	Boc-Ala-Onp[33] MeO-Suc-Ala-Ala-Pro-Val-nitroanilide[33] MeO-Suc-Ala-Ala-Pro-Met-nitroanilide[33]	α_1-PI[33] α_2-M[33] Elafin[34]	Chloromethylketones[32] Methylsulphonyl succinamide derivative[35,36]
Proteinase 4	30[37]	Serine	Fibrin[37]	Boc-Ala-Onp[37]	α_2-M[37]	
Cathepsin B	37–40[38]	Cysteine	Proteoglycan[38]	Z-Arg-Arg-NH-nitrophenol[38]	Cystatin[38] α_2-M[38]	
Cathepsin D	42[39]	Aspartic acid	Haemoglobin[40,41]	—	—	Gly-Glu-Gly-Phe-Leu-Gly-d-Phe-Leu[42]

References: [1]Bieth (1989); [2]Groutas, (1987); [3]Travis (1988); [4]Baugh and Travis (1976); [5]McDonald and Kelley (1980); [6]Malemud and Janoff (1975); [7]Janoff et al. (1976); [8]Kaiser et al. (1976); [9]Starkey et al. (1977); [10]Mainardi et al. (1980); [11]Bieth (1989); [12]Nakajima et al. (1979); [13]Travis and Salvesen (1983); [14]Thompson and Ohlsson (1986); [15]Eisenberg et al. (1990); [16]Wiedow et al. (1990); [17]Shenvi and Kettner (1984); [18]Williams et al. (1991); [19]Hassal et al. (1985); [20]Angelastro et al. (1990); [21]Powers et al. (1977); [22]Powers (1983); [23]Doherty et al. (1986); [24]Fletcher et al. (1990); [25]Salvesen et al. (1987); [26]Hohn et al. (1989); [27]Suter et al. (1988); [28]Mehdi et al. (1990); [30]Peet et al. (1990); [31]Campanelli et al. (1990b); [32]Kao et al. (1988); [33]Rao et al. (1991); [34]Wiedow et al. (1991); [35]Groutas et al. (1989); [36]Groutas et al. (1990); [37]Ohlsson et al. (1990); [38]Buttle et al. (1991); [39]Ishikawa and Cimasoni (1977); [40]Levy et al. (1989); [41]Ichimanu et al. (1990); [42]Lauritzen et al. (1984).

19 arginines and only nine acidic amino-acid residues (Bode *et al.*, 1989). Comparison of the amino-acid sequences of HNE with other serine proteinases reveals a 43% homology with pancreatic elastase and 37% homology with cathepsin G.

The mRNA for HNE is not present in mature neutrophils. HNE is transcribed in bone marrow progenitor cells and packaged into the primary granules at the promyelocyte stage (Takahashi *et al.*, 1988a) The primary translation product is inactive, processing to active HNE occurring during or after storage in granules (Takahashi *et al.*, 1988a). Once inside the primary granule, the highly cationic HNE associates with the negatively charged glycosaminoglycans present to form an inactive complex (Avila and Convit, 1976; Travis, 1988). In addition, a cytosolic protein present in human monocytes, macrophages and neutrophils has been described that is a potent inhibitor of HNE (Remold-O'Donnell *et al.*, 1989, 1992). This protein has an *Mr* of 42 kD and was identified as a member of the serpin superfamily by sequence homology (Remold-O'Donnell *et al.*, 1989). These mechanisms ensure that HNE is maintained in an inactive form until it is discharged into phagosomes or to the exterior of the cell.

HNE can be released into the external environment by leakage from the phagolysosome or by cell death. Normally this is not a problem because of the presence of abundant levels of endogenous inhibitors in the external milieu. However, when there is an imbalance favouring the active enzyme over the endogenous inhibitor, connective tissue damage may occur. Recent data suggest that during degranulation a significant proportion of the HNE released to the cell exterior becomes bound to the external surface of the plasma membrane (Travis *et al.*, 1992). It appears to be bound by ionic interactions between the acidic sialic acid residues on cell-surface glycoproteins and the very basic arginine residues of HNE (Travis *et al.*, 1992), however, specific cell-surface receptors for HNE have also been reported (Dwenger *et al.*, 1986).

Proteinase inhibitors constitute approximately 10% of the total protein in plasma (Travis and Salvesen, 1983). There are several proteinase inhibitors that are capable of inhibiting HNE. α_1-PI is a plasma protein that can inhibit most serine proteinases but inactivates HNE at a much faster rate than other enzymes (Beatty et al., 1980). Human α_1-PI is a glycoprotein with an Mr of approximately 52 000 and consists of a single polypeptide chain (Crawford, 1973; Pannell et al., 1974) containing 394 amino-acid residues (Kurachi et al., 1981). It is a member of the class of macromolecular protease inhibitors known as serpins (SERine Protease INhibitors). The importance of α_1-PI in the protection from HNE-induced connective tissue damage is supported by the fact that individuals with low amounts of plasma α_1-PI have the tendency to develop emphysema at an early age (Laurell and Eriksson, 1963). Patients with an inherited deficiency of α_1-PI (referred to as Pi$_{zz}$) have circulating levels of α_1-PI of about 15% that of normals owing to a mutation in the protein chain that modifies post-translational glycosylation leading to reduced secretion (Travis and Salvesen, 1983). Thus, in these genetically predisposed patients an imbalance between HNE and the endogenous proteinase inhibitor α_1-PI can occur.

It has also been postulated that HNE-mediated connective tissue damage can occur in normal individuals when intensive neutrophil infiltration or other factors, such as cigarette smoke or environmental pollutants, interfere with the proteinase–antiproteinase balance. α_1-PI contains an active site associated methionine at residue 358 (Johnson and Travis, 1978) that is readily oxidized resulting in functional inactivation of inhibitor (Carp et al., 1982). Thus, an increase in HNE burden coupled with inactivation of α_1-PI by oxidants (or enzymes, see Section 4.1) generated by inflammatory cells or from the environment may result in a proteinase–inhibitor imbalance and tissue destruction.

Travis et al. (1992) have postulated that the oxidative inactivation of α_1-PI could also have an important physiological role. These authors suggest that the HNE bound to the cell surface (see above) would be protected by a "halo of oxidizing agents around the cell" generated by the oxidative burst, which would destroy the inhibitory activity of α_1-PI. Thus, expression of the catalytic activity of HNE would be confined to substrates in direct contact with the cell membrane. This local expression of catalytic activity could be an important component of the neutrophil's ability to migrate through tissues, particularly through the basement membrane during extravasation, despite the presence of an apparent excess of α_1-PI.

SLPI, also known as anti-leucoprotease (ALP), is an endogenous inhibitor of elastase and cathepsin G that is secreted from bronchial serous cells. SLPI is a low molecular weight non-glycosylated protein containing 107 amino-acid residues with an Mr of 11 726 (Thompson and Ohlsson, 1986). The amino-acid sequence revealed that SLPI consists of two homologous but distinct domains and suggested that one contained the HNE-inhibiting site, the other the cathepsin G site. However, site-directed mutagenesis studies of SLPI have

shown that the HNE, chymotrypsin and trypsin inhibitory sites are all in the carboxyterminal domain (Eisenberg et al., 1990). The relatively low Mr of SLPI may be important in the physiological role of this inhibitor, allowing it access to regions where the higher Mr α_1-PI and α_2-M cannot penetrate. In fact, two reports indicate that SLPI does inhibit protein degradation at the cell–substratum interface under conditions where other inhibitors are ineffective or much less effective (Rice and Weiss, 1990: Stolk et al., 1992). However, SLPI does contain a methionine in the region of the active site and, therefore, is subject to oxidative inactivation (Travis and Fritz, 1991).

Elafin is an endogenous inhibitor of HNE isolated from the scales of patients with psoriasis. Amino-acid analysis of elafin shows that the inhibitor is composed of 57 amino acids and has a predicted Mr of 7017 (Wiedow et al., 1990). The structure of elafin appears to be unique with only 38% amino-acid homology with the C-terminal end of SLPI and about 13% homology with the N-terminal end (Wiedow et al., 1990). Elafin inhibits HNE and pancreatic elastase with a high affinity but, unlike some of the other endogenous inhibitors, does not inhibit plasmin, trypsin, chymotrypsin or cathepsin G. The high affinity and specificity of elafin for HNE suggests that this protein may play an important role in regulating HNE activity in the skin.

α_2-M is a glycoprotein with an Mr of 725 000 and a plasma concentration of 250 mg per 100 ml (Travis and Salvesen, 1983). α_2-M inhibits all classes of proteinases by a unique mechanism that involves trapping the enzyme (Travis and Salvesen, 1983). The contribution of α_2-M to regulation of HNE and other serine proteases is not clear, but complexes of α_2-M and proteinases are rapidly cleared from the circulation, suggesting that it may function by targeting excess proteinase activity for endocytosis and destruction by the liver and spleen (Travis and Salvesen, 1983). α_2-M appears to play a major role in the control of metalloproteinases and is discussed more fully in that context (Sections 4.1 and 4.2).

HNE has been implicated in the pathology associated with numerous diseases including emphysema, ARDS, cystic fibrosis and chronic bronchitis. The imbalance between proteinase and anti-proteinase is a central theme in the hypothesis linking neutrophil proteinases to connective tissue damage. Supporting this hypothesis is the high incidence of early-onset pulmonary emphysema in people with a genetic deficiency that leads to reduced levels of α_1-PI (Eriksson, 1965: Kueppers and Black, 1974; Larsson, 1978). In addition, cigarette smokers have increased neutrophil infiltration of the lung, increased proteinase burden and a decrease in α_1-PI function (Gadek et al., 1979; Carp et al., 1982; Hunninghake and Crystal 1983; Janoff et al., 1983; Fera et al., 1986). However, only a low percentage of cigarette smokers develop emphysema (Janoff, 1985) nor do they all display inactivated α_1-PI (Stone *et al.*, 1983; Abboud *et al.*, 1985). The slow development of emphysema in humans (30–40 years) makes it difficult to prove a direct causative effect of HNE. However, proteinase–anti-proteinase imbalance in animals can lead to emphysematous changes in the lung. Emphysema in rats treated with endotoxin is exacerbated by depressing the synthesis of α_1-PI with galactosamine (Blackwood *et al.*, 1984). Likewise inactivation of α_1-PI in dogs with chloramine-T is associated with emphysema-like lesions (Abrams *et al.*, 1981). Beige mice, which lack both elastase and cathepsin G in their neutrophils, showed no histological evidence of lung injury when endotoxin instillation was used to produce a neutrophil infiltration into the lung (Starcher and Williams, 1989). These and numerous other animal and human studies are suggestive of a role of HNE in the connective tissue destruction in emphysema but direct proof remains elusive.

Cystic fibrosis is another disease where the proteinase–antiproteinase hypothesis may be relevant. Free HNE has been isolated from patients with cystic fibrosis (Davis *et al.*, 1983; Goldstein and Doring, 1986: Suter *et al.*, 1986). Although serum levels of α_1-PI were also elevated in cystic fibrosis patients, little functional α_1-PI was found in sputum (Goldstein and Doring, 1986) or bronchial lavage fluids of these patients (Wewers, 1989). Connective tissue destruction has been observed in the lungs of patients with cystic fibrosis (Bruce *et al.*, 1985). HNE has been shown to increase secretions from airway submucosal serous cells (Sommerhoff *et al.*, 1990) suggesting a role for this enzyme in disorders associated with mucus hypersecretion, such as cystic fibrosis. This HNE induced hypersecretion has been shown to be inhibited by a specific synthetic inhibitor of HNE (ICI 200,355) (Sommerhoff *et al.*, 1991; Schuster *et al.*, 1992). HNE cleavage of immunoglobulin and complement has been suggested to play a role in the depression in phagocytosis of *P. aeruginosa* seen in cystic fibrosis patients (Fick *et al.*, 1984). Treatment with aerosolized α_1-PI improved the ability of inflammatory cells from cystic fibrosis patients to kill *P. aeruginosa* (McElvaney *et al.*, 1991). Recently, it has been shown that the ELF from patients with cystic fibrosis stimulated IL-8 mRNA synthesis in a human bronchial epithelial cell line, whereas normal ELF did not have this effect (Nakamura *et al.*, 1992). ELF-induced IL-8 gene expression was inhibited by various HNE inhibitors including α_1-PI, SLPI, PMSF and a peptidyl chloromethylketone. Incubation of the bronchial epithelial cell line with purified HNE resulted in an increase in IL-8 transcription and release of IL-8-like neutrophil chemotactic activity. These data suggest that in cystic fibrosis there is an imbalance between HNE and the anti-protease screen which may result in some of the morbidity associated with this disorder.

ARDS is an acute life-threatening disease characterized by pulmonary oedema and a massive neutrophil infiltration

(Weiland *et al.*, 1986; Repine and Beehler 1991). Patients with ARDS have increased levels of oxidized α_1-PI suggesting that a proteinase inhibitor imbalance may be an important feature of this disease (Cochrane *et al.*, 1983). There is some controversy about whether the increased level of HNE brought about by the massive infiltration of neutrophils in ARDS is complexed to endogenous inhibitor and therefore inactive. Both α_1-PI and α_2-M are greatly increased in the bronchial lavage fluids of patients with ARDS (Wewers *et al.*, 1988; Wewers, 1989). In several studies the lavage fluid was able to cleave a low molecular weight substrate specific for HNE (Wewers, 1989; Lee *et al.*, 1981; McGuire *et al.*, 1982) but this was not the case in other studies (Idell *et al.*, 1985; Weiland *et al.*, 1986). Some of these discrepancies may be due to the unique nature of α_2-M which can block HNE cleavage of a macromolecular substrate such as elastin but allow cleavage of low molecular weight substrates (Travis and Salvesen, 1983). In at least one study, ARDS lavage fluid was able to cleave low molecular weight substrates but not insoluble elastin (Wewers, 1989). Therefore, a clear role for free HNE in the pathology of ARDS has not yet been established.

Increased neutrophil recruitment in response to repeated infections is thought to play a role in the connective tissue changes seen in chronic bronchitis. Lung secretions from patients with bronchiectasis degrade elastin *in vitro* and this degradation can be blocked with a synthetic elastase inhibitor (Stockley *et al.*, 1990a). Further studies are needed to demonstrate a direct role of HNE in the pathology of chronic bronchitis.

As discussed in the preceding paragraphs, connective tissue damage can occur in diseases where there is an intense neutrophil infiltration and release of proteolytic enzymes. HNE can cause connective tissue damage if present in quantities that exceed the endogenous proteinase inhibitors or if these proteinase inhibitors are rendered ineffective by oxidation. However, neutrophil proteinases possess an additional mechanism for eluding inhibition by endogenous anti-proteinases. There is considerable *in vitro* evidence that stimulated neutrophils can tightly bind to their connective tissue substrates such that serum anti-proteinases are excluded from the microenvironment of tight cell–substrate contact (Campbell *et al.*, 1982; Weiss and Regiani, 1984; Weitz *et al.*, 1987; Campbell and Campbell, 1988; Rice and Weiss, 1990; Janusz and Doherty, 1991). The influx of large numbers of neutrophils to an inflammatory site may result in significant tissue damage due to proteolysis that occurs in this protected microenvironment. It is still unclear which neutrophil proteases play a role in this situation but HNE is obviously an important candidate. The use of selective inhibitors could greatly assist in answering this question.

In addition to a possible role in neutrophil-mediated proteolytic damage to tissue components, HNE may make an additional contribution to the inflammatory response, i.e. induction of increased vascular permeability. Under certain conditions, the extravasation of neutrophils in response to a chemotactic stimulus is accompanied by leakage of plasma proteins from the vasculature (Bjork *et al.*, 1982). It has been known for a long time that strongly cationic proteins (e.g. polylysine, protamine), including some found in neutrophil granules (e.g. HNE, cathepsin G), can induce vascular leak when injected into animals (reviewed in Henson and Johnston, 1987; Wasi and Movat, 1979; Needham *et al.*, 1988). Recent *in vivo* studies showed that local administration of HNE or polylysine to the hamster cheek pouch induced vascular leak which occurred only in the venules and was not associated with neutrophil accumulation, arteriolar constriction/dilation or overt signs of damage to the vasculature (Rosengren and Arfors, 1991). When the HNE was incubated *in vitro* with an irreversible elastase inhibitor (L658,758) prior to administration, the ability to induce vascular leak was not abolished despite complete inhibition of its catalytic activity. In contrast, dextran sulphate (a polyanion which also inhibits the catalytic activity of HNE) was able to block the vascular leak induced by both HNE and polylysine (Rosengren and Arfors, 1991). These *in vivo* results suggest that it is the cationic property of HNE and not its proteolytic activity that is responsible for its ability to induce vascular leak. However, not all *in vivo* data support this contention and, in a considerable number of studies, the intratracheal administration of HNE has been shown to cause increased vascular leak, accompanied by damage to the vasculature and haemorrhage, which was abolished by inhibition of the catalytic activity of HNE (Powers, 1983; Bonney *et al.*, 1989; Fletcher *et al.*, 1990, 1991; Williams *et al.*, 1991; Herbert *et al.*, 1992; Skiles *et al.*, 1992). It may be that the low dose of HNE (approximately 0.1 μg) used in the hamster cheek pouch experiments was insufficient to cause proteolytic damage to the vasculature which could obscure a non-proteolyic mechanism. Some *in vitro* studies also support a non-proteolytic mechanism for HNE-induced vascular leak. HNE induced an increase in the permeability of endothelial cell monolayers to protein; this activity was associated with toxicity to the endothelial cells, was retained when the catalytic activity of HNE was destroyed by heat inactivation or incubation with an irreversible inhibitor (Suc-Ala-Ala-Pro-Val-chloromethylketone), but was blocked by the polyanion, heparin (Peterson *et al.*, 1987). Although this *in vitro* activity of HNE does not require the proteolytic activity of HNE, it could be abolished by the presence of α_1-PI. Interestingly, although α_1-PI can inactivate the proteolytic activity of HNE, the enzyme–inhibitor complex is also much less cationic than HNE itself (Baugh and Travis, 1976). This observation, plus the finding that α_1-PI also blocked the ability of protamine, a polycation without proteolytic activity, to increase the permeability of endothelial cell monolayers to protein *in vitro* (Peterson *et al.*, 1987), is consistent with positive charge

being the major mechanism involved. The relevance of these phenomena to neutrophil-mediated vascular leakage is not proven but it has been shown that dextran sulphate, but not low molecular weight elastase inhibitors, blocked the neutrophil-dependent vascular leak induced in the hamster cheek pouch by LTB$_4$ (Rosengren and Arfors, 1990). It therefore seems plausible that, at areas of contact between neutrophil and endothelial cell membranes from which α_1-PI would be excluded, the surface expression of HNE (Travis *et al.*, 1992) and other polycations from the neutrophil granules could induce vascular leak. This hypothesis does not, however, adequately explain the absence from most sites of neutrophil accumulation *in vivo* of the endothelial cell toxicity seen with polycations *in vitro* (Peterson, *et al.*,1987; Needham *et al.*, 1988).

Numerous synthetic and natural HNE inhibitors have been proposed as therapeutic entities to restore proteinase/anti-proteinase balance in a number of connective tissue diseases (Table 4.3). Recently, a review of the numerous synthetic inhibitors of HNE has been published (Trainor, 1987). Synthetic inhibitors of HNE are designed to interfere with the catalytic triad of aspartic acid, histidine and serine. These inhibitors are of many different types including the reversible peptidyl trifluoromethylketones (Williams *et al.*, 1991), aldehydes (Hassal *et al.*, 1985), diketones (Angelastro *et al.*, 1990), keto-esters (Peet *et al.*, 1990) and boronic acids (Shenvi and Kettner, 1984). The peptidyl chloromethylketones are irreversible inhibitors of HNE (Powers *et al.*, 1977). There are also a number of non-peptide-based inhibitors of HNE including the cephalosporins (Doherty *et al.*, 1986), chloroisocoumarins (Harper and Powers, 1985; Harper *et al.*, 1985), ynenol lactones (Copp *et al.*, 1989) and a tetrahydrothieno pyridine derivative (Herbert *et al.*, 1992). A number of these inhibitors have been tested in rodents for their ability to block HNE-induced lung damage in both acute and chronic models. When administered intratracheally or by aerosol, peptidyl chloromethylketones (Powers, 1983), trifluoromethylketones (Fletcher *et al.*, 1990; Williams *et al.*, 1991) and cephalosporin derivatives (Bonney *et al.*, 1989; Fletcher *et al.*, 1990) have been shown to inhibit HNE-induced acute lung haemorrhage and/or emphysema in rodents. Replacement of the P2 proline in peptidyl trifluoromethylketones with non-naturally occurring N-substituted glycine residues resulted in a HNE inhibitor with an increased duration of action when administered intratracheally (Skiles *et al.*, 1992). In contrast, there have been few published data on orally active inhibitors of HNE. Recently there have been several publications describing in detail orally active β-lactam inhibitors of human neutrophil elastase (Shah *et al.* 1992; Hagmann *et al.* 1993). A potent orally active cephalosporin derivative was shown to inhibit HNE-induced lung haemorrhage in hamsters with an ED$_{50}$ of 1.5 mg/kg (Fletcher *et al.*, 1991) while a tetrahydrothieno pyridine derivative displayed an ED$_{50}$ of approximately

100 mg/kg in a similar model in rats (Herbert *et al.*, 1992).

Recombinant versions of the endogenous inhibitors α_1-PI and SLPI are also undergoing evaluation as therapeutic agents to restore proteinase–anti-proteinase balance. Recombinant SLPI has been shown to augment the anti-HNE capacity of epithelial lining fluid of sheep (Vogelmeier *et al.*, 1990) and to reduce the emphysema-like changes caused by HNE instillation in hamsters (Lucey *et al.*, 1990; Rudolphus *et al.*, 1991). Similarly, administration of aerosolized α_1-PI to sheep resulted in an increase in the anti-HNE levels in the epithelial lining fluid (Hubbard *et al.*, 1989).

3.2 CATHEPSIN G

Another major proteinase of the human neutrophil primary granule is cathepsin G (EC 3.4.21.20). Cathepsin G (CatG) is a very basic protein that usually hydrolyses substrates after methionine, leucine or phenylalanine residues. CatG is capable of degrading a number of connective tissue macromolecules including laminin (Heck *et al.*, 1990), fibronectin (Suter *et al.*, 1988) and proteoglycan (Kaiser *et al.*, 1976; Roughley, 1977). CatG can also degrade elastin and collagen but at a very slow rate (Travis, 1988). The cloning at CatG using the human leukaemia cell line U-937 revealed that the mature protein contains 235 amino acids, three disulphide bonds, a single glycosylation site and an 18 amino-acid signal peptide (Salvesen *et al.*, 1987). The gene organization of cathepsin G resembles that of other serine proteinases with the active site histidine, aspartic acid and serine residues located on three separate exons of a five exon gene (Hohn *et al.*, 1989). Sequence homology exists between CatG and rat mast cell protease II (47%) and a protein from activated mouse cytotoxic T-lymphocytes (56%) (Salvesen *et al.*, 1987).

CatG has antimicrobial properties that are independent from its catalytic activity (Odeberg and Ohlsson, 1975). Recently, the antimicrobial activity of CatG has been found to reside in two distinct peptides corresponding to residues 1–5 (IIGGR) and 77–83 (HPQYNQR) (Bangalore *et al.*, 1990). In addition, synthetic peptides corresponding to these sequences were found to exhibit antimicrobial activity *in vitro* (Bangalore *et al.*, 1990). Therefore, CatG appears to be able to both kill and digest bacteria. In addition, after release during degranulation, a proportion of the CatG appears to bind via ionic interactions to the external surface of the neutrophil plasma membrane (Travis *et al.*, 1992), in which location it may have additional roles (as discussed for HNE in Section 3.1).

As with HNE, CatG has been implicated as participating in connective tissue degradation in inflammatory lesions. Although the exact role of CatG in tissue pathology is not known, CatG is capable of degrading a variety of connective tissue macromolecules. However, CatG was shown not to be effective in producing emphysema in hamsters. It is possible that CatG may contribute to connective tissue degradation by acting in concert with other proteinases. CatG together with hypochlorous acid released by neutrophils has been shown to activate neutrophil procollagenase to collagenase (Capodici and Berg, 1989a; Capodici *et al.*, 1989) which may contribute to connective tissue degradation. There has been some controversy as to whether CatG might augment elastin degradation by HNE. An equimolar mixture of HNE and CatG resulted in a greater than five-fold increase in the degradation of human lung elastin compared to HNE alone (Boudier *et al.*, 1981). However, others found that a combination of HNE and CatG resulted in only a two-fold increase in elastin degradation (Reilly *et al.*, 1984). In addition, CatG did not potentiate HNE-induced emphysema in hamsters (Lucey *et al.*, 1985). This later result may be due to the lack of synergism of these two proteinases against hamster lung elastin (Lucey *et al.*, 1985). Recently, using cryostat sections of human skin a mixture of HNE and CatG was shown to result in a 1.9-fold increase over the sum of the individual enzymes in the amount of elastic fibre degradation (Boudier *et al.*, 1991).

Studies with substrates other than elastin have shown that inhibition of both HNE and CatG was required to block neutrophil or neutrophil granular extract-mediated connective tissue degradation completely. Degradation of azure hide powder, a complex connective tissue substrate, by human neutrophil extract was completely inhibited only when a combination of CatG and HNE inhibitors were used (Doherty *et al.*, 1990; Mehdi *et al.*, 1990). Similarly, a combination of an HNE and CatG inhibitor was required to block cartilage proteoglycan degradation by stimulated neutrophils or neutrophil lysate (Janusz and Doherty, 1991). These studies suggest that inhibitors of both HNE and CatG are required to block neutrophil degradation of certain connective tissue substrates but does not imply that these enzymes act synergistically.

CatG has other biological properties that may contribute to an inflammatory response. Platelet aggregation induced by activated neutrophils was found to be inhibited by a peptidyl chloromethylketone CatG inhibitor, by a specific antibody to CatG (Selak *et al.*, 1988) and by recombinant eglin C (Renesto *et al.*, 1990). Pretreatment of neutrophils with TNF-α has been shown to increase CatG release and enhance platelet aggregation (Renesto and Chignard, 1991). This TNF-enhanced platelet aggregation by activated neutrophils was inhibited by α_1-ACT, an endogenous inhibitor of CatG, further implicating this enzyme in neutrophil-mediated platelet aggregation (Renesto and Chignard, 1991). CatG and HNE have been shown to increase secretion from airway submucosal serous cells suggesting a role for CatG in pulmonary disorders associated with mucus hypersecretion such as chronic bronchitis and cystic fibrosis (Sommerhoff *et al.*, 1990). In addition free CatG has been detected in the sputum of patients with cystic fibrosis (Goldstein and Doring, 1986).

The plasma protein α_1-ACT is an acute-phase protein which is a potent endogenous inhibitor of CatG and a member of the serpin family (Travis *et al.*, 1978). In addition to its role as an endogenous proteinase inhibitor, α_1-ACT exhibits other potentially important biological activities. Natural and recombinant α_1-ACT as well as α_1-ACT–CatG complexes have been shown to inhibit superoxide generation by activated human neutrophils (Kilpatrick *et al.*, 1991). Amino-acid substitutions into the active site of α_1-ACT indicated that antiproteolytic activity was not required for inhibition of superoxide generation (Kilpatrick *et al.*, 1991). Therefore, α_1-ACT contains several domains with different biological activities which regulate neutrophil function. α_1-ACT–CatG complexes have also been shown to induce the synthesis of IL-6 from lung fibroblasts (Kurdowska and Travis, 1990). Conditioned media from α_1-ACT–CatG-stimulated fibroblasts was shown to stimulate acute phase protein synthesis from a human hepatocyte cell line, suggesting that proteinase–serpin complexes produced in inflammatory foci may induce acute phase synthesis (Kurdowska and Travis, 1990). Indeed, Travis *et al.* (1992) propose that the α_1-ACT–CatG complexes provide the earliest signal for initiating the acute phase response. Section 7.2 contains further discussion of the pharmacological activities of inhibitors of CatG-like enzymes.

CatG is inhibited by several different classes of synthetic inhibitors. Azapeptides (Gupton *et al.*, 1984), sulphonyl fluorides (Yoshimura *et al.*, 1982), certain heterocycles such as 2-substituted 4H-3,1-benzoxazinones (Teshima *et al.*, 1982) and peptide chloromethylketones (Powers *et al.*, 1977) are inhibitors of CatG. The extended substrate binding site of CatG has been mapped using series of peptide 4-nitroanilide substrates (Tanaka *et al.*, 1985; Nakajima *et al.*, 1979). The preferred amino acid in the P_1 site was found to be Phe with Pro or Met best at P_2 and Val Thr optimal at P_3. No significant improvement was seen with substitutions at the P_4 site. Using the peptide recognition sequence Val-Pro-Phe, the trifluoromethylketone, diketone and keto ester derivatives were synthesized and found to be inhibitors of CatG (Mehdi *et al.*, 1990; Peet *et al.*, 1990). Two of these inhibitors *N*-[(4-chlorophenyl)sulphonylaminocarbonyl]-phenyl carbonyl-Val-Pro-Val diketone and keto ester had K_i values of 800 and 440 nM respectively.

3.3   PROTEINASE 3

Baggiolini and co-workers (1978) initially described a third major serine proteinase of neutrophil primary granules. This enzyme, PR-3, was purified from human neutrophils and was found to produce emphysema in hamsters of comparable severity to that produced by an equal amount of HNE (Kao *et al.*, 1988). Initially there was some confusion as to the identity of PR-3 and several other neutrophil serine proteinases. The N-terminal

amino-acid sequence of PR-3 was found to be similar but not identical to a 29 kD neutrophil serine proteinase with antimicrobial activity (p29b) and a cDNA for a proteinase termed myeloblastin that was down-regulated in differentiated human leukaemia HL-60 cells (Bories *et al.*, 1989; Campanelli *et al.*, 1990a). A cDNA for the complete p29b protein (Campanelli *et al.*, 1990b) showed identity with the cDNA for myeloblastin (Bories *et al.*, 1989) and the partial amino-acid sequence from PR-3 (Rao *et al.*, 1991) suggesting that these three proteins derive from a single gene product. PR-3 is a 29 kD serine proteinase with a sequence that is highly homologous to HNE, CatG and T-cell granzymes and contains the Ser, Asp, His catalytic triad of serine proteinases (Campanelli *et al.*, 1990a). Analysis using synthetic peptide substrates indicated that, like HNE, PR-3 preferred small aliphatic amino acids Val, Ala and Ser at the P_1 position (Rao *et al.*, 1991). Using immuno-histochemical techniques, PR-3 has been found to reside mainly in the neutrophil primary granules with small amounts in the plasma membrane (Csernok *et al.*, 1990).

The association constants for PR-3 with a number of the endogenous inhibitors of HNE and CatG were determined (Rao *et al.*, 1991). The interaction of α_1-PI with PR-3 occurred with K_a approximately one order of magnitude lower than that for its interaction with HNE. The K_a for α_2-M and PR-3 was found to be comparable to that for HNE. However, PR-3 was not inhibited by α_1-ACT or SLPI. Elafin, an endogenous inhibitor of HNE located in human skin was found to be a potent inhibitor of PR-3 (Wiedow *et al.*, 1991).

Since PR-3 is more abundant in human neutrophils than HNE and can induce emphysema in rodents, it is possible that this enzyme may play a role in the connective tissue degradation associated with various diseases. Therefore, there has been interest in developing inhibitors to PR-3. An irreversible inhibitor of HNE, MeO-Suc-Ala-Ala-Pro-Val-CH$_2$Cl was found to inhibit PR-3 but was approximately two logs less potent than against HNE (Rao *et al.*, 1991). Derivatives of 3-benzyl-[(methylsulphonyl)oxy]succinimide were found to be moderately potent inhibitors of PR-3 (Groutas *et al.*, 1989, 1990). Much work still needs to be done in the development of specific potent inhibitors of PR-3.

Another protein found in neutrophil primary granules that is closely related to HNE, CatG and PR-3 is the antimicrobial protein azurocidin. The cDNA of azurocidin displays extensive cDNA homology to HNE, CatG and PR-3 but contains Gly instead of Ser and His substitutions in the catalytic triad (Almeida *et al.*, 1991). Therefore, azurocidin is the only one of these four granule antimicrobial proteins named that is not a proteinase (Campanelli *et al.*, 1990a; Almeida *et al.*, 1991).

3.4   PROTEINASE 4

Recently, another serine proteinase (proteinase 4) was

isolated from human neutrophil primary granules using a monoclonal antibody affinity column (Ohlsson *et al.*, 1990). This serine proteinase had an *Mr* of 30 000 on SDS–PAGE and was inhibited by α_1-PI and α_2-M. Proteinase 4 can digest fibrin but not elastin (Ohlsson *et al.*, 1990). The N-terminal amino-acid sequence of proteinase 4 showed that this enzyme was distinct from but closely related to both HNE and CatG (Ohlsson *et al.*, 1990; Lundberg *et al.*, 1991). The function of this enzyme at present is unknown.

3.5 CATHEPSIN B

Cathepsin B is a cysteine proteinase that is a constituent of neutrophil primary granules (Bainton, 1988). Although neutrophils contain cathepsin B, the macrophage is probably the more relevant source of this enzyme at inflammatory loci. In human lung lavage fluid the specific activity of neutrophil cathepsin B was found to be much lower than that of the macrophage enzyme (Orlowski *et al.*, 1991). Cathepsin B can exist in a number of different forms at various steps in its biosynthetic pathway. The cloning of human cathepsin B from hepatoma cells has yielded information on the processing pathway of cathepsin B (Chan *et al.*, 1986). The preprocathepsin B was cloned and found to code for a 35.9 kD protein containing 339 amino acids with a single glycosylation site (Chan *et al.*, 1986).

The preprocathepsin B gene codes for a 17-residue amino-terminal prepropeptide sequence followed by a 62-residue propeptide sequence, a 254-residue mature cathepsin B (single chain form) and a 6-residue carboxy-terminal extension. The single chain active cathepsin B can also be processed to a double chain active form found in lysosomes (Gal *et al.*, 1985; Hannewinkel *et al.*, 1987). Adding to this complexity is the purification of an alkali-stable high molecular weight (37 kD) form of cathepsin B from purulent human sputum (Buttle *et al.*, 1991).

Cathepsin B is capable of degrading a number of connective tissue macromolecules including proteoglycan and collagen (Barrett *et al.*, 1982). Transcription of cathepsin B is increased in arthritic synovial fibroblasts compared to normal fibroblasts (Trabandt *et al.*, 1991). Also, instillation of cathepsin B into the lungs of hamsters results in degradation of lung elastin and emphysema-like connective tissue changes (Lesser *et al.*, 1992).

Cathepsin B is inhibited by the general endogenous proteinase inhibitor α_2-M and cystatins (Barrett *et al.*, 1988). Synthetic inhibitors of cysteine proteinases including cathepsin B have been recently extensively reviewed (Shaw, 1990) and will be only briefly mentioned here. Several naturally occurring, low molecular weight cysteine proteinase inhibitors including leupeptin (acetyl-Leu-Leu-Argal) (Shaw, 1990) and E-64 (L-trans-epoxysuccinylleucylamido(4-guanidino)butane) (Barrett

et al., 1982) are widely used as general cysteine proteinase inhibitors. Synthetic inhibitors of cysteine proteinases, and cathepsin B in particular, include the irreversible peptide chloromethylketones (Barrett 1973), peptidyl fluoromethylketones (Rasnick, 1985) and their acyloxymethyl derivatives (Smith *et al.*, 1988) and peptidyl sulphonium salts (Shaw, 1988). Peptide aldehydes (O'Connor-Westerik and Wolfenden, 1972) and trifluoromethylketones are reversible inhibitors of cathepsin B (Smith *et al.*, 1988). However, unlike the case with serine proteinases which are inhibited better by trifluoromethylketones than aldehydes: the opposite is true for the cysteine proteinases (Smith *et al.*, 1988). Recently, cathepsin B has been shown to be inhibited by peptide α-keto esters, α-keto amides, α-diketones and α-keto acids (Hu and Abeles, 1990). In the antigen-induced arthritis model, the fluoromethylketone Z-Phe-Ala-CH_2F decreased the severity of arthritis as measured histologically (van Noorden *et al.*, 1988). These data suggested that cathepsin B from neutrophils, chondrocytes and/or fibroblasts may be important in the tissue damage associated with arthritis.

3.6 CATHEPSIN D

Cathepsin D is an aspartic acid proteinase with optimal catalytic activity at an acid pH (3.5–4.0) (Ichimanu *et al.*, 1990) that suggests the physiological site of action of this enzyme is the lysosome. Cathepsin D isolated from human neutrophil granule preparation has a molecular weight of 42 kD (Ishikawa and Cimasoni, 1977). Radiolabelled haemoglobin is generally used as a substrate for cathepsin D (Levy *et al.*, 1989). This enzyme is inhibited by pepstatin A, a general aspartic acid proteinase inhibitor, and by Gly-Glu-Gly-Phe-Leu-Gly-(D)Phe-Leu, a specific competitive inhibitor of cathepsin D (Gubensek *et al.*, 1976; Lauritzen *et al.*, 1984). Cathepsin D appears to function as a lysosomal proteinase and whether this enzyme is involved in significant tissue pathology is unclear.

4. *Secondary/tertiary Granules*

In view of the ongoing controversy concerning the existence of the tertiary granules (see Section 2), the proteases associated with both secondary and tertiary granules will be discussed together. The enzymes to be discussed are matrix metalloproteinases and this class in general has been the subject of a number of recent reviews (Matrisian, 1990, 1992; Woessner, 1991; Birkedal-Hansen *et al.*, 1992; Docherty *et al.*, 1992).

4.1 HUMAN NEUTROPHIL COLLAGENASE

Neutrophils have long been known to contain a

collagenolytic metalloproteinase (HNC) with similarities to the connective tissue degrading metalloproteinases secreted by other cell types (reviewed in Weiss and Peppin, 1986; Matrisian, 1990, 1992; Docherty et al., 1992; Woessner, 1992). A standardized nomenclature for this family of proteases has recently been proposed and EC numbers assigned (International Union of Biochemistry and Molecular Biology, 1992; Nagase et al., 1992). They are collectively known as matrixins or matrix metalloproteinases, i.e. MMP followed by a number to indicate the individual family member (Woessner, 1991; Nagase et al., 1992). HNC is MMP-8, EC 3.4.24.34, but the term HNC will be used here since it accurately and unambiguously identifies this particular MMP. The properties of HNC are summarized in Table 4.4.

HNC shares certain properties with the other members of the MMP family, i.e. it is a metalloprotease which contains zinc bound in the active site, requires the presence of calcium in the medium for activity, has a neutral pH optimum and is synthesized as a catalytically inactive proenzyme (proHNC) (Mookhtiar et al., 1986; reviewed in Weiss and Peppin, 1986; Woessner, 1991). Much controversy has appeared in the literature concerning the size, structure and activation mechanisms for HNC and it is only in recent years with the cloning of the gene (Hasty et al., 1990; Devarajan et al., 1991), that it has become possible to resolve most of these conflicts (Table 4.4). The gene contains untranslated sequences of unknown function at both the 5′-end (70 nucleotides) and 3′-end (751 or 900 nucleotides) (Hasty et al., 1990; Devarajan et al., 1991). The amino-acid sequence

exhibits considerable homology with other MMPs (e.g. 58% identity and 72% chemical similarity when compared to human fibroblast collagenase, MMP-1) and can be divided into similar domains (Figure 4.1).

The N-terminal 20 amino-acid signal peptide (the pre-domain of preproHNC) is presumably involved in transporting the protein across the membrane of the endoplasmic reticulum, from where it is directed to the secondary granules as they are formed during neutrophil maturation in the bone marrow. The signal peptide is rapidly removed as it is not found in the stored pro-enzyme. A sequence of 80 amino acids (residues 21–100, the pro-domain of proHNC) is found in the latent but not the active forms of the enzyme. By analogy with other MMPs it can be inferred that this domain keeps the latent form catalytically inactive via coordination of the sulphydryl of Cys^{91} to the zinc in the active site, thus making this essential coordination site unavailable for catalysis. All methods of activating HNC result in replacement of the sulphydryl ligand by water. This is the so-called "cysteine switch" mechanism (Springman et al., 1990: van Wart and Birkedal-Hansen, 1990) which is believed to occur in the activation of all MMPs and is associated with the highly conserved sequence, PRCGVPDVA, around the implicated cysteine residue (van Wart and Birkedal-Hansen, 1990). Residues 101–262 contain the active site including the conserved zinc-binding region (residues 214–224). The sequence of residues from 263 to the C-terminus (residue 467) is homologous to hemopexin (a haem-binding plasma protein) and vitronectin. This domain is thought to be involved in substrate binding (Clark and Cawston,

Table 4.4 The matrix metalloproteinases of human neutrophils

Enzyme		Molecular mass (kD)	Protease class	Biological substrates	Synthetic substrates	Endogenous inhibitors	Selected synthetic inhibitors
Human neutrophil collagenase (HNC, MMP-8, EC 3.4.24.34)[1]	Pro Mature	$58-105^{2,3,4,5}$ 58^2	Metallo(Zn)	Collagen types I, II and III[6] α_2-M, α_1-PI, α_1-ACT, C1 inhibitor[7,8,9,10]	DNP-Pro-Leu-Ala-Tyr-Trp-Ala-Arg[11]	α_2-M, TIMP-1, TIMP-2[12]	Hydroxamates, thiols, phosphonamidates, phosphinates[13,14,15]
Human neutrophil gelatinase (HNG, MMP-9, EC 3.4.24.35) aka: gelatinase B, 92 kD gelatinase, type IV collagenase, type V collagenase[1]	Pro Mature	92^{16} 82^{16}	Metallo(Zn)	Gelatin, collagen types IV, V, VII and X,[17,18] elastin,[19] proteoglycan[20]	DNP-Pro-Leu-Gly-Met-Trp-Ser-Arg[11]	α_2-M, TIMP-1, TIMP-2[12]	Hydroxamates, thiols, phosphonamidates, phosphinates[13,14,15]

References: [1]Nagase et al. (1992); [2]Mallya et al. (1990); [3]Hasty et al. (1990); [4]Williams and Lin (1984); [5]Hasty et al. (1986); [6]Netzel-Arnett et al., (1991a); [7]Knauper et al. (1990); [8]Desrochers et al. (1992); [9]Vissers et al. (1988); [10]Knauper et al. (1991); [11]Netzel-Arnett et al. (1991b); [12]Woessner (1991); [13]Johnson (1990); [14]Henderson et al. (1990); [15]Wahl et al. (1989); [16]Ogata et al. (1992); [17]Docherty et al. (1992); [18]Murphy et al. (1982); [19]Senior et al. (1991); [20]Murphy et al. (1991).

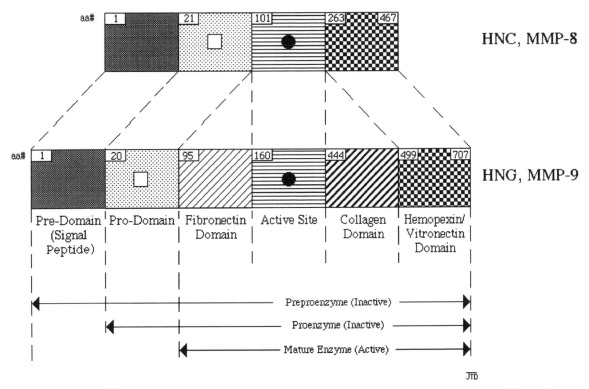

Figure 4.1 The domain structure of human neutrophil collagenase (MMP-8) and human neutrophil gelatinase (MMP-9).

1989). A similar hemopexin-like domain occurs in all other MMPs (Matrisian, 1990, 1992; Woessner, 1991; Docherty *et al.*, 1992). Six potential glycosylation sites can be identified and some appear to be used since deglycosylation causes a reduction in M_r of 32 000 (Knauper *et al.*, 1990a). Variable glycosylation may make some contribution to the range of molecular weights which have been reported for the proenzyme (58–105 kD) (Williams and Lin, 1984; Hasty *et al.*, 1986). Some reports of high molecular weight forms of proHNC may be due to the formation of stable complexes with endogenous inhibitors (Blaser *et al.*, 1991).

HNC is released with other granule constituents when the cell is appropriately stimulated (Hibbs *et al.*, 1984; Weiss and Peppin, 1986). The MMPs in other cells are not stored but are secreted immediately upon synthesis. This difference from other cell types is consistent with the fact that once neutrophil differentiation has been completed in the bone marrow and the mature neutrophil released into the circulation, it loses a large proportion of its capacity for protein synthesis (Beaulieu *et al.*, 1987). When the HNC gene was expressed in COS-7 cells, proHNC was secreted and not stored (Hasty *et al.*, 1990), indicating that the signal peptide of preproHNC does not contain a message which targets it to intracellular storage. It has been suggested that the additional

glycosylation of proHNC compared to human fibroblast collagenase (MMP-1) may be responsible for its targeting to the secondary granule (Mallya *et al.*, 1990).

Activation of latent HNC (opening of the "cysteine switch") can be achieved by diverse mechanisms: heavy metals, chaotropic agents, proteases and oxidizing agents (Weiss and Peppin, 1986; Springman *et al.*, 1990; van Wart and Birkedal-Hansen, 1990). The common feature of all these mechanisms is that they remove Cys[91] from the coordination sphere of the active site zinc. As a result, active enzyme can be obtained with or without cleavage of peptide bonds and a reduction in molecular weight. However, once the enzyme has been activated by non-proteolytic means (e.g. (4 aminophenyl)mercuric acetate, APMA) it undergoes autocatalytic cleavage in three steps to yield the most active form in which the Phe[99]–Met[100] or Met[100]–Leu[101] bond of proHNC has been cleaved; intermediate forms with less than maximal activity can be detected during the autoactivation process (Blaser *et al.*, 1991). Cleavage by other proteases (typsin, CatG, elastase) can lead to active forms of various molecular weights (Knauper *et al.*, 1990a) but further cleavage can lead to inactivation (Murphy *et al.*, 1980).

The above studies of activation in cell-free systems do not identify the important activation mechanisms used *in vivo*. Weiss reviewed the available evidence on this question and has convincingly implicated the oxidizing agents generated from the oxygen burst (Weiss *et al.*, 1985). Since neutrophils stimulated to release the contents of their secondary granules also generate reactive oxygen species (superoxide, hydrogen peroxide, hydroxyl radicals, chloramines), both of the ingredients required for such an activation process are produced in the same place at the same time. Support for this mechanism comes from data on patients with chronic granulomatous disease whose neutrophils are unable to generate reactive oxygen species and, unlike neutrophils from normal individuals, released only latent enzyme when stimulated with phorbol esters (Weiss *et al.*, 1985). Identifying which of the many products formed in the cascade of reactions induced by the oxidative burst actually perform the activation step has been difficult. Several oxidation reactions could be effective in removing Cys^{91} from the active site zinc: reaction of the sulphydryl with chloramines, formation of disulphides or oxidative damage to tertiary structure (Springman *et al.*, 1990; van Wart and Birkedal-Hansen, 1990). A contribution from cleavage of the pro-domain by other proteases cannot be excluded and some reports have combined both mechanisms by suggesting that it is CatG that is activated by oxidation and it subsequently cleaves latent HNC to an active form (Capodici and Berg, 1989b, 1991; Capodici *et al.*, 1989). It may be that several of these mechanisms operate in parallel in the *in vivo* environment.

HNC was named for its ability to cleave collagen in the triple helix domain but is now recognized to be active on a range of other substrates. It cleaves all three chains of helical type I, II and III collagen at a single site three-quarters of the way from the N-terminus, between residues 775 (Gly) and 776 (Leu or Ile) (Netzel-Arnett *et al.*, 1991a). The conformation at this site is essential for susceptibility to HNC since the same sequences occur elsewhere in collagen but are not cleaved (Netzel-Arnett *et al.*, 1991a). In contrast to human fibroblast collagenase, which preferentially cleaves soluble type III collagen over soluble type I, HNC exhibits the opposite preference (Hasty *et al.*, 1987; Mallya *et al.*, 1990). However, these differences are largely lost when the collagen substrates are in the form of fibrils. HNC does not cleave types IV and V collagen but is effective against the type II collagen found in cartilage (Hasty *et al.*, 1987). Non-collagen proteins cleaved by HNC include a number of protease inhibitors (human and rat α_2-M, human and rat α_1-PI, human α_1-ACT, human C1-inhibitor, rat α_1-inhibitory protein-III, ovostatin) (Vissers *et al.*, 1988; Knauper *et al.*, 1990b, 1991; Desrochers *et al.*, 1992). A detailed analysis of the cleavage sites in protein substrates plus a range of synthetic peptides demonstrated that the specificity of HNC is distinctly different from fibroblast collagenase (Netzel-Arnett *et al.*, 1991a). In particular, HNC accommodates aromatic residues in subsite P_1' much better than human fibroblast collagenase. Based on these observations, a series of peptide substrates were optimized to produce continuously recording fluorescent

assays for each of five human MMPs (Netzel-Arnett *et al.*, 1991b). The hydrolysis rates for the HNC substrate (DNP-Pro-Leu-Ala-Tyr-Trp-Ala-Arg, k_{cat}/K_m = 1400 $\mu M^{-1} h^{-1}$) exceeds that of collagen itself ($k_{cat}/K_m = 690 \mu M^{-1} h^{-1}$) while cleavage of this peptide by human fibroblast collagenase (MMP-1) is considerably slower ($k_{cat}/K_m = 9.7 \mu M^{-1} h^{-1}$) (data calculated from Netzel-Arnett *et al.* (1991b)). Because of the likelihood that this peptide will be cleaved by other proteinases it was not recommended for use with impure enzyme preparations.

The bulk (>95%) of the endogenous inhibitory activity in serum against metalloproteinases can be attributed to α_2-M. As described in Section 3.1, α_2-M is a large ($Mr = 725\,000$) glycoprotein (8–10% carbohydrate) (Travis and Salvesen, 1983; Cawston, 1986). The inhibitory activity of α_2-M is initiated by cleavage of the inhibitor by the target protease in a domain known as the "bait" region which contains sequences which can act as substrates for diverse proteases of all classes. Once the protease has been lured into cleaving the "bait" region, this triggers a conformational change in α_2-M which results in the entrapment of the protease within the inhibitor structure to form a complex which has no catalytic activity against macromolecular substrates but can cleave small peptides which diffuse into the complex and find the active site (Barrett and Starkey, 1973; Travis and Salvesen, 1983). Subsequently, a thiol ester linkage is formed between the enzyme and inhibitor in a proportion of the complexes, resulting in loss of all catalytic activity (Travis and Salvesen, 1983). The complexes are recognized and endocytosed by macrophages via a specific cell surface receptor resulting in their rapid clearance (Travis and Salvesen, 1983). Although α_2-M is the major endogenous metalloproteinase inhibitor in the circulation, because of its large size it is relatively excluded from normal tissues (Cawston, 1986). However, vascular permeability is increased in inflammatory lesions and α_2-M can be found in such situations (Cawston *et al.*, 1990), presumably where and when it is most needed.

It was originally reported that α_1-PI was an effective inhibitor of collagenases (Ohlsson and Ohlsson, 1973) but this was subsequently found to be incorrect (Woolley *et al.*, 1975). In contrast to α_2-M, where cleavage is an integral part of the mechanism by which this antiprotease inhibits proteases, cleavage of the serpins (α_1-PI, α_1-ACT) by HNC does not result in inhibition of HNC. Instead, products are formed which have lost their ability to inhibit serine proteases such as HNE and CatG (Vissers *et al.*, 1988; Knauper *et al.*, 1990b; Desrochers *et al.*, 1992). This ability to cleave and inactivate serpins suggests that HNC could contribute to a breakdown in the antiprotease screen and permit the unregulated cleavage of host proteins by serine proteases from the neutrophil or other sources. In addition, it has been reported that proteolytically inactivated α_1-PI is chemotactic for neutrophils and may thus recruit more cells which could exacerbate loss of the antiprotease screen (Banda *et al.*, 1986).

A family of metalloprotease inhibitors known as TIMPs are produced locally in tissues and found in the circulation. The first such inhibitor discovered was given the acronym TIMP but is now known as TIMP-1 to distinguish it from other members of the family. TIMP-1 is produced by many cell types, but not neutrophils (Welgus and Stricklin, 1983; Cooper *et al.*, 1985), and is a 184 amino-acid protein (calculated $Mr = 21\ 000$) which is heavily glycosylated, bringing its observed Mr up to 28 500 (Cawston, 1986). It contains 12 cysteines, all of which are involved in the formation of six internal disulphide bridges. The mechanism of inhibition is not precisely known but a 1:1 complex of TIMP-1:protease is formed in which the TIMP-1 is not cleaved (Cawston, 1986). TIMP-1 only binds to active HNC and does not recognize proHNC (Osthues *et al.*, 1992). In connective tissue cells such as fibroblasts, chondrocytes and macrophages, many of the stimuli which induce the secretion of metalloproteinases also induce the secretion of TIMP-1. Although at first sight it appears to be a self-defeating exercise to produce both the protease and its inhibitor at the same time, Matrisian (1992) has suggested that since TIMP-1 does not inhibit autocatalytic activation there would be a brief period of metalloprotease activity prior to its inhibition, thus producing a tightly controlled, self-limiting reaction. The relevance of this hypothesis to HNC is uncertain since neutrophils do not produce TIMP-1. However, tissue fluids constitutively contain TIMP-1 and this presumably limits the action of HNC. Neutrophil elastase can cleave and inactivate TIMP-1 (Okada *et al.*, 1988), providing a means by which neutrophils could overcome the inhibition of MMPs in inflammatory foci. This phenomenon is analogous to the ability of HNC to inactivate the serpins (see above) and suggests that these complex interactions of proteases and their inhibitors could enable the proteases to express their activity in a restricted fashion (locally and temporally) in the face of a highly effective battery of inhibitors. There is a small amount of TIMP-1 in the plasma (approximately 1 μg/ml) but it makes only a small contribution (1–2%) to the total circulating antimetalloproteinase screen (Welgus and Stricklin, 1983). TIMP-1 is identical to a protein with erythroid potentiating activity (EPA) (Stricklin and Welgus, 1986) but the significance of this property is uncertain. TIMP-2 is an inhibitor of HNC, which is structurally related to TIMP-1 (41% amino-acid identity, 12 cysteines forming six disulphide bridges) (Stetler-Stevenson *et al.*, 1989) but is not heavily glycosylated resulting in a lower observed Mr of 21 000. TIMP-2 (also known as metalloproteinase inhibitor) exhibits erythroid-potentiating activity (Stetler-Stevenson *et al.*, 1992) but differs from TIMP-1 in that it can inhibit the autoproteolytic activation process of collagenases (de Clerk *et al.*, 1991). The relative importance of

TIMP-2 and a variety of less well-characterized metalloproteinase inhibitors (Cawston, 1986) in the control of HNC activity is far from clear.

The physiological role of HNC is not immediately obvious. The major role of the neutrophil is host defence against bacteria and fungi, and these microorganisms do not contain collagen. However, since HNC has activity on substrates other than collagen (as described above), there may be an undetected role for HNC in the killing or destruction of invading microorganisms. Weiss has suggested that the primary role of the MMPs of the neutrophil may be to enable these cells to digest their way through the basement membrane of blood vessels and through the matrix of tissues in order to reach the site of an infection or inflammation (Weiss and Peppin, 1986). Subsequently, these authors provided *in vitro* evidence that emigration of neutrophils involves local damage to the basement membrane followed by repair of the damage by the overlying endothelial cells. However, the use of a range of endogenous and synthetic proteinase inhibitors, including TIMP-1, failed to identify the proteinases involved (Huber and Weiss, 1989). In contrast, Bakowski and Tschesche recently provided *in vitro* morphological evidence that TIMP-1 inhibited the ability of stimulated neutrophils to penetrate human amniotic membrane (used as a model of extravasation and migration through tissues) thus implicating an MMP but not identifying which one (Bakowski and Tchesche, 1992); quantitative analysis of this data is underway. There is a considerable body of evidence from other studies demonstrating that neutrophils can create an environment at the interface of the cell with substratum that is shielded from the action of endogenous macromolecular inhibitors (Campbell *et al.*, 1982; Weiss and Regiani, 1984; Weitz *et al.*, 1987; Campbell and Campbell, 1988; Rice and Weiss, 1990; Janusz and Doherty, 1991) (see also Section 3.1). The endogenous proteinase inhibitors do not have the specificity or ability to penetrate this environment which would enable the enzymes involved to be identified. Synthetic inhibitors with the desired properties may be available in the near future. The composition of the vascular basement membrane (type IV and V collagens, laminin, proteoglycans etc.) does not include HNC substrates, and neutrophil gelatinase (MMP-9, see Section 4.2) is a more likely candidate than HNC for a role in penetration of the basement membrane. If dissolution of matrix is required for migration through tissues, HNC has the required ability to digest fibrillar collagen, although there is little evidence to support such a mechanism. The physiological role of HNC remains a mystery.

In any inflammatory condition where neutrophils are found at the site of connective tissue damage, HNC could potentially be a mediator of such damage by directly attacking collagen and/or inactivating the antiproteases that hold serine proteases in check, and/or recruiting more leucocytes via chemotactic fragments formed from cleaved collagen (Laskin *et al.*, 1986; Riley *et al.*, 1988). However, direct evidence for such a role is hard to find since there are many other cells and proteases present. Elevated levels of active HNC were found in mouth-rinse samples from periodontitis patients and the levels were lowered by successful treatment (scaling, tetracyclines) (Gangbar *et al.*, 1990; Sorsa *et al.*, 1990; Uitto *et al.*, 1990). Tetracyclines were found to be more potent inhibitors of HNC than of fibroblast collagenase (MMP-1) and it has been suggested that this is the mechanism underlying their efficacy in periodontal disease (Suomalainen *et al.*, 1992). Tetracyclines also inhibit neutrophil functions such as superoxide anion production, degranulation and migration (Gabler and Creamer, 1991) so their efficacy in this condition cannot be considered proof of a primary role for HNC in periodontal disease. Extensive damage to cartilage collagen (type II) occurs in the presence of an influx of neutrophils in inflammatory arthritis. It has been shown that the latent collagenase in rheumatoid synovium is MMP-1 (fibroblast collagenase), not HNC (Konttinen *et al.*, 1991). In the synovial fluids from rheumatoid arthritis patients there have been contradictory reports of the presence of active collagenase, and whether it is of fibroblast (MMP-1) or neutrophil (MMP-8) origin (Cawston *et al.*, 1984; Peltonen, 1978). Complexes of collagenases with α_2-M and TIMPs do occur in synovial fluids from rheumatoid arthritis patients (Cawston *et al.*, 1984; Osthues *et al.*, 1992) but the antiprotease screen still appears to be effective in the fluid phase. The total collagenase reserve of neutrophils from synovial fluids of rheumatoid arthritis patients was not reduced compared to neutrophils from the blood of the same patients (Konttinen *et al.*, 1991), suggesting that no collagenase had been released from these cells while on their way into the synovial cavity or while there (Sorsa *et al.*, 1992). It may be that only those neutrophils which adhere to an opsonized surface (e.g. antibody-coated collagen/ cartilage) release and activate MMPs. Within the secluded environment at the interface of neutrophil and sub-stratum, the neutrophil may exclude macromolecular antiproteases (Chatham *et al.*, 1990a, 1990b; Sorsa *et al.*, 1992) leading to cartilage damage at the cell/cartilage interface without detectable collagenase activity in synovial fluid or significant loss of collagenase from neutrophils free in the synovial fluid. It is noteworthy that the gold compounds used in the therapy of rheumatoid arthritis can inhibit HNC (e.g. the IC_{50} for myocrysin is 3.5 nM) leading to the suggestion that this activity may contribute to their therapeutic effects (Mallya and van Wart, 1987; Mallya and van Wart, 1989). However, other reports have demonstrated that gold compound, like other heavy-metal containing compounds, can activate proHNC (Saari *et al.*, 1990; Sorsa *et al.*, 1989b, 1990; Suomalainen *et al.*, 1991) and it is not clear whether the overall *in vivo* effect of these two conflicting activities will be an increase or a decrease in collagenase activity (Sorsa *et al.*, 1989a). Synovial fluids taken prior to therapy from patients with septic arthritis contained active metalloproteinases and no antiprotease activity was found (Cawston *et al.*, 1990). Presumably the vast influx of neutrophils had been activated by potent bacterial stimuli and released enough active enzyme to overwhelm the antiprotease screen (α_2-M, TIMP). Active HNC was found in bronchoalveolar lavage fluids from patients with rheumatoid interstitial lung disease, idiopathic pulmonary fibrosis (Weiland *et al.*, 1986; Gilligan *et al.*, 1990), bronchiolitis (Kindt *et al.*, 1989) and adult respiratory distress syndrome (Christner *et al.*, 1985) and may contribute to the pathogenesis of these diseases. The development of bioavailable, synthetic inhibitors with the ability to inhibit HNC at the cell/substratum interface should provide the means to evaluate the role of HNC in disease and could prove to be valuable therapeutic agents in a number of diseases.

The primary focus of the extensive ongoing search for synthetic inhibitors of matrix metalloproteinases with good oral absorption and useful pharmacokinetics has been on fibroblast collagenase (MMP-1) and stromelysin (MMP-3) rather than HNC (Johnson *et al.*, 1987; Wahl *et al.*, 1989; Henderson, *et al.*, 1990; Johnson, 1990). However, most available inhibitors display considerable overlap of activity against other members of the MMP family. Most of the potent inhibitors reported to date are at least partially peptidic and contain residues mimicking the residues on the P′ side, or both the P and P′ sides of the scissile bond. Compounds containing P-side residues only do not result in potent inhibitors. All inhibitors contain a ligand for the active site zinc and a variety of functional groups have been found to be effective: hydroxamates, thiols, phosphonamidates, phosphonates, phosphinates. Some extremely potent inhibitors have been identified, e.g. the hydroxamates SC-44,463 (Delaisse *et al.*, 1985, 1988) and Ro31-4724 (Nixon *et al.*, 1991), and the phosphinic acid Ro31-7467 (Nixon *et al.*, 1991), but compounds with good oral absorption and useful pharmacokinetics have been difficult to find. It will be particularly useful to exploit the differences in substrate specificity seen within this class of proteases to develop highly selective inhibitors which would enable the individual roles of the various MMPs to be determined. For example, Ro31-7467 is 12-fold more potent as an inhibitor of collagenase (MMP-1) than stromelysin (MMP-3) and inhibits loss of collagen, but not loss of proteoglycan, from IL-1 stimulated bovine nasal cartilage *in vitro* (Nixon *et al.*, 1991).

4.2 GELATINASE

The second MMP in neutrophils is a gelatinase which has had a large number of other names: MMP-9, EC 3.4.24.35, gelatinase B, 92 kD gelatinase, type IV collagenase, type V collagenase (Nagase *et al.*, 1992). For this review the descriptive trivial name, HNG, will be used.

HNG has certain features characteristic of all MMPs (Table 4.4) but shares with HNC a feature which distinguishes these two neutrophil MMPs from the other members of the family, i.e. they are stored in granules and released by degranulation rather than synthesized and secreted upon demand. In contrast to the HNC gene which is expressed only in neutrophils, the HNG gene is expressed in a number of other cell types (macrophages, keratinocytes, tumour cells) (Wilhelm *et al.*, 1989) which also express a second gelatinase, MMP-2 (also known as gelatinase A, 72 kD gelatinase, 72 kD type IV collagenase; Nagase *et al.*, 1992). Despite its name, therefore, not all HNG found *in vivo* can be assumed to come from neutrophils. It had been thought that once differentiation of the neutrophil had been completed and the mature cell released into the circulation, all gene expression for granule contents ceased. Interestingly, it has been demonstrated that in neutrophils from an inflammatory lesion the HNG gene is reactivated (newly synthesized HNG was detected) (Beaulieu *et al.*, 1987). It may be that any gelatinase synthesized by mature neutrophils is secreted rather than stored since secondary granule formation is over by the time the neutrophil leaves the bone marrow.

The latent form of HNG, proHNG, has an *Mr* of 92 000; the protein component comprises *Mr* 82 000, the rest being carbohydrate. The domain structure of HNG (Figure 4.1) resembles that of HNC but contains two additional domains: a proline-rich domain of unknown function with homology to collagen; a domain with homology to fibronectin which provides the molecule with a binding site for gelatin in addition to the binding that occurs via the active site (Wilhelm *et al.*, 1989). This additional interaction with substrate may allow the active site to move from one scissile bond to another without the enzyme losing contact with a macromolecular substrate. Such a phenomenon could protect the active site from inhibitors present in the fluid phase and allow local proteolysis to proceed while enzyme diffusing off the substrate would be inhibited. The predomain has the characteristics of a signal peptide and presumably directs preproHNC to the endoplasmic reticulum where other signals direct it to secondary/ tertiary granules in differentiating neutrophils. The conserved zinc binding region and the "cysteine switch" sequence are also present.

Activation of proHNG after release from degranulating neutrophils resembles that of HNC (see Section 4.1). A "cysteine switch" is also involved but there is evidence of additional autocatalytic cleavage sites in the C-terminal region. Stromelysin (MMP-3) is a particularly effective activator of HNG (Ogata *et al.*, 1992). In contrast to the proHNG released from neutrophils during degranulation, the proenzyme synthesized and secreted by fibroblasts, macrophages, etc. leaves the cell as a complex with

TIMP-1. Although neutrophils do not contain TIMP-1, complexes of HNG and proHNG can form with the TIMPs secreted by other cells. The ability of TIMP-1 to associate with the pro-form of HNG implies the presence on HNG of a second binding site for TIMP-1 other than the active site since the active site is masked in the pro-form. Such a site is clearly not present in proHNC. This binding site has been localized to the C-terminal domain of proHNG. Binding of TIMP-1 to this site prevents autocatalytic activation of HNG but does not prevent activation by other means. Once the "cysteine switch" of HNG has been opened, the enzyme expresses catalytic activity despite the presence of TIMP-1 bound to the second site. A second molecule of TIMP-1 or TIMP-2 is needed to interact with the active site in order to inhibit degradation of substrate (Murphy *et al.*, 1982; Murphy *et al.*, 1991; Docherty *et al.*, 1992). It has recently been shown that the 72 kD gelatinase (MMP-2) can be activated by interaction with the membrane of activated cells and that TIMP-2 blocks this interaction by competing for a membrane binding site in the C-terminal domain of MMP-2 which is distinct from the catalytic site; this binding also inhibits autocatalytic activation (Ward *et al.*, 1991). To date, a similar membrane-based mechanism of activation has not been identified for HNG, although Weiss pointed out the potential advantages of such a scheme in 1986 (Weiss and Peppin, 1986). The major physiological inhibitors of HNG are α_2-M, TIMP-1 and TIMP-2. Inhibition of MMPs by α_2-M and TIMPs has also been discussed in Section 4.1.

The substrate specificity of HNG is markedly different from that of HNC. Thus, HNG cannot cleave the triple helical region of native types I, II or III collagen but can digest the denatured forms of these substrates, i.e. gelatin (Murphy *et al.*, 1982). HNG can, however, digest the native triple helical regions of type IV, V, VII and X collagens plus cartilage proteoglycans (Murphy *et al.*, 1982, 1991; Docherty *et al.*, 1992). It has very low activity against casein and albumin but has been shown to have significant elastolytic activity (on a molar basis it is 30% as active as human leucocyte elastase) (Murphy *et al.*, 1991; Senior *et al.*, 1991). In a study of cleavage of synthetic peptides, Netzel-Arnett *et al.* (1991b) predicted that the best substrates for HNG should have Met in the P'_1 position, Leu in P_2 and Ser in P'_3. A substrate suitable for continuously recording fluorescent assays (DNP-Pro-Leu-Gly-Met-Trp-Ser-Arg) was prepared which exhibited a $k_{cat}/K_m = 46.8\ \mu M^{-1}\ h^{-1}$ (calculated from Netzel-Arnett *et al.*, 1991b).

The physiological role of HNG in neutrophil function, like that of HNC, remains controversial. The most plausible hypothesis is that HNG is necessary for the neutrophils to digest their way through vascular basement membrane in order to extravasate and reach the site of an inflammatory stimulus (Weiss and Peppin, 1986; Woessner, 1992). This hypothesis is particularly attractive since release of gelatinase and transfer of adhesion molecules to the plasma membrane are responses that occur at lower concentrations of chemotactic factors than the release of other secondary granule contents or release of primary granule components (Dewald *et al.*, 1982). It is thus possible to envisage (Weiss and Peppin, 1986) neutrophils within the vasculature being at the distal end of a concentration gradient where the low levels of chemotactic factors induce the responses needed for adherence to vascular endothelial cells (via adhesion molecule expression) and penetration of the basement membrane (release and activation of gelatinase). Upon extravasation and movement up the concentration gradient, higher concentrations of chemotactic factors would induce the activation of microbicidal functions (release of lactoferrin, myeloperoxidase, cationic proteins). Despite the attractions of this hypothesis there are very few supporting data. This is caused by the absence of inhibitors which can discriminate between the various metalloproteinases and can be demonstrated to inhibit proteolysis at the cell–substratum interface.

If, as discussed above, HNG is required for neutrophil extravasation, it implies a role in both the host defence functions of neutrophils and their contribution to all inflammatory diseases in which neutrophils are involved. HNG has been found in high levels in a number of inflammatory lesions (rheumatoid synovial fluids, gingival crevicular fluid periodontitis patients, etc.) but proof of a pathological role is lacking.

4.3   PLASMINOGEN ACTIVATOR

A proteolytic activity with the properties of plasminogen activator of the urokinase type has been identified in the secondary granules of human neutrophils (Heiple and Ossowski, 1986). This activity was translocated to the cell surface when degranulation was induced by phorbol esters indicating that it was a membrane-associated enzyme. Interestingly, the recovery of activity was increased 100-fold in the presence of DFP suggesting that it is stored in an inactive form which is DFP-insensitive, and that it can be degraded by other, active, DFP-sensitive, neutrophil serine proteases. These observations are consistent with the report that larger amounts of plasminogen activator can be recovered from the neutrophils of patients with a deficiency in their serine protease activity (Chediak–Higashi syndrome) than from the neutrophils of normals (de Saint Basile *et al.*, 1985). The data of Granelli-Piperno *et al.* (1977), however, conflict with the above reports. These authors found that plasminogen activator was constitutively secreted into the culture medium by human neutrophils *in vitro*. Secretion was enhanced by low concentrations of phorbol ester and Con A which did not induce release of primary or secondary granule contents and was inhibited by glucocorticoids and inhibitors of RNA or protein synthesis (Granelli-Piperno *et al.*, 1977). Resolution of this conflict would be well worthwhile since release of

plasminogen activator from neutrophils, and its regulation could play an important physiological/pathological role, not only in terms of fibrinolysis but also the activation of proMMPs to their catalytically active forms.

5.   *Kininogenases*

These proteases are assumed to be located in granules but it is not known in which population. Kininogenase or kallikrein are terms used to describe an extensive family of proteases which have the capacity to release kinins from their precursors, kininogens. Kinins are potent inducers of oedema, pain and vasodilatation so that the presence of such activity in neutrophils could contribute to both their role in host defence and their ability to elicit an inflammatory response. This topic has been comprehensively reviewed and will only be summarized here (Bhoola *et al.*, 1992). Three classes of kininogenases have been reported in human neutrophils:

1. A membrane-associated or granule protease with an acid pH optimum which liberated kinin-like activity from a plasma protein precursor (Greenbaum, 1972, 1979). Neither the kinin precursor protein (leukokininogen), nor the kinins generated (leukokinins), are related to the classical kininogens or kinins (bradykinin, Lys-bradykinin, Met-Lys-bradykinin) (Chang *et al.*, 1972; Freer *et al.*, 1972; Greenbaum, 1979). It is possible that this kininogenase is cathepsin D but no work on the topic has been published for some years.

2. A number of authors have reported neutrophil neutral proteases, probably serine proteases, which can liberate kinin activity from kininogens (Movat *et al.*, 1973, 1976; Wendt and Blumel, 1979; Lupke *et al.*, 1982, 1983). The activity appears to reside in primary granules but has not been assigned, as yet, to any of the currently identified primary granule proteases. Once again, this does not appear to be under investigation at present.

3. Immunohistological studies of the distribution of tissue kallikrein in infected human kidneys and psoriatic skin showed intense granular staining of infiltrating neutrophils; no immunoreactivity was seen in other blood cells (Bhoola *et al.*, 1992). This activity appears to be located in the primary granules but further data are needed. Although release of tissue kallikrein could not be induced by FMLP, thrombin released both enzyme activity and immunoreactivity (Cohen *et al.*, 1991; Bhoola *et al.*, 1992). The prior incorporation of [^{35}S]-methionine into the released material suggests that it was synthesized by the neutrophils themselves (Cohen *et al.*, 1991) but it is possible that some proportion of the intracellular material was endocytosed in the form of a complex with α_1-PI (Bhoola *et al.*, 1992). This situation is complicated by the presence of kallikrein substrates (high molecular weight and low molecular weight

kininogens) and plasma prekallikrein bound to a receptor on the neutrophil surface (Bhoola *et al.*, 1992; Gustafson *et al.*, 1989).

It has been suggested that the role of the kinin-forming system in neutrophils could be to generate kinins in close proximity to endothelial cells during extravasation. The ability of kinins to cause endothelial cell retraction and gap formation could create a route for the neutrophil through the endothelial cell barrier (Bhoola *et al.*, 1992). However, no direct evidence for such a role is available as yet. It is clear that the ability of neutrophils to generate kinins could have a major physiological and pathological role. Further investigation of this phenomenon is required to assess its importance and potential as a target for therapeutic intervention.

6.   *Cytoplasmic Enzymes*

There has been increasing interest in the role of intra-cellular proteinases that exist outside the granules/lysosomes. These proteinases play a role in a number of cellular functions including degradation of proteins to control their duration of action or concentration, post-translational maturation of proteins, and proteolytic modifications of membrane-associated proteins and receptors (Pontremoli and Melloni, 1986). A cytosolic enzyme that has received considerable attention is a calcium-dependent cysteine proteinase known as calpain. Calpain is found in virtually all mammalian cell types. The precise biological role of calpain is unclear but this enzyme has been implicated in cell membrane fusion and in post-synaptic membrane remodelling in the hippocampus after long-term potentiation (Mellgren, 1987). The structure and function of calpain has been the subject of a number of reviews (Mellgren, 1987; Suzuki, 1987); therefore, we will restrict discussion to neutrophil-specific aspects of calpain.

Another cytoplasmic enzyme that has received considerable attention lately is the ICE. IL-1 is a major mediator in inflammation and exists in an α and β form. IL-1β is synthesized in an inactive pro-form and is processed to biologically active IL-1β by ICE. Although the majority of published studies have been performed in monocytes/macrophages, there is some evidence that ICE may be present in neutrophils.

6.1   HUMAN NEUTROPHIL CALPAIN

Calpain (EC 3.4.22.17) is a cytosolic cysteine proteinase, present in virtually all cell types including neutrophils (Legendre and Jones, 1988), which has a neutral pH optimum and an absolute Ca^{2+} dependence. Calpain is a heterodimer consisting of a large catalytic (Mr 80 000) and a small regulatory subunit (Mr 28 000). Two different forms of calpain exist as determined by calcium

sensitivity; calpain I is activated by low concentrations of Ca^{2+} (micromolar) and calpain II by high concentrations of Ca^{2+} (millimolar). The 80 kD subunits of the two forms of calpain are different, whereas the 28 kD subunits are identical (Suzuki, 1987). The amino-acid sequence of the large subunit of calpain I as deduced from its cDNA revealed a four-domain structure composed of 714 amino-acid residues (Aoki *et al.*, 1986). The function of two of the four domains is known: proteolytic activity is associated with residues 81–330 of domain two and the calcium-binding properties with domain four (Suzuki, 1987). Recently, a possible function for domain one has been reported. Autodigestion of calpain I resulted in the release of a peptide that was chemotactic for neutrophils (Kunimatsu *et al.*, 1989) and was found to be identical to the N-terminal nine amino acids of domain one except that the peptide lacked a methionine and was acetylated at the N-terminus (Kunimatsu *et al.*, 1989). The biological significance of this chemotactic peptide, presumably derived intracellularly from domain one, is unclear at this time.

Activation of neutrophils with PMA or FMLP results in enhanced production of superoxide and release of granule contents (Smolen *et al.*, 1981; McPhail and Snyderman, 1983; Pozzan *et al.*, 1983). PKC appears to be involved in the signal transduction leading to neutrophil activation in response to PMA and FMLP (Melloni *et al.*, 1986; Pontremoli *et al.*, 1986). The primary response of neutrophils to low concentrations of PMA is the production of superoxide with little degranulation whereas stimulation with FMLP or higher concentrations of PMA results in both superoxide production and exocytosis of neutrophil granules (Pontremoli *et al.*, 1986, 1987, 1988). Treatment of neutrophils with the cysteine proteinase inhibitor leupeptin enhanced the oxidative burst but inhibited degranulation mediated by PMA or FMLP stimulation (Pontremoli *et al.*, 1986). Identical results were seen when a monoclonal antibody against calpain was used in place of leupeptin (Pontremoli *et al.*, 1988). These results led to the suggestion that calpain cleaves the membrane-associated calcium-dependent form of PKC which is involved in the activation of superoxide production, converting it to the calcium- and phospholipid-independent soluble form of PKC which phosphorylates specific cytoskeletal proteins involved in degranulation (Melloni *et al.*, 1985). Inhibition of calpain would therefore prevent the formation of the soluble form of PKC and result in its continued association with the plasma membrane, enhancing superoxide production, and render the PKC ineffective for signal transduction in the cytosol, resulting in inhibition of granule exocytosis. It is difficult to accept this hypothesis at face value given the evidence that leupeptin does not penetrate cell membranes (Mehdi, 1991) and the unlikely proposal (Pontremoli *et al.*, 1988) that a monoclonal antibody to calpain enters the neutrophil cytosol.

Calpain has been implicated as the enzyme in human and murine macrophages which processes proIL-1α (33 kD) to the mature form (17 kD) (Kobayashi *et al.*, 1990; Carruth *et al.*, 1991). Corresponding data are not yet available for neutrophils, although they do release IL-1α (see Chapter 5). The significance of proIL-1α processing is uncertain since, unlike IL-1β where the pro-form is not biologically active, both pro- and mature IL-1α have full activity. The processing of proIL-1β to its mature form is described in Section 6.2 of this chapter.

Although thought to be an intracellular proteinase, calpain and its endogenous inhibitor calpastatin have been detected in the synovial fluids of patients with osteoarthritis (Suzuki *et al.*, 1990). The calpain activity in the synovial fluids was detected as caseinolytic activity and by Western blot using specific affinity-purified antibodies to calpain. The synovial fluid calpain was able to degrade cartilage proteoglycan suggesting a possible role in cartilage matrix degradation.

The activity of calpain is closely regulated by its endogenous inhibitor calpastatin. Two types of calpastatin have been described. A 68 kD liver type and a 46 kD form isolated from erythrocytes (Wang, 1990). Calpastatin is highly specific for calpain and inhibition is Ca^{2+} dependent.

Synthetic inhibitors of calpain can be divided into several classes and have been the subject of several recent reviews (Wang, 1990; Mehdi, 1991) so will be mentioned only briefly. Leupeptin, a microbial peptide aldehyde, is a reversible inhibitor of calpain and other cysteine proteinases but also inhibits some serine proteinases. The oxirane inhibitor, E-64, is an irreversible inhibitor of calpain but again is not selective for this enzyme since it also inhibits other cysteine proteinases (Parkes *et al.*, 1985). Highly selective and potent tripeptidyl chloromethyl ketones were synthesized as irreversible inhibitors of calpain (Sasaki *et al.*, 1986). The most potent inhibitor was Leu-Leu-Phe CH_2Cl which was 14 times more potent than E-64 (Sasaki *et al.*, 1986). However, a useful inhibitor of an intracellular enzyme must penetrate the plasma membrane. Neither leupeptin nor E-64 can penetrate into the cell. Recently, a derivative of E-64 containing no charged groups (E-64-d) was found to be orally active and to penetrate the cell membrane (Shoji-Kasai *et al.*, 1988). Several peptide aldehyde inhibitors of calpain that penetrate into cells have been reported. The dipeptide aldehydes Cbz-Val-Phe-H (Mehdi *et al.*, 1988) and Cbz-Leu-nLeu-H (calpeptin) (Tsujinaka *et al.*, 1988) have been both shown to be cell-penetrating inhibitors of calpain. These dipeptide aldehydes do not inhibit trypsin-like serine proteinases but they do inhibit the cysteine proteinase cathepsin B (Mehdi, 1991).

6.2 INTERLEUKIN-1β CONVERTING ENZYME

IL-1 is a cytokine that exists in two forms, α and β, and is a major mediator of the inflammatory process. IL-1β is generated as a 31 kD inactive pro-form which is subsequently proteolytically processed to an active 17.5 kD mature protein (Mosley *et al.*, 1987; Black *et al.*, 1988; Hazuda *et al.*, 1989). ProIL-1β is processed by cleavage at the Asp[116]–Ala[117] bond by an ICE isolated from the human monocytic leukaemia cell line THP-1 and peripheral blood monocytes (Black *et al.*, 1989; Kostura *et al.*, 1989; Howard *et al.*, 1991). This enzyme also cleaves proIL-1β at the Asp$_{27}$–Gly$_{28}$ bond to yield a 28 kD protein whose function is unknown (Black *et al.*, 1989; Howard *et al.*, 1991). ICE from THP-1 has been purified and cloned, and shown to be a cysteine proteinase with a unique preference for the cleavage of Asp-X linkages (where X is a small hydrophobic residue) (Thornberry *et al.*, 1992). ICE is a heterodimer transcribed as a proenzyme with an Mr of 45 kD that is processed to subunits of 20 and 10 kD (Thornberry *et al.*, 1992). In contrast to IL-1β, both proIL-1α and the mature form have full biological activity. Processing of IL-1α is less well understood but calpain has been implicated as the processing enzyme (see Section 6.1).

IL-1β is a major product of activated monocytic cells. However, many different cell types with appropriate stimulation can produce IL-1α and/or β mRNA *in vitro* (Oppenheim *et al.*, 1986). Human, mouse and rabbit neutrophils have been shown to produce a factor with the biological activity (mouse thymocyte proliferating activity), Mr and pH profile consistent with that of IL-1 (Goto *et al.*, 1984; Tiku *et al.*, 1986; Goh *et al.*, 1989). Human neutrophils have also been shown to translate and transcribe the IL-1α and β genes (Lindemann *et al.*, 1988, 1989; Marucha *et al.*, 1990, 1991; Roberge *et al.*, 1991; see Chapter 5). However, production of IL-1β by neutrophils does not necessarily mean that ICE is present. Certain cells such as the keratinocyte produce 31 kD proIL-1β but do not secrete active 17.5 kD IL-1β (Mizutani *et al.*, 1991). In addition, neutrophil proteinases such as elastase and cathepsin G are capable of cleaving proIL-1β to an active form of similar size and specific activity as that produced by ICE processing in monocytes (Hazuda *et al.*, 1990). However, it has been recently reported that peripheral blood neutrophils express mRNA for ICE (Black *et al.*, 1991). Therefore, neutrophils may possess multiple proteolytic pathways for the processing of proIL-1β.

7. Plasma Membrane Proteases

The proteases on the external surface of the plasma membrane are part of a dynamic population of cell surface proteins, the composition of which can be rapidly altered in response to a variety of stimuli. For example, membrane proteins can be: (a) shed from the surface via cleavage of the covalent bonds which anchor them in the membrane; (b) removed from or added to the surface along with the membrane itself (endocytosis/exocytosis); or (c) added to membrane by increased synthesis or acquired by binding non-covalently to cell surface receptors. Many of these mechanisms are used in the regulation of cell surface proteases, thus providing the neutrophil with the means to adapt its complement of membrane proteases rapidly to changes in its environment. One consequence of this adaptability is that the characteristics of neutrophils used in *in vitro* studies (e.g. levels of enzyme present in granules versus on the cell surface, amount of enzyme internalized and degraded) can be highly dependent on their past history – either while in the donor or during the isolation process. One example of this is the patient described by Veys whose neutrophils initially appeared to be FcγRIII negative. A comparison of this individual's neutrophils prepared using three different methods of isolation revealed that, although they were FcγRIII deficient when isolated over Ficoll-Hypaque or by dextran sedimentation, they expressed normal FcγRIII when isolated by whole blood lysis (Veys *et al.*, 1991). This individual clearly had an unusual sensitivity and selectivity for FcγRIII loss during isolation which, although it may not be expressed *in vivo*, could contribute confusion in interpretation of *in vitro* data. Some of the apparently contradictory data in the literature concerning neutrophil membrane proteases may be a consequence of using populations of cells which, due to their history or the isolation technique used, are not equivalent.

The nature and functions ascribed to plasma membrane proteases are diverse and, in many cases, still ill-defined. The following discussion includes proteases ranging from well-characterized proteins with clearly identified roles to uncharacterized activities whose existence is inferred from a physiological function and its regulation by protease inhibitors.

7.1 NEUTRAL ENDOPEPTIDASE (Table 4.5)

NEP (EC 3.4.24.11) cleaves peptides on the amino side of a hydrophobic amino acid. This specificity means that it can cleave a wide range of substrate peptides (Boileau *et al.*, 1989). However, because of its importance in the inactivation of enkephalin, it is widely known as enkephalinase (Boileau *et al.*, 1989). The common lymphoblastic leukaemia antigen (CALLA, CD10) has been found to be identical to NEP. This enzyme is widely distributed in the body: brush border membranes of the renal proximal tubules, intestine and placenta, specific areas of the brain, neutrophils (but not other leucocytes) (Iwamoto *et al.*, 1990a; Kimura *et al.*, 1990). The NEP gene has been cloned, expressed, and its structure and function extensively analysed by genetic manipulation (Boileau *et al.*, 1989; Le Moual *et al.*, 1991). NEP is a zinc metalloprotease which consists of a single chain anchored in the plasma membrane by a hydrophobic sequence towards the N-terminus of the molecule (Boileau *et al.*, 1989). A soluble form of NEP is found in urine where it is the major kininase.

NEP inhibitors have revealed an important role for this enzyme in regulating the response of neutrophils to those neutrophil stimuli which are NEP substrates, e.g. FMLP, substance P, enkephalin and bradykinin. For example, the polarization, migration, and adhesion molecule expression/shedding responses to FMLP and substance P (Iwamoto *et al.*, 1990b; Shipp *et al.*, 1991; Skidgel *et al.*, 1991) and the ability of Met-enkephalin to enhance the ADCC activity of neutrophils (Shipp *et al.*, 1990) were enhanced by inhibition of NEP. Based on these results it appears that NEP on neutrophil membranes normally reduces the response to these peptides by inactivating them before they have had the opportunity to elicit their

Table 4.5 Neutral endopeptidase

Name(s)	Neutral endopeptidase (NEP, enkephalinase, CALLA, CD10, membrane metallo-endopeptidase)
EC number	3.4.24.11
Mol. wt	90 kD, but can differ due to variable glycosylation[1]
Sub-units	Single chain[2]
Sequence homologies	Active site is homologous to that of thermolysin[1,2]
Type	Metalloendopeptidase (Zn)[1,2]
pH optimum	7.0[2]
Physiological substrates	Peptides less than about 3 kD, on the amino side of a hydrophobic amino acid (enkephalins, substance P, fMet-Leu-Phe, kinins, atrial naturetic peptide)[1,2]
Synthetic substrates	Ant-Ala-Gly-Leu-Ala-NH-Nb[3]
Natural inhibitors	None reported
Synthetic inhibitors	Phosphoramidon, thiorphan[1]

References: [1]Erdos and Skidgel (1989); [2]Boileau *et al.* (1989); [3]Yuli and Lelkes (1991).

maximal effect. Indeed, it has been shown that intact neutrophils or membrane preparations from neutrophils can cleave these substrates and that this cleavage can be inhibited by NEP inhibitors (Painter *et al.*, 1988; Yuli and Snyderman, 1988; Iwamoto *et al.*, 1990b; Kimura *et al.*, 1990; Yuli and Lelkes, 1991) or anti-NEP antibodies (Painter *et al.*, 1988). Immunocytochemistry has localized high concentrations of NEP to the neutrophil plasma membrane (Iwamoto *et al.*, 1990a; Kimura *et al.*, 1990).

When neutrophils were activated with PMA, the NEP activity on the cell surface was dramatically reduced (Erdos *et al.*, 1989; Skidgel *et al.*, 1991). This was shown to be caused by internalization of the enzyme, since activity could be recovered if the cells were lysed within 5 min. If, however, lysis was delayed for 30 min the NEP activity could no longer be recovered, presumably because of intracellular proteolytic degradation (Erdos *et al.*, 1989). It is therefore apparent that the amount of NEP present on neutrophils can be rapidly down-regulated by PMA-induced endocytosis and that such changes could have a profound effect on neutrophil function. However, although this PMA-induced phenomenon was confirmed (Shipp *et al.*, 1991), other agonists have been reported to produce contradictory results; either an increase (FMLP, TNF, GM-CSF, A23187) (Shipp *et al.*, 1991) or a slight decrease (FMLP) (Painter, personal communication) in cell surface NEP activity. The data themselves offer a means of resolving the contradiction: if the cells used in the experiment have been subject to an unplanned stimulus, e.g. endotoxin during isolation, a significant proportion of the cell surface NEP could have already been internalized and degraded, and therefore be unavailable for translocation to the surface in response to another stimulus. Indeed, a second stimulus would continue the internalization process and further decrease cell surface NEP. In contrast, quiescent cells may contain a reservoir of NEP stored in granules which can be brought to the surface when the cell is stimulated, thus counteracting the losses due to internalization and perhaps producing a net increase. Resolution of these contradictions is required in order to fully understand the role of NEP in regulation of neutrophil function.

An additional controversy has been identified concerning the role of NEP in neutrophil responses to one particular agonist – FMLP. As described above, several groups have demonstrated that inhibition of NEP potentiates neutrophil responses to peptide agonists that are NEP substrates. However, Yuli and Lelkes (1991) postulated that cleavage by NEP of FMLP bound to its receptor may be involved in amplification of the gradient perception mechanism of neutrophils and also in regulating the clearance of ligand from receptor, and thus the rate at which unoccupied receptors become available for further cycles of FMLP binding. This hypothesis was put forward to explain the anomalous non-Michaelis–

Menten kinetics of FMLP hydrolysis at the low concentrations which induce chemotaxis and predicts that inhibition of NEP should inhibit some neutrophil functions, particularly migration and/or chemotaxis. It has recently been reported (Painter, 1991) that chemotaxis towards FMLP is blocked by the NEP inhibitor phosphoramidon while the rapid (<1 min) responses to FMLP, i.e. shape change, actin polymerization and superoxide anion production, were unimpaired. Although the rapid down-regulation (by internalization) of its own receptor by FMLP was not inhibited, the re-expression of the receptor at the surface was inhibited more than 90% by phosphoramidon. This inhibition of FMLP receptor recycling by phosphoramidon could explain its reported (Painter, 1991) inhibition of chemotaxis (which requires sustained responses to the chemotactic agent, perhaps involving receptor recycling) but not the spectrum of rapid responses (shape change, actin polymerization and superoxide anion production, down-regulation of the FMLP receptor; which require only a brief exposure to agonist with minimal opportunity for receptor recycling). Further studies are required to determine the significance of this phenomenon and whether it applies to other peptide agonists.

The above observations relate to inactivation of peptides by NEP. However, many biologically active peptides are generated by cleavage from an inactive precursor. Neutrophils can generate the potent vaso-constrictor, endothelin-1, from its inactive precursor, big endothelin. Inhibition of this process by the NEP inhibitor phosphoramidon, but not other protease inhibitors, suggests that the responsible enzyme is NEP (Sessa *et al.*, 1991).

No natural deficiencies of NEP have been reported so the "natural" experiment is not available. No endogenous inhibitors have been reported to date, suggesting that regulation of NEP activity is performed by rapidly changing the amount of enzyme present on the cell surface (see above). However, *in vivo* studies are consistent with a role for NEP in limiting those inflammatory responses in which the mediators involved are NEP substrates, e.g. neurogenic inflammation/tachykinins. NEP inhibitors potentiated the inflammatory and contractile response to exogenously administered tachykinins (Honda *et al.*, 1991; Cheung *et al.*, 1992) and potentiated a number of neurogenic inflammatory responses (Umeno *et al.*, 1989, 1990; reviewed in Nadel, 1991; Nadel and Borson, 1991). Furthermore, administration of exogenous NEP itself reduces the response to exogenous tachykinins (Kohrogi *et al.*, 1989; Murlas *et al.*, 1992). Although these data suggest that NEP plays a role in inflammation, the interesting question of whether it is NEP on neutrophils, as opposed to on other cell types, remains open. The intriguing observation of measurable levels of soluble NEP in synovial fluids from patients with a variety of arthritides suggests a possible role in these conditions, although the cell source and mechanism of its release are unknown (Appelbloom *et al.*, 1991).

7.2 MEMBRANE SERINE PROTEASES AND SIGNAL TRANSDUCTION

For some years there has been considerable interest in the hypothesis that a serine protease located on the plasma membrane of neutrophils is involved in the signal transduction process elicited by various neutrophil stimuli (see below for references). However, the literature on the subject is full of contradictions and no clear picture has yet emerged. A major contributing factor to the conflict is the variety of methodological differences encountered, such that few of the studies have been rigorously repeated in independent laboratories. The divergence in methodology includes such components as: the species from which neutrophils are taken, the stimuli used, the functional or biochemical responses monitored and the protease inhibitors employed. Furthermore, the substrate of the putative "second messenger" protease has not been identified, leaving a major weakness in the hypothesis. Rather than present an exhaustive review of the extensive literature on this subject, a selection from the more recent studies will be provided (which contains references to earlier work).

Ward and Becker (1970) were amongst the earliest to propose that serine proteases were involved in the signal transduction process of neutrophils. However, many of their supporting data came from studies in which phosphonic acid derivatives were used as inhibitors (Ward and Becker, 1970). The use of these compounds has been criticized on the grounds that their detergent-like effects on membranes, and not their ability to inhibit serine proteases, could be enough to explain the observed inhibitory activity on neutrophil function (reviewed in Wilkinson, 1982). Furthermore, the original studies which identified the enzymes with putative roles in signal transduction were performed using rabbit cells; the equivalent enzymes are not found in human neutrophils (reviewed in Wilkinson, 1982).

More recent suggestions have focused on a membrane-associated chymotrypsin-like serine protease. In a series of publications, King and co-workers have demonstrated that exogenous CatG can prime neutrophils to respond to agonists (e.g. the generation of superoxide anion in response to FMLP or PMA), but not stimulate them directly (Kusner and King, 1989; Kusner *et al.*, 1991) and that a monoclonal antibody (mAb 1-15) to a chymotrypsin-like enzyme in neutrophil membranes strongly inhibits the superoxide anion response to FMLP or PMA (King *et al.*, 1986, 1987, 1991). Although purification and structural characterization of the protease is underway (King *et al.*, 1991), definitive demonstration of its physiological or pathological role requires identification of its substrate.

Other data supporting a role for a chymotrypsin- or CatG-like enzyme in signal transduction come from studies with the natural inhibitors of serine proteases. Human α_1-PI has been shown to inhibit chemotaxis of human neutrophils *in vitro* (Goetzl, 1975; Stockley *et al.*, 1990b). This seems to be a species-specific effect since human α_1-PI had little effect on rat neutrophils (Hornbeck *et al.*, 1987). Stockley *et al.* (1990b) also showed that the potencies of three human, macromolecular anti-proteases (α_1-PI, α_1-ACT, SLPI) as inhibitors of chemotaxis correlated with their association rate constants for CatG. However, studies with α_1-ACT strongly suggest that this serpin has a number of activities independent of protease inhibition. In particular, recombinant forms of α_1-ACT have been prepared which are devoid of antiprotease activity but retain the ability to inhibit superoxide production (Kilpatrick *et al.*, 1991). In addition, it appears that cleaved or complexed α_1-ACT has chemotactic activity, induces the synthesis of IL-6 and interacts directly with the enzyme system responsible for superoxide generation to produce inhibition (Rubin, 1992). Therefore, its ability to inhibit neutrophil function does not necessarily implicate a chymotrypsin-like protease in signal transduction. An antibody directed against CatG, but not one directed against cathepsin B, inhibited the chemotactic response to FMLP (Lomas *et al.*, 1991). There is evidence for the presence of CatG and HNE on the surface of neutrophils (Travis *et al.*, 1992), however, the effects of antibodies should be interpreted with caution since antibody to CatG would form immune complexes on the surface of neutrophils; such complexes will not be formed with antibodies to cathepsin B if this enzyme is not present on the neutrophil surface. Surface-bound immune complexes could lead to functional effects via activation of Fc receptors or via steric hindrance; mechanisms which are independent of a functional role for CatG in signal transduction. However, Stockley and co-workers also reported that chloromethylketone inhibitors of CatG and chymotrypsin (Gly-Leu-Phe-CH$_2$Cl, Gly-Gly-Phe-CH$_2$Cl), but not trypsin (TLCK), also inhibited chemotaxis (Lomas *et al.*, 1991). The apparent specificity of the different chloromethylketones goes some way to ruling out their non-specific thiol reactivity as the mechanism of action. Furthermore, Gervaix *et al.* (1991) have shown that carboxybenzyl-Leu-Tyr-CH$_2$Cl (zLYCK), a chymotrypsin inhibitor, produced parallel inhibition of the chymotrypsin-like peptidase activity on the surface of intact human neutrophils and their ability to generate superoxide anion in response to FMLP. In contrast, PMA-induced superoxide production was relatively resistant and phagocytosis of endotoxin-coated oil particles was completely resistant to inhibition by zLYCK. The insensitivity of PMA-induced neutrophil superoxide anion production to a serine esterase inhibitor (DFP) was also noted by Tsan and Jiang (1985), despite complete inhibition of cell surface serine protease activity. Although the interpretation of the effects of zLYCK are complicated by its non-specific thiol reactivity, a similar inhibitory profile was observed with N-benzoyl-Tyr-p-nitroanilide (Gervaix et al., 1991), a non-reactive chymotrypsin substrate which could compete with the unidentified natural substrate.

In contrast to the above data, TPCK and TLCK were shown to inhibit PMA-induced superoxide anion production by human neutrophils (Conseiller and Lederer, 1989). They showed that there was no detectable loss of total intracellular non-protein thiols, eliminating non-specific thiol depletion as the mechanism of action. Furthermore, although TPCK and TLCK inhibit PKC in cell-free assays, they did not inhibit the activity in intact neutrophils. However, they also noted that other serine protease inhibitors (PMSF, leupeptin) with similar specificities were without effect on superoxide anion production, casting doubt on the identity of the target for TPCK and TLCK as a protease. They subsequently identified a 15 kD protein on the neutrophil surface which was covalently labelled by tritiated TPCK and TLCK (Conseiller et al., 1990). This protein has not yet been characterized but is unlikely to be a serine protease because of its low molecular weight – serine proteases are usually greater than 20 kD. It should be noted that this body of work involved the use of PMA as the neutrophil stimulus and even if the mechanism of action of TLCK and TPCK does not involve a serine protease in this situation, stimuli operating through cell surface receptors may be different.

The accumulated data on this topic provides considerable circumstantial evidence in favour of a role for a serine protease in the signal transduction process in neutrophils. However, the case will not be complete until the enzyme and its substrate are identified and details of a specific mechanism delineated.

7.3   MEMBRANE PROTEASES AND RECEPTOR SHEDDING

Neutrophils can express on their surfaces a wide range of receptors which play important roles in their ability to respond to signals from the environment. The function of neutrophils can be regulated by changes in the levels of expression of these surface receptors. Membrane expression can be increased by synthesis of new receptors or translocation to the surface of stored receptors and can be decreased by internalization of receptors (e.g. the IL-1 receptor; Rhyne et al., 1988) or by shedding them from the surface. The shedding process has additional regulatory potential since it can release soluble receptor which may still bind ligand to form either an inactive complex (e.g TNFα, IL-1) or a biologically active complex (e.g. IL-6). If the complex is biologically inactive, this would reduce the amount of ligand available to interact with cell-bound receptors and could provide

a natural control mechanism for attenuating the response to certain neutrophil stimulants. In fact, soluble receptors are currently being investigated as potential therapeutic agents (Janson and Arend, 1992). Shedding of receptors has been demonstrated for a number of neutrophil stimuli, as shown in Table 4.6. It seems more than likely that cell surface proteases will be involved in the shedding of some receptors but other mechanisms are possible (see below) and there are only limited data available to date (summarized in Table 4.6).

TNF receptors are anchored in the plasma membrane of neutrophils by a membrane-spanning sequence of amino acids and are rapidly shed when neutrophils are exposed to physiological (FMLP, C5a, GM-CSF) and pharmacological agonists (PMA, A23187) (Porteu and Nathan, 1991; Porteu et al., 1991). The shed TNF receptor is a truncated form of the membrane-associated receptor, suggesting the involvement of a protease. Shedding of the TNF receptor could not be inhibited by inhibitors of serine or thiol proteases (Porteu and Nathan, 1991). Exposure of neutrophils to exogenous neutrophil elastase did cause shedding but this enzyme is not the one involved in agonist-induced shedding since elastase preferentially released the p75 compared to the p55 TNF receptor while cell activation induces shedding of both forms of the receptor and agonist-induced shedding is completely resistant to a serine protease inhibitor (DFP) and an elastase inhibitor (methoxysuccinyl-Ala-Ala-Pro-ValCH$_2$Cl) (Porteu and Nathan, 1991; Porteu et al., 1991).

Neutrophils express a low affinity receptor for the Fc region of IgG that is linked to the membrane via a phosphatidylinositol-glycan anchor (FcγRIII-1, also known as CD16-1) (see Chapter 7). This receptor is lost from the surface of neutrophils when they are exposed to PMA or FMLP (Huizinga et al., 1988; Harrison et al., 1991). On NK cells a different form of this receptor (FcγRIII-2, also known as CD16-2) is anchored in the membrane by a membrane spanning sequence of amino acids and shedding could be blocked by 1,10-phenanthroline (suggesting the involvement of a metallo-protease). In contrast, shedding from neutrophils was not blocked by this inhibitor (Harrison et al., 1991). It is uncertain what the mechanism of FcγRIII-1 shedding is in neutrophils; since it possesses a phosphatidylinositol-glycan anchor it need not involve a protease and the involvement of a phospholipase C has been suggested (Huizinga et al., 1988).

In murine neutrophils, the adhesion molecule L-selectin (also known as MEL-14 antigen; see Chapters 7 and 10) is anchored in the membrane by a membrane-spanning sequence of amino acids and is shed within minutes after exposure to chemotactic stimuli such as C5a and LTB$_4$. The shed form is about 5–10 kD smaller than the membrane-bound form, consistent with protease mediated cleavage. While treatment of neutrophils with elastase, trypsin or collagenase had no effect on

Table 4.6 Shedding of neutrophil receptors

Receptor	Membrane anchor	Protease implicated	Reference
TNF	Peptide[a]	Yes	Porteu et al. (1991), Porteu and Nathan (1991)
FcγRIII-1	PIG[b]	(Phospholipase C)?	Huizinga et al. (1988), Harrison et al. (1991)
L-selectin (murine)	Peptide	Yes (chymotrypsin-like)	Jutila et al. (1991)
L-selectin	Peptide	No	Campanero et al. (1991)
CD44		Yes	Campanero et al. (1991), Jackson et al. (1992)
CD43	Peptide	Yes	Campanero et al. (1991), Remold-O'Donnell and Rosen (1990)
CR1	Peptide	?	Holers et al. (1992)
CR3	Peptide	?	Holers et al. (1992)

[a] Membrane spanning sequence of amino acids.
[b] Phosphatidylinositol glycan anchor.

L-selectin expression and CatG had only a slight effect, chymotrypsin produced marked loss of L-selectin antigen (staining with MEL-14 antibody) and function *in vitro* (binding to high endothelial venules) and *in vivo* (ability of treated neutrophils injected back into mice to accumulate in the inflamed peritoneal cavity) (Jutila *et al.*, 1991). Chymotrypsin treatment did not cause the shedding of four other cell-surface antigens studied (Mac-1, LFA-1, RB6-8C5 antigen, SK 105 antigen); these antigens are not lost in response to chemotactic stimuli (Jutila *et al.*, 1991). However, although these data do make a compelling case for the involvement of a chymotrypsin-like protease in the shedding of L-selectin, the enzyme itself has not been identified and the evidence remains circumstantial. Data for the human homologue of the MEL-14 antigen are described below.

Campanero *et al.* (1991) performed studies on the changes in adhesion molecule expression on human neutrophils induced by TNFα, FMLP, A23187 and PMA. These stimuli caused the down-regulation of CD44 (Hermes-1, the hyaluronate receptor), L-selectin (LAM-1, LECAM-1, Leu 8, DREG-56 antigen; the human equivalent of the murine MEL-14 antigen) and CD43 (sialophorin) while up-regulating the expression of CD45 and CD11b. Serine protease inhibitors (PMSF plus aprotinin) abrogated the down-regulation of CD43 and CD44, but not that of L-selectin (Campanero *et al.*, 1991), however, the identities of the proteases involved remain unknown. Down-regulation of cell surface receptors has been observed in a clinical setting, i.e. down-regulation of L-selectin on the circulating leucocytes of patients with sepsis (Hasslen *et al.*, 1991).

The above studies suggest that proteases are involved in the shedding of certain receptors from the surface of neutrophils and that this phenomenon plays an important role in the regulation of neutrophil function. However, the case for the involvement of proteases will not be conclusive until the specific enzymes involved are identified. It is even possible that non-enzymatic mechanisms may operate in certain cases. For example, it has been suggested that loss of membrane surface tension as cell volume decreases in hyperosmolar media (as occurs during freezing) may be sufficient to cause shedding of Fc receptors, CR1 and CR3, from neutrophils (Takahashi *et al.*, 1985). A similar loss of surface tension may occur in stimulated neutrophils as a result of addition of membrane to the plasma membrane through degranulation. Alternatively, it has been suggested the shedding of CR3 from phorbol ester-treated human neutrophils occurs through the loss from the membrane of vesicles containing intact CR3, a mechanism which does not necessarily involve a protease (Pryzwansky *et al.*, 1991). However, if protease(s) are found to be involved, the development of specific inhibitors should be possible. It is difficult at this time to predict what impact the inhibition of shedding *in vivo* would have on neutrophil function.

7.4 CELL SURFACE RECEPTORS FOR PROTEASES

There are examples already mentioned in this review of situations where the activities of proteases are regulated at the neutrophil surface by binding to specific membrane-anchored receptors: the membrane activation of pro-72 kD gelatinase (MMP-2) (Section 4.2) and the binding of kallikrein and its substrate, kininogen (Section 5). Additional examples include homologous members of the regulators of complement activation gene family (Holers *et al.*, 1992). MCP (CD46, gp45-70) (Matsumoto *et al.*, 1992) is present on many cell types, including neutrophils, and regulates the activity of the complement cascade by binding iC3/C3b and iC4/C4b, and acting as a cofactor for the plasma protease, factor I, in the inactivation of C3b/C4b by proteolysis, thus contributing to the protection of host cells against complement attack. DAF and CR1 are structurally related molecules with similar functional roles (Holers *et al.*, 1992). An additional cell-surface protease receptor (effector cell protease receptor-1, EPR-1) is found on neutrophils and other leucocytes and binds the serine protease, clotting factor Xa (Altieri and Edgington, 1990). The physiological role of EPR-1 was not defined but these authors proposed that such surface receptors could be functionally important in a number of ways, including: local activation or inactivation of a protease at the cell surface; assembly of multicomponent systems on membrane surfaces; and sequestration of a protease away from ambient inhibitors. These mechanisms could have a broad range of utilities and EPR-2, -3, etc. may yet be identified.

8.   Miscellaneous Proteases

Recent studies implicate an unidentified serine protease in the cleavage of the acute phase protein, C-reactive protein, to peptides which inhibit neutrophil generation of superoxide (Shephard et al., 1989, 1990). The data suggest that this phenomenon could be a regulatory mechanism operative in inflammatory lesions.

ACE has long been recognized to have an important role in the cardiovascular system as a result of its ability to convert the inactive peptide, angiotensin I, to a potent vasoconstrictor, angiotensin II. However, ACE can also cleave a number of other biologically important peptides, converting them to biologically inactive products (Alhenc-Gelas et al., 1990; Beneteau-Burnat and Baudin, 1991). The location of ACE on the luminal surface of vascular endothelial cells, anchored by a short hydrophobic region near the C-terminal end of the molecule, presents the active site of the enzyme to blood-borne vasoactive peptide substrates such as angiotensin I and bradykinin. In addition, however, ACE is also found at other locations: seminiferous tubules, sperm, epididymal tubules, epithelial cells of the renal proximal tubules, chromaffin cells of the adrenal gland, glucocorticoid treated monocytes and macrophages (Beneteau-Burnat and Baudin, 1991). To date, the evidence indicates that neutrophils do not possess ACE, although a number of reports exist which may cause confusion. For example, an enzyme which converted angiotensin I to angiotensin II was reported in neutrophils (Klickstein et al., 1982; Wintroub et al., 1984; Dzau et al., 1987) and a human monocyte-derived cell-line (U937) under conditions which induced differentiation along a neutrophil pathway (Snyder et al., 1985): this activity is attributable to CatG, not ACE. It is uncertain to what extent the ability of CatG to masquerade as ACE in enzyme assays may contribute to the correlation observed in patients with certain inflammatory lung diseases (allergic alveolitis, sarcoidosis) between ACE activity and numbers of neutrophils in bronchoalveolar lavage fluids (Prior et al., 1990; Larsson et al., 1992).

Synthetic inhibitors of ACE have many effects on inflammation and lung function (Rinaldo and Dauber, 1985; Lindgren et al., 1987; Lindgren and Andersson, 1989). Many of these effects can be explained by their ability to interfere with the metabolism by ACE of biologically active peptides such as bradykinin and substance P. However, it has recently been realized that captopril, but not other ACE inhibitors, can inhibit both of the catalytic activities possessed by a neutrophil enzyme known as LTA4 hydrolase or aminopeptidase (Orning et al., 1991a, 1991b). The biological role of the aminopeptidase activity is not known but LTA4 hydrolase is required for the synthesis of the potent neutrophil chemotactic factor LTB4. It is therefore possible that inhibition of LTB4 synthesis by captopril contributes to some of its anti-inflammatory effects. In particular, captopril has been shown to reduce the damage to heart tissue in models of ischaemia/reperfusion injury and its radical scavenging activity was suggested as a possible mechanism (McMurray and Chopra, 1991). However, since the injury is thought to be mediated by neutrophil accumulation, inhibition of LTB4 could also be a factor in these pharmacological activities of captopril, if it occurs under in vivo conditions.

9.   Discussion

Neutrophils provide an essential function in host defence against bacterial and fungal infections. Upon phagocytosis of a microorganism, neutrophil granule proteinases play a role in the killing and digestion of these invaders. The granules contain numerous proteinases capable of digesting a wide variety of substrates. However, when released into the extracellular environment these enzymes are capable of destroying the extracellular matrix. Normally the substantial antiproteinase screen of endogenous inhibitors is sufficient to confine the activity of extracellularly released proteinases to the restricted location and/or period of time required for their physiological functions. However, in some disease states there is evidence for a proteinase–inhibitor imbalance. In animal models of connective tissue damage there is evidence for tissue damage by HNE, PR-3 and cathepsin B. In addition to their direct effects on connective tissue degradation, neutrophil granule proteinases have other proinflammatory properties. HNE has been shown to stimulate production of the chemotactic cytokine IL-8 from a bronchial epithelial cell line which suggests that this enzyme can function to perpetuate the inflammatory process by recruiting more neutrophils. The complex of neutrophil proteinases with their endogenous inhibitors have also been shown to stimulate cytokine production. Also, HNE and CatG have been shown to stimulate secretion of mucus components from submucosal gland cells which may contribute to the morbidity of diseases in which mucus is a feature. There is evidence that HNE is a contributing factor in some human diseases but a role for the other granule proteinases cannot be excluded. In particular, HNC and HNG have properties which could make them villains in some disease situations despite their likely essential roles in host defence.

Numerous natural and synthetic inhibitors of neutrophil granule proteinases have been described. Some of these have been shown to inhibit significantly tissue damage mediated by the administration of granule proteases in animal models but they have been less effective against the damage mediated by the release of endogenous enzymes. It will be a real challenge to develop inhibitors of the granule proteases which are effective at the cell–substratum interface where conditions will not favour the inhibitors, i.e. penetration to this location could be difficult, concentrations of both enzyme and substrate are high, the proteinases could have multiple binding sites for substratum which keep them bound, while cleaving multiple bonds and shielding the active site from fluid-phase inhibitors. The evaluation of specific non-toxic inhibitors of HNE is currently underway in humans. The results of such clinical trials will help define the role of neutrophil granule proteinases in human diseases and the scientific community eagerly awaits the outcome of these studies.

The potential roles in disease states of neutrophil proteases in other subcellular compartments is even less clearly understood. It is an area which is ripe for further study and offers the possibility of regulating neutrophil function at points prior to the release of granule proteases and other inflammatory mediators. Inhibition at these earlier points could lead to more effective control of neutrophil-mediated tissue damage than the direct inhibition of a granule protease after its release from the neutrophil.

10. Acknowledgements

The authors wish to thank the following: C.A. Gabel, P.G. Mitchell, R. Painter, E.R. Pettipher, L.A. Reiter, H.J. Showell, J. Travis and F. Woessner for their valuable input; S. Gaskey for secretarial assistance and J. Doherty for preparing Figure 4.1.

11. References

Abboud, R.T., Fera, T., Richter, A., Tabona, M.Z. and Joha, S. (1985). Acute effect of smoking on the functional activity of α_1-protease inhibitor in bronchoalveolar lavage fluid. Am. Rev. Respir. Dis. 131, 79–85.

Abrams, W.R., Cohen, A.B., Damiano, V.V., Eliraz, A., Kimbel, P., Meranze, D.R. and Weinbaum, G. (1981). A model of decreased functional α_1-proteinase inhibitor: pulmonary pathology of dogs exposed to chloramine T. J. Clin. Invest. 68, 1132–1139.

Alhenc-Gelas, F., Soubrier, F., Hubert, C., Allegrini, J., Lattion, A.L. and Corvol, P. (1990). The angiotensin I-converting enzyme (kininase II): progress in molecular and genetic structure. J. Cardiovasc. Pharmacol. 15 (Suppl. 6), S25–S29.

Almeida, R.P., Melchior, M., Campanelli, D., Nathan, C. and Gabay, J. (1991). Complementary DNA sequence of human neutrophil azurocidin, an antibiotic with extensive homology to serine proteases. Biochem. Biophys. Res. Comm. 177, 688–695.

Altieri, D.C. and Edgington, T.S. (1990). Identification of effector cell protease receptor-1. A leukocyte-distributed receptor for the serine protease factor Xa. J. Immunol. 145, 246–253.

Angelastro, M.R., Mehdi, S., Burkhart, J.P., Peet, N.P. and Bey, P. (1990). α-Diketone and α-keto ester derivatives of N-protected amino acids and peptides as novel inhibitors of cysteine and serine proteinases. J. Med. Chem. 33, 11–13.

Aoki, Y. (1978). Crystallization and characterization of a new protease in mitochondria of bone marrow cells. J. Biol. Chem. 253, 2026–2032.

Aoki, Y. (1992). Medullasin; a new target for anti-inflammatory drug design. Drug News Perspect. 5, 534–541.

Aoki, Y., Urata, G., Takaku, F. and Katunuma, N. (1975). A new protease inactivating delta-amino-levulinic acid synthase in mitochondria of human bone marrow cells. Biochem. Biophys. Res. Comm. 65, 567–574.

Aoki, K., Imajoh, S., Ohno, S., Yasufumi, E., Koike, M., Kosaki, G. and Suzuki, K. (1986). Complete amino acid sequence of the large subunit of the low-Ca^{++}-requiring form of human Ca^{++}-activated neutral protease (mCANP) deduced from its cDNA sequence. FEBS Lett. 205, 313–317.

Appelbloom, T., de Maertelaer, V., de Prez, E., Hauzeur, J.P. and Deschodt-Lanckman, M. (1991). Enkephalinase: a physiologic neuroimmunomodulator detected in synovial fluid. Arthritis Rheum. 34, 1048–1051.

Avila, J.L. and Convit, J. (1976). Physiochemical characterization of the glycosaminoglycan–lysosomal enzyme interaction in vitro: a model of control of leukocyte lysosomal activity. Biochem. J. 160, 129–136.

Baggiolini, M. (1980). In "The Cell Biology of Inflammation" (ed. G. Weissman), pp. 163–187. Elsevier/North Holland, New York.

Baggiolini, M., Bretz, U., Dewald, B. and Feigenson, M.E. (1978). The polymorphonuclear leukocyte. Agents Actions 8, 3–10.

Bainton, D.F. (1988). In "Inflammation: Basic Principles and Clinical Correlates" (eds J.I. Gallin, I.M. Goldstein and R. Snyderman) pp. 265–280. Raven Press, New York.

Bainton, D.F., Miller, L.J., Kishimoto, T.K. and Springer, T.A. (1987). Leukocyte adhesion receptors are stored in peroxidase-negative granules of human neutrophils. J. Exp. Med. 166, 1641–1653.

Bakowski, B. and Tschesche, H. (1992). Migration of polymorphonuclear leukocytes through human amnion membrane – a scanning electron microscopic study. Biol. Chem. Hoppe-Seyler 373, 529–546.

Banda, M.J., Griffin, G.L., Clark, E.J. and Senior, R.M. (1986). Chemotactic activity for neutrophils is generated by the proteolysis of α_1-proteinase inhibitor by a metalloproteinase. Fed. Proc. 45, 636.

Bangalore, N., Travis, J., Onunka, V.C., Pohl, J. and Shafer, W.M. (1990). Identification of the primary antimicrobial domains in human neutrophil cathepsin G. J. Biol. Chem. 265, 13584–13588.

Barrett, A.J. (1973). Human cathepsin B1: purification and some properties of the enzyme. Biochem. J. 131, 809–822.

Barrett, A.J. and Starkey, P.M. (1973). The interactions of α_2-macroglobulin with proteinases. Characteristics and specificity of the reaction, and a hypothesis concerning its molecular mechanism. Biochem. J. 133, 709–724.

Barrett, A.J., Kembhavi, A.A., Brown, M.A., Kirschke, H., Knight, C.G., Tamai, K. and Hanada, K. (1982). L-trans-Epoxysuccinyl leucylamido (4-guanidino) butane (E-64) and its analogues as inhibitors of cysteine proteinases including cathepsins B, H and L. Biochem. J. 201, 189–198.

Barrett, A.J., Buttle, D.J. and Mason, R.W. (1988). Lysosomal cysteine proteinases. ISI Atlas Sci. 1, 256–260.

Baugh, R.J, and Travis, J. (1976). Human leukocyte granule elastase: rapid isolation and characterization. Biochemistry 15, 836–841.

Beatty, K., Bieth, J. and Travis, J. (1980). Kinetics of association of serine proteinases with native and oxidized α_1-proteinase inhibitor and α_1-antichymotrypsin. J. Biol. Chem. 255, 3931–3934.

Beaulieu, A.D., Lang, F., Belles-Isles, M. and Poubelle, P. (1987). Protein biosynthetic activity of polymorphonuclear leukocytes in inflammatory arthropathies. Increased synthesis and release of fibronectin. J. Rheumatol. 14, 656–661.

Beneteau-Burnat, B. and Baudin, B. (1991). Angiotensin-converting enzyme: clinical applications and laboratory investigations on serum and other biological fluids. Crit. Rev. Lab. Sci. 28, 337–356.

Bhoola, K.D., Figueroa, C.D. and Worthy, K. (1992). Bioregulation of kinins: kallikreins, kininogens, and kininases. Pharmacol. Rev. 44, 1–80.

Bieth, J.G. (1989). In "Elastin and Elastases" (eds R. Ladislas and R. Hornebeck) pp. 24–31. CRC Press, Inc., Boca Raton.

Birkedal-Hansen, H., Werb, Z., Welgus, H.G. and van Wart, H.E. (eds) (1992). "Matrix Metalloproteinases and Inhibitors". Proceedings of the Matrix Metalloproteinase Conference held at Sandestin Beach, Florida, 1989. Gustav Fischer Verlag, Stuttgart, Germany.

Bjork. J., Hedqvist, P. and Arfors, K.-E. (1982). Increase in vascular permeability induced by leukotriene LTB$_4$ and the role of polymorphonuclear leukocytes. Inflammation 6, 189–200.

Black. R.A., Kronheim, S.R., Cantrell, M., Deeley, M.C., March, C.J., Prickett, K.S., Wignall, J., Conlon, P.J., Cosman, D. and Hopp, T.P. (1988). Generation of biologically active interleukin-1β by proteolytic cleavage of the inactive precursor. J. Biol. Chem. 263, 9437–9442.

Black, R.A., Kronheim, S.R. and Sleath, P.R. (1989). Activation of interleukin-1β by a co-induced protease. FEBS Lett. 247, 386–390.

Black, R.A., Sleath, P.R. and Kronheim, S.R. (1991). International Patent Application, PCT/US91/02339.

Blackwood, R.A., Moret, J., Mandl, I. and Turino, G.M. (1984). Emphysema induced by intravenously administered endotoxin in an α_1-antitrypsin deficient rat model. Am. Rev. Respir. Dis. 130, 231–236.

Blaser, J., Knauper, V., Osthues, A., Reinke, H. and Tschesche, H. (1991). Mercurial activation of human polymorphonuclear leucocyte procollagenase. Eur. J. Biochem. 202, 1223–1230.

Bode, W., Meyer, E.J. and Powers, J.C. (1989). Human leukocyte and porcine pancreatic elastase: X-ray crystal structures, mechanism, substrate specificity, and mechanism-based inhibitors. Biochemistry 28, 1951–1963.

Boileau, G., Crine, P. and Devault, A. (1989). In "UCLA Symposium on Cellular and Molecular Biology", new series, Vol. 104, "Cellular Proteases and Control Mechanisms" (ed. T.E. Hugli) pp. 159–168. A.R. Liss, Inc., New York.

Bonney, R.J.. Ashe, B., Maycock., A., Dellea, P., Hand, K., Osinga, D., Fletcher, D., Mumford, R., Davies, P., Frankenfield, D., Nolan, T., Schaeffer, L., Hagmann, W., Finke, P., Shah, S., Dorn. C. and Doherty, J. (1989). Pharmacological profile of the substituted beta-lactam L659.286: a member of a new class of human PMN elastase inhibitors. J. Cell Biochem. 39, 47–53.

Bories, D., Raynal. M.-C., Solomon, D.H., Darzynkiewicz, Z. and Cayre, Y.E. (1989). Down-regulation of a serine protease, myeloblastin, causes growth arrest and differentiation of promyelocytic leukemia cells. Cell 59, 959–968.

Borregaard, N., Heiple, J., Simons, E.R. and Clark, R.A. (1983). Subcellular localization of the b-cytochrome component of the human neutrophil microbicidal oxidase. Translocation during activation. J. Cell Biol. 97, 52–61.

Borregaard, N., Christensen, L., Bjerrum, O.W., Birgens, H.S. and Clemmensen, I. (1990). Identification of a highly mobilizable subset of human neutrophil intracellular vesicles that contain tetranectin and latent alkaline phosphatase. J. Clin. Invest. 85, 408–416.

Borregaard, N., Kjeldsen, L., Rygaard, K., Bastholm, L., Nielsen, M.H., Sengelov, H., Bjerrum, O.W. and Johnsen, A.H. (1992). Stimulus-dependent secretion of plasma proteins from human neutrophils. J. Clin. Invest. 90, 86–96.

Boudier, C., Holle, C. and Bieth, J.G. (1981). Stimulation of the elastinolytic activity of leukocyte elastase by leukocyte cathepsin G. J. Biol. Chem. 256, 10256–10258.

Boudier, C., Godeau, G., Hornebeck, W., Robert, L. and Bieth, J.G. (1991). The elastolytic activity of cathepsin G: an ex vivo study with dermal elastin. Am. J. Respir. Cell Mol. Biol. 4, 497–503.

Brederoo, P., van der Meulen, J. and Mommaas-Kienhuis, A.M. (1983). Development of the granule population in neutrophil granulocytes from human bone marrow. Cell Tissue Res. 234, 469–496.

Bretz, U. and Baggiolini, M. (1982). Biochemical and morphological characterization of azurophil and specific granules of human neutrophilic polymorphonuclear leukocytes. J. Cell Biol. 63, 251–269.

Bruce, M.C., Ponce. L.. Klinger, J.D., Stern, R.C., Tomashelshi, J.F. and Dearborn, D.G. (1985). Biochemical and pathological evidence for proteolytic destruction of lung connective tissue in cystic fibrosis. Am. Rev. Resp. Dis. 132, 529–535.

Buttle, D.J., Abrahamson, M., Burnett, D., Mort, J.S., Barrett, A.J., Dando, P.M. and Hill, S.L. (1991). Human sputum cathepsin B degrades proteoglycan, is inhibited by α_2-macroglobulin and is modulated by neutrophil elastase cleavage of cathepsin B precursor and cystatin C. Biochem. J. 276, 325–331.

Campanelli, D., Detmers, P.A., Nathan, C.F. and Gabay, J.E. (1990a). Azurocidin and a homologous serine protease from neutrophils. Differential antimicrobial and proteolytic properties. J. Clin. Invest. 85, 904–915.

Campanelli, D., Melchior, M., Fu, Y., Nakata, M., Shuman, H., Nathan, C. and Gabay, J.E. (1990b). Cloning of cDNA for proteinase 3: a serine protease, antibiotic, and autoantigen from human neutrophils. J. Exp. Med. 172, 1709–1715.

Campanero, M.R., Pulido, R., Alonso, J.L., Pivel, J.P., Pimentel, M.F., Fresno, M. and Sanchez, M.F. (1991). Down-regulation by tumor necrosis factor-alpha of neutrophil cell surface expression of the sialophorin CD43 and the hyaluronate receptor CD44 through a proteolytic mechanism. Eur. J. Immunol. 21, 3045–3048.

Campbell, E.J. and Campbell, M.A. (1988). Pericellular proteolysis by neutrophils in the presence of proteinase inhibitors: effects of substrate opsonization. J. Cell Biol. 106, 667–676.

Campbell, E.J., Senior, R.M., McDonald, J.A. and Cox., D.L. (1982). Proteolysis by neutrophils. Relative importance of cell-substrate contact and oxidative inactivation of proteinase inhibitors in vitro. J. Clin. Invest. 70, 845–852.

Capodici, C. and Berg, R.A. (1989a). Cathepsin G degrades denatured collagen. Inflammation 13, 137–145.

Capodici, C. and Berg, R.A. (1989b). Hypochlorous acid (HOCl) activation of neutrophil collagenase requires cathepsin G. Agents Actions 27, 481–484.

Capodici, C. and Berg, R.A. (1991). Neutrophil collagenase activation: the role of oxidants and cathepsin G. Agents Actions 34, 8–10.

Capodici, C., Muthukumaran, G., Amoruso, M.A. and Berg, R.A. (1989). Activation of neutrophil collagenase by cathepsin G. Inflammation 13, 245–258.

Carp, H., Miller, F., Hoidal, J.R. and Janoff, A. (1982). Potential mechanism of emphysema: α_1-proteinase inhibitor recovered from the lungs of cigarette smokers contains oxidized methionine and has decreased elastase inhibitory capacity. Proc. Natl Acad. Sci. USA 79, 2041–2045.

Carruth, L.M., Demczuk, S. and Mizel, S.B. (1991). Involvement of a calpain-like protease in the processing of the murine interleukin 1 alpha precursor. J. Biol. Chem. 266, 12162–12167.

Cawston, T.E. (1986). In "Proteinase inhibitors" (eds A.J. Barrett and G. Salvesen) pp. 589–610. Elsevier, Amsterdam.

Cawston, T.E., Mercer, E., de Silva, M. and Hazelman, B.L. (1984). Metalloproteinases and collagenase inhibitors in rheumatoid synovial fluid. Arthritis Rheum. 27, 285–290.

Cawston, T., McLaughlin, P., Coughlan, R., Kyle, V. and Hazleman, B. (1990). Synovial fluids from infected joints contain metalloproteinase-tissue inhibitor of metalloproteinase (TIMP) complexes. Biochim. Biophys. Acta 1033, 96–102.

Chan, S.J., Segundo, B.S., McCormick, M.B. and Steiner, D.F. (1986). Nucleotide and predicted amino acid sequences of cloned human and mouse preprocathepsin B cDNAs. Proc. Natl Acad. Sci. USA 83, 7721–7725.

Chang, J., Freer, R., Stella, R. and Greenbaum, L.M. (1972). Studies on leukokinins. II. Studies on the formation, partial amino acid sequence and chemical properties of leukokinins M and PMN. Biochem. Pharmacol. 21, 3095–3106.

Chatham, W.W., Heck, L.W. and Blackburn, W.D.J. (1990a). Ligand-dependent release of active neutrophil collagenase. Arthritis Rheum. 33, 228–234.

Chatham, W.W., Heck, L.W. and Blackburn, W.D.J. (1990b). Lysis of fibrillar collagen by neutrophils in synovial fluid. A role for surface-bound immunoglobulins. Arthritis Rheum. 33, 1333–1339.

Cheung, D., Bel, E.H., Den Hartigh, J., Dijkman, J.H. and

Sterk, P.J. (1992). The effect of an inhaled neutral endopeptidase inhibitor, thiorphan, on airway responses to neurokinin A in normal humans in vivo. Am. Rev. Respir. Dis. 145, 1275–1280.

Christner, P., Fein, A., Goldberg, S., Lippmann, M., Abrams, W. and Weinbaum, G. (1985). Collagenase in the lower respiratory tract of patients with adult respiratory distress syndrome. Am. Rev. Respir. Dis. 131, 690–695.

Clark, I.M. and Cawston, T.E. (1989). Fragments of human fibroblast collagenase. Purification and characterization. Biochem. J. 263, 201–206.

Cochrane, C.G., Spragg, R. and Revak, S.D. (1983). Pathogenesis of the adult respiratory distress syndrome. Evidence of oxidant activity in bronchoalveolar lavage fluid. J. Clin. Invest. 71, 754–761.

Cohen, W.M., Wu, H.F., Featherstone, G.L., Jenzano, J.W. and Lundblad, R.L. (1991). Linkage between blood coagulation and inflammation. Stimulation of neutrophil tissue kallikrein release by thrombin. Biochem. Biophys. Res. Comm. 176, 315–320.

Conseiller, E.C. and Lederer, F. (1989). Inhibition of NADPH oxidase by aminoacyl chloromethane protease inhibitors in phorbol-ester-stimulated human neutrophils: a reinvestigation. Are proteases really involved in the activation process? Eur. J. Biochem. 183, 107–114.

Conseiller, E.C., Schott, D. and Lederer, F. (1990). Inhibition by aminoacyl-chloromethane protease inhibitors of superoxide anion production by phorbol-ester-stimulated human neutrophils. The labeled target is a membrane protein. Eur. J. Biochem. 193, 345–350.

Cooper, T.W., Eisen, A.Z., Stricklin, G.P. and Welgus, H.G. (1985). Platelet derived collagenase inhibitor – characterization and subcellular location. Proc. Natl Acad. Sci. USA 82, 2779–2783.

Copp, L.J., Krantz, A. and Spencer, R.W. (1989). Kinetics and mechanism of human leukocyte elastase inactivation by ynenol lactones. Biochemistry 26, 169–178.

Crawford, I.P. (1973). Purification and properties of normal human α_1-antitrypsin. Arch. Biochem. Biophys. 156, 215–222.

Csernok, E., Ludemann, J., Gross, W.L. and Bainton, D.F. (1990). Ultrastructural localization of proteinase 3, the target antigen of anti-cytoplasmic antibodies circulating in Wegener's granulomatosis. Am. J. Path. 137, 1113–1120.

Damiano, V.V., Kucich, U., Murer, E., Laudenslager, N. and Weinbaum, G. (1988). Ultrastructural quantitation of peroxidase and elastase-containing granules in human neutrophils. Am. J. Path. 131, 235–245.

Davis, W.B., Fells, G.A., Chernick, M.S., diSant'Agnese, P.A. and Crystal, R.G. (1983). A role for neutrophils in the derangements of the bronchial wall characteristic of cystic fibrosis. Am. Rev. Resp. Dis. 127, 207A.

de Clerk, Y.A., Yean, T.-D., Lu, H.S., Ting, J. and Langley, K.E. (1991). Inhibition of the autoproteolytic activation of interstitial procollagenase by recombinant metalloproteinase inhibitor MI/TIMP-2. J. Biol. Chem. 266, 3893–3899.

Delaisse, J.-M., Eeckhout, Y., Sear, C., Galloway, A., McCullagh, K. and Vaes, G. (1985). A new synthetic inhibitor of mammalian tissue collagenase inhibits bone resorption in culture. Biochem. Biophys. Res. Comm. 133, 483–490.

Delaisse, J.-M., Eeckhout, Y. and Vaes, G. (1988). Bone resorbing agents affect the production and distribution of procollagenase as well as the activity of collagenase in bone. Endocrinology 123, 264–276.

de Saint Basile. G., Fischer, A., Dautzenberg, M.D., Durandy, A., le Deist, F., Angles-Cano, E. and Griscelli, C. (1985). Enhanced plasminogen-activator production by leukocytes in human and murine Chediak–Higashi syndrome. Blood 65, 1275–1281.

Desrochers, P.E., Mookhtiar, K., van Wart, H.E., Hasty, K.A. and Weiss, S.J. (1992). Proteolytic inactivation of α_1-proteinase inhibitor and α_1-antichymotrypsin by oxidatively activated human neutrophil metalloproteinases. J. Biol. Chem. 267, 5005–5012.

Devarajan, P., Mookhtiar, K., van Wart, H. and Berliner, N. (1991). Structure and expression of the cDNA encoding human neutrophil collagenase. Blood 77, 2731–2738.

Dewald, B., Brenz, U. and Baggiolini, M. (1982). Release of gelatinase from a novel secretory compartment of neutrophils. J. Clin. Invest. 70, 518–525.

Docherty, A.J.P., O'Connell, J., Crabbe, T., Angal, S. and Murphy, G. (1992). The matrix metalloproteinases and their natural inhibitors: prospects for treating degenerative tissue diseases. Trends Biotech. 10, 200–207.

Doherty, J.B., Ashe, B.M., Argenbright, L.W., Barker, P.L., Bonney, R.J., Chandler, G.O., Dahlgren, M.E., Dorn, C.P., Finke, P.E., Firestone, R.A., Fletcher, D., Hagmann, W.K., Mumford, R., O'Grady, L., Maycock, A.L., Pisano, J.M., Shah, S.K., Thompson, K.R. and Zimmerman, M. (1986). Cephalosporin antibiotics can be modified to inhibit human leukocyte elastase. Nature 322, 192–194.

Doherty, N.S., Dinerstein, R.J. and Mehdi, S. (1990). Novel inhibitors of polymorphonuclear neutrophil (PMN) elastase and cathepsin G: evaluation in vitro of their potential for the treatment of inflammatory connective tissue damage. Int. J. Immunopharmac. 12, 787–795.

Dwenger, A., Tost, P. and Hole, W. (1986). Evaluation of elastase and alpha-1-proteinase inhibitor–elastase uptake by polymorphonuclear leukocytes and evidence of an elastase specific receptor. J. Clin. Chem. Clin. Biochem. 24, 299–308.

Dzau, V.J., Gonzales, D., Kaempfer, C., Dubin, D. and Wintroub, B.U. (1987). Human neutrophils release serine proteases capable of activating prorenin. Circ. Res. 60, 595–601.

Eisenberg, S.P., Hale, K.K., Heimdal, P. and Thompson, R.C. (1990). Location of the protease-inhibitory region of secretory leukocyte protease inhibitors. J. Biol. Chem. 265, 7976–7981.

Erdos, E.G. and Skidgel, R.A. (1989). In "Neurochemical Pharmacology – A Tribute to B.B. Brodie" (ed. E. Costa) pp. 47–54. Raven Press, New York.

Erdos, E.G., Wagner, B., Harbury, C.B., Painter, R.G., Skidgel, R.A. and Fa, X.G. (1989). Down-regulation and inactivation of neutral endopeptidase 24.11 (enkephalinase) in human neutrophils. J. Biol. Chem. 264, 14519–14523.

Eriksson, S. (1965). Studies in α_1-antitrypsin deficiency. Acta Med. Scand. 177 (Suppl. 432), 1–85.

Farley, D., Salvesen, G. and Travis, J. (1988). Molecular cloning of human elastase. Biol. Chem. Hoppe Seyler 369 (Suppl.), 3–7.

Fera, T., Abboud, R.T., Richter, A. and Johal, S.S. (1986).

Acute effect of smoking on elastase-like esterase activity and immunological neutrophil elastase levels in bronchoalveolar lavage fluid. Am. Rev. Respir. Dis. 133, 568–573.

Fick, R.B., Naegel, G.P., Squier, S., Wood, R.E., Gee, J.B.L. and Reynolds, H.Y. (1984). Proteins of the cystic fibrosis respiratory tract: fragmented immunoglobulin G opsonic antibody causing defective opsonophagocytosis. J. Clin. Invest. 74, 236–248.

Fletcher, D.S., Osinga, D.G., Hand, K.M., Dellea, P.S., Ashe, B.M., Mumford, R.A., Davies, P., Hagmann, W., Finke, P.E., Doherty, J.B. and Bonney, R.J. (1990). A comparison of α_1-proteinase inhibitor, Methoxysuccinyl-Ala-Ala-Pro-Val-Chloromethyl ketone and specific β-lactam inhibitors in an acute model of human polymorphonuclear leukocyte elastase induced lung hemorrhage in the hamster. Am. Rev. Respir. Dis. 141, 672–677.

Fletcher, D., Hand, K., Osinga, D., Dellea, P., Doherty, J. and Dorn, C. (1991). L-680,833: A potent, orally active inhibitor of human PMN elastase in a model of elastase-induced lung damage in the hamster. Pharmacologist 33, 156.

Freer, R., Chang, J. and Greenbaum, L.M. (1972). Studies on leukokinins. III, Pharmacological activities of leukokinins M and PMN. Biochem. Pharmacol. 21, 3107–3110.

Gabler, W.L. and Creamer, H.R. (1991). Suppression of human neutrophil functions by tetracyclines. J. Periodont. Res. 26, 52–58.

Gadek, J.E., Fells, G.A. and Crystal, R.G. (1979). Cigarette smoking induces functional antiproteinase deficiency in the lower respiratory tract of humans. Science 206, 1315–1316.

Gal, S., Willingham, M.C. and Gottesman, M.M. (1985). Processing and lysosomal localization of a glycoprotein whose secretion is transformation stimulated. J. Cell Biol. 100, 535–544.

Gangbar, S., Overall, C.M., McCulloch, C.A. and Sodek, J. (1990). Identification of polymorphonuclear leukocyte collagenase and gelatinase activities in mouthrinse samples: correlation with periodontal disease activity in adult and juvenile periodontitis. J. Periodont. Res. 25, 257–267.

Gervaix, A., Kessels, G.C., Suter, S., Lew, P.D. and Verhoeven, A.J. (1991). The chymotrypsin inhibitor carbobenzyloxy-leucine-tyrosine-chloromethylketone interferes with the neutrophil respiratory burst mediated by a signaling pathway independent of PtdInsP$_2$ breakdown and cytosolic free calcium. J. Immunol. 147, 1912–1919.

Gilligan, D.M., O'Connor, C.M., Ward. K., Moloney, D., Bresnihan. B. and FitzGerald, M.X. (1990). Bronchoalveolar lavage in patients with mild and severe rheumatoid lung disease. Thorax 45, 591–596.

Goetzl, E.J. (1975). Modulation of human neutrophil polymorphonuclear leucocyte migration by human plasma alpha-globulin inhibitor and synthetic esterase inhibitors. Immunology 29, 163–174.

Goh, K., Furusawa, S., Kawa, Y., Neigishi-Okitsu, S. and Mizoguchi, M. (1989). Production of interleukin-1α and -β by human peripheral polymorphonuclear neutrophils. Int. Arch. Allergy Appl. Immunol. 88, 297–303.

Goldstein, W. and Doring, G. (1986). Lysosomal enzymes from polymorphonuclear leukocytes and proteinase inhibitors in patients with cystic fibrosis. Am. Rev. Respir. Dis. 134, 49–56.

Goto, F., Nakamura, S., Goto, K. and Yoshinaga, M. (1984). Production of a lymphocyte proliferation potentiating factor by purified polymorphonuclear leucocytes from mice and rabbits. Immunology 53, 683–692.

Granelli-Piperno, A., Vassali, J.-D. and Reich, E. (1977). Secretion of plasminogen activator by human polymorphonuclear leukocytes. J. Exp. Med. 146, 1693–1706.

Greenbaum, L.M. (1972). Leukocyte kininogenases and leukokinins from normal and malignant cells. Am. J. Pathol. 68, 613–623.

Greenbaum, L.M. (1979). In "Bradykinin, Kallidin and Kallikrein" (ed. E.G. Erdos) pp. 91–102. Springer-Verlag, Berlin.

Groutas, W.C. (1987). Inhibitors of leukocyte elastase and leukocyte cathespin G. Agents for the treatment of emphysema and related ailments. Medicinal Res. Rev. 7, 227–241.

Groutas, W.C., Stanga, M.A. and Brubaker, M.J. (1989). ^{13}C NMR evidence for an enzyme-induced lossen rearrangement in the mechanism-based inactivation of chymotrypsin by 3-benzyl-N((methylsulfonyl)oxy) succinimide. J. Am. Chem. Soc. 111, 1931–1932.

Groutas, W.C., Hoidal, J.R., Brubaker, M.J., Stanga, M.A., Venkataraman, R., Gray, B.H. and Rao, N.V. (1990). Inhibitors of human leukocyte proteinase-3. J. Med. Chem. 33, 1085–1087.

Gubensek, F., Barstow, L., Kregar, I. and Turk, V. (1976). Rapid isolation of cathepsin D by affinity chromatography on the immobilized synthetic inhibitor. FEBS Lett. 71, 42–46.

Gupton, B.F., Carroll, D.L., Tuhy, P.M., Kam, C.-M. and Powers, J.C. (1984). Reaction of azapeptides with chymotrypsin-like enzymes. New inhibitors and active site titrants for chymotrypsin Aa, subtilisin BPN, subtilisin Carlsberg, and human leukocyte cathepsin G. J. Biol. Chem. 259, 4279–4287.

Gustafson, E.J., Sehmaier, A.H., Wachfogel, Y.T., Kaufman, N., Kulieh, U. and Colman, R.W. (1989). Human neutrophils contain and bind high molecular weight kininogen. J. Clin. Invest. 84, 28–35.

Hagmann, W.K., Kissinger, A.L., Shah, S.K., Finke, P.E., Dorn, C.P., Brause, K.A., Ashe, B.M., Weston, H., Maycock, A.L., Knight, W.B., Dellea, P.S., Fletcher, D.S., Hand, K.M., Osinga, D., Davies, P. and Doherty, J.B. (1993) Orally active β-lactam inhibitors of human leukocyte elastase. 2. Effect of C-4 substitution. J. Med. Chem. 36, 771–777.

Hannewinkel, H., Glossl, J. and Kneese, H. (1987). Biosynthesis of cathepsin B in cultured normal and I-cell fibroblasts. J. Biol. Chem. 262, 12351–12355.

Harper, J.W. and Powers, J.C. (1985). Reaction of serine proteases with substituted 3-alkoxychloroisocoumarins and 3-alkoxyamino 4-chloroisocoumarins: new reactive mechanism-based inhibitors. Biochemistry 24, 7200–7213.

Harper, J.W., Hemmi, K. and Powers, J.C. (1985). Reaction of serine proteases with substituted isocoumarins: discovery of 3,4-dichloroisocoumarin, a new general mechanism based serine protease inhibitor. Biochemistry 24, 1831–1841.

Harrison, D., Phillips, J.H. and Lanier, L.L. (1991). Involvement of a metalloprotease in spontaneous and phorbol ester-induced release of natural killer cell-associated FcγRIII (CD16-II). J. Immunol. 147, 3459–3465.

Hassal, C.H., Johnson, W.H., Kennedy, A.J. and Roberts, N.A. (1985). A new class of inhibitors of human leukocyte elastase. FEBS Lett. 183, 201–205.

Hasslen, S.R., Nelson, R.D., Kishimoto, T.K., Warren, W.E., Ahrenholz, D.H. and Solem, L.D. (1991). Down-regulation of homing receptors: a mechanism for impaired recruitment of human phagocytes in sepsis. J. Trauma 31, 645–652.

Hasty, K.A., Hibbs, M.S., Kang, A.H. and Mainardi, C.L. (1986). Secreted forms of human neutrophil collagenase. J. Biol. Chem. 261, 5645–5650.

Hasty, K.A., Jeffrey, J.J., Hibbs, M.S. and Welgus, H.G. (1987). The collagen substrate specificity of human neutrophil collagenase. J. Biol. Chem. 262, 10048–10052.

Hasty, K.A., Pourmotabbed, T.F., Goldberg, G.I., Thompson, J.P., Spinella, D.G., Stevens, R.M. and Mainardi, C.L. (1990). Human neutrophil collagenase. A distinct gene product with homology to other matrix metalloproteinases. J. Biol. Chem. 265, 11421–11424.

Hazuda, D., Webb, R.L., Simon, P. and Young, P. (1989). Purification and characterization of human recombinant precursor interleukin 1β. J. Biol. Chem. 264, 1689–1693.

Hazuda, D.J., Strickler, J., Kueppers, F., Simon, P.L. and Young, P.R. (1990). Processing of precursor interleukin 1β and inflammatory disease. J. Biol. Chem. 265, 6318–6322.

Heck, L.W., Blackburn, W.D., Irwin, M.H. and Abrahamson, D.R. (1990). Degradation of basement membrane laminin by human neutrophil elastase and cathepsin G. Am. J. Path. 136, 1267–1274.

Heiple, J.M. and Ossowski, J.M. (1986). Human neutrophil plasminogen activator is localized in specific granules and is translocated to the cell surface by exocytosis. J. Exp. Med. 164, 826–840.

Henderson, B., Docherty, A.J.P. and Beeley, N.R.A. (1990). Design of inhibitors of articular cartilage destruction. Drugs Future 15, 495–508.

Henson, P.M. and Johnston, R.B. (1987). Tissue injury and inflammation: oxidants, proteinases and cationic proteins. J. Clin. Invest. 79, 669–674.

Herbert, J.M., Frehel, D., Rosso, M.P., Seban, E., Castet, C., Pepin, O., Maffrand, J.P. and Le Fur, G. (1992). Biochemical and pharmacological activities of SR 26831, a potent and selective elastase inhibitor. J. Pharmcol. Exp. Ther. 260, 809–816.

Hibbs, M. and Bainton, D.F. (1989). Human neutrophil gelatinase is a component of specific granules. J. Clin. Invest. 84, 1395–1402.

Hibbs, M.S., Hasty, K.A., Kang, A.H. and Mainardi, C.L. (1984). Secretion of collagenolytic enzymes by human polymorphonuclear leukocytes. Coll. Relat. Res. 4, 467–477.

Hohn, P.A., Popescu, N.C., Hanson, R.D., Salvesen, G. and Ley, T.J. (1989). Genomic organization and chromosomal localization of the human cathepsin G gene. J. Biol. Chem. 264, 13412–13419.

Holers, V.M., Kinoshita, T. and Molina. H. (1992). The evolution of mouse and human complement C3-binding proteins: divergency of form but conservation of function. Immunol. Today 13, 231–236.

Honda. I., Kohrogi, H., Yamaguchi. T., Ando, M. and Araki, S. (1991). Enkephalinase inhibitor potentiates substance P- and capsaicin-induced bronchial smooth muscle contractions in humans. Am. Rev. Resp. Dis. 143, 1416–1418.

Hornbeck, W., Soleilhac, J.M.. Tixier, J.M., Moczar, E. and Robert. L. (1987). Inhibition by elastase inhibitors of the formyl-Met-Leu-Phe-induced chemotaxis of rat polymorphonuclear leukocytes. Cell Biochem. Funct. 5, 113–122.

Howard, A.D., Kostura, M.J., Thornberry, N., Ding, G.J.F., Limjuco, G., Weidner, J., Salley, J.P., Hogquist, K.A., Chaplin, D.D., Mumford, R.A., Schmidt, J.A. and Tocci, M.J. (1991). IL-1-converting enzyme requires aspartic acid residues for processing of the IL-1β precursor at two distinct sites and does not cleave 31-kDa IL-1α. J. Immunol. 147, 2964–2969.

Hu, L.-Y. and Abeles, R.H. (1990). Inhibition of cathepsin B and papain by peptidyl α-keto esters, α-keto amides, α-diketones, and α-keto acids. Arch. Biochem. Biophys. 281, 271–274.

Hubbard, R.C., Casolaro, M.A., Mitchell, M., Sellers, S.E., Arabia, F., Matthay, M.A. and Crystal, R.G. (1989). Fate of aerosolized recombinant DNA-produced α_1-antitrypsin: use of the epithelial surface of the lower respiratory tract to administer proteins of therapeutic importance. Proc. Natl Acad. Sci. USA 86, 680–684.

Huber, A.R. and Weiss, S.J. (1989). Disruption of the sub-endothelial basement membrane during neutrophil diapedesis in an in vitro construct of a blood vessel wall. J. Clin. Invest. 83, 1122–1136.

Huizinga, T.W.J., van der Schoot, C.E., Jost, C., Klaassen, R., Kleijer, M., von dem Borne, A.E.G.K., Roos, D. and Tetteroo, P.A.T. (1988) The PI-linked receptor FcRIII is released on stimulation of neutrophils. Nature 333, 667–669.

Hunninghake, G.W. and Crystal, R.G. (1983). Cigarette smoking and lung destruction: accumulation of neutrophils in the lungs of cigarette smokers. Am. Rev. Respir. Dis. 128, 833–838.

Ichimanu, E., Sakai, H., Saku, T., Kunimatsu, K., Kato, Y., Kato, I. and Yamamoto, K. (1990). Characterization of hemoglobin-hydrolyzing acidic proteinases in human and rat neutrophils. J. Biochem. (Tokyo) 108, 1009–1015.

Idell S., Kucich, U., Fein, A., Kueppers, F., James, H.L., Walsh, P.N., Weinbaum, G., Colman, R.W. and Cohen, A.B. (1985). Neulrophil elastase-releasing factors in broncho-alveolar lavage from patients with adult respiratory distress syndrome. Am. Rev. Respir. Dis. 132, 1098–1105.

International Union of Biochemistry and Molecular Biology (1992). "Enzyme Nomenclature 1991. Recommendations of the Nomenclature Committee of the International Union of Biochemtistry and Molecular Biology on the Nomenclature and Classification of Enzymes". Academic Press, New York.

Ishikawa, I. and Cimasoni, G. (1977). Isolation of cathepsin D from human leukocytes. Biochim. Biophys. Acta 480, 228–240.

Iwamoto, I., Kimura, A., Ochiai, K., Tomioka, H. and Yoshida, S. (1990a). Distribution of neutral endopeptidase activity in human blood leukocytes. J. Leukocyte Biol. 49, 116–125.

Iwamoto, I., Kimura, A., Yamazaki, H., Nakagawa, N., Tomioka, H. and Yoshida, S. (1990b). Neutral endo-peptidase modulates substance P-induced activation of human neutrophils. Int. Arch Allergy Appl. Immunol. 93, 133–138.

Jackson, D.G., Buckley, J. and Bell, J.I. (1992). Multiple variants of the human lymphocyte homing receptor CD44 generated by insertions at a single site in the extracellular domain. J. Biol. Chem. 267, 4732–4739.

Janoff, A. (1985). Elastases and emphysema: current assessment of the protease–antiprotease hypothesis. Am. Rev. Respir. Dis. 132, 417–433.

Janoff, A.G.F., Malemud, C.V. and Elias, J.M. (1976). Degradation of cartilage proteoglycan by human leukocyte granule neutral proteases – a model of joint injury. I. Penetration of enzyme into rabbit articular cartilage and release of $^{35}SO_4$-labeled material from the tissue. J. Clin. Invest. 57, 615–624.

Janoff, A., Raju, L. and Dearing, R. (1983). Levels of elastase activity in bronchoalvcolar lavage fluids of healthy smokers and nonsmokers. Am. Rev. Respir. Dis. 127, 540–544.

Janson, R.W. and Arend, W.P. (1992). Receptor-targeted immunotherapy. Bull. Rheum, Dis. 41, 6–8.

Janusz, M.J. and Doherty, N.S. (1991). Degradation of cartilage matrix proteoglycan by human neutrophils involves both elastase and cathepsin G. J. Immunol. 146, 3922–3928.

Johnson, D. and Travis, J. (1978). Structural evidence for methionine at the reactive site of human α_1-antiproteinase inhibitor. J. Biol. Chem. 253, 7142–7144.

Johnson, W.H. (1990). Collagenase inhibitors: a new class of disease-modifying antirheumatic drugs. Drug News Perspect. 3, 453–458.

Johnson, W.H., Roberts, N.A. and Borkakoti, N. (1987). Collagenase inhibitors: their design and potential therapeutic use. J. Enzyme Inhibition 2, 1–22.

Jutila, M.A., Kishimoto, T.K. and Finken, M. (1991). Low-dose chymotrypsin treatment inhibits neutrophil migration into sites of inflammation in vivo: effects on Mac-1 and MEL-14 adhesion protein expression and function. Cell Immunol. 132, 201–214.

Kaiser, H., Greenwald, R.A., Finestein, G. and Janoff, A. (1976). Degradation of cartilage proteoglycan by human leukocyte granule neutral proteases – a model of joint injury degradation of isolated bovine nasal cartilage proteoglycan. J. Clin. Invest. 57, 625–632.

Kao, R.C., Wehner, N.G., Skubitz, K.M., Gray, B.H. and Hoidal, J.R. (1988). Proteinase 3. A distinct human polymorphonuclear leukocyte proteinase that produces emphysema in hamsters. J. Clin. Invest. 82, 1963–1973.

Kilpatrick, L., Johnson, J.L., Nickbarg, E.B., Wang, Z.M., Clifford, T.F., Banach, M., Cooperman, B.S., Douglas, S.D. and Rubin, H. (1991). Inhibition of human neutrophil superoxide generation by α_1-antichymotrypsin. J. Immunol. 146, 2388–2393.

Kimura, A., Iwamoto, I., Ochiai, K., Nakagawa, N., Tomioka, H. and Yoshida. S. (1990). Neutral endopeptidase activity in human peripheral blood leukocytes. Jpn J. Allergol. 39, 307–312.

Kindt, G.C., Weiland, J.E., Davis, W.B., Gadek, J.E. and Dorinsky, P.M. (1989). Bronchiolitis in adults. A reversible cause of airway obstruction associated with airway neutrophils and neutrophil products. Am. Rev. Respir. Dis. 140, 483–492.

King, C.H., Peck, C.A., Haimes, C.S., Kazura, J.W., Spagnuolo, P.J., Sawer, J.A., Olds, G.R. and Mahmoud, A.A.F. (1986). Modulation of human neutrophil effector functions by monoclonal antibodies against surface membrane molecules of 94,000 and 180,000 molecular weight. Blood 67, 188–194.

King, C.H., Goralnik, C.H., Kleinhenz, P.J., Marino, J.A., Sedor, J.R. and Mahmoud, A.A.F. (1987). Monoclonal antibody characterization of a chymotrypsin-like molecule on neutrophil membrane associated with cellular activation. J. Clin. Invest. 79, 1091–1098.

King, C.H., Hull, A., Kleinhenz, P.J., Phillips, N.F.B. and Marino, J.A. (1991). Structural and functional characterization of the human neutrophil 1-15 antigen, an Mr 65,000 to 70,000 activation-associated membrane protease. J. Immunol. 146, 3115–3123.

Kjeldson, L., Bjerrum, O.W., Askaa, J. and Borregard, N. (1992). Subcellular localization and release of human neutrophil gelatinase, confirming the existence of separate gelatinase containing granules. Biochem. J. 287, 603–610.

Klickstein. L.B., Kaempfer, C.E. and Wintroub, B.U. (1982). The granulocyte angiotensin system: Angiotensin I converting activity of cathepsin G. J. Biol. Chem. 257, 1504–1506.

Knauper, V., Kramer, S., Reinke, H. and Tschesche. H. (1990a). Characterization and activation of procollagenase from human polymorphonuclear leucocytes. N-terminal sequence determination of the proenzyme and various proteolytically activated forms. Eur. J. Biochem. 189, 295–300.

Knauper, V., Reinke, H. and Tschesche, H. (1990b). Inactivation of human plasma α_1-proteinase inhibitor by human PMN leucocyte collagenase. FEBS Lett. 263, 355–357.

Knauper, V., Triebel, S., Reinke, H. and Tschesche, H. (1991). Inactivation of human plasma C1-inhibitor by human PMN leucocyte matrix metalloproteinases. FEBS Lett. 290, 99–102.

Kobayashi, T. and Robinson, J.M. (1991). A novel intracellular compartment with unusual secretory properties in human neutrophils. J. Cell Biol. 113, 743–756.

Kobayashi, Y., Yamamoto, K., Saido, T., Kawasaki, H., Oppenheim, J.J. and Matsushima, K. (1990). Identification of calcium-activated neutral protease as a processing enzyme of human interleukin-1α. Proc. Natl Acad. Sci. USA 87, 5548–5552.

Kohrogi, H., Nadel, J.A., Malfroy, B., Gorman, C., Bridenbaugh, R., Patton, J.S. and Borson. D.B. (1989). Recombinant human enkephalinase (neutral endopeptidase) prevents cough induced by tachykinins in awake guinea pigs. J. Clin. Invest. 84, 781–786.

Konttinen, Y.T., Lindy, O., Kemppinen, P., Saari, H., Suomalainen, K., Vauhkonen, M., Lindy, S. and Sorsa, T. (1991). Collagenase reserves in polymorphonuclear neutrophil leucocytes from synovial fluid and peripheral blood of patients with rheumatoid arthritis. Matrix 11, 296–301.

Kostura, M.J., Tocci, M.J., Limjuco, G., Chin, J., Cameron, P., Hillman, A.G., Chartrain. N.A. and Schmidt, J.A. (1989). Identification of a monocyte specific pre-interleukin 1β convertase activity. Proc. Natl Acad. Sci. USA 86, 5227–5231.

Kueppers, F. and Black, L.F. (1974). Alpha$_1$-antitrypsin and its deficiency. Am. Rev. Resp. Dis. 110, 176–194.

Kunimatsu, M., Higashiyama, S., Sato, K., Ohkubo, I. and Sasaki, M. (1989). Calcium-dependent cysteine proteinase is a precursor of a chemotactic factor for neutrophils. Biochem. Biophys. Res. Comm. 164, 875–882.

Kurachi, K., Chandra, T., Friezner Degen, S.J., White, T.T., Marchioro, S., Woo, L.C. and Davie, E.W. (1981). Cloning and cDNA coding for α_1-antitrypsin. Proc. Natl Acad. Sci. USA 78, 6826–6830.

Kurdowska, A. and Travis, J. (1990). Acute phase protein stimulation by antichymotrypsin-cathepsin G complexes. Evidence for the involvement of interleukin-6. J. Biol. Chem. 265, 21023–21026.

Kusner, D.J. and King, C.H. (1989). Protease-modulation of neutrophil superoxide response. J. Immunol. 143, 1696–1702.

Kusner, D.J., Aucott, J.N., Franceschi, D., Sarasua, M.M., Spagnuolo, P.J. and King, C.H. (1991). Protease priming of neutrophil superoxide production. Effects on membrane lipid order and lateral mobility. J. Biol. Chem. 266, 16465–16471.

Larsson, C. (1978). Natural history and life expectancy in severe α_1-antitrypsin deficiency, Piz. Acta Med. Scand. 204, 345–355.

Larsson, K., Eklund, A., Malmberg, P., Bjermer, L., Lundgren, R. and Belin, L. (1992). Hyaluronic acid (hyaluronan) in BAL fluid distinguishes farmers with allergic alveolitis from farmers with asymptomatic alveolitis. Chest 101, 109–114.

Laskin, D.L., Kimura, T., Sakakibara. S., Riley, D.J. and Berg, R.A. (1986). Chemotactic activity of collagen-like poly-peptides for human peripheral blood neutrophils. J. Leukocyte Biol. 39, 255–266.

Laurell, C.B. and Eriksson, S. (1963). The electrophoretic α_1-globulin pattern of serum in α_1-antitrypsin deficiency. Scand. J. Clin. Lab. Invest. 15, 132–140.

Lauritzen, E., Moller, S. and Leerhoy, S. (1984). Leukocyte migration inhibition in vitro with inhibitors of aspartic and sulphhydryl proteinases. Acta Pathol. Microbiol. Immunol. Scand. 92C, 107–112.

Lee, C.T., Fein, A.M., Lippmann. M., Holtzman, H., Kimbel. P. and Weinbaum. G. (1981). Elastolytic activity in pulmonary lavage fluid from patients with adult respiratory distress syndrome. N. Engl. J. Med. 304, 192–196.

Legendre, J.L. and Jones, H.P. (1988). Purification and characterization of calpain from human polymorphonuclear leukocytes. Inflammation 12, 51–65.

Le Moual, H., Devault, A., Roques, B.P. and Crine, P. (1991). Identification of glutamic acid 646 as a zinc-coordinating residue in endopeptidase-24.11. J. Biol. Chem. 266, 15670–15674.

Lesser, M., Padilla, M.L. and Cardozo, C. (1992). Induction of emphysema in hamsters by intratracheal instillation of cathepsin B. Am. Rev. Respir. Dis. 145, 661–668.

Levy, J., Kolshi, G.B. and Douglas, S.D. (1989). Cathepsin D-like activity in neutrophils and monocytes. Infect. Immun. 57, 1632–1634.

Lew, P.D., Monod, A., Waldvogel, F.A., Dewald, B. and Baggiolini, M. (1986). Quantitative analysis of the cytosolic free calcium dependency of exocytosis from three subcellular compartments in intact human neutrophils. J. Cell Biol. 102, 2197–2204.

Lindemann, A., Riedel, D., Oster, W., Meuer, S.C., Blohm, D., Mertelsmann, R.H. and Hermann, F. (1988). Granulocyte–macrophage colony-stimulating factor induces IL-1 production by human polymorphonuclear neutrophils. J. Immunol. 140, 837–839.

Lindemann, A., Riedel, D., Oster, W., Ziegler-Heitbrock, H.W.L., Mertelsmann, R. and Hermann, F. (1989). Granulocyte–macrophage colony-stimulating factor induces cytokine secretion by human polymorphonuclear leukocytes. J. Clin. Invest. 83, 1308–1312.

Lindgren, B.R. and Andersson, R.G. (1989). Angiotensin-converting enzyme inhibitors and their influence on inflammation, bronchial reactivity and cough. A research review. Med. Toxicol. Adverse Drug Exp. 4, 369–380.

Lindgren, B.R., Andersson, C.D. and Andersson, R.G. (1987). Potentiation of inflammatory reactions in guinea-pig skin by an angiotensin converting enzyme inhibitor (MK 422). Eur. J. Pharmacol. 135, 383–387.

Lomas, D.A., Afford, S.C. and Stockley, R.A. (1991). Modulation of neutrophil chemotaxis by cell surface serine proteases. Am. Rev. Resp. Dis. 143, A323.

Lucey, E.C., Stone, P.J., Breuer, R., Christensen, T.G., Calore, J.D., Catanese, A., Franzblau, C. and Snider, G.L. (1985). Effect of combined human neutrophil cathepsin G and elastase on induction of secretory cell metaplasia and emphysema in hamsters, with in vitro observations on elastolysis by these enzymes. Am. Rev. Respir. Dis. 132, 362–366.

Lucey, E.C., Stone, P.J., Ciccolella, D.E., Breuer, R., Christensen, T.G., Thompson, R.C. and Snider, G.L. (1990). Recombinant human secretory leukocyte–protease inhibitor: in vitro properties, and amelioration of human neutrophil elastase-induced emphysema and secretory cell metaplasia in the hamster. J. Lab. Clin. Med. 115, 224–232.

Lundberg, E., Bergenfeldt, M. and Ohlsson, K. (1991). Release of immunoreactive human neutrophil proteinase 4, normally and in peritonitis. Scand. J. Clin. Lab. Invest. 51, 23–30.

Lupke, U., Rautenberg, W. and Tschesche, H. (1982). Kininogenases from human polymorphonuclear leukocytes. Agents Actions 9 (Suppl.), 308–314.

Lupke, U., Meyer, K., Geiger, R. and Tschesche, H. (1983). Isolation of two kallikreins from human leukocytes. Hoppe-Seylers Z. Physiol. Chem. 364, 1174–1175.

Mainardi, C.L., Hasty, D.L., Sayer, J.M. and Kang, A.H. (1980). Specific cleavage of human type III collagen by human polymorphonuclear leukocyte elastase. J. Biol. Chem. 255, 12006–12010.

Malemud, C.J. and Janoff, A. (1975). Identification of neutral proteases in human neutrophil granules that degrade articular proteoglycan. Arthritis Rheum. 18, 361–368.

Mallya, S.K. and Van Wart, H.E. (1987). Inhibition of human neutrophil collagenase by gold(I) salts used in chrysotherapy. Biochem. Biophys. Res. Comm. 144, 101–108.

Mallya, S.K. and Van Wart, H.E. (1989). Mechanism of inhibition of human neutrophil collagenase by gold(I) chrysotherapeutic compounds. Interaction at a heavy metal binding site. J. Biol. Chem. 264, 1594–1601.

Mallya, S.K., Mookhtiar, K.A., Gao, Y., Brew, K., Dioszegi, M., Birkedal-Hansen. H. and Van Wart, H.E. (1990). Characterization of 58-kilodalton human neutrophil collagenase: comparison with human fibroblast collagenase. Biochemistry 29, 10628–10634.

Marucha, P.T., Zeff, R.A. and Kreutzer, D.L. (1990). Cytokine regulation of IL-1β gene expression in the human polymorphonuclear leukocyte. J. Immunol. 145, 2932–2937.

Marucha, P.T., Zeff, R.A. and Kreutzer, D.L. (1991). Cytokine induced IL-1β gene expression in the human polymorphonuclear leukocyte: transcriptional and post-translational regulation by tumor necrosis factor and IL-1. J. Immunol. 147, 2603–2608.

Matrisian, L.M. (1990). Metalloproteinases and their inhibitors in matrix remodeling. Trends Genetics 6, 121–125.

Matrisian, L.M. (1992). The matrix-degrading metalloproteinases. BioEssays 14, 455–463.

Matsumoto, M., Seya, T. and Nagasawa, S. (1992). Polymorphism and proteolytic fragments of granulocyte membrane cofactor protein (MCP, CD46) of complement. Biochem. J. 281, 493–499.

McDonald, J.A. and Kelley, D.G. (1980). Degradation of fibronectin by human leukocyte elastase. Release of biologically active fragments. J. Biol. Chem. 255, 8848–8858.

McElvaney, N.G., Hubbard, R.C., Birrer, P., Chernick, M.S., Caplan, D.B., Frank, M.M. and Crystal, R.G. (1991). Aerosol α1-antitrypsin treatment for cystic fibrosis. Lancet 337, 392–394.

McGuire, W.W., Spragg, R.G., Cohen, A.B. and Cochrane, C.G. (1982). Studies on the pathogenesis of the adult respiratory distress syndrome. J. Clin. Invest. 69, 543–553.

McMurray, J. and Chopra, M. (1991). Influence of ACE inhibitors on free radicals and reperfusion injury: pharmacological curiosity or therapeutic hope? Br. J. Clin. Pharmacol. 31, 373–379.

McPhail, L.C. and Snyderman, R. (1983). Activation of the respiratory burst enzyme in human polymorphonuclear leukocytes by chemoattractants and other soluble stimuli. Evidence that the same oxidase is activated by different transductional mechanisms. J. Clin. Invest. 72, 192–200.

Mehdi, S. (1991). Cell-penetrating inhibitors of calpain. Trends Biochem. Sci. 16, 150–153.

Mehdi, S., Angelastro, M.R., Wiseman, J.S. and Bey, P. (1988). Inhibition of the proteolysis of rat erythrocyte membrane proteins by a synthetic inhibitor of calpain. Biochem. Biophys. Res. Comm. 157, 1117–1123.

Mehdi, S., Angelastro, M.R., Burkhart, J.P., Koehl, J.R., Peet, N.P. and Bey, P. (1990). The inhibition of human neutrophil elastase and cathepsin G by peptidyl 1,2-dicarbonyl derivatives. Biochem. Biophys. Res. Comm. 166, 595–600.

Mellgren, R.L. (1987). Calcium-dependent proteases: an enzyme system active at cellular membranes. FASEB J. 1, 110–115.

Melloni, E., Pontremoli, S., Michetti, M., Sacco, O., Sparatore, B., Salamino, F. and Horecker, B.L. (1985). Binding of protein kinase C to neutrophil membranes in the presence of Ca++ and its activation by a Ca++-requiring proteinase. Proc. Natl Acad. Sci. USA 82, 6435–6439.

Melloni, E., Pontremoli, S., Michetti, M., Sacco, O., Sparatore, B. and Horecker, B.L. (1986). The involvement of calpain in the activation of protein kinase C in neutrophils stimulated by phorbol myristic acid. J. Biol. Chem. 261, 4101–4105.

Mizutani, H., Black, R. and Kupper, T.S. (1991). Human keratinocytes produce but do not process pro-interleukin-1 (IL-1) beta. Different strategies of IL-1 production and processing in monocytes and keratinocytes. J. Clin. Invest. 87, 1066–1071.

Mollinedo, F. and Schneider, D.L. (1984). Subcellular localization of cytochrome b and ubiquinone in a tertiary granule of resting human neutrophils and evidence for a proton pump ATPase. J. Biol. Chem. 259, 7143–7150.

Mookhtiar, K.A., Wang, F. and Van Wart, H.E. (1986). Functional constituents of the active site of human neutrophil collagenase. Arch. Biochem. Biophys. 246, 645–649.

Mosley, B., Dower, S.K., Gillis, S. and Cosman, D. (1987). Determination of the minimum polypeptide lengths of the functionally active sites of human interleukins 1α and 1β. Proc. Natl Acad. Sci. USA 84, 4572–4576.

Movat, H.Z., Steinberg, S.G., Habal, F.M. and Ramadive, N.S. (1973). Demonstration of a kinin-generating enzyme in the lysosomes of human polymorphonuclear leukocytes. Lab. Invest. 29, 669–684.

Movat, H.Z., Habal, F.M. and Macmorine, D.R.L. (1976). Neutral proteases of human PMN leukocytes with kininogenase activity. Int. Arch. Allergy Appl. Immunol. 50, 257–281.

Murlas, C.G., Lang, Z., Williams, G.J. and Chodimella, V. (1992). Aerosolized neutral endopeptidase reverses ozone-induced airway hyperreactivity to substance P. J. Appl. Physiol. 72, 1133–1141.

Murphy, G., Bretz, B., Baggiolini, M. and Reynolds, J.J. (1980). The latent collagenase and gelatinase of human polymorphonuclear neutrophil leucocytes. Biochem. J. 192, 517–525.

Murphy, G., Reynolds, J.J., Bretz, U. and Baggiolini, M. (1982). Partial purification of collagenase and gelatinase from human polymorphonuclear leucocytes. Biochem. J. 203, 209–221.

Murphy, G., Crockett, M.I., Ward. R.V. and Docherty, A.J.P. (1991). Matrix metalloproteinase degradation of elastin, type IV collagen and proteoglycan: a quantitative comparison of the activities of 95 kDa and 72 kDa gelatinases, stromelysins-1 and -2 and punctuated metalloproteinase (PUMP). Biochem. J. 277, 277–279.

Nadel, J. (1991). Neutral endopeptidase modulates neurogenic inflammation. Eur. Respir. J. 4, 745–754.

Nadel, J.A. and Borson, D.B. (1991). Modulation of neurogenic inflammation by neutral endopeptidase. Am. Rev. Respir. Dis. 143, S33–S36.

Nagase, H., Barrett, A.J. and Woessner, J.F.J. (1992). Nomenclature and glossary of the matrix metalloproteinases. Matrix (Suppl. 1), 421–424.

Nakajima, K., Powers, J.C., Ashe, B.M. and Zimmerman, M. (1979). Mapping the extended substrate binding site of cathepsin G and human leukocyte elastase. J. Biol. Chem. 254, 4027–4032.

Nakamura, H., Okano, K., Aoki, Y. Shimizu, H. and Naruto, M. (1987). Nucleotide sequence of bone marrow serine protease (human medullasin) gene. Nucleic Acid Res. 15, 9601–9602.

Nakamura, A., Yoshimura, H.K., McElvaney, N.G. and Crystal, R.G. (1992). Neutrophil elastase in respiratory epithelial lining fluid of individuals with cystic fibrosis induces interleukin-8 gene expression in a human bronchial epithelial cell line. J. Clin. Invest. 89, 1478–1484.

Needham, L., Hellewell, P.G., Williams, T.J. and Gordon, J.L. (1988). Endothelial cell functional responses and increased vascular permeability induced by polycations. Lab. Invest. 59, 538–548.

Netzel-Arnett, S., Fields, G.B., Birkedal-Hansen, H. and Van Wart, H.E. (1991a). Sequence specificities of human fibroblast and neutrophil collagenases. J. Biol. Chem. 266, 6747–6755.

Netzel-Arnett, S., Mallya, S.K., Nagase. H., Birkedal-Hansen, H. and Van Wart, H.E. (1991b). Continuously recording fluorescent assays optimized for five human matrix metalloproteinases. Anal. Biochem. 195, 86–92.

Nixon, J.S., Bottomley, K.M., Broadhurst, M.J., Brown, P.A., Johnson, W.H., Lawton, G., Marley, J., Sedgwick, A.D. and Wilkinson, S.E. (1991). Potent collagenase inhibitors prevent interleukin-1-induced cartilage damage in vitro. Int. J. Tissue React. 13, 237–241.

O'Connor-Westerik, J. and Wolfenden, R. (1972). Aldehydes as inhibitors of papain. J. Biol. Chem. 247, 8195–8197.

Odeberg, H. and Ohlsson, I. (1975). Antibacterial activity of cationic proteins from human granulocytes. J. Clin. Invest. 56, 1118–1124.

Ogata, Y., Enghild, J.J. and Nagase, H. (1992). Matrix metalloproteinase 3 (stromelysin) activates the precursor for the human matrix metalloproteinase 9. J. Biol. Chem. 267, 3581–3584.

Ohlsson, K. and Ohlsson, I. (1973). The neutral proteases of human granulocytes. Eur. J. Biochem. 36, 473–481.

Ohlsson, K., Linder, C. and Rosengren, M. (1990). Monoclonal antibodies specific for neutrophil proteinase 4: production and use for isolation of the enzyme. Biol. Chem. Hoppe-Seyler 371, 549–556.

Okada, Y., Watanabe, S., Nakanishi, I., Kishi, J.-I., Hayakawa, T., Watorek, W., Travis, J. and Nagase, H. (1988). Inactivation of tissue inhibitor of metalloproteinases by neutrophil elastase and other serine proteases. FEBS Lett. 229, 157–160.

Okano, K., Aoki, Y., Sakurai, Kajitani, M., Kanai, S., Shimazu, T. and Naruto, M. (1987). Molecular cloning of complementary DNA for human medullasin: an inflammatory serine protease in bone marrow cells. J. Biochem. 102, 13–16.

Oppenheim, J.J.. Kovacs, E.J., Matsushima, K. and Durum, S.K. (1986). There is more than one interleukin 1. Immunol. Today 7, 45–55.

Orlowski, M., Orlowski, J., Lesser, M. and Kilburn, K.H. (1991). Proteolytic enzymes in bronchopulmonary lavage fluids: cathepsin B-like activity and prolyl endopeptidase. J. Lab. Clin. Med. 97, 467–476.

Orning, L., Krivi, G., Bild, G., Gierse, J., Aykent, S. and Fitzpatrick, F.A. (1991a). Inhibition of leukotriene A$_4$ hydrolase/aminopeptidase by captopril. J. Biol. Chem. 266, 16507–16511.

Orning, L., Krivi, G. and Fitzpatrick, F.A. (1991b). Leukotriene A4 hydrolase. Inhibition by bestatin and intrinsic aminopeptidase activity establish its functional resemblance to metallohydrolase enzymes. J. Biol. Chem. 266, 1375–1378.

Osthues, A., Knauper, V., Oberhoff, R., Reinke, H. and Tschesche, H. (1992). Isolation and characterization of tissue inhibitors of metalloproteinases (TIMP-1 and TIMP-2) from human rheumatoid synovial fluid. FEBS Lett. 296, 16–20.

Painter, R.G. (1991). Inhibition of neutrophil neutral endopeptidase by phosphoramidon blocks recycling of formyl-Met-Leu-Phe receptors. FASEB J. 5, A1352.

Painter, R.G., Dukes, R., Sullivan, J., Carter, R. and Erdos, E.G. (1988). Function of neutral endopeptidase on the cell membrane of human neutrophils. J. Biol. Chem. 263, 9456–9461.

Pannell, R., Johnson, D. and Travis, J. (1974). Isolation and properties of human plasma α_1-proteinase inhibitor. Biochemistry 13, 5439–5445.

Parkes, C., Kembhavi, A.A. and Barrett, A.J. (1985). Calpain inhibition by peptide epoxides. Biochem. J. 230, 509–516.

Peet, N.P., Burkhart, J.P., Angelastro, M.R., Giroux, E.L., Mehdi, S., Bey, P., Kolb, M., Neises, B. and Schirlin, D. (1990). Synthesis of peptidyl fluoromethyl ketones and peptidyl α-keto esters as inhibitors of porcine pancreatic elastase, human neutrophil elastase, and rat and human neutrophil cathepsin G. J. Med. Chem. 33, 394–407.

Peltonen, L. (1978). Collagenase in synovial fluid. Scand. J. Rheumatol. 7, 49–54.

Perez, H.D., Marder, S., Elfman, F. and Ives, H.E. (1987). Human neutrophils contain subpopulations of specific granules exhibiting different sensitivities to changes in cytosolic free calcium. Biochem. Biophys. Res. Comm. 145, 976–981.

Peterson, M.W., Stone, P. and Shasby, D.M. (1987). Cationic neutrophil proteins increase transendothelial albumin movement. J. Appl. Physiol. 62, 1521–1530.

Pontremoli, S. and Melloni, E. (1986). Extralysosomal proteinase degradation. Ann. Rev. Biochem. 55, 455–481.

Pontremoli, S., Melloni, E., Michetti, M., Sacco, O., Sparatore, B., Salamino, F., Damiani, G. and Horecker, B.L. (1986). Cytolytic effects of neutrophils: role for a membrane-bound neutral proteinase. Proc. Natl Acad. Sci. USA 83, 1685–1689.

Pontremoli, S., Molloni, E., Michetti, M., Sparatore. B., Salamino, F., Sacco, O. and Horecker, B.L. (1987). Phosphorylation and proteolytic modification of specific cytoskeletal proteins in human neutrophils stimulated by phorbol 12-myristate-13-acetate. Proc. Natl Acad. Sci. USA 84, 3604–3608.

Pontremoli, S., Molloni, E., Damiani, G., Salamino, F., Sparatore, B., Michetti, M. and Horecker, B.L. (1988). Effects of a monoclonal anti-calpain antibody on responses of stimulated human neutrophils. Evidence for a role for proteolytically modified protein kinase C. J. Biol. Chem. 263, 1915–1919.

Porteu, F., Brockhaus, M., Wallach, D., Engelmann, H. and Nathan, C.F. (1991). Human neutrophil elastase releases a ligand-binding fragment from the 75-kDa tumor necrosis factor (TNF) receptor. Comparison with the proteolytic activity responsible for shedding of TNF receptors from stimulated neutrophils. J. Biol. Chem. 266, 18846–18853.

Porteu, F. and Nathan, C. (1991). Shedding of tumor necrosis factor receptors by activated human neutrophils. J. Exp. Med. 172, 599–607.

Powers, J.C. (1983). Synthetic elastase inhibitors: prospects for use in the treatment of emphysema. Am. Rev. Respir. Dis. 127, 554–558.

Powers, J.C., Gupton, B.F., Harley, A.D., Nishino, N. and Whitley, R.J. (1977). Specificity of porcine pancreatic elastase, human leukocyte elastase and cathepsin G. Inhibition with peptide chloromethyl ketones. Biochim. Biophys. Acta 485, 156–166.

Pozzan. T., Lew, D.P., Wollheim, C.B. and Tsein, R.Y. (1983). Is cytosolic ionized calcium regulating neutrophil activation? Science 221, 1413–1415.

Prior, C., Barbee, R.A., Evans, P.M., Townsend, P.J., Primett, Z.S., Fyhrquist, F., Gronhagen-Riska, C. and Haslam, P.L. (1990). Lavage versus serum measurements of lysozyme, angiotensin converting enzyme and other inflammatory markers in pulmonary sarcoidosis. Eur. Respir. J. 3, 1146–1154.

Pryzwansky, K.B., Wyatt, T., Reed, W. and Ross, G.D. (1991). Phorbol ester induces transient focal concentrations of functional, newly expressed CR3 in neutrophils at sites of specific granule exocytosis. Eur. J. Cell Biol. 54, 61–75.

Rao, N.V., Wehner, N.G., Marshall, B.C., Gray, W.R., Gray, B.H. and Hoidal, J.R. (1991). Characterization of Proteinase 3 (PR-3), a neutrophil serine proteinase. J. Biol. Chem. 266, 9540–9548.

Rasnick, D. (1985). Synthesis of peptide fluoromethyl ketones and the inhibition of human cathepsin B. Anal. Biochem. 149, 461–465.

Reilly, C.F., Fukunaga, Y., Powers, J.C. and Travis, J. (1984). Effect of neutrophil cathepsin G on elastin degradation by neutrophil elastase. Hoppe-Seyler's Z. Physiol. Chem. 365, 1131–1135.

Remold-O'Donnell, E. and Rosen, F.S. (1990). Proteolytic fragmentation of sialophorin: localization of the activation-inducing site and examination of the role of sialic acid. J. Immunol. 145, 3372–3378.

Remold-O'Donnell, E., Nixon, J.C. and Rose, R.M. (1989). Characterization of the human elastase inhibitor molecule associated with monocytes, macrophages and neutrophils. J. Exp. Med. 169, 1071–1086.

Remold-O'Donnell, E., Chin, J. and Alberts, M. (1992). Sequence and molecular characterization of human monocyte/neutrophil elastase inhibitor. Proc. Natl Acad. Sci. USA 89, 5635–5639.

Renesto, P. and Chignard, M. (1991). Tumor necrosis factor-α enhances platelet activation via cathepsin G released from neutrophils. J. Immunol. 146, 2305–2309.

Renesto, P., Ferrer, L.P. and Chignard, M. (1990). Interference of recombinant eglin C, a proteinase inhibitor extracted from leeches, with neutrophil-mediated platelet activation. Lab. Invest. 62, 409–416.

Repine, J.E. and Beehler, C.J. (1991). Neutrophils and adult respiratory distress syndrome, two interlocking perspectives in 1991. Am. Rev. Respir. Dis. 144, 251–252.

Rhyne, J.A., Mizel, S.B., Taylor, R.G., Chedid, M. and McCall, M. (1988). Characterization of the human interleukin 1 receptor on human polymorphonuclear leukocytes. Clin. Immunol. Immunopathol. 48, 354–361.

Rice, W.G. and Weiss, S.J. (1990). Regulation of proteolysis at the neutrophil–substrate interface by secretory leukoprotease inhibitor. Science 249, 178–181.

Rice, W.G., Kinkade, J.M. and Parmley, R.T. (1986). High resolution of heterogeneity among human neutrophil granules: physical, biochemical and ultrastructural properties of isolated fractions. Blood 68, 541–555.

Riley, D.J., Berg, R.A., Soltys, R.A., Kerr, J.S., Guss, H.N., Curran, S.F. and Laskin, D.L. (1988). Neutrophil response following intratracheal instillation of collagen peptides into rat lungs. Exp. Lung Res. 14, 549–563.

Rinaldo, J.E. and Dauber, J.H. (1985). Modulation of endotoxin-induced neutrophil alveolitis by captopril and by hyperoxia. J. Leukocyte Biol. 37, 87–99.

Roberge, C.J., Grassi, J., De Medicis, R., Frobert, Y., Lussier, A., Naccache, P.H. and Poubelle, P.E. (1991). Crystal–neutrophil interactions lead to interleukin-1 synthesis. Agents Actions 34, 38–41.

Rosengren, S. and Arfors, K.-E. (1990). Neutrophil-mediated vascular leakage is not suppressed by leukocyte elastase inhibitors. Am. J. Physiol. 259 (Heart Circ. Physiol. 28), H1288–H1294.

Rosengren, S. and Arfors, K.-E. (1991). Polycations induce microvascular leakage of macromolecules in hamster cheek pouch. Inflammation 15, 159–172.

Rothe, G., Klingel, S., Assflag-Machleidt, I., Machleidt, W., Zirkelbach, C., Banati, R.B., Mangel, W.F. and Valet, G. (1992). Flow cytometric analysis of protease activities in vital cells. Biol. Chem. Hoppe-Seyler 373, 547–554.

Roughley, P.J. (1977). The degradation of cartilage proteoglycans by tissue proteases. Proteoglycan heterogeneity and the pathway of proteolytic degradation. Biochem. J. 167, 639–647.

Rubin, H. (1992). The biology and biochemistry of antichymotrypsin and its potential role as a therapeutic agent. Biol. Chem. Hoppe-Seyler 373, 497–502.

Rudolphus, A., Kramps, J.A. and Dijkman, J.H. (1991). Effect of human antileukoprotease on experimental emphysema. Eur. Respir. J. 4, 31–39.

Saari, H., Suomalainen, K., Lindy, O., Konttinen, Y.T. and Sorsa, T. (1990). Activation of latent human neutrophil collagenase by reactive oxygen species and serine proteases. Biochem. Biophys. Res. Comm. 171, 979–987.

Salvesen, G., Farley, D., Shuman, J., Przybyla, A., Reilly, C. and Travis, J. (1987). Molecular cloning of human cathepsin G: structural similarity to mast cell and cytotoxic T lymphocyte proteinases. Biochemistry 26, 2289–2293.

Sasaki. T., Kikuchi, T., Fukui, I. and Murachi, T. (1986). Inactivation of calpain I and calpain II by specificity-oriented tripeptidyl chloromethyl ketones. J. Biochem. 99, 173–179.

Schettler, A., Thorn, H., Jockusch, B.M. and Tschesche, H. (1991). Release of proteinases from stimulated polymorphonuclear leukocytes. Evidence for subclasses of the main granule types and their association with cytoskeletal components. Eur. J. Biochem. 197, 197–202.

Schuster, A., Ueki, I. and Nadel, J. (1992). Neutrophil elastase stimulates tracheal submucosal gland secretion that is inhibited by ICI 200,355. Am. J. Physiol. 262 (Lung Cell Mol. Physiol. 6), L86–91.

Selak, M.A., Chignard, M. and Smith, J.B. (1988). Cathepsin G is a strong platelet agonist released by neutrophils. Biochem. J. 251, 293–299.

Sengelov, H., Nielsen, M. H. and Borregaard, N. (1992). Separation of human neutrophil plasma membrane from intracellular vesicles containing alkaline phosphatase and NADPH oxidase activity by free flow electrophoresis. J. Biol. Chem. 267, 14912–14917.

Senior, R.M., Griffin, G.L., Fliszar, C.J., Shapiro, S.D., Goldberg, G.I. and Welgus, H.G. (1991). Human 92- and 72-kilodalton type IV collagenases are elastases. J. Biol. Chem. 266, 7870–7875.

Sessa, W.C., Kaw, S., Hecker, M. and Vane, J.R. (1991). The biosynthesis of endothelin-1 by human polymorphonuclear leukocytes. Biochem. Biophys. Res. Comm. 174, 613–618.

Shah, S.K., Dorn, C.P., Finke, P.E., Hale, J.J., Hagmann, W.K., Brause, K.A., Chandler, G.O., Kissinger, A.L., Ashe, B.M., Weston, H., Knight, W.B., Maycock, A.L., Dellea, P.S., Fletcher, D.S., Hand, K.M., Mumford, R.A., Underwood, D.J. and Doherty, J.B. (1992) Orally active β-lactam inhibitors of human leukocyte elastase-1. Activity of 3,3-Diethyl-2-azetidinones. J. Med. Chem. 35, 3745–3754.

Shaw, E. (1988). Peptidyl sulfonium salts: a new class of protease inhibitors. J. Biol. Chem. 263, 2768–2772.

Shaw, E. (1990). Cysteinyl proteinases and their selective inactivation. Adv. Enzymol. Relat. Areas Mol. Biol. 63, 271–347.

Shenvi, A.B. and Kettner, C. (1984). Inhibition of the serine proteases leukocyte elastase, pancreatic elastase, cathepsin G and chymotrypsin by peptide boronic acids. J. Biol. Chem. 259, 15106–15114.

Shephard, E.G., Beer, S.M., Anderson, R., Strachan, A.F., Nel, A.E. and de Beer, F.C. (1989). Generation of biologically active C-reactive protein peptides by a neutral protease on the membrane of phorbol myristate acetate-stimulated neutrophils. J. Immunol. 143, 2974–2981.

Shephard, E.G., Anderson, R., Rosen, O., Myer, M.S., Fridkin, M., Strachan, A.F. and de Beer, F.C. (1990). Peptides generated from C-reactive protein by a neutrophil membrane protease. Amino acid sequence and effects of peptides on neutrophil oxidative metabolism and chemotaxis. J. Immunol. 145, 1469–1476.

Shipp, M.A., Stefano, G.B., D'Adamio, L., Switzer, S.N., Howard, F.D., Sinisterra, J., Scharrer, B. and Reinhertz, E.L. (1990). Down-regulation of enkephalin mediated inflammatory responses by CD10/neutral endopeptidase 24.11. Nature 347, 394–396.

Shipp, M.A., Stefano, G.B., Switzer, S.N., Griffin, J.D. and Reinherz, E.L. (1991). CD10, CALLA, neutral endopeptidase 24.11 modulates inflammatory peptide-induced changes in neutrophil morphology, migration and adhesion proteins and is itself regulated by neutrophil activation. Blood 78, 1834–1841.

Shoji-Kasai, Y., Senshu, M., Iwashita, S. and Imahori, K. (1988). Thiol protease-specific inhibitor E-64 arrests human epidermoid carcinoma A431 cells at mitotic metaphase. Proc. Natl. Acad. Sci. USA 85, 146–150.

Singer, I.I., Scott, S., Kawka, D.W. and Kazazis, D.M. (1989). Adhesomes: specific granules containing receptors for laminin, C3bi/fibrinogen, fibronectin and vitronectin in human polymorphonuclear leukocytes and monocytes. J. Cell Biol. 109, 3169–3182.

Sinha, S., Watorek, W., Karr, S., Giles, J., Bode, W. and Travis, J. (1987). Primary structure of human neutrophil elastase. Proc. Natl Acad. Sci. USA 84, 2228–2232.

Skidgel, R.A., Jackman, H.L. and Erdos, E.G. (1991). Metabolism of substance P and bradykinin by human neutrophils. Biochem. Pharmacol. 41, 1335–1344.

Skiles. J.W., Fuchs, V., Miao, C., Sorcek, R., Grozinger, K.G., Mauldin, S.C., Vitous, J., Mui. P.W., Jacober, S., Chow, G., Matteo, M., Skoog, M., Weldon, S. M., Possanza, G., Keirns, J., Letts, G. and Rosenthal, A.S. (1992). Inhibition of human leukocyte elastase (HLE) by N-substituted peptidyl trifluoromethyl ketones. J. Med. Chem. 35, 641–661.

Smith, G.P., Sharp, G. and Peters, T.J. (1985). Isolation and characterization of alkaline phosphatase-containing granules (phosphasomes) from human polymorphonuclear leucocytes. J. Cell Sci. 76, 167–178.

Smith, R.A., Copp, L.J., Coles, P.J., Pauls, H.W., Robinson, V.J., Spencer, R.W., Heard, S.B. and Krantz, A. (1988). New inhibitors of cysteine proteinases. Peptidyl acyloxymethyl ketones and the quiescent nucleofuge strategy. J. Am. Chem. Soc. 110, 4429–4431.

Smolen, J.E. (1989). In "The Neutrophil: Cellular Biochemistry and Physiology" (ed. M.B. Hallett). pp. 23–61. CRC Press Inc., Boca Raton.

Smolen, J.E., Korchak, H.M. and Weissmann, G. (1981). The roles of extracellular and intracellular calcium in lysosomal enzyme release and superoxide anion generation by human neutrophils. Biochim. Biophys. Acta 677, 512–520.

Snyder, R. A., Kaempfer, C. E. and Wintroub, B. U. (1985). Chemistry of a human monocyte-derived cell line (U937): identification of the angiotensin I converting enzyme activity as leukocyte cathepsin G. Blood 65, 176–182.

Sommerhoff, C.P., Nadel, J.A., Basbaum, C.B. and Caughey, G.H. (1990). Neutrophil elastase and cathepsin G stimulate secretion from cultured bovine airway gland serous cells. J. Clin. Invest. 85, 682–689.

Sommerhoff, C.P., Krell, R.D., Williams, J.L., Gomes, B.C., Strimpler, A. M. and Nadel, J. (1991). Inhibition of human elastase by ICI 200,355. Eur. J. Pharm. 193, 153–158.

Sorsa, T., Konttinen, Y.T., Lauhio, A., Saari, H., Suomalainen, K. and Lindy, S. (1989a). Gold(I) compounds and human neutrophil collagenase [letter; comment]. J. Rheumatol., 16, 1009–1010.

Sorsa. T., Saaari, H., Konttinen, Y. T., Suomalainen, K., Lindy, S. and Uitto, V. J. (1989b). Non-proteolytic activation of latent human neutrophil collagenase and its role in matrix destruction in periodontal diseases. Int. J. Tissue React. 11, 153–159.

Sorsa, T., Suomalainen, K. and Uitto, V.J. (1990). The role of gingival crevicular fluid and salivary interstitial collagenases in human periodontal diseases. Arch. Oral Biol. 35, (Suppl.), 193S–196S.

Sorsa. T.. Konttinen. Y., Lindy, O., Ritchlin, C., Saari, H., Suomalainen, K., Eklund. K.K. and Santavirta, S. (1992). Collagenase in synovitis of rheumatoid arthritis. Semin. Arthritis Rheum. 22, 44–53.

Springman, E.B., Angleton, E.L., Birkedal-Hansen, H. and Van Wart, H. E. (1990). Multiple modes of activation of latent human fibroblast collagenase: Evidence for the role of a Cys_{73} active-site zinc complex in latency and a "cysteine switch" mechanism for activation. Proc. Natl Acad. Sci. USA 87, 364–368.

Starcher, B. and Williams, I. (1989). The beige mouse: role of neutrophil elastase in the development of pulmonary emphysema. Exp. Lung Res. 15, 785–800.

Starkey, P.M., Barrett, A.J. and Burleigh, M.C. (1977). The degradation of articular collagen by neutrophil proteinases. Biochim. Biophys. Acta 483, 386–397.

Stetler-Stevenson. W.G., Krutzsch, H.C. and Liotta, L. (1989). Tissue inhibitor of metalloproteinase (TIMP-2): a new member of the metalloproteinase inhibitor family. J. Biol. Chem. 264, 17374–17378.

Stetler-Stevenson, W.G., Bersch, N. and Golde, D.W. (1992). Tissue inhibitor of metalloproteinase-2 (TIMP-2) has erythroid potentiating activity. FEBS Lett. 296, 231–234.

Stockley, R.A., Hill, S.L. and Burnett, D. (1990a). Proteinases in chronic lung infection. Ann. N.Y. Acad. Sci. 624, 257–266.

Stockley, R.A., Shaw, J., Afford, S.C., Morrison, H.M. and Burnett, D. (1990b). Effect of α_1-protease inhibitor on neutrophil chemotaxis. Am. J. Respir. Cell Mol. Biol. 2, 163–170.

Stolk, J., Davies, P., Kramps, J.A., Dijkman, J.H., Humes, J.J., Knight, W.B., Green, B.G., Mumford, R., Bonney, R.J. and Hanlon, W.A. (1992). Potency of antileukoprotease and α_1-antitrypsin to inhibit degradation of fibrinogen by adherent polymorphonuclear leukocytes from normal subjects and patients with chronic granulomatous disease. Am. J. Respir. Cell Mol. Biol. 521–526.

Stone, P.J., Calore, J.D., McGowan, S.E., Bernardo, J., Snider, G.L. and Franzblau, C. (1983). Functional α_1-protease inhibitor in the lower respiratory tract of cigarette smokers is not decreased. Science 221, 1187–1189.

Stricklin, G.P. and Welgus, H.G. (1986). Physiological relevance of the erythroid-potentiating activity of TIMP. Nature 321, 628.

Suomalainen, K., Sorsa, T., Lindy, O., Saari, H., Konttinen, Y.T. and Uitto, V. J. (1991). Hypochlorous acid induced activation of human neutrophil and gingival crevicular fluid collagenase can be inhibited by ascorbate. Scand. J. Dent. Res. 99, 397–405.

Suomalainen, K., Sorsa, T., Golub, L.M., Ramamurthy, N., Lee, H.M., Uitto, V.J., Saari, H. and Konttinen. Y.T. (1992). Specificity of the anticollagenase action of tetra-

cyclines: relevance to their anti-inflammatory potential. Animicrob. Agents Chemother. 36, 227–229.

Suter, S., Schaad, U. B., Tegner, H., Ohlsson, K., Desgrandchamps, D. and Wardvogel, F.A. (1986). Levels of free granulocytc elastase in bronchial secretions from patients with cystic fibrosis: effect of antimicrobial treatment against *Pseudomonas aeruginosa*. J. Infect. Dis. 153, 902–909.

Suter, S., Schaad, U.B., Morgenthaler, J.J., Chevallier, I. and Schnebli, H.P. (1988). Fibronectin-cleaving actively in bronchial secretions of patients with cystic fibrosis. J. Infect. Dis. 158, 89–100.

Suzuki. K. (1987). Calcium activated neutral protease: domain structure and activity regulation. Trends Biochem. Sci. 12, 103–105.

Suzuki, K., Shimizu, K., Hamamoto, T., Nakagawa, Y., Hamakubo, T. and Yamamuro, T. (1990). Biochemical demonstration of calpains and calpastatin in osteoarthritic synovial fluid. Arthritis Rheum. 33, 728–732.

Takahashi, T., Inada, S., Pommier, C.G., O'Shea, J.J. and Brown, E.J. (1985). Osmotic stress and the freeze–thaw cycle cause shedding of Fc and C3b receptors by human polymorphonuclear leukocytes. J. Immunol. 134, 4062–4068.

Takahashi, H., Nukiwa, T., Basset, P. and Crystal, R. G. (1988a). Myelomonocytic cell lineage expression of the neutrophil elastase gene. J. Biol. Chem. 263, 2543–2547.

Takahashi, H., Nukiwa, T., Yoshimura, K., Quick, C.D., States, D.J., Holmes, M.D., Whang-Peng, J., Knutsen, T. and Crystal, R.G. (1988b). Structure of the human neutrophil elastase gene. J. Biol. Chem. 263, 14739–14747.

Tanaka, T., Minematsu, Y., Reilly, C.F., Travis, J. and Powers, J.C. (1985). Human leukocyte cathepsin G. Subsite mapping with 4-nitroanilides, chemical modification, and effect of possible cofactors. Biochemistry, 24, 2040–2047.

Teshima, T., Griffin, J.C. and Powers, J.C. (1982). A new class of heterocyclic serine protease inhibitors. Inhibition of human leukocyte elastase, porcine pancreatic elastase, cathepsin G, and bovine chymotrypsin Aa with substituted benzoxazinones, quinazolines, and anthranilates J. Biol. Chem. 257, 5085–5091.

Thompson, R.C. and Ohlsson, K. (1986). Isolation, properties, and complete amino acid sequence of human secretory leukocyte protease inhibitor, a potent inhibitor of leukocyte elastase. Proc. Natl Acad. Sci. USA 83, 6692–6696.

Thornberry, N., Bull, H.G., Calaycay, J.R., Chapman. K.T., Howard, A.D., Kostura, M.J., Miller, D.K., Molineaux, S.M., Weidner, J.R., Aunins, J., Elliston, K.O., Ayala, J.M., Casano. F.J., Chin, J., Ding, G.J.-F., Egger, L.A., Gaffney, E.P., Limjuco, G., Palyha, O.C., Raju, S.M., Rolando, A.M., Salley, J.P., Yamin, T.T., Lee, T.D., Shively, J.E., MacCross, M., Mumford, R.A., Schmidt, J.A. and Tocci, M.J. (1992). A novel heterodimeric cysteine protease is required for interleukin-1β processing in monocytes. Nature 356, 768–774.

Tiku, K., Tiku, M.L. and Skosey, J.L. (1986). Interleukin 1 production by human polymorphonuclear neutrophils. J. Immunol. 136, 3677–3685.

Trabandt, A., Gay, R.E., Fassbender, H.-G. and Gay, S. (1991). Cathepsin B in synovial cells at the site of joint destruction in rheumatoid arthritis. Arthritis Rheum. 34, 1444–1451.

Trainor, D.A. (1987). Synthetic inhibitors of human neutrophil elastase. Trends Pharmacol. Sci. 8, 303–307.

Travis, J. (1988). Structure, function, and control of neutrophil proteinases. Am. J. Med. 84, 37–42.

Travis, J. and Fritz, H. (1991). Potential problems in designing elastase inhibitors for therapy. Am. Rev. Respir. Dis. 143 1412–1415.

Travis, J. and Salvesen, G.S. (1983). Human plasma proteinase inhibitors. Ann. Rev. Biochem. 52, 655–709.

Travis, J., Bowen, J. and Baugh, R. (1978). Human α_1-antichymotrypsin: interaction with chymotrypsin-like proteases. Biochemistry 17, 5651–5656.

Travis, J., Potempa, J., Bangalore, N. and Kurdowska, A. (1992). In "Current Topics in Rehabilitation: Biochemistry of Pulmonary Emphysema" (ed. C. Grassi, J. Travis, L. Casali and M. Luisetti) pp. 71–79. Springer Verlag, London.

Tsan, M.-F. and Jiang, M.-S. (1985). Membrane endo-peptidases of human neutrophil. Inflammation 9, 113–126.

Tsujinaka, T., Kajiwara, Y., Kambayashi, J., Sakon. M., Higuchi, N., Tanaka, T. and Mori, T. (1988). Synthesis of a new cell penetrating calpain inhibitor (Calpeptin). Biochem. Biophys. Res. Comm. 153, 1201–1208.

Uitto, V.J., Suomalainen, K. and Sorsa, T. (1990). Salivary collagenase. Origin, characteristics and relationship to periodontal health. J. Periodont. Res. 25, 135–142.

Umeno, E., Nadel, J.A., Huang, H.T. and McDonald, D.M. (1989). Inhibition of neutral endopeptidase potentiates neurogenic inflammation in the rat trachea. J. Appl. Physiol. 66, 2647–2652.

Umeno, E., Nadel, J.A. and McDonald, D.M. (1990). Neuro-genic inflammation of the rat trachea; fate of neutrophils that adhere to venules. J. Appl. Physiol. 69, 2131–2136.

van Noorden, C.J.F., Smith, R.E. and Rasnick, D. (1988). Cysteine proteinase activity in arthritic rat knee joints and the effects of a selective systemic inhibitor, Z-Phe-AlaCH$_2$F. J. Rheumatol. 15, 1525–1535.

Van Wart, H.E. and Birkedal-Hansen, H. (1990). The cysteine switch: a principle of regulation of metalloproteinase activity with potential applicability to the entire matrix metallo-proteinase family. Proc. Natl Acad. Sci. USA, 87, 5578–5582.

Veys, P.A., Wilkes, S. and Hoffbrand, A.V. (1991). Deficiency of neutrophil FcR III. Blood 78, 852–853.

Vissers, M.C., George, P.M., Bathurst, I.C., Brennan, S.O. and Winterbourn, C.C. (1988). Cleavage and inactivation of α_1-antitrypsin by metalloproteinases released from neutro-phils. J. Clin. Invest. 82, 706–711.

Vogelmeier, C., Buhl, R., Hoyt, R.F., Wilson, E., Fells, G.A., Hubbard. R.C., Schnebli, H.P., Thompson, R.C. and Crystal, R.G. (1990). Aerosolization of recombinant SLPI to augment antineutrophil elastase protection of pulmonary epithelium. J. Appl. Physiol. 69, 1843–1848.

Volpe, P., Krause, K.-H., Hashimoto, S., Zorzato, F., Pozzan, T. Meldolesi, J. and Lew, D.P. (1988). "Calciosome," a cytoplasmic organelle: the inositol 1,4,5-triphosphate-sensitive Ca^{2+} store of nonmuscle cells? Proc. Natl Acad. Sci. USA 85, 1091–1095.

Wahl, R.C., Dunlap, R.P. and Morgan, B. (1989). Biochemistry and inhibition of collagenase and stromelysin. Ann. Rep. Med. Chem. 25, 177–184.

Wang, K.W. (1990). Developing selective inhibitors of calpain. Trends Pharm. Sci. 11, 139–142.

Ward, P.A. and Becker, E.L. (1970). Biochemical demon-stration of the activatable esterase of the rabbit neutrophil involved in the chemotactic response. J. Immunol. 105, 1057–1067.

Ward, R.V., Atkinson, S.J., Slocombe, P.M., Docherty, A.J.P., Reynolds, J.J. and Murphy, G. (1991). Tissue inhibitor of metalloproteinases-2 inhibits the activation of 72kDa progelatinase by fibroblast membranes. Biochim. Biophys. Acta 1078, 242–246.

Wasi, S. and Movat, H. Z. (1979). Phlogistic substances in neutrophil leukocyte lysosomes: their possible role in vivo and their in vitro properties. Curr. Topics Pathol. 68, 213–237.

Weiland, J.E., Davis, W.B., Holter, J.F., Mohammed, J.R., Dorinsky, P.M. and Gadek, J. E. (1986). Lung neutrophils in the adult respiratory distress syndrome. Clinical and patho-logical significance. Am. Rev. Respir. Dis. 133, 218–225.

Weiss, S.J. and Peppin, G.J. (1986). Collagenolytic metallo-enzymes of the human neutrophil. Characteristics, regulation and potential function in vivo. Biochem. Pharmacol. 35, 3189–3197.

Weiss, S.J. and Regiani, S. (1984). Neurophils degrade sub-endothelial matrices in the presence of α_1-proteinase inhibitor. Cooperative use of lysosomal proteinases and oxygen metabolites. J. Clin. Invest. 73, 1297–1303.

Weiss, S.J., Peppin, G., Ortiz, X., Ragsdale, C. and Test, S.T. (1985). Oxidative autoactivation of latent collagenase by human neutrophils. Science 227, 747–749.

Weitz, J.I., Huang, A.J., Landman, S.L., Nicholson, S.C. and Silverstein, S.C. (1987). Elastase-mediated fibrinogenolysis by chemoattractant-stimulated neutrophils occurs in the presence of physiologic concentrations of antiproteinases. J. Exp. Med 166, 1836–1850.

Welgus, H.G. and Stricklin, G.P. (1983). Human skin fibro-blast collagenase inhibitor. Comparative studies in human connective tissues, serum, and amniotic fluid. J. Biol. Chem. 258, 12259–12264.

Wendt, P. and Blumel, G. (1979). In "Current Concepts in Kinin Research" (eds G.J. Haberland and U. Hamberg) pp. 73–81. Pergamon Press, Oxford.

Wewers, M. (1989). Pathogenesis of emphysema. Assessment of basic science concepts through clinical investigation. Chest 95, 190–195.

Wewers, M.D., Herzyk, D.J. and Gadek, J.E. (1988). Alveolar fluid neutrophil elastase activity in the adult respiratory distress syndrome is complexed to α_2-macroglobulin. J. Clin. Invest. 82, 1260–1267.

Wiedow, O., Schroder, J.-M., Gregory, H., Young, J.A. and Christopher, E. (1990). Elafin: an elastase-specific inhibitor of human skin. J. Biol. Chem. 265, 14791–14795.

Wiedow. O., Luedemann, J. and Utecht. B. (1991). Elafin is a potent inhibitor of proteinase 3. Biochem. Biophys. Res. Comm. 174, 6–10.

Wilhelm, S.M., Collier, I.E., Marmer, B.L., Eisen, A.Z., Grant, G.A. and Goldberg, G.I. (1989). SV40-transformed human lung fibroblasts secrete a 92-kDa type IV collagenase which is identical to that secreted by normal human macrophages. J. Biol. Chem. 264, 17213–17221.

Wilkinson, P.C. (1982). "Chemotaxis and Inflammation", 2nd edn. Churchill Livingstone, Edinburgh.

Williams, H.R. and Lin, T.Y. (1984). Human polymorpho-nuclear leukocyte collagenase and gelatinase. Comparison of certain enzymatic properties. Int. J. Biochem. 16, 1321–1329.

Williams, J.C., Falcone, R.C., Knee, C., Stein, R.L., Stimpler, A.M., Reeves, B., Giles, R.E. and Knell, R.D. (1991).

Biological characterization of ICI 200,880 and ICI 200,355, novel inhibitors of human neutrophil elastase. Am. Rev. Respir. Dis. 144, 875–883.

Wintroub, B.U., Klickstein, L.B., Dzau, V.J. and Watt, K.W. (1984). Granulocyte–angiotensin system: identification of angiotensinogen as the plasma protein substrate of leukocyte cathepsin G. Biochemisry 23, 227–232.

Woessner, J.F. (1991). Matrix metalloproteinases and their inhibitors in connective tissue remodeling. FASEB J. 5, 2145–2154.

Woessner, J.F. (1992). In "Biochemistry of Inflammation" (eds J.T. Whicher and S.W. Evans) pp. 57–89. Klewer Academic Publishers, Dordrecht.

Woolley, D.E., Roberts, D.R. and Evanson, J.M. (1975). Inhibition of human collagenase activity by a small molecular weight serum protein. Biochem. Biophys. Res. Comm. 66, 747–754.

Yoshimura, T., Barker, L.N. and Powers, J.C. (1982). Specificity and reactivity of human leukocyte elastase, porcine pancreatic elastase, human granulocyte cathepsin G and bovine pancreatic chymotrypsin with arylsulfonyl fluorides. Discovery of a new series of potent and specific irreversible elastase inhibitors. J. Biol. Chem. 257, 577–584.

Yuli, I. and Lelkes, P.I. (1991). Neutral endopeptidase activity in the interaction of N-formyl-L-Methionyl-L-Leucyl-L-Phenylalanine with human polymorphonuclear leukocytes. Eur. J. Biochem. 201, 421–430.

Yuli, I. and Snyderman, R. (1988). Extensive hydrolysis of N-formyl-L-Methionyl-L-Leucyl-L-[^{3}H]Phenylalanine by human polymorphonuclear leukocytes; a potential mechanism for modulation of the chemoattractant signal. J. Immunol. 261, 4902–4908.

5. Neutrophil-derived Inflammatory Mediators

Shaun R. McColl and Henry J. Showell

1. Introduction

The pathophysiological role of neutrophils in both acute and chronic inflammatory processes is well documented. However, as recently discussed by Lloyd and Oppenheim (1992) and in contrast to the well-accepted efferent effector function (via the release of preformed mediators) of neutrophils in inflammatory processes, the recognition of potential afferent effector function (via *de novo* synthesis and release of bioactive lipids and cytokines) has only recently come to be appreciated. In the past, any afferent role of neutrophils on immune processes was summarily dismissed owing to the prevailing wisdom that neutrophils were end-stage, short-lived cells incapable of significant protein synthesis. Clearly, at this juncture we believe this latter perception to be incorrect, and there is now compelling evidence that neutrophils should be seriously considered in the context of the afferent limb of the immune response. Below we will review current evidence supporting this potentially extremely important function.

2. Eicosanoids

2.1 INTRODUCTION

Major developments in the field of eicosanoid research can be temporally divided into two major parts. The first part, which took place from the 1930s to 1970, involved the discovery and characterization of the major prostaglandins and the discovery of the SRS-A. The second part occurred along with the development of technology such as gas-chromatography mass-spectrometry in the mid–1970s, which enabled the discovery of the labile prostaglandins, elucidation of the structure of SRS-A, and characterization of the lipoxygenase arm of the arachidonic acid cascade.

The eicosanoids are a group of potent pro-inflammatory lipids which mediate a wide variety of intra- and extracellular responses. Under normal dietary conditions, these compounds are derived from the 20-carbon polyunsaturated fatty acid arachidonic acid, which is stored in membrane phospholipids. Arachidonic acid release is

Immunopharmacology of Neutrophils
ISBN 0–12–339250–0

controlled by one or more phospholipases A_2 which specifically cleave this fatty acid from position 2 of phospholipids. The principal source of free arachidonic acid in neutrophils is thought to be phosphatidyl choline, which predominantly contains arachidonic acid in position 2. Once released, free arachidonic acid is either rapidly re-esterified into membrane phospholipids, or is metabolized by one of several oxygenases which may be present in neutrophils. In the case of metabolism by lipoxygenases, synthesis of either LTs or lipoxins will result. In the case of metabolism by cyclooxygenase, prostaglandins will be produced. In the following several pages, the ability of neutrophils to produce eicosanoids is described. Readers interested in more detail are encouraged to refer to the reviews cited in each of the following sections.

2.2   5-Lipoxygenase

While conducting the experiments which eventually led to the isolation of TXA_2, Samuelsson and his colleagues found that platelets produced two other major AA metabolites, HHT, the hemiacetal derivative of PHD, (now known as TXB_2) and 12-HETE (Hamberg and Samuelsson, 1974). Extension of these studies eventually uncovered the 5-lipoxygenase pathway in leucocytes.

The 5-LO catalyses the specific dioxygenation of arachidonic acid at position 5, thereby initiating LT synthesis (for detailed reviews see Lewis and Austen, 1984; Stjerschantz, 1984; Johnson et al., 1986; Samuelsson et al., 1987; Borgeat, 1988; Borgeat and Naccache, 1990; Lewis et al., 1990; Musser and Kreft, 1992). The resultant compound, known as 5-HPETE, is rapidly reduced to 5-HETE (Borgeat et al., 1976), or 5S,6S-5(6)-oxido-7,9,11,14-eicosatetraenoic acid LTA_4 (Borgeat and Samuelsson, 1979a). It is believed that 5-HETE production is the result of the action of a peroxidase, whereas LTA_4 formation is catalysed by the second enzymatic activity inherent in the 5-lipoxygenase, known as LTA synthetase (Rouzer et al., 1986). LTA_4 is highly unstable and may be non-enzymatically hydrolysed to compounds with little or no biological activity. In several cell types, including monocyte/macrophages and eosinophils, LTA_4 may also be enzymatically metabolized by a glutathione peroxidase to 5S,6R-5-hydroxy-6-S-glutathionyl-7,9,11,14-eicosatetraenoic acid (LTC_4), however, this pathway does not exist in neutrophils. LTA_4, may also be metabolized to 5S,12R-5,12-dihydroxy-6,8,10,14-eicosatetraenoic acid (LTB_4), the most potent product of this pathway in neutrophils (Borgeat and Samuelsson, 1979b). The enzyme responsible for this step in the pathway is known as the LTA hydrolase (Radmark et al., 1984). LTB_4 may further be metabolized by Ω-oxidation into 20-hydroxy- and 20-carboxy-LTB_4, which are considerably less active than LTB_4 (Dahinden et al., 1984; Nadeau et al., 1984). In addition, recent studies have shown that 20-hydroxy

LTB_4 may be a potent antagonist of LTB_4 in vivo (Pettipher et al., 1993).

As mentioned above, neutrophils are capable of synthesizing several 5-LO products. However, in terms of biological significance, LTB_4 is by far the most potent metabolite (for a detailed review, see Borgeat and Naccache, 1990). LTB_4 is a potent stereospecific phagocyte activator which was originally characterized as an endogenous neutrophil chemotactic factor (Ford-Hutchinson et al., 1980; Palmer et al., 1980; Palmblad et al., 1981). It has since been shown to stimulate many other neutrophil functions including degranulation (Bokoch and Reed, 1981; Serhan et al., 1982; Showell et al., 1982), aggregation (Ford-Hutchinson et al., 1980; O'Flaherty et al., 1981), adherence (Palmblad et al., 1981; Gimbrone et al., 1984; Hoover et al., 1984), and calcium mobilization (Naccache and Sha'afi, 1983; Naccache et al., 1989). It also modifies the activity of other cells of the immune system such as eosinophils, monocytes and lymphocytes (Rola-Plesczynski, 1985; Rola-Plesczynski and Stankova, 1992).

Neutrophils synthesize LTB_4 and related compounds in response to a variety of stimuli, notably, the calcium ionophore A23187 (Borgeat and Samuelsson, 1979c), urate and calcium pyrophosphate crystals (Poubelle et al., 1987), opsonized and unopsonized zymosan (Claesson et al., 1981), and chemotactic factors such as FMLP (Clancy et al., 1983; Salari et al., 1985), C5a (Clancy et al., 1983), PAF (Chilton et al., 1982; Lin et al., 1982) and IL-8 (Schroeder, 1989). In addition, it has recently been shown that pretreatment of neutrophils with the cytokine GM-CSF dramatically enhances LTB_4 synthesis in response to subsequent activation by chemotactic factors such as FMLP, C5a, PAF (Dahinden et al., 1988; DiPersio et al., 1988a, 1988b; McColl et al., 1991) as well as IL-8 (McDonald et al., 1993). The potential physiological importance of the latter observation becomes more evident when one considers that neutrophils migrating from the peripheral blood to sites of inflammation and infection are likely to be exposed to combinations of both chemotactic factors and cytokines as the neutrophils approach these sites. More recently, it has been shown that the priming effect of GM-CSF is mediated at both the level of substrate availability (arachidonic acid) and activation of the 5-LO (McColl et al., 1991). Studies at the molecular level have begun to shed significant light on the mechanism by which GM-CSF primes neutrophils for increased LTB_4 synthesis (see below). However, further studies will be required specifically to address the question as to whether upregulation of the 5LO and/or FLAP at the molecular level is required for the priming effect of GM-CSF. In addition, no studies to date have evaluated the mechanism by which GM-CSF modulates the activity of the PLA_2.

Our understanding of the cellular mechanisms controlling leukotriene synthesis have recently taken a great leap forward by virtue of several biochemical and molecular biological breakthroughs. Attempts to purify this enzyme came to fruition several years ago (Rouzer and Samuelsson, 1985; Rouzer et al., 1986) and led to the discovery that for leukotriene synthesis to occur in a physiological setting (i.e. an intact cell), the 5-LO needed to be translocated to cell membranes (Rouzer and Samuelsson, 1987; Rouzer and Kargman, 1988). This finding provided the first significant insight obtained for many years, into the process by which the 5-LO is activated. The 5-LO, a 78 kD protein, was subsequently cloned (Dixon et al., 1988). Further molecular biological studies revealed that the gene encoding the 5-LO spans more than 82 kb and consists of 14 exons (Funk et al., 1989). The messenger RNA is approximately 2.7 kb (Dixon et al., 1988). It has been reported that the 5'-regulatory region of the 5-LO is similar in appearance to those of several well-characterized housekeeping genes and is therefore not expected to be subjected to significant regulation at the transcriptional level (Funk et al., 1989). However, the same laboratory subsequently reported a possible site for the Sp1 transcription factor (Hoshiko et al., 1990). To date, no reports on regulation of the 5-LO gene in mature leucocytes have been reported. However, recent studies have shown that treatment of neutrophils with GM-CSF increases de novo synthesis of the 5-LO without modulating the level of 5-LO mRNA, implying that GM-CSF stimulates 5-LO expression at the translation level in neutrophils (Pouliot et al., 1992a).

A second major breakthrough concerning the mechanisms controlling LT synthesis occurred with the discovery of a small membrane-bound protein which appears to serve as a docking-site for the 5-LO (Dixon et al., 1990). This protein, which was sequenced and cloned in 1990, was termed the FLAP (Miller et al., 1990). This title may be a little premature inasmuch as it is still not known whether FLAP actually activates the 5-LO or whether its major function is to enable the 5-LO to bind to membranes, which are an area rich in substrate (arachidonic acid) and low in peroxidases, which would enable activation of the 5-LO in a physiological setting. FLAP is an 18 kD protein with a 1.0 kb mRNA (Miller et al., 1990). The 5'-regulatory region of the FLAP gene has also recently been characterized and two putative transcription factor binding sites have been reported: one for activator protein-2 and the other, a glucocorticoid-responsive element (Kennedy et al., 1991). Treatment of neutrophils with either GM-CSF or TNFα, stimulates a rapid up-regulation of FLAP gene expression which appears to be due to effects at both the transcriptional and translational levels (Pouliot et al., 1992b).

2.3 15-LIPOXYGENASE

The 15-LO is the second of the three mammalian lipoxygenases, the third being the platelet 12-LO. For many years, little attention was paid to this enzyme in neutrophils since its major products were believed to be 15-HPETE and 15-HETE and these compounds were assumed to be less interesting biologically than the LTs. However, it was recently established that the combined actions of the neutrophil 15-LO and 5-LO can lead to a class of metabolites known as the LXs (for detailed reviews, see Samuelsson et al., 1987; Rokach and Fitzsimmons, 1988; Serhan, 1991). As with the 5-LO cascade, several different metabolites may be produced. Two of these metabolites in particular, LXA4 and LXB4 appear to possess a range of biological activities unique amongst the eicosanoids (Samuelsson et al., 1987; Serhan, 1991).

Although LXA4 and LXB4 share several actions, this is not the case for all of their effects. Both LXs exert effects on the microcirculation and induce vaso- and bronchoconstriction in vivo, but the effects of LXA4 are better characterized. LXA4 elicits several effects on neutrophils including chemotaxis, although this is not a potent effect and may not be biologically relevant, and release of arachidonic acid. Interestingly, the latter effect does not appear to involve activation of the 5-LO and therefore presumably does not involve calcium mobilization. In addition, LXA4 inhibits the ability of FMLP to stimulate chemotaxis, calcium mobilization and generation of IP3, but does not inhibit superoxide production induced by FMLP. Other cellular targets for these compounds include endothelial cells (prostacyclin formation) and natural killer cells (inhibition of cytotoxicity) (all reviewed in Serhan, 1991).

A human 15-LO was recently purified from an eosinophil-enriched leucocyte population. SDS–PAGE revealed a single band having an estimated molecular weight of approximately 70 kD (Sigal et al., 1988, 1990). The 15-LO was subsequently cloned from a human reticulocyte cDNA library (Sigal et al., 1990). Although no studies concerning the regulation of 15-LO gene expression in neutrophils have been reported as yet, the results of a recent study in human monocytes shows that the 15-LO gene may be regulated at the transcriptional level (Conrad et al., 1992). In that study, it was shown that, of a large number of cytokines, including IL-1 to IL-6, GM-CSF and M-CSF, TNFα, TGFβ, IFNγ and PDGF, only IL-4 was capable of stimulating up-regulation of the 15-LO gene. This was observed at the mRNA level, the protein level (by immunofluorescence in whole cells) and at the functional level. Of further interest was the observation that this up-regulation by IL-4 was completely inhibited when the cells were coincubated with IFNγ indicating the existence of both positive and negative signals involved in the control of synthesis and function of this enzyme. In light of these observations in monocytes, it will be of considerable interest to document the regulation of the 15-LO in human neutrophils.

2.4 Cyclooxygenase

The CO, also known as PGG/H synthetase, is the key enzyme in the cascade leading to the production of the PGs (for detailed reviews, see Moncada and Vane 1978; Wolfe, 1982; Johnson et al., 1986; Needleman et al., 1986). This enzyme catalyses the conversion of free arachidonic acid to the unstable endoperoxides, PGG_2 and PGH_2 whose synthesis is the gateway to the more biologically active PGs, including PGE_2, prostacyclin PGI_2 and TXA_2. The latter two compounds have been implicated in the control of blood coagulation (Willis and Smith, 1981; Johnson et al., 1986), whereas PGE_2 possesses a multitude of biological actions including effects on the cardiovascular system (vasodilation, smooth muscle relaxation) and the central nervous system (pyrogenic), and activates intracellular messenger pathways within responsive cells by stimulating adenylate cyclase (Johnson et al., 1986; Needleman et al., 1986).

Whether or not neutrophils have the ability to synthesize prostaglandins has been the subject of considerable debate for many years. While several studies in the 1970s reported production of PGE_2 and TXB_2 in response to chemotactic factors and phagocytic activation (Goldstein et al., 1978; Palmer and Salmon, 1983), many investigators could not reproduce these observations. However, the recent discovery of the existence of multiple CO genes may have shed some light on this conundrum. One of these genes has a 2.8 kb mRNA, is constitutively expressed, and does not appear to be significantly regulated at the transcriptional level (O'Banion et al., 1991). The second, however, has a 4.0 kb mRNA. Its expression in fibroblasts is up-regulated in response to stimulation with either serum or phorbol ester but could only be demonstrated if the cells were pretreated with cycloheximide, indicating that the mRNA is likely to be extremely unstable (O'Banion et al., 1991; for review see Xie et al., 1992). In spite of this instability, stimulation with serum or phorbol ester resulted in an increase in the level of CO protein having an estimated molecular weight of approximately 70 kD. O'Sullivan et al. (1992) have recently shown that up-regulation of prostanoid synthesis in alveolar macrophages by LPS involves increased gene expression of a CO with an mRNA of approximately 4.0 kb. Although neither of these two genes has yet been demonstrated in neutrophils, a recent study has shown that stimulation of neutrophils with GM-CSF leads to the production of prostaglandins by these cells (Hermann et al., 1990). In addition, this phenomenon is protein synthesis-dependent since treatment of the cells with cycloheximide prior to stimulation with GM-CSF inhibited the release of prostaglandins implying that GM-CSF may upregulate CO gene expression in these cells. It will therefore be of great interest to confirm these results at the molecular level.

3. Platelet-activating Factor

3.1 Introduction

Over two decades ago, PAF was first identified as a potential contributing factor involved in hypersensitivity reactions (Henson, 1969, 1970a, 1970b, 1971; Siriganian and Osler, 1971; Benveniste et al., 1972). PAF became the adopted name for this fluid-phase substance, released from antigen-stimulated (IgE-mediated) basophils, based on its ability to activate naive platelets. In 1979 the chemical nature of PAF was elucidated by three independent groups as 1-alkyl-2-acetyl-sn-glycero-3-phosphocholine (Benveniste et al., 1979; Blank et al., 1979; Demopoulus et al., 1979). Demopoulus et al. and Benveniste et al. focussed on the biochemical characterization of the IgE-dependent PAF, whereas Blank et al. isolated PAF from renal medulla, a tissue previously shown to contain an anti-hypertensive polar renal lipid (APRL). Soon after the structural elucidation of PAF, it became clear that platelets were not the only responsive cell but many other cells including neutrophils, eosinophils, monocytes–macrophages were, in addition to being sensitive to the actions of exogenous PAF, also capable of synthesizing PAF. Several recent reviews have covered many aspects of the state of the art of PAF research (e.g. Pinckard et al., 1988; Saito and Hanahan, 1989; Snyder, 1990; Evans et al., 1991; Koltai et al., 1991a, 1991b; Chung, 1992; Page, 1992). In this section we will specifically focus on neutrophils both as a source and a target of PAF.

3.2 PAF Biosynthesis and Release

Many independent reports have provided evidence that neutrophils are a likely source of PAF in inflammatory reactions (Lynch et al., 1979; Betz and Henson, 1980; Clark et al., 1980; Lotner et al., 1980; Camussi et al., 1981; Alonso et al., 1982; Mueller et al., 1983, 1984; Chilton et al., 1984; Clay et al., 1984; Jouvin-Marche et al., 1984; Pinckard et al., 1984; Oda et al., 1985; Weintraub et al., 1985; Ramesha and Pickett, 1987; Bussolino et al., 1992; Tufano et al., 1992). Human neutrophils are thought to synthesize PAF predominantly via a deacylation–reacylation pathway involving transfer of acetate from acetyl CoA to lyso PAF formed from the initial action of a 1-O-alkyl PC-specific PLA_2 on pre-existing intracellular precursor pools of PC (Chilton et al., 1984; Mueller et al., 1984). Interestingly, the fatty acid in the sn2 position that is released from the precursor pool of 1-O-alkyl PC by the action of PLA_2 appears to be in the main part, arachidonic acid (Chilton, 1989). Therefore, in neutrophils, upon appropriate activation, two highly potent lipid mediators, i.e. PAF and LTB_4 (see above), can be formed from one precursor molecule. While LTB_4 appears to be released from neutrophils to the extracellular space via a highly specific transport mechanism (Lam *et al.*, 1990), the mechanism whereby PAF is released from neutrophils is still poorly understood. *In vitro* – as was first shown in the basophil system (Benveniste *et al.*, 1972) – albumin appears to be necessary for PAF to be recovered extracellularly from neutrophils (Ludwig *et al.*, 1985; Cluzel *et al.*, 1989). However, in a recent report where human plasma deficient in PAF acetylhydrolase (see below) was used in the incubation medium, PAF release from neutrophils appeared not to be dependent on albumin, but rather a factor of a larger MW ~ 240 kD. It is presently unclear whether this factor is related to lipoproteins previously reported to have high capacity binding for PAF (Benveniste *et al.*, 1988). Irrespective of the extracellular fate of PAF, significant amounts of PAF have also been shown to remain cell-associated (Lynch and Henson, 1986; Roubin *et al.*, 1986; Sisson *et al.*, 1987; Riches *et al.*, 1990). The function of cell-associated PAF remains to be established, however, both second messenger (Worthen *et al.*, 1988; Riches *et al.*, 1990; Stewart *et al.*, 1990) and intercellular signal roles have been proposed (Zhou *et al.*, 1992).

3.3 PAF BIOLOGICAL ACTIVITY AND METABOLIC FATE

PAF, when added exogenously to neutrophils *in vitro*, appears to activate functional responses (e.g. chemotaxis, exocytosis, oxidase priming/activation, homotypic aggregation, increased surface expression of the $\beta 2$ integrin CD11b/CD18, and Fc receptor expression, consistent with a profile observed with other chemotactic factors (e.g. FMLP, C5a, LTB₄, IL-8) (O'Flaherty *et al.*, 1981; Shaw *et al.*, 1981; Smith *et al.*, 1984; Dewald and Baggiolini, 1985; Gay *et al.*, 1986; Shalit *et al.*, 1987, 1988; Gay and Stitt, 1988; Vercellotti *et al.*, 1988; Koenderman *et al.*, 1989; Fukuchi *et al.*, 1992; Pinckard *et al.*, 1992). Evidence for a specific high-affinity binding-site on neutrophils was obtained using radiolabelled PAF and PAF antagonists (Valone and Goetzl, 1983; Ng and Wong, 1986; Hwang, 1988; Marquis *et al.*, 1988; O'Flaherty *et al.*, 1988; Stewart and Dusting, 1988; Paulson *et al.*, 1990). More recently cloning of the PAF receptor was achieved (Honda *et al.*, 1991; Ye *et al.*, 1991; Kunz *et al.*, 1992). For a detailed review of the structure of the PAF receptor and other chemotactic factor receptors see Chapter 6.

PAF synthesized by neutrophils is a heterogeneous mixture of homologous forms, the predominant species being 16:0-, 18:0 and 18:1 (1-O-alkyl PAF) with lesser amounts of other phosphocholine and ethanolamine species (Weintraub *et al.*, 1985; Ludwig and Pinckard, 1987). A full characterization of the *in vitro* biological activities of all of the various isoforms of PAF on neutrophils has yet to be undertaken. However, recent work of Pinckard and co-workers (1992) have provided evidence that the potency and efficacy of the three main isoforms (i.e., C16-, C18- and C18-1 alkyl PAF) do not necessarily conform to a one to one relationship among the various bioassays examined, i.e. exocytosis, (activation and desensitization) chemotaxis, oxidase priming. While not proving the existence of subfamilies of PAF receptors, these findings nonetheless provide evidence that such may exist. Interestingly, 1-acyl-2-acetyl-*sn*-glycero-3-phosphocholine (1-O-acyl PC) analogues of PAF, which are also synthesized by neutrophils (Mueller *et al.*, 1984; Satouchi *et al.*, 1985, 1987; Sturk *et al.*, 1989) also appear to be able to interact with neutrophils in a productive fashion. While exhibiting weak intrinsic activity as direct neutrophil agonists, these compounds at nanomolar concentrations, however, are capable of both blocking secretory responses mediated by PAF and priming the oxidase for activation by secondary stimuli such as C5a and FMLP (Triggiani *et al.*, 1991b; Pinckard *et al.*, 1992). It is interesting to note that these 1-O-acyl PAF analogues are the major species synthesized by activated mast cells and endothelial cells (Triggiani *et al.*, 1990; Vercellotti *et al.*, 1990; Zimmerman *et al.*, 1990; Clay *et al.* 1991; Kuijpers *et al.*, 1991, 1992; Lorant *et al.*, 1991; Mueller, *et al.*,1991) implying that this membrane-bound lipid is potentially capable of modulating neutrophil function in both a positive and negative fashion. PAF is inactivated in neutrophils by the action of a PAF acetyl hydrolase resulting in the formation of lyso PAF which is then rapidly reacylated with long chain fatty acids, arachidonate being the preferred species (Chilton *et al.*, 1983; Triggiani *et al.*, 1991a). In contrast to PAF, the acyl analogues of PAF appear to be predominantly metabolized via an alternative pathway involving removal of the long-chain fatty acid at the *sn*-1 position (Triggiani *et al.*, 1991a). Extracellular PAF is metabolized via the action of a highly specific AH associated with the low-density lipoproteins (Stafforini *et al.*, 1987) and thus when added to plasma, PAF exhibits a very short half-life. Interestingly, PAF previously bound to its releasing factor isolated from the plasma of AH-deficient patients is resistant to the action of AH but is still capable of activating neutrophils, implying a potentially important role for this molecule (Miwa *et al.*, 1992). It will be interesting to see in future studies whether the PAF-releasing factor described above bears any relationship to the PAF-binding proteins previously described by Benveniste *et al.* (1988). In a recent publication, this form of PAF was reported to be present in plasma and synovial fluid obtained from arthritic patients (Hilliquin *et al.*, 1992).

4. *Cationic Proteins*

Neutrophils contain within azurophil granules, an impressive armamentarium of cationic proteins ranging in molecular weight from < 4 to 60 kD which appear to be intimately involved in oxygen-independent killing of microorganisms by these cells. Currently, four classes of cationic proteins have been identified in human neutrophils and they are: the defensins (HNP-1, HNP-2, HNP-3 and HNP-4); CatG; CAP37/azurocidin; and BPI/CAP57/BP. (For recent reviews on the nature of these proteins, see Lehrer and Ganz, 1990; Spitznagel, 1990; Ganz et al., 1990). That neutrophil-derived proteins were pro-inflammatory was first demonstrated by Janoff and Zweifach (1964) following up on earlier observations of Spitznagel and Chi (1963) and Frimmer and Hegner (1963). Golub and Spitznagel (1965) and Ranadive and Cochrane (1968) subsequently provided evidence of the existence of subfractions of cationic proteins isolated from rabbit neutrophil granules that had oedema inducing properties which were both dependent on and independent from effects related to mast cell activation. Specific secretion of granule constituents, including cationic proteins, has been shown to occur *in vitro* when neutrophils are exposed to immune complexes (Weissman et al., 1971; Henson et al., 1972; and Ranadive et al., 1973). Therefore, in addition to lytic mechanisms mediated, for example, by various bacterial toxins, the selective secretion of cationic proteins from neutrophils is likely to occur when cells encounter appropriate immune stimuli. Evidence in support of this idea was provided by Camussi et al. (1982) where in renal biopsies taken from SLE patients with glomerulo-nephritis, deposits of neutrophil cationic proteins (NCP) were detected in glomerular capillary walls. In addition, neutrophils obtained from the circulation were markedly depleted of NCP. In a more recent study, exogenous administration of PAF to rabbits induced a proteinuria with the attendant deposition of both neutrophil and platelet-derived cationic proteins in the glomerular capillaries (Camussi et al., 1984). Thus, in some non-infectious inflammatory diseases there is compelling evidence that the inappropriate release of neutrophil cationic proteins is likely to be a contributing factor leading to tissue injury. What remains to be better defined is whether or not cationic proteins are directly involved in mediating non-pathological inflammatory processes. In this regard, several *in vitro* and *in vivo* studies have pointed to endothelial cells as being a likely target for the action of cationic protein as well as other synthetic polycations (DeVries et al., 1953; Stein et al., 1956; Skutelsky and Danon, 1976; Pelikan et al., 1979; Vehaskari et al., 1984; Peterson et al., 1987; Sunnergren et al., 1987; Needham et al., 1988). While not definitely proving the involvement of neutrophil-derived cationic proteins, the recent findings of suppression of neutrophil-dependent vascular leak by dextran sulphate (a potential surrogate for heparin) provided evidence that release of such proteins may be occurring as neutrophils diapedese through endothelial cells in response to a chemotactic stimulus (Rosengren et al., 1989). Previous

demonstrations of neutrophil-dependent oedema using similar experimental animal models led to the suggestion that the increased vascular permeability observed in this setting is likely to be a physiological process important for optimal delivery of humoral components necessary for host defence (Issekutz, 1981; Wedmore and Williams, 1981; Hellewell and Williams, 1986). Therefore, it would appear that cationic proteins released from neutrophils in response to soluble (e.g. the chemotactic factors C5a, LTB$_4$, PAF) and insoluble (e.g. immune complexes) stimuli can influence the integrity of the vascular endothelium in both a physiological and pathophysiological manner. As reagents become available that will allow specific detection of each of the various neutrophil cationic proteins that have now been purified and chemically characterized, it will be interesting to determine which of these proteins are detectable either individually or collectively in either of the above-described scenarios. Furthermore, having purified material in hand will facilitate a broader understanding of other potentially important inflammatory properties of these proteins. For example, the defensins HNP-1 and HNP-2 (Territo et al., 1989), as well as CAP37 (Pereira et al., 1990; Pohl et al., 1990) have recently been reported to be chemotactic for monocytes *in vitro*.

5. Cytokines

5.1 Introduction

Over the last few years, increasing attention has been paid to the investigation of RNA synthesis, protein synthesis and protein secretion by neutrophils. It has been a long-held belief that these cells are terminally differentiated phagocytes which arrive on the scene of acute inflammation possessing all the weapons required to perform their primary role – that of phagocytosis and destruction of invading organisms and unwanted cellular debris. However, the fact that these cells are capable of gene transcription and significant protein synthesis under appropriate stimulatory conditions is becoming increasingly apparent. In fact, it is now known that neutrophils actively synthesize membrane and cytoskeletal proteins such as CR1, CR3, C3, MHC class I molecules, actin and several cationic proteins (Neuman et al., 1990; Waksman et al., 1990; Botto et al., 1992). In addition, it has been recently documented that these cells are capable of synthesizing and secreting extracellular matrix proteins such as fibronectin and thrombospondin (LaFleur et al., 1987; Kreis et al., 1989). Of particular interest is the fact that the synthesis and secretion of the latter two proteins is significantly up-regulated in neutrophils taken from an inflammatory milieu – the synovial fluid of patients suffering from rheumatoid arthritis.

A recent report has clearly documented the ability of neutrophils to up-regulate total RNA synthesis in response to a select number of agonists (Beaulieu *et al.*, 1992). The most potent agonists were the chemotactic oligopeptide FMLP, and the cytokines GM-CSF and TNFα. Of further significance is the observation that TNF and GM-CSF have the ability to stimulate c-fos mRNA accumulation in neutrophils (Colotta *et al.*, 1987; McColl *et al.* 1989). The protein product of this gene forms the homo- and heterodimers comprising the nuclear transcription factor AP-1 which is one of the major transcriptional regulators involved in cytokine gene regulation (Ransome and Verma, 1990). In addition to producing the proteins mentioned above, neutrophils are capable of synthesizing and secreting a large array of cytokines and are thus capable of up-regulating the immune response at inflammatory sites. These products are the focus of this section of the chapter.

5.2 INTERLEUKINS-1α and β

IL-1α and β, TNFα and IL-6 are produced by many of the cells in the body and act on almost as many different cells stimulating a variety of functions. Indeed, these cytokines are loosely termed "multifunctional cytokines" (Akira *et al.*, 1990). The first "interleukin" to be discovered and named, IL-1, actually consists of two closely related polypeptides known as IL-1α and β (for an extensive review, see Dinarello, 1991). These polypeptides have assumed great importance in the field of immunology because of their broad spectrum of activity on the immune system. IL-1α and β are the products of separate genes, which bind to and activate the same cell receptors (a similar situation exists for TNFα, and TNFβ). These proteins are initially produced as a 31 kD precursor which is cleaved and subsequently secreted as a 17 kD active cytokine, although several studies suggest that the 31 kD protein can be secreted and then cleaved by enzymes which may be present at specific inflammatory sites, including collagenase, CatG and elastase (Black *et al.*, 1988; Beuscher *et al.*, 1990). IL-1 is produced by many different cells in the body, including vascular endothelial cells and fibroblasts (Libby *et al.*, 1986; Warner *et al.*, 1987; Yamoto *et al.*, 1989). Amongst the myeloid cells, monocyte/macrophages (Sisson and Dinarello, 1988; Lonnemann *et al.*, 1989), T lymphocytes (Numerof *et al.*, 1990) as well as neutrophils (Tiku *et al.*, 1986; Lindemann *et al.*, 1988; Marucha *et al.*, 1990, 1991; Roberge *et al.*, 1991) are all capable of synthesizing and secreting active IL-1 in response to a variety of agonists.

While both IL-1α and β undergo the same post-translational processing, their production and secretion are not linked. Indeed, most cells produce between 5 and 10 times more IL-1β than IL-1α and neutrophils are no exception to this (Roberge *et al.*, 1991). This difference at the level of protein synthesis is also apparent at the mRNA level (Demczuk *et al.*, 1987). Indeed, it is here where an explanation for the predominance of IL-1β

expression may be found. The 3'-untranslated region of the mRNA of cytokine genes characteristically contains "AUUUA" repeats which appears to confer instability on the mRNA (Shaw and Kamen, 1986; Wilson and Treisman, 1988). This is believed to be one of the major mechanisms by which cytokine synthesis is regulated. The IL-1α gene contains six such repeats, whereas only two of these sequences are present in the IL-1β gene (March *et al.*, 1985). This potentially makes the IL-1α mRNA more unstable than that for IL-1β, and therefore less translation may occur and lower levels of protein may be produced.

The production of IL-1 by neutrophils has now been well documented. These cells produce relatively low levels of both IL-1α and β in response to stimulation with LPS, opsonized and unopsonized particles (e.g. zymosan), microcrystals, as well as GM-CSF and TNFα (Tiku *et al.*, 1986; Lindemann *et al.*, 1988; Roberge *et al.*, 1991). The highest levels of IL-1 production result from activation of neutrophils by phagocytic stimuli such as zymosan or microcrystals (Roberge *et al.*, 1991). In addition, under these conditions, the majority of IL-1 produced (between 70–90%) is released by the cells. In contrast, when neutrophils are stimulated with cytokines such as GM-CSF or TNFα, smaller levels are produced overall, and the majority (90–95%) is retained inside the cell. The significance of the retention of IL-1 by neutrophils is not yet well understood, although it has also been reported for other cell types. Perhaps the answer lies with the possibility that IL-1 is also involved in intracellular signalling.

While it is now clear that neutrophils produce and secrete both IL-1α and β, the relative contribution of neutrophils to the synthesis of IL-1 is small when compared to that by monocyte/macrophages. For example, monocytes synthesize approximately 50–100 times more IL-1 than do neutrophils stimulated under similar conditions. This in no way diminishes the importance of IL-1 synthesis by neutrophils for two major reasons. First, IL-1 is a potent cytokine and therefore relatively small amounts of this cytokine are sufficient to have a large impact on the immune response. Second, the number of neutrophils present at certain inflammatory sites may be of sufficient magnitude to mount a relatively large synthesis and secretion of IL-1, particularly where phagocytosis is involved.

5.3 TUMOUR NECROSIS FACTOR α

TNFα, as the name implies, was originally characterized as a cytokine possessing the ability to induce tumour necrosis. However, it is now realized that this cytokine plays important roles in host defence against infections and also exerts important effects on a variety of different cells of the immune system (Akira *et al.*, 1990; Fiers, 1991). For example, TNFα is capable of directly activating and priming mature phagocytes such as neutrophils and monocytes *in vitro*, and may therefore play critical amplification roles in the inflammatory response. For example, TNFα stimulates neutrophil degranulation (Richter *et al.*, 1989), enhances arachidonic acid release (DiPersio *et al.*, 1988a), leukotriene synthesis (Roubin *et al.*, 1987) and the neutrophil respiratory burst (Atkinson *et al.*, 1988; McColl *et al.*, 1990a).

TNFα synthesis by neutrophils has been documented by two separate groups in which the possible contribution by monocytes to the detection of TNFα was also carefully examined and ruled out. In one study, Dubravek *et al.* (1990) demonstrated that peripheral blood neutrophils stimulated with LPS release relatively large quantities of TNFα compared to human monocytes. Levels of TNFα in resting monocytes were roughly five-fold greater than that in neutrophils, however, TNFα production by neutrophils was stimulated to a greater extent upon incubation of the cells with LPS. Interestingly, bioassay indicated levels of TNFα far below those detected by ELISA, suggesting the co-release of an inhibitor of TNFα bioactivity. In a separate study, LPS and the opportunistic fungus *Candida albicans* was shown to induce TNFα production in neutrophils (Djeu *et al.*, 1990). Although it is impossible to compare the amounts of TNFα detected with those reported in the previous study because no indication of the definition of TNFα activity was given in the second report, the overall results support those of the previous study. That the release of TNFα by neutrophils requires up-regulation of gene expression was demonstrated in two ways. First, LPS induced an accumulation of TNFα mRNA in neutrophils, and second, prior treatment of neutrophils with either the transcription inhibitor actinomycin D or the protein synthesis inhibitors emitine or cycloheximide prevented the release of TNFα. These observations imply that TNFα is not stored in neutrophils and released upon appropriate stimulation.

5.4   INTERLEUKIN-6

IL-6 is another important multifunctional cytokine (Akira *et al.*, 1990). It stimulates differentiation of B cells and induces antibody production (Hirano *et al.*, 1986). IL-6 also stimulates acute-phase protein release by hepatocytes and growth of T cells, hybridomas and melanomas (Gauldie *et al.*, 1987; Van Damme *et al.*, 1987; Kawano *et al.*, 1988; Lotz *et al.*, 1988). In addition, this cytokine, in conjunction with IL-3 and IL-1, stimulates growth of myeloid precursors (Ikebuchi *et al.*, 1987). Recently, a study reporting the production of IL-6 by peripheral blood neutrophils has been published (Cicco *et al.*, 1990). Of a large array of cytokines, including G- and M-CSF, IL-3 and IFN, only GM-CSF and TNFα were found to release significant quantities of IL-6 as determined by bioassay. In addition, Northern blot analysis revealed an accumulation of IL-6

mRNA within 4 h of stimulation by TNFα thereby indicating that *de novo* expression of the IL-6 gene was probably required.

5.5   INTERFERON α

Of further interest is a recent report documenting the ability of human peripheral blood neutrophils to synthesize and secrete IFNα in response to G-CSF (Shirafuji *et al.*, 1990). This response was also observed at both the level of transcription and translation. Although no other agonist was examined, the use of G-CSF as a stimulus effectively eliminated the possibility that contaminating mononuclear cells may have been responsible for the observed production of IFNα since these cells do not respond to G-CSF (Nienhuis, 1988; Weisbart and Golde, 1989). It has been postulated that the ability of peripheral blood neutrophils to produce this cytokine in response to G-CSF may have significant biological importance since it is known that *in vivo* administration of G-CSF increases neutrophil production (Bronchud *et al.*, 1988; Nienhuis, 1988) and several previous studies have suggested that neutrophil production *in vivo* may be controlled by circulating levels of G-CSF. On the other hand, it has been shown that IFNα inhibits neutrophil colony formation *in vitro* (Greenberg and Mosny, 1977). Therefore, it is possible that neutrophil production may be haemostatically controlled by the balance between circulating G-CSF and IFNα produced in response to G-CSF.

5.6   COLONY-STIMULATING FACTORS

Neutrophils are also capable of producing CSFs under appropriate conditions. Lindemann *et al.* (1989) stimulated peripheral blood neutrophils with GM-CSF and measured subsequent release of G-CSF and M-CSF. A murine bioassay which is responsive to these two cytokines but not GM-CSF, was used to determine the quantity of G- and M-CSF secreted. In addition, accumulation of mRNA for both G- and M-CSF was observed in GM-CSF-treated neutrophils. The potential contribution of contaminating monocytes was ruled out by probing the Northern blots with a c-*fms* cDNA. The product of this proto-oncogene is the M-CSF receptor which is expressed by monocytes but not neutrophils (Sariban *et al.*, 1985; Sherr *et al.*, 1985). Under conditions where mRNA for G- and M-CSF were observed, no c-*fms* mRNA transcripts were detected.

5.7   TRANSFORMING GROWTH FACTOR β

It has recently been shown that TGF is a potent neutrophil activating factor, stimulating neutrophil chemotaxis in the fM range (Fava *et al.*, 1991; Reibman et al., 1991). This makes TGFβ the most potent neutrophil chemoattractant yet found, approximately 100 000-fold more potent than FMLP. In addition, it appears that this cytokine is unique amongst neutrophil chemotactic factors since it activates these cells in a calcium-independent, protein synthesis-dependent manner. Another highly unusual feature of the relationship between neutrophils and TGFβ is the manner in which neutrophils produce and release TGFβ (Fava et al., 1991). Whereas other cell types appear to up-regulate TGFβ gene expression and subsequent translation and secretion, neutrophils appear to store this cytokine and secrete it from storage sites upon appropriate stimulation. This phenomenon has been reported in several separate studies. For instance, Carrington et al. (1988), showed that subpopulations of bone marrow neutrophils contain significant levels of TGFβ. A subsequent study showed that both human peripheral blood monocytes and neutrophils contain TGFβ but, unlike monocytes, neutrophils do not release this cytokine in response to LPS (Grotendorst et al., 1989). In that study, it was shown that both monocytes and neutrophils contain TGFβ mRNA in the resting state, but do not up-regulate this level upon stimulation with LPS. This latter observation led to the proposal that TGFβ production in these cells is regulated at a post-transcriptional level (Grotendorst et al., 1989). The puzzle as to why neutrophils store this cytokine but do not appear to release it, was addressed recently when Fava et al. (1991) showed that incubation of neutrophils with PMA for 30 min was sufficient to induce the release of relatively large quantities of TGFβ (100 ng/$1-2 \times 10^7$ neutrophils) implying that TGFβ may be stored in granules in these cells. The biological significance of these observations remains be adequately explored.

5.8 INTERLEUKIN-8

IL-8, also known as NAP-1, neutrophil-activating factor 1 (NAF-1), monocyte-derived NAP, and lymphocyte-derived NAP, is a prominent member of a recently discovered family of small molecular weight inflammatory cytokines known as the PF4 superfamily, and is also referred to as the intercrine or the chemokine family (for reviews, see Stoeckle and Barker, 1990; Oppenheim et al., 1991; Schall, 1991). The various members of this gene superfamily are related by primary amino-acid sequence similarity and possession of a highly conserved four-cysteine motif. The members of this superfamily may be further subdivided into two subfamilies depending on the arrangement of the first two cysteines in the four-cysteine motif. The C-X-C subfamily which includes PF$_4$ (Deuel et al., 1977), IL-8, NAP-2 and melanocyte growth-stimulatory activity is characterized by having the first two cysteines separated by an intervening amino acid (Oppenheim et al., 1991). In the second subfamily, which includes the cytokines RANTES

(Schall et al., 1988), MCP-1 (Furutani et al., 1989; Matsushima et al., 1989; Yoshimura et al., 1987), the macrophage inflammatory proteins-1α and β (Obaru et al., 1986; Sherry et al., 1988; Brown et al., 1989; Wolfe and Cerami, 1989), HC-14 (Chang et al., 1989) and I-309 (Brown et al., 1989), the first two cysteines are directly adjacent (Schall, 1991). The potential importance of these cytokines in immune regulation and inflammatory reactions stems from the fact that they are chemotactic and activating factors for leukocytes with different degrees of specificity, with the pro-inflammatory actions of the members of the C-C branch being directed more towards mononuclear cells, and those of the C-X-C branch, towards neutrophils. Indeed, IL-8 stimulates neutrophil chemotaxis both in vitro and in vivo (Peveri et al., 1988). In addition, it activates a variety of neutrophil functions including calcium mobilization, the respiratory burst, degranulation (Peveri et al., 1988), adhesion (Carveth et al., 1989; Detmers et al., 1990) and leukotriene synthesis (Schroeder, 1989). Since its discovery almost 5 years ago, detailed studies have shown that this cytokine is synthesized and secreted by many different cell types, notably monocyte/macrophages (Matsushima et al., 1988; Peveri et al., 1988), endothelial cells (Strieter et al., 1989a; Schroeder and Christophers, 1989) and fibroblasts (Strieter et al., 1989b; Schroeder et al., 1990). However, recently, it has been shown that phagocytosing neutrophils may also be a significant source of IL-8 (Bazzoni et al., 1991). In fact, it appears that IL-8 may be one of the major protein products secreted by these cells since the secretion of IL-8 by neutrophils is of the same magnitude as that by mononuclear cells under the same conditions. Recent studies in our laboratory (SRM) have shown that neutrophils stimulated with GM-CSF or TNFα do not contain detectable levels of mRNA for RANTES, MCP-1, cytokines of the C-C subfamily whereas under the same conditions, large quantities of IL-8 mRNA accumulate (see Figure 5.1). This implies that neutrophils are only capable of producing chemokines to which they respond (e.g. IL-8) and not factors which activate monocytes and lymphocytes. In terms of the role of neutrophils in acute inflammation, these observations make biological sense, since they suggest that migrating and phagocytosing neutrophils are able to secrete large quantities of a chemotactic cytokine to which they can respond, yet they do not produce factors which could attract and activate large numbers of monocytes and lymphocytes, an event which could rapidly lead to chronic inflammation.

5.9 INTERLEUKIN-1 RECEPTOR ANTAGONIST

In addition to synthesizing and releasing pro-inflammatory cytokines, recent studies have shown that

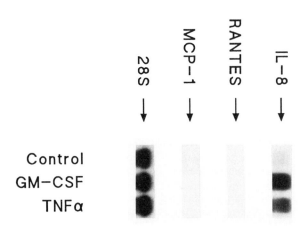

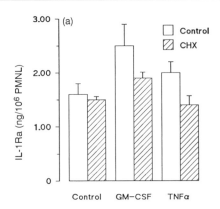

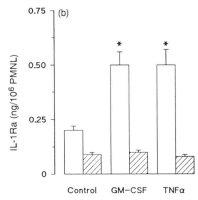

Figure 5.1 The expression of chemokine mRNA in human peripheral blood neutrophils stimulated with GM-CSF or TNFα. Neutrophils were isolated from the peripheral blood of normal donors and incubated for 2 h at 37°C with diluent (0.01% BSA in PBS), 1 nM GM-CSF or 100 ng/ml TNFα. Total RNA was then isolated and Northern blots were performed as described in McColl et al. (1992). To confirm equal loading and integrity of the RNA, the filters were also hybridized with an oligonucleotide which binds to 28S RNA. The cDNAs used in this study were provided by Dr Thomas Schall at Genentech Incorporated.

Figure 5.2 The synthesis of human IL-1Ra by human neutrophils stimulated with GM-CSF or TNFα. Neutrophils were isolated from the peripheral blood of normal donors and incubated for 24 h at 37°C with diluent (0.01% BSA in PBS), 1 nM GM-CSF or 100 ng/ml TNFα following pretreatment for 1 h with cycloheximide (10 μg/ml). IL-1Ra was then measured by ELISA in the cell lysates (a) and supernatants (b) as described in McColl et al. (1992). *Significantly different from control as $P < 0.006$ (Student t-test). The values are the mean ± SEM of duplicate determinations from three separate donors.

neutrophils are also a major source of the recently discovered IL-1Ra (McColl *et al.*, 1992). As its name implies, this molecule binds to but does not activate IL-1 receptors, thereby acting as a specific IL-1Ra (Carter *et al.*, 1990; Eisenberg *et al.*, 1990; Dinarello, 1991). In terms of *de novo* protein synthesis, as measured by incorporation of ^{35}S-methionine during protein synthesis, IL-1Ra is the major neutrophil protein secreted in response to either GM-CSF or TNFα (McColl *et al.*, 1990b, 1992). No other cytokine tested, including G-CSF, IL-1, PDGF, TGFβ, IL-4, IL-6, IL-8 or IFNγ, stimulated production of this cytokine in neutrophils. The up-regulation of IL-1Ra secretion by neutrophils involves stimulation of gene expression, since GM-CSF and TNFα also rapidly induced IL-1Ra mRNA in neutrophils, with maximum induction being observed within 1 h of stimulation. Quantitative measurements by ELISA showed that there is approximately eight times more intracellular IL-1Ra than extracellular IL-1Ra in resting neutrophils. This drops to a four to five-fold excess when the cells are stimulated with either GM-CSF or TNFα, with most of the newly synthesized IL-1Ra being secreted. In activated cells, intracellular IL-1Ra is approximately 2–2.5 ng/10^6 cells with approximately 0.5 ng/10^6 cells being secreted. As is the case with TGFβ (Grotendorst *et al.*, 1989; Fava *et al.*, 1991), it appears that neutrophils contain stored, or preformed IL-1Ra (see Figure 5.2). Indeed, incubation of the cells with

cycloheximide has no effect on the level of IL-1Ra in the intracellular compartment. Overall, these figures imply that neutrophils are capable of producing IL-1Ra in approximately 100-fold excess to that of IL-1. This is an important observation when considering that such an excess is required to inhibit the proinflammatory effects of IL-1 *in vivo* (Seckinger *et al.*, 1990; Wakabayashi *et al.*, 1991). As mentioned above, while all of the newly synthesized IL-1Ra in neutrophils is secreted, the majority of the IL-1Ra found in neutrophils is preformed, but is not released in response to cytokine stimulation. Although the reasons for this are not yet clear, it is possible that significant amounts of IL-1Ra could be released at sites of inflammation when neutrophils are either lysed, for example, by bacterial toxins, or undergo apoptosis (Savill *et al.*, 1989; Hogquist *et al.*, 1991).

5.10 SUMMARY

Protein synthesis and secretion by neutrophils can be elicited by a variety of agonists including endotoxins, phorbol esters, phagocytic activators such as yeast particles and microcrystals, and several cytokines including GM-CSF and TNFα. From the studies published to date, it appears that neutrophils are capable of producing many different cytokines. However, they generally make cytokines that monocyte/macrophages also produce. In addition, the production of these cytokines, if taken on a cell for cell basis, is generally far lower than that produced by monocyte/macrophages under equivalent conditions, although there are certain exceptions to this rule (IL-8, TNFα, IL-1Ra). As mentioned above, this by no means reduces the biological impact of cytokine production by neutrophils which are often present at sites of inflammation in numbers far in excess of those of monocytes or tissue-based macrophages. The potential contribution by neutrophils may therefore by highly significant both physiologically and pathophysiologically.

Another interesting point is that, although all of the neutrophil-derived cytokines reported to date are also made by mononuclear phagocytes, there may be several monocyte/macrophage products which neutrophils do not synthesize (e.g. MCP-1). This observation implies the existence either of specific gene repressors in neutrophils, or the lack of a specific transcriptional control mechanism in neutrophils which is present in mononuclear phagocytes. Future studies specifically focusing on transcriptional activation of specific genes in neutrophils will be required to address this hypothesis.

6. *References*

Akira, S., Hirano, T., Taga, T. and Kishimoto, T. (1990). Biology of multifunctional cytokines: IL-6 and related molecules (IL-1 and TNF). FASEB J. 4, 2860–2867.

Alonso, F., Gil, M.G., Sanchez-Crespo, M. and Mato, J.M. (1982). Activation of 1-alkyl-2-lyso-glycero-3-phosphocholine acetyl-CoA transferase during phagocytosis in human polymorphonuclear leukocytes. J. Biol. Chem. 257, 3376–3378.

Atkinson, Y.H., Marasco, W.A., Lopez, A.F. and Vadas, M.A. (1988). Recombinant human tumor necrosis factor-α. Regulation of N-formylmethionylleucylphenylalanine receptor affinity and function on human neutrophils. J. Clin. Invest. 81, 759–765.

Bazzoni, F., Cassatella, M.A., Rossi, F., Ceska, M., Dewald, B. and Baggiolini, M. (1991). Phagocytosing neutrophils produce and release high amounts of the neutrophil-activating peptide 1/interleukin 8. J. Exp. Med. 173, 771–774.

Beaulieu, A.D., Paquin, R., Rathanaswami, P. and McColl, S.R. (1992). Nuclear signaling in neutrophils: stimulation of RNA synthesis is a response to a limited number of pro-inflammatory agonists. J. Biol. Chem. 267, 426–432.

Benveniste, J., Henson, P.M. and Cochrane, C.G. (1972). Leukocyte-dependent histamine release from rabbit platelets. The role of IgE, basophils and a platelet-activating factor. J. Exp. Med. 136, 1356–1377.

Benveniste, J., Tence, M., Varenne, P., Bidault, J., Boulet, C. and Polonsky, J. (1979). Semi-synthese et structure purposee du facteur activant les plaquettes (PAF); PAF-acether, un alkyl ether analogue de la lysophosphatidylcholine. C.R. Acad. Sci. (Paris) 289, 1037–1040.

Benveniste, J., Nunez, D., Duriez, P., Kurth, R., Bidault, J. and Fruchart, J.-C. (1988). Preformed PAF-acether and lyso PAF-acether are bound to lipoproteins. FEBS Lett. 226, 371–376.

Betz, S.J. and Henson, P.M. (1980). Production and release of platelet-activating factor (PAF); dissociation from degranulation and superoxide production in the human neutrophil. J. Immunol. 125, 2756–2763.

Beuscher, H.U., Guenther, C. and Roellinghoff, M. (1990). IL-1 beta secreted by activated murine macrophages as a biologically inactive precursor. J. Immunol. 144, 2179–2183.

Black, R.A., Kronheim, S.R., Cantrell, M., Deeley, M.C., March, C.J., Pricket, K.S., Wignall, J., Conlon, P.J., Cosman, D., Hopp, T.P. and Mochizuki, D.Y. (1988). Generation of biologically-active interleukin-1 beta by proteolytic cleavage of the inactive precursor. J. Biol. Chem. 263, 9437–9442.

Blank, M.L., Snyder, F., Byers, L.W., Brooks. B. and Muirhead, E.E. (1979). Antihypertensive activity of an alkyl ether analog of phosphatidylcholine. Biochem Biophys. Res. Comm. 90, 1194–1200.

Bokoch, G.M. and Reed, P.Q. (1981). Effect of various lipoxygenase metabolites of arachidonic acid on degranulation of polymorphonuclear leukocytes. J. Biol. Chem. 256, 5317–5320.

Borgeat, P. (1988). Biochemistry of the lipoxygenase pathways in neutrophils. Can. J. Physiol. Pharmacol. 67, 936–942.

Borgeat, P. and Naccache, P.H. (1990). Biosynthesis and biological activity of leukotriene B₄. Clin. Biochem. 23, 459–468.

Borgeat, P. and Samuelsson, B. (1979a). Metabolism of arachidonic acid in polymorphonuclear leukocytes: unstable intermediate in the formation of dihydroxy acids. Proc. Natl Acad. Sci. USA 17, 3213–3217.

Borgeat, P. and Samuelsson, B. (1979b). Metabolism of arachidonic acid in polymorphonuclear leukocytes: structural analysis of novel hydroxylated compounds. J. Biol. Chem. 254, 7865–7869.

Borgeat, P. and Samuelsson, B. (1979c). Metabolism of arachidonic acid in polymorphonuclear leukocytes: effects of the ionophore A23187. Proc. Natl Acad. Sci. USA 76, 2148–2152.

Borgeat P., Hamberg, M. and Samuelsson, B. (1976). Transformation of arachidonic acid and homo-gamma-linolenic acid in rabbit polymorphonuclear leukocytes. J. Biol. Chem. 251, 7816–7820.

Botto, M., Lissandrini, D., Sorio, C. and Walport, M.J. (1992). Biosynthesis and secretion of complement component (C3) by activated human polymorphonuclear leukocytes. J. Immunol. 149, 1348–1355.

Bronchud, M.H., Potter, M.R., Morgenstern, G., Blasco, M.J., Scarffe, J.H., Thatcher, N., Crowther, D., Souza, L.M., Alton, N.K., Testa, N.G. and Dexter, T.M. (1988). In vitro and in vivo analysis of the effects of recombinant human granulocyte colony-stimulating factor in patients. Br. J. Cancer 58, 64–69.

Brown, K.D., Zurawski, S.M., Mosmann, T. and Zurawski, G. (1989). A family of small inducible proteins secreted by leukocytes are members of a new superfamily that includes leukocyte- and fibroblast-derived inflammatory agents, growth factors, and indicators of various inflammatory activation processes. J. Immunol. 142, 679–687.

Bussolino, F., Sironi, M., Bocchietto, E. and Mantovani, A. (1992). Synthesis of platelet-activating factor by polymorphonuclear neutrophils stimulated with interleukin-8. J. Biol. Chem. 207, 14598–14603.

Camussi, G., Aglietta, M., Coda, R., Bussolino, F., Piacibello, W. and Tetta, C. (1981). Release of platelet-activating factor (PAF) and histamine. II. The cellular origin of human PAF: monocytes, polymorphonuclear neutrophils and basophils. Immunology 42, 191–199.

Camussi, G., Tetta, C., Segoloni, G., Coda, R. and Vercellone, A. (1982). Localization of neutrophil cationic proteins and loss of anionic charges in glomeruli of patients with systemic lupus erythematosus glomerulonephritis. Clin. Immunol. Immunopath. 24, 299–314.

Camussi, G., Tetta, C., Coda, R., Segoloni, G.P. and Vercellone, A. (1984). Platelet-activating factor-induced loss of glomerular anionic charges. Kidney Int. 25, 73–81.

Carrington, J.L., Roberst, A.B., Flanders, K.C., Roche, N.S. and Reddi, A.H. (1988). Accumulation, localization and compartmentation of transforming growth factor β during endochondral bone development. J. Cell. Biol. 107, 1969–1975.

Carter, D.B., Diebel, M.R., Dunn, C.J., Tomich, C.S.C., Laborde, A.L., Slighton, A.E., Berger, A.E., Bienkowski, M.J., Sun, F.F., McEwan, R.N., Harris, P.K.W., Yem, A.W., Waszak, G.A., Chosay, J.G., Sieu, L.C., Hardee, M.M., Zurcher-Neely, H.A., Reardon, I.M., Heinrikson, R.L., Truesdell, S.E., Shelly, J.A., Eessalu, T.E., Taylor, B.M. and Tracey, D.E. (1990). Purification, cloning, expression and biological characterization of an interleukin-1 receptor antagonist protein. Nature 344, 633–637.

Carveth, H.J., Bohnsack, J.F., McIntyre, T.M., Baggiolini, M., Prescott, S.M. and Zimmerman, G.A. (1989). Neutrophil activating factor (NAF) induces polymorphonuclear leukocyte adherence to endothelial cells and to subendothelial matrix proteins. Biochem. Biophys. Res. Comm. 162, 387–393.

Chang, H.C., Hsu, F., Freeman, G.J., Griffin, J.D. and Reinherz, E.L. (1989). Cloning and expression of a γ-inteferon-inducible gene in monocytes: a new member of a cytokine gene family. Int. Immunol. 1, 388–399.

Chilton, F.H. (1989). Potential phospholipid source(s) of arachidonate used for the synthesis of leukotrienes by the neutrophil. Biochem. J. 258, 327–333.

Chilton, F.H., O'Flaherty, J.T., Walsh, C.E., Thomas, M.J., Wykle, R.L., DeChaletet, R. and Waite, B.M. (1982). Platelet-activating factor. Stimulation of the lipoxygenase pathway in polymorphonuclear leukocytes by 1-O-alkyl-2-O-acetyl-sn-glycero-3-phosphocholine. J. Biol. Chem 257, 5402–5407.

Chilton, F.H., O'Flaherty, J.T., Ellis, J.M., Swendsen, C.L. and Wykle, R.L. (1983). Selective acylation of lyso platelet activating factor by arachidonate in human neutrophils. J. Biol. Chem. 258, 7268–7271.

Chilton, F.H., Ellis, J.M., Olson, S.C. and Wykle, R.L. (1984). 1-O-Alkyl-2-arachidonoyl-sn-glycero-3-phosphocholine. A common source of platelet-activating factor and arachidonate in human polymorphonuclear leukocytes. J. Biol. Chem. 259, 12014–12019.

Chung, K.F. (1992). Platelet-activating factor in inflammation and pulmonary disorders. Clin. Sci. 83, 127–138.

Cicco, N., Lindemann, A., Content, J., Vandenbussche, P., Lubbert, M., Gauss, J., Mertelsmann, R. and Hermann, F. (1990). Inducible production of interleukin-6 by human polymorphonuclear neutrophils: role of granulocyte-macrophage colony-stimulating factor and tumor necrosis factor-alpha. Blood 75, 2049–2052.

Claesson, H.E., Lundberg, U. and Malmsten, C. (1981). Serum coated zymosan stimulates the synthesis of leukotriene B4 in human polymorphonuclear leukocytes. Inhibition by cyclic AMP. Biochem. Biophys. Res. Comm. 99, 1230–1237.

Clancy, R.M., Dahinden, C.A. and Hugli, T.E. (1983). Arachidonate metabolism by human polymorphonuclear leukocytes stimulated by N-formyl-Met-Leu-Phe or complement component C5a is independent of phospholipase activation. Proc. Natl Acad. Sci. USA 80, 7200–7204.

Clark. P.O., Hanahan, D.J. and Pinckard, R.N. (1980). Physical and chemical properties of platelet-activating factor obtained from human neutrophils and monocytes and rabbit neutrophils and basophils. Biochim. Biophys. Acta 628, 69–75.

Clay, K.L., Murphy, R.C., Andres, J.L., Lynch, J. and Henson, P.M. (1984). Structure elucidation of platelet activating factor derived from human neutrophils. Biochem. Biophys. Res. Comm. 121, 815–825.

Clay, K.L., Johnson, C. and Worthen, G.S. (1991). Biosynthesis of platelet activating factor and 1-O-acyl analogues by endothelial cells. Biochim. Biophys. Acta. 1094, 43–50.

Cluzel, M., Undem, B.J. and Chilton, F.H. (1989). Release of platelet-activating factor and the metabolism of leukotriene B4 the human neutrophil when studied in a cell superfusion model. J. Immunol. 143, 3659–3665.

Colotta, F., Wang, J.M., Polentarutti, N. and Mantovani, A. (1987). Expression of c-fos protoncogene in normal human peripheral blood granulocytes. J. Exp. Med. 165, 1224–1229.

Conrad, D.J., Kuhn, H., Mulkins, M., Highland, E. and Sigal, E. (1992). Specific inflammatory cytokines regulate the expression of human monocyte 15-lipoxygenase. Proc. Natl Acad. Sci. USA 89, 217–221.

Dahinden, C.A., Clancy, R.M. and Hugli, T.E. (1984). Stereospecificity of leukotriene B4 and structure–function relationship for chemotaxis of human neutrophils. J. Immunol. 133, 1477–1482.

Dahinden, C.A., Zingg, J., Maly, F.E. and de Wick, A.L. (1988). Leukotriene production in human neutrophils primed by recombinant human granulocyte–macrophage colony-stimulating factor and stimulated with the complement component C5a and FMLP as second signals. J. Exp. Med. 167, 1281–1295.

Demczuk, S., Baumberger, C., Mach, B. and Dayer, J.M. (1987). Expression of human IL-1 alpha and beta messenger RNAs and IL-1 activity in human peripheral blood mononuclear cells. J. Mol. Cell. Immunol. 3, 255–262.

Demopoulus, C.A., Pinckard, R.N. and Hanahan, D.J. (1979). Platelet-activating factor. Evidence for 1-O-alkyl-2-acetyl-sn-glycero-3-phosphocholine as the active component. A new class of lipid chemical mediators. J. Biol. Chem. 254, 9355–9358.

Detmers, P.A., Lo, S.K., Olsen-Egbert, E., Walz, A., Baggiolini, M. and Cohn, Z.A. (1990). Neutrophil activating protein 1/interleukin 8 stimulates the binding activity of the leukocyte adhesion receptor CD11b/CD18. J. Exp. Med. 171, 1151–1162.

Deuel, T.F., Keim, P.S., Farmer, M. and Heinrikson, R.L. (1977). Amino acid sequence of platelet factor 4. Proc. Natl Acad. Sci. USA 74, 2256–2258.

DeVries, A.J., Feldman, J.O., Stein, O., Stein, Y. and Katchalski, E. (1953). Effects of intravenously administered poly-D-L-lysine in rats. Proc. Soc. Exp. Biol. Med. 82, 237–240.

Dewald, B. and Baggiolini, M. (1985). Activation of NADPH oxidase in human neutrophils. Synergism between FMLP and neutrophil products PAF and LTB$_4$. Biochem. Biophys. Res. Commun. 128, 297–304.

Dinarello, C.A. (1991). Interleukin-1 and interleukin-1 antagonism. Blood 77, 1627–1652.

DiPersio, J.F., Billing, P., Williams, R. and Gasson, J.C. (1988a). Human granulocyte–macrophage colony-stimulating factor and other cytokines prime human neutrophils for enhanced arachidonic acid release and leukotriene B$_4$ synthesis. J. Immunol. 140, 4315–4322.

DiPersio, J.F., Naccache. P.H., Borgeat, P., Gasson, J.C., Nguyen, M.H. and McColl, S.R. (1988b). Characterization of the priming effects of human granulocyte–macrophage colony-stimulating factor on human neutrophil leukotriene synthesis. Prostaglandins 36, 673–691.

Dixon, R.A.F., Jones, R.E., Diehl, R.E., Bennet, C.D., Kargman, S. and Rouzer, C.A. (1988). Cloning of the cDNA for human 5-lipoxygenase. Proc. Natl Acad. Sci. USA 85 416–420.

Dixon, R.A.F., Diehl, R.E., Opas, E., Rands, E., Vickers, P.J., Evans, J.F., Gillard, J.W. and Miller, D.K. (1990). Requirement of a 5-lipoxygenase-activating protein for leukotriene synthesis. Nature 343, 282–284.

Djeu, J.Y., Serbousek, D. and Blanchard, D.K. (1990). Release of tumor necrosis factor by human polymorphonuclear leukocytes. Blood 76, 1405–1409.

Dubravek, D.B., Spriggs, D.R., Mannick, J.A. and Rodrick, M.L. (1990). Circulating human peripheral blood granulocytes synthesize and secrete tumor necrosis factor α. Proc. Natl Acad. Sci. USA 87, 6758–6761.

Eisenberg, S.P., Evans, R.J., Arend, W.P., Verderder, E., Brewer, C.H., Hannum, C.H. and Thompson, R.C. (1990). Primary structure and functional expression from complementary DNA of a human interleukin-1 receptor antagonist. Nature 343, 341–346.

Evans, R.D., Lund, P. and Williamson, D.H. (1991). Platelet-activating factor and its metabolic effects. Prost. Leuk. Ess. Fatty Acids 44, 1–10.

Fava, R.A., Olsen, N.J., Postlethwaite, A.E., Broadley, K.N., Davidson, J.M., Nanney, L.R., Lucas, C. and Townes, A.S. (1991). Transforming growth factor β1 (TGFβ1)-induced neutrophil recruitment to synovial tissues: implications for TGFβ-driven synovial inflammation and hyperplasia. J. Exp. Med. 173, 1121–1132.

Fiers, W. (1991). Tumor necrosis factor. Characterization at the molecular, cellular and in vivo level. FEBS Lett. 285, 199–212.

Ford-Hutchinson, A.W., Bray, M.A., Doig, M.V., Shipley, M.E. and Smith, M.J.H. (1980). Leukotriene B$_4$, a potent chemokinetic and aggregating substance released from polymorphonuclear leukocytes. Nature 286, 254–265.

Frimmer, M. and Hegner, D. (1963). Isolierung eines basischen polypeptids mit leukotaktischer und permeationsfordernder wirkung. Arch. Exp. Path. Pharmakol. 245, 355–373.

Fukuchi, Y., Sato, M., Yamashita, T. and Koyama, J. (1992). Low ligand binding activities of two distinct types of Fcγ receptor guinea pig peripheral blood polymorphonuclear leukocytes are differentially improved by proteolysis or platelet activating factor. Mol. Pharm. 29, 583–592.

Funk, C.D., Hoshiko, S., Matsumoto, T., Radmark, O. and Samuelsson, B. (1989). Characterization of the human 5-lipoxygenase. Proc. Natl Acad. Sci. USA 86, 2587–2591.

Furutani, Y., Mormura, H., Notake, M., Oyamada, Y., Fukue, T., Yamada, M., Larsen, C.G.. Oppenheim, J.J. and Matsushima, K. (1989). Cloning and sequencing of the cDNA for human monocyte chemotactic and activating factor (MCAF). Biochem. Biophys. Res. Comm. 159, 249–255.

Ganz, T., Selsted, M.E. and Lehrer, R.l. (1990). Defensins. Eur J. Haematol. 44, 1–8.

Gauldie, J., Richards, C., Harnish, D., Lansdorp, P. and Baumann, H. (1987). Interferon beta 2/B-cell stimulatory factor type 2 shares identity with monocyte-derived hepatocyte-stimulating factor and regulates the major acute-phase protein response in the liver. Proc. Natl Acad. Sci. USA, 84, 7251–7255.

Gay, J.C. and Stitt, E.S. (1988). Enhancement of phorbol ester-induced protein kinase activity in human neutrophils by platelet-activating factor. J. Cell. Physiol. 137, 439–447.

Gay, J.C., Beckman, J.K., Zabog, K.A. and Lukens, J.N. (1986). Modulation of neutrophil oxidative responses to soluble stimuli by PAF. Blood 67, 931–936.

Gimbrone, M.A., Brock, A.F. and Schafer, A.I. (1984). Leukotriene stimulates polymorphonuclear leukocyte adhesion to cultured endothelial cells. J. Clin. Invest. 74, 1552–1555.

Goldstein, I.M., Malmsten, C.L., Kundahl, H., Kaplan, H.B., Radmark, O., Samuelsson, B. and Weissmann, G.A. (1978). Thromboxane generation by human peripheral blood polymorphonuclear leukocytes. J. Exp. Med. 148, 7887–7892.

Golub, E.S. and Spitznagel, J.K. (1965). The role of lysosomes in hypersensitivity reactions. Tissue damage by polymorphonuclear neutrophil lysosomes. J. Immunol. 95, 1060–1066.

Greenberg, P.L. and Mosny, S.A. (1977). Cytotoxic effects of interferon in vitro on granulocytic progenitor cells. Cancer Res. 37, 1794–1799.

Grotendorst, G.R., Smale, G. and Pencev, D. (1989). Production of transforming growth factor beta by human peripheral blood monocytes and neutrophils. J. Cell. Physiol. 140, 396–402.

Hamberg, M. and Samuelsson, B. (1974). Prostaglandin endoperoxides: novel transformations of arachidonic acid in human platelets. Proc. Natl Acad. Sci. USA 71, 3400–3404.

Hellewell, P.G. and Williams, T.J. (1986). A specific antagonist of platelet-activating factor suppresses edema formation in an Arthus reaction but not edema induced by leukocyte chemoattractants in rabbit skin. J. Immunol. 137, 302–307.

Henson, P.M. (1969). Role of complement and leukocytes in immunologic release of vasoactive amines from platelets. Fed. Proc. 28, 1721–1728.

Henson, P.M. (1970a). Release of vasoactive amines from rabbit platelets induced by sensitized mononuclear leukocytes and antigen. J. Exp. Med. 131, 287–306.

Henson, P.M. (1970b). Mechanisms of release of constituents from rabbit platelets by antigen-antibody complexes and complement. II. Interaction of platelets with neutrophils. J. Immunol. 105, 490–501.

Henson, P.M. (1971). The immunologic release of constituents from neutrophil leukocytes. I. The role of antibody and complement on non-phagocytosable surfaces or phagocytosable particles. J. Immunol. 107, 1535–1546.

Henson, P.M., Johnson, H.B. and Spiegelberg, H.L. (1972). The release of granule enzymes from human neutrophils stimulated by aggregated immunoglobulin of different classes and sub-classes. J. Immunol. 109, 1182–1192.

Hermann, F., Lindemann, A., Gauss, J. and Mertelsmann, R. (1990). Cytokine-stimulation of prostaglandin synthesis from endogenous and exogenous arachidonic acids in polymorphonuclear leukocytes involving activation and new synthesis of cyclooxygenase. Eur. J. Immunol. 20, 2513–2516.

Hilliquin, P., Menkes, C.J., Laoussadi, S., Benveniste, J. and Arnoux, B. (1992). Presence of PAF-acether in rheumatic disease. Ann. Rheum. Dis. 51, 29–31.

Hirano, T., Yasukawa, K., Harada, H., Taga, T., Watanabe, Y., Matsuda, T., Kashiwamura, S., Nakajima, K., Koyama, K., Iwamatu, A., Tsunasawa, S., Sakiyama, K., Takhara, Y., Taniguchi, T. and Kishimoto, T. (1986). Complementary DNA for a novel human interleukin (BSF-2) that induces B lymphocytes to produce immunoglobulin. Nature 324, 73–76.

Hogquist, K.A., Nett, M.A., Unanue, E.R. and Chaplin, D.D. (1991). Interleukin-1 is processed and released during apoptosis. Proc. Natl Acad. Sci. USA 88, 8485–8489.

Honda, Z.-I., Nakamura, M., Miki, I., Minami, M., Watanabe, T., Seyama, Y., Okudo, H., Toh, H., Ito, K., Miyamoto, T. and Shimuzu, T. (1991). Cloning by functional expression of platelet-activating factor receptor from guinea-pig lung. Nature 349, 342–346.

Hoover, R.L., Karnovsky, M.J., Austen, K.F., Corey, E.J. and Lewis, R.A. (1984). Leukotriene B4 action on endothelium mediates augmented neutrophil/endothelial adhesion. Proc. Natl Acad. Sci. USA 81, 2191–2193.

Hoshiko, S., Radmark, O. and Samuelsson, B. (1990). Characterization of the human 5-lipoxygenase gene promoter. Proc. Natl Acad. Sci. USA 87, 9073–9077.

Hwang, S.B. (1988). Identification of a second receptor of platelet-activating factor from human polymorphonuclear leukocytes. J. Biol. Chem. 263, 3225–3233.

Ikebuchi, K., Wong, G.G., Clark, S.C., Ihle, J.N., Hirai, Y. and Ogawa, M. (1987). Interleukin 6 enhancement of interleukin 3-dependent proliferation of multipotential hemopoietic progenitors. Proc. Natl Acad. Sci. USA 84, 9035–9039.

Issekutz, A.C. (1981). Vascular responses during acute neutrophilic inflammation: their relationship to in vivo neutrophil emigration. Lab. Invest. 45, 435–441.

Janoff, A. and Zweifach, B.W. (1964). Production of inflammatory changes in the microcirculation by cationic proteins extracted from lysosomes. J. Exp. Med. 120, 747–764.

Johnson, M.M., Carey, F. and MacMillan, R.M. (1986). Alternative pathways of arachidonate metabolism: prostaglandins, thromboxane and leukotrienes. Essays Biochem. 19, 41–141.

Jouvin-Marche, E., Ninio, E., Beauvain, G., Tence, M., Niaudet, P. and Benveniste, J. (1984). Biosynthesis of Paf-acether (platelet-activating factor). VII. Precursors of Paf-acether and acetyl transferase activity in human leukocytes. J. Immunol. 133, 892–898.

Kawano, M., Hirano, T., Matsuda, T., Taga, T., Horii, Y., Iwato, K., Asaoka, H., Tang, B., Tanabe, O., Tanaka, H., Kuramoto, A. and Kishimoto, T. (1988). Autocrine generation and requirement of BSF-2/IL-6 for human multiple myelomas. Nature 332, 83–85.

Kennedy, B.P., Diehl, R.E., Boie, Y., Adam, M. and Dixon, R.A.F. (1991). Gene characterization and promoter analysis of the human 5-lipoxygenase-activating protein (FLAP). J. Biol. Chem. 266, 8511–8516.

Koenderman, L., Yazdombakksh, M., Roos, D. and Verhoeven, A.J. (1989). Dual mechanisms in priming of chemoattractant-induced respiratory burst in human granulocytes. J. Immunol. 142, 623–628.

Koltai, M., Hosford, D., Guinot, P, Esanu, A. and Braquet, P. (1991a). Platelet activating factor (PAF). A review of its effects, antagonists and future clinical implications. (Part 1). Drugs 42, 9–29.

Koltai, M., Hosford, D., Grinot, P., Esanu, A. and Braquet, P. (1991b). Platelet activating factor (PAF). A review of its effects, antagonists and possible future clinical implications. (Part II). Drugs 42, 174–204.

Kreis, C., LaFleur, M., Ménard, C., Paquin, R. and Beaulieu, A.D. (1989). Thrombospondin and fibronectin are synthesized by neutrophils in human inflammatory joint disease and in a rabbit model of in vivo neutrophil activating. J. Immunol. 143, 1961–1968.

Kuijpers, T.W., Hakkert, B.C., Hoogerwerf, M., Verhoeven, A.J. and Roos, D. (1991). The role of endothelial leukocyte-adhesion molecule-1 (ELAM-1) and platelet-activating factor (PAF) in neutrophil adherence to IL-1-prestimulated endothelial cells: ELAM-1-mediated CD18 activation. J. Immunol. 147 1369–1376.

Kuijpers, T.W., Hakkert, B.C., Hart, M.H.L. and Roos, D. (1992). Neutrophil migration across monolayers of cytokine-prestimulated endothelial cells: a role for platelet-activating factor and IL-8. J. Cell Biol. 117, 565–572.

Kunz, D., Gerard, N. and Gerard, C. (1992). The human leukocyte platelet-activating factor receptor. J. Biol. Chem. 287, 9101–9106.

LaFleur, M., Beaulieu, A.D., Kreis, C. and Poubelle, P.E. (1987). Fibronectin gene expression in polymorphonuclear leukocytes. Accumulation of mRNA in inflammatory cells. J. Biol. Chem. 262, 2111–2115.

Lam, B.K., Gagnon, L., Austen, K.F. and Soberman, R.J. (1990). The mechanism of leukotriene B4 export from human polymorphonuclear leukocytes. J. Biol. Chem. 265, 13438–13441.

Lehrer, R.I. and Ganz, T. (1990). Antimicrobial polypeptides of human neutrophils. Blood 76, 2169–2181.

Lewis, R.A. and Austen, K.F. (1984). The biologically active leukotrienes. J. Clin. Invest. 73, 889–897.

Lewis, R.A., Austen, K.F. and Soberman, R.J. (1990). Leuko-trienes and other products of the 5-lipoxygenase pathway. N. Engl. J. Med. 323, 645–655.

Libby, P., Ordovas, J.M., Auger, K.R., Robbins, A.H., Birimyi, L.K. and Dinarello, C.A. (1986). Endotoxin and tumor necrosis factor induce interleukin-1 gene expression in adult human vascular endothelial cells. Am J. Pathol. 124, 179–185.

Lin, A.H., Morton, D.R. and Gorman, R.R. (1982). Acetyl glyceryl ether phosphorylcholine stimulates leukotriene B4 synthesis in human polymorphonuclear leukocytes. J. Clin. Invest. 70, 1058–1065.

Lindemann, A., Riedel, D., Oster, W., Meuer, S.C., Blohm, D., Mertelsmann, R.H. and Hermann, F. (1988). Granulocyte–macrophage colony-stimulating factor induces interleukin 1 production by human polymorphonuclear neutrophils. J. Immunol. 140, 837–839.

Lindemann, A., Riedel, D., Oster, W., Ziegler-Heitbrock, H.W.L., Mertelsmann, R. and Hermann, F. (1989). Granulocyte–macrophage colony-stimulating factor induces cytokine secretion by human polymorphonuclear leukocytes. J. Clin. Invest. 83, 1308–1312.

Lloyd, A.R. and Oppenheim, J.J. (1992). Poly's lament: the neglected role of the polymorphonuclear neutrophil in the afferent limb of the immune response. Immunol. Today 13, 169–172.

Lonnemann, G., Endres, S., van der Meer, J.W., Cannon, J.G., Koch, K.M. and Dinarello, C.A. (1989). Differences in the synthesis and kinetics of release of interleukin 1 alpha, interleukin 1 beta and tumor necrosis factor from human mononuclear cells. Eur. J. Immunol. 19, 1531–1536.

Lorant, D.E.K., Patel, K.D., McIntyre, T.M., McEver, R.P., Prescott, S.M. and Zimmerman, G.A. (1991). Coexpression of GMP-140 and PAF by endothelium stimulated by histamine and thrombin: a juxtacrine system for adhesion and activation for neutrophils. J. Cell Biol. 115, 223–234.

Lotner, G.Z., Lynch, J.M., Betz, S.J. and Henson, P.M. (1980). Human neutrophil-derived platelet activating factor. J. Immunol. 124, 676–684.

Lotz, M., Jirik, F., Kabourdis, R., Tsoukas, C., Hirano, T.K.T. and Carson, D.A. (1988). B cell-stimulating factor 2/interleukin 6 is a costimulant for human thymocytes and T lymphocytes. J. Exp. Med. 167, 1253–1258.

Ludwig, J.C. and Pinckard, R.N. (1987). In "New Horizons in Platelet Activating Factor Research" (ed. C.M. Winslow and M.L. Lee) pp 59–71. John Wiley & Sons, New York.

Ludwig, J.C., Hoppens, C.L., McManus, L.M., Mott, G.E. and Pinckard, R.N. (1985). Modulation of platelet-activating factor (PAF) synthesis and release from human polymorpho-nuclear leukocytes (PMN): role of albumin. Arch. Biochem. Biophys. 241, 337–347.

Lynch, J.M. and Henson, P.M. (1986). The intracellular retention of newly synthesized platelet-activating factor. J. Immunol. 137, 2653–2661.

Lynch, J.M., Lotner, G.Z., Betz, S.J. and Henson, P.M. (1979). The release of platelet-activating factor by stimulated rabbit neutrophils. J. Immunol. 123, 1219–1226.

March, C.J., Mosley, B., Larsen, A., Cerretti, D.P., Braedt, G., Price, V., Gillis, S., Henney, C.S., Kronheim, S.R., Grabstein, K., Conlon, P.J., Hopp, T.P. and Cosman, D.

(1985). Cloning, sequence and expression of two distinct human interleukin-1 complementary DNAs. Nature 315, 641–647.

Marquis, O., Robaut, C. and Cavero, I. (1988). [^{3}H] 52770 RP, a platelet-activating factor receptor antagonist, and tritiated platelet-activating factor label a common specific binding site in human polymorphonuclear leukocytes. J. Pharmacol. Exp. Ther. 244, 709–715.

Marucha, P.T., Zeff, R.A. and Kreutzer, D.L. (1990). Cytokine regulation of IL-1β gene expression in the human poly-morphonuclear leukocyte. J. Immunol. 145, 2932–2937.

Marucha, P.T., Zeff, R.A. and Kreutzer, D.L. (1991). Cytokine-induced IL-1β gene expression in the human polymorphonuclear leukocyte: Transcriptional and post-transcriptional regulation by tumor necrosis factor and IL-1 J. Immunol. 147, 2603–2608.

Matsushima, K., Morishita, K., Yoshimura, T., Lavu, S., Kobayashi, Y., Lew, W., Appella, E., Kung, H.F., Leonard, E.J. and Oppenheim, J.J. (1988). Molecular cloning of a human monocyte-derived neutrophil chemotactic factor (MDNCF) and the induction of MDNCF mRNA by inter-leukin 1 and tumor necrosis factor. J. Exp. Med. 167, 1883–1893.

Matsushima, K., Larsen, C.G., DuBois, G.C. and Oppenheim, J.J. (1989). Purification and characterization of a novel mono-cyte chemotactic and activating factor produced by a human myelomonocytic cell line. J. Exp. Med. 169, 1485–1490.

McColl, S.R., Kreis, C., Borgeat, P., Di Persio, J.F. and Naccache, P.H. (1989) Involvement of G proteins in neutrophil activation and priming by granulocyte macrophage colony stimulating factor. Blood 73, 588–591.

McColl, S.R., Beausiegle, D., Gilbert, C. and Naccache, P.H. (1990a). Priming of the human neutrophil respiratory burst by granulocyte–macrophage colony-stimulating factor and tumor necrosis factor involves regulation at a post-receptor level. Enhancement of the effect of agents which directly activate G proteins. J. Immunol. 145, 3047–3053.

McColl, S.R., Paquin, R. and Beaulieu, A.D. (1990b). Selective synthesis and secretion of a 23 kD protein by neutrophils following stimulation with granulocyte–macrophage colony-stimulating factor and tumor necrosis factor α. Biochem. Biophys. Res. Comm. 172, 1209–1216.

McColl, S.R., Krump, E., Naccache, P.H., Poubelle, P.E., Braquet, M. and Borgeat, P. (1991). Granulocyte–macrophage colony-stimulating factor enhances the synthesis of leuko-triene B4 by human neutrophils in response to PAF-acether. Enhancement of both arachidonic acid release and 5-lipoxygenase activation. J. Immunol. 146, 1204–1211.

McColl, S.R., Paquin, R., Ménard, C. and Beaulieu, A.D. (1992). Human neutrophils produce high levels of the interleukin 1 receptor antagonist in response to granulocyte/macrophage colony-stimulating factor and tumor necrosis factor α. J. Exp. Med. 176, 593–598.

McDonald, P.P., Pouliot, M., Borgeat, P. and McColl, S.R. (1993). Induction by chemokines of lipid mediator synthesis in GM-CSF-treated human neutrophils. J. Immunol. 151, 6399–6409.

Miller, D.K., Gillard, J.W., Vickers, P.J., Sadowski, S., Léveille, C., Mancini, J.A., Charleson, P., Dixon, R.A.F., Ford-Hutchinson, A.W., Fortin, R., Gauthier, J.Y., Rodkey, J., Rosen, R., Rouzer, C., Sigal, I.S., Strader, C.D. and Evans, J.F. (1990). Identification and isolation of a membrane protein necessary for leukotriene production. Nature 343, 278–281.

Miwa, M., Sugatani, J., Ikemura, T., Okamoto, Y., Ino, M., Saito, K., Suzuki, Y. and Matsumoto, M. (1992). Release of newly synthesized platelet-activating factor (PAF) from human polymorphonuclear leukocytes under *in vivo* conditions: contribution of PAF-releasing factor in serum. J. Immunol. 148, 872–880.

Moncada, S. and Vane, J.R. (1978). Pharmacology and endogenous roles of prostaglandin endoperoxides thromboxane A_2 and prostacyclin. Pharm. Rev. 30, 293–331.

Mueller, H.W., O'Flaherty, J.T. and Wykle, R.L. (1983). Biosynthesis of platelet activating factor in rabbit polymorphonuclear neutrophils. J. Biol. Chem. 258, 6213–6218.

Mueller, H.W., O'Flaherty, J.T. and Wykle, R.L. (1984). The molecular species distribution of platelet-activating factor synthesized by rabbit and human neutrophils. J. Biol. Chem. 259, 14554–14559.

Mueller, H.W., Nollert, M.U. and Eskin, S.G. (1991). Synthesis of 1-acyl-2-[^{3}H]acetyl-*sn*-glycero-3-phosphocholine, a structural analog of platelet activating factor by vascular endothelial cells. Biochem. Biophys. Res. Comm. 176, 1557–1564.

Musser, J.H. and Kreft, A.F. (1992). 5-Lipoxygenase: properties, pharmacology, and the quinolinyl(bridged)aryl class of inhibitors. J. Med. Chem. 35, 2501–2524.

Naccache, P.H. and Sha'afi, R.I. (1983). Arachidonic acid, leukotriene B_4, and neutrophil activation. Ann. N.Y. Acad. Sci. 414, 125–139.

Naccache, P.H., Sha'afi, R.I. and Borgeat, P. (1989). In "The Neutrophil: Cellular Biochemistry and Physiology" (ed. M.B. Hallet) pp. 116–140.

Nadeau, M., Fruteau de Laclos, B., Picard, S., Braquet, P. and Borgeat, P. (1984). Studies on leukotriene B_4 Ω-oxidation in human leukocytes. Can. J. Biochem. Cell. Biol. 62, 1321–1326.

Needham, L., Hellewell, P.G., Williams, T.J., and Gordon, J.L. (1988). Endothelial functional responses and increased vascular permeability induced by polycations. Lab. Invest. 59, 538–548.

Needleman, P., Turk, J., Jakschik, B.A., Morrison, A.R. and Lefkowith, J.B. (1986). Arachidonic acid metabolism. Ann. Rev. Biochem. 55, 69–102.

Neuman, E., Huleatt, J.W. and Jack, R.M. (1990). Granulocyte–macrophage colony-stimulating factor increases synthesis and expression of CR1 and CR3 by human peripheral blood neutrophils. J. Immunol. 145, 3325–3332.

Ng, D.J. and Wong, K. (1986). GTP regulation of platelet-activating factor binding to human neutrophil membranes. Biochem. Biophys. Res. Comm. 141, 353–359.

Nienhuis, A.W. (1988). Hematopoietic growth factors. Biological complexity and clinical promise. N. Engl. J. Med. 318, 916–918.

Numerof, R.P., Kotich, A.N., Dinarello, C.A. and Mier, J.W. (1990). Pro-interleukin 1β production by a subpopulation of human T cells, but not NK cells, in response to interleukin 2. Cell. Immunol. 130, 118–128.

O'Banion, M.K., Sadowski, H.B., Winn, V. and Young, D.A. (1991). A serum- and glucocorticoid-regulated 4-kilobase mRNA encodes a cyclooxygenase-related protein. J. Biol. Chem. 266, 23261–23267.

Obaru, K., Fukuda, M., Maeda, S. and Shimada, K. (1986). A cDNA clone used to study mRNA inducible in human tonsillar lymphocytes by a tumor promoter. J. Biochem. 99, 885–894.

Oda, M.K., Satouchi, K., Yasunga, K. and Saito, K. (1985). Molecular species of platelet-activating factor generated by human neutrophils challenged with ionophore A23187. J. Immunol. 134, 1090–1093.

O'Flaherty, J.T., Miller, C.H., Lewis, J.C., Wykle, R.L., Bass, D.A. and McCall, C.E. (1981). 1-O-Alkyl-*sn*-glyceryl-3-phosphorylcholines. A novel class of neutrophil stimulants. Am. J. Pathol. 103, 70–78.

O'Flaherty, J.T., Surles, J.R., Redman, J., Jacobson, D., Piantadosi, C. and Wykle, R.L. (1988). Binding and metabolism of platelet-activating factor by human neutrophils. J. Clin. Invest. 78, 381–388.

Oppenheim, J.J., Zachariae, C.O.C., Mukaida, N. and Matsushima, K. (1991). Properties of the novel proinflammatory supergene "intercrine" cytokine family. Ann. Rev. Immunol. 9, 617–648.

O'Sullivan, M.G., Chilton, F.H., Huggins, E.M. and McCall, C.E. (1992). Lipopolysaccharide priming of alveolar macrophages for enhanced synthesis of prostanoids involves induction of a novel prostaglandin H synthase. J. Biol. Chem. 267, 14547–14550.

Page, C.P. (1992). Mechanisms of hyperresponsiveness: platelet-activating factor. Am. Rev. Resp. Dis. 145, S31–S33.

Palmblad, J., Malmsten, C.L., Uden, A.M., Radmark, O., Engstedt, L. and Samuelsson, B. (1981). Leukotriene B_4 is a potent and stereospecific activator of neutrophil chemotaxis and adherence. Blood 58, 658–661.

Palmer, R.M.J., Stepney, R.J., Higgs, G.A. and Eakins, K.E. (1980). Chemokinetic activity of arachidonic lipoxygenase activities on leukocytes from different species. Prostaglandins 20, 411–418.

Palmer, R.M.J. and Salmon, J.A. (1983). Release of leukotriene B_4 from human neutrophils and its relationship to degranulation induced by N-formyl-methionyl-leucyl-phenylalanine, serum-treated zymosan and the ionophore A23187. Immunology 50, 65–73.

Paulson, S.K., Wolf, J.L., Novotney-Barry, A. and Cox, C.P. (1990). Pharmacologic characterization of the rabbit neutrophil receptor for platelet-activating receptor. Proc. Soc. Exp. Biol. Med. 195, 247–254.

Pelikan, P., Gimbrone, M.A. and Cotran, R.S. (1979). Distribution and movement of anionic cell surface sites in cultured human vascular endothelial cells. Atherosclerosis 32, 69–80.

Pereira, H.A., Shafer, W.M., Pohl, J., Martin, L.E. and Spitznagel, J.K. (1990). CAP 37, a human neutrophil-derived chemotactic factor with monocyte specific activity. J. Clin. Invest. 85, 1468–1476.

Peterson, M.W., Stone, P. and Shasby, P.M. (1987). Cationic neutrophil proteins increase transendothelial albumin movement. J. Appl. Physiol. 62, 1521–1530.

Pettipher, E.R., Salter, E.R., Breslow, R., Raycroft, L. and Showell, H.J. (1993). Specific inhibition of leukotriene B_4 (LTB$_4$)-induced neutrophil emigration by 20-hydroxy LTB$_4$: implications for the regulation of inflammatory responses. Br. J. Pharmacol. 423–427.

Peveri, P., Walz, A., Dewald, B. and Baggiolini, M. (1988). A novel neutrophil activating factor produced by human mononuclear phagocytes. J. Exp. Med. 167, 1547–1559.

Pinckard, R.N., Jackson, E.M., Hoppens, C., Weintraub, S.T., Ludwig, J.C., McManus, L.M. and Mott, G.E. (1984). Molecular heterogeneity of platelet-activating factor produced by stimulated human polymorphonuclear leukocytes. Biochem. Biophys. Res. Comm. 122, 325–332.

Pinckard, R.N., Ludwig, J.C. and McManus, M. (1988). In "Inflammation: Basic Principles and Clinical Correlates" (eds. J.I. Gallin, I.M. Goldstein and R. Snyderman), pp. 139–167. Raven Press, New York.

Pinckard, R.N., Showell, H.J., Castillo, R., Lear, C., Breslow, R., McManus, L.M., Woodard, D.S. and Ludwig, J.C. (1992). Differential responsiveness of human neutrophils to the autocrine actions of 1-O-akyl-homologs and 1-acyl analogs of platelet-activating factor. J. Immunol. 148, 3528–3535.

Pohl, J., Pereira, H.A., Martin, N.M. and Spitznagel, J.K. (1990). Amino acid sequence of CAP37, a human neutrophil granule-derived antibacterial and monocyte-specific chemotactic glycoprotein structurally similar to neutrophil elastase. FEBS Lett. 272, 200–204.

Poubelle, P.E., De Medicis, R. and Naccache, P.H. (1987). Monosodium rate and calcium pyrophosphate crystals differentially activate the excitation–response coupling sequence of human neutrophils. Biochem. Biophys. Res. Comm. 149, 649–657.

Pouliot, M., McDonald, P.P., Borgeat, P. and McColl, S.R. (1992a). Recombinant human granulocyte–macrophage colony-stimulating factor enhances 5-lipoxygenase levels in human polymorphonuclear leukocytes. J. Immunol., in press.

Pouliot, M., McDonald, P.P., Borgeat, P. and McColl, S.R. (1992b). Recombinant human granulocyte–macrophage colony-stimulating factor stimulates five lipoxygenase-activating protein gene expression in neutrophils. (Submitted for publication).

Radmark, O., Shimizu. T., Jornvall, H. and Samuelsson, B. (1984). Leukotriene A4 hydrolase in human leukocytes: purification and properties. J. Biol. Chem. 259, 12339–12345.

Ramesha, C.S. and Pickett, W. (1987). Species-specific variations in the molecular heterogeneity of platelet-activating factor. J. Immunol. 138, 1559–1563.

Ranadive, N.S. and Cochrane, C.G. (1968). Isolation and characterization of permeability factors from rabbit neutrophils. J. Exp. Med. 128, 605–622.

Ranadive, N.S., Sajnani, A.N., Alimurka, K. and Movat, H.Z. (1973). Release of basic proteins and lysosomal enzymes from neutrophil leukocytes of the rabbit. Int. Arch. All. 45, 880–898.

Ransome, L.J. and Verma, I.M. (1990). Nuclear proto-oncogenes FOS and JUN. Ann. Rev. Cell Biol. 6, 539–557.

Reibman, J., Meixler, S., Lee, T.C., Gold, L.I., Cronstein, B.N., Haines, K.A., Kolasinski, S.L. and Weissmann, G.A. (1991). Transforming growth factor β1, a potent chemoattractant for human neutrophils, bypasses classic signal-transduction pathways. Proc. Natl Acad. Sci. USA 88, 6805–6809.

Riches, D.W.H., Young, S.K., Seccombe, J.F., Henson, J.E., Clay, K.L. and Henson, P.M. (1990). The subcellular distribution of platelet-activating factor in stimulated neutrophils. J. Immunol. 145, 3062–3070.

Richter, J., Andersson, T. and Olsson, I. (1989). Effect of tumor necrosis factor and granulocyte–macrophage colony-stimulating factor on neutrophil degranulation. J. Immunol. 142, 3199–3205.

Roberge, C.J., Grassi, J., De Medicis, R., Frobert, Y., Lussier, A., Naccache, P.H. and Poubelle, P.E. (1991). Crystal–neutrophil interactions lead to interleukin-1 synthesis. Agents Actions 34, 38–41.

Rokach, J. and Fitzsimmons, B. (1988). The lipoxins. Int. J. Biochem. 20, 753–758.

Rola-Plesczynski, M. (1985). Immunoregulation by leukotrienes and other lipoxygenase products. Immunol. Today 6, 302–308.

Rola-Plesczynski, M. and Stankova, J. (1992). Cytokine gene regulation by PGE2, LTB4 and PAF. Mediators inflammation 1, 5–8.

Rosengren, S., Ley, K. and Arfors, K.-E. (1989). Dextran sulfate prevents LTB4-induced permeability increase, but not neutrophil emigration, in the hamster cheek pouch. Microvasc. Res. 38, 243–254.

Roubin, R., Dulioust, A., Haye-Legrand, I., Ninio, E. and Benveniste, J. (1986). Biosynthesis of PAF-acether: VIII: Impairment of PAF-acether production in activated macrophages does not depend upon acetyl transferase activity. J. Immunol. 136, 1796–1802.

Roubin, R., Elsas, P.P., Fiers, W. and Dessin, A.J. (1987). Recombinant human tumor necrosis factor (rTNF) enhances leukotriene biosynthesis in neutrophils and eosinophils stimulated with the Ca2+ ionophore A23187. Clin. Exp. Immunol. 70, 484–490.

Rouzer, C.A. and Kargman, S. (1988). Translocation of 5-lipoxygenase to the membrane in leukocytes challenged with ionophore A23187. J. Biol Chem. 263, 10980–10988.

Rouzer, C.A. and Samuelsson, B. (1985). On the nature of the 5-lipoxygenase reaction in human leukocytes: enzyme purification and requirement for multiple stimulatory factors. Proc. Natl Acad. Sci. USA 82, 6040–6044.

Rouzer, C.A. and Samuelsson, B. (1987). Reversible, calcium-dependent membrane association of human leukocyte 5-lipoxygenase. Proc. Natl Acad. Sci. USA 84, 7393–7397.

Rouzer, C.A., Matsumoto, T. and Samuelsson, B. (1986). Single protein from human leukocytes possesses 5-lipoxygenase and LTA4 synthase activities. Proc. Natl Acad. Sci. USA 83, 857–861.

Saito, K. and Hanahan, D.J. (1989). "Platelet-activating Factor and Diseases". International Medical Publishers, Tokyo.

Salari, H., Braquet, P., Naccache, P.H. and Borgeat, P. (1985). Characterization of the effect of N-formyl-methionyl-leucyl-phenylalanine on leukotriene synthesis in human polymorphonuclear leukocytes. Inflammation 9, 127–138.

Samuelsson, B., Dahlen, S.V., Londgren, J.A., Rouzer, C.A. and Serhan, C.N. (1987). Leukotrienes and lipoxins: Structures, biosynthesis, and biological effects. Science 237, 1171–1176.

Sariban, E., Mitchell, T. and Kufe, D. (1985). Expression of c-fms proto-oncogene during human monocyte differentiation. Nature 316, 64–66.

Satouchi, K., Oda. M., Yascinaga, K. and Saito, K. (1985). Evidence for the production of 1-acyl-2-acetyl-sn-glyceryl-3-phosphorycholine concomitantly with platelet-activating factor. Biochem. Biophys. Res. Comm. 128, 1409–1417.

Satouchi, K., Oda, M. and Saito. K. (1987). 1-Acyl-2-acetyl-sn-glycero-3-phosphocholine from stimulated human polymorphonuclear leukocytes. Lipids 22, 285–287.

Savill, J.S., Wyllie, A.H., Henson, J.E., Walport, M.J., Henson, P.M. and Haslett, C. (1989). Macrophage phagocytosis of aging neutrophils in inflammation. Programmed cell death in the neutrophil leads to recognition by macrophages. J. Clin. Invest. 83, 865–875.

Schall, T.J. (1991). Biology of the RANTES/SIS cytokine family. Cytokine 3, 165–183.

Schall, T.J., Jongstra, J., Dyer, B.J., Jorgensen, J., Clayberger, C., Davis, M.M. and Krensky, A.M. (1988). A human T cell-specific molecule is a member of a new gene family. J. Immunol. 141, 1018–1025.

Schroeder, J.M. (1989). The monocyte-derived neutrophil-activating peptide (Nap/Interleukin 8) stimulates the human neutrophil 5-lipoxygenase but not the release of cellular arachidonate. J. Exp. Med. 170, 847–863.

Schroeder, J.M. and Christophers, E. (1989). Secretion of novel and homologous neutrophil-activating peptides by LPS-stimulated human endothelial cells. J. Immunol. 142, 244–251.

Schroeder, J.M., Sticherling, M., Hennicke, H.H., Preissner, W.C. and Christophers, E. (1990). IL 1α, or tumor necrosis factorα stimulate release of three NAP 1/IL 8-related neutrophil chemotactic proteins in human dermal fibroblasts. J. Immunol. 144, 2223–2232.

Seckinger, P., Klein-Nulend, J., Alander, C., Thompson, R.C., Dayer, J.M. and Raisz, L.G. (1990). Natural and recombinant human IL-1 receptor antagonists block the effects of IL-1 on bone resorption and prostaglandin production. J. Immunol. 145, 4181–4184.

Serhan, C.N. (1991). Lipoxins: eicosanoids carrying intra- and intercellular messages. J. Bioen. Biomem. 23, 105–122.

Serhan, C.N., Radin, A., Smolen, J.E., Korchak, H., Samuelsson, B. and Weissmann, G. (1982). Leukotriene B4 is a complete secretagogue in human neutrophils: a kinetic analysis. Biochem. Biophys. Res. Comm. 107, 1006–1010.

Shalit, M., Dabini, G.A. and Southwick, F.S. (1987). Platelet-activating factor both stimulates and "primes" human polymorphonuclear leukocyte active filament assembly. Blood 70, 1921–1927.

Shalit, M., Allman, C.V., Akkin, P.C. and Zweiman, B. (1988). Platelet activating factor increases expression of complement receptors on human neutrophils. J. Leukoc. Biol. 44, 212–217.

Shaw, G. and Kamen, R. (1986). A conserved AU sequence from the 3′-untranslated region of GM-CSF mRNA that mediates selective mRNA degradation. Cell 46, 659–667.

Shaw, J.O., Pinckard, R.N., Ferrigni, K.S., McManus, L.M. and Hanahan, D.J. (1981). Activation of human neutrophils with 1-O-hexadecyl/octadecyl-2-acetyl-sn-glyceryl-3-phosphorylcholine (platelet activating factor). J. Immunol. 127, 1250–1255.

Sherr, C.J., Rettenmier, C.W., Sacca, R., Roussel, M.F., Look, A.T. and Stanley, E.R. (1985). The c-fms proto-oncogene product is related to the receptor for the mononuclear phagocyte growth factor, CSF-1. Cell 41, 665–676.

Sherry, B., Tekamp-Olson, P., Gallegos, C., Bauer, D., Davatelis, G., Wolpe, S.D., Masiarz, A., Coit, D. and Cerami, A. (1988). Resolution of the two components of macrophage inflammatory protein 1, and cloning and characterization of one of those components, macrophage inflammatory protein 1β. J. Exp. Med. 168, 2251–2259.

Shirafuji, N., Matsuda, S., Ogura, H., Tani, K., Kodo, H., Ozawa, K., Nagata, S., Asuno, S. and Takaku, F. (1990). Granulocyte colony-stimulating factor stimulates mature neutrophilic granulocytes to produce interferon α. Blood 75, 17–19.

Showell, H.J., Naccache, P.H., Borgeat, P., Picard, S., Vallerand, P., Becker, E.L. and Sha'afi, R.I. (1982). Characterization of the secretory activity of leukotriene B4 towards rabbit neutrophils. J. Immunol. 128, 811–816.

Sigal, E., Craik, C.S., Highland, E., Grunberger, D., Costello, L.L., Dixon, R.A.F. and Nadel, J.A. (1988). Molecular cloning and primary structure of human 15-lipoxygenase. Biochem. Biophys. Res. Comm. 157, 457–464.

Sigal, E., Grunberger, D., Highland, E., Gross, C., Dixon, R.A.F. and Craik, C.S. (1990). Expression of cloned human reticulocyte 15-lipoxygenase and immunological evidence that 15-lipoxygenases of different cell types are related. J. Biol. Chem 265, 5113–5120.

Siriganian, R.P. and Osler, A.G. (1971). Destruction of rabbit platelets in the allergic response of sensitized leukocytes. I. Demonstration of a fluid phase intermediate. J. Immunol. 106, 1244–1251.

Sisson, S.D. and Dinarello, C.A. (1988). Production of interleukin-1 alpha, interleukin-1 beta and tumor necrosis factor by human mononuclear cells stimulated with granulocyte–macrophage colony-stimulating factor. Blood 72, 1368–1374.

Sisson, J.H., Prescott, S.M., McIntyre, T.M. and Zimmerman, G.A. (1987). Production of platelet-activating factor by stimulated human polymorphonuclear leukocytes. Correlation of synthesis with release, functional events and leukotriene B4 metabolism. J. Immunol. 138, 3918–3926.

Skutelsky, E. and Danon, D. (1976). Redistribution of surface anionic sites on the luminal front of blood vessel endothelium after interaction with polycationic ligand. J. Cell. Biol. 71, 232–241.

Smith, R.J., Bowman, B.J. and Iden, S.S. (1984). Stimulation of the human neutrophil superoxide anion-generating system with 1-O-hexadecyl/octadecyl-2-acetyl-sn-glyceryl-3-phosphorylcholine. Biochem. Pharm. 33, 973–978.

Snyder, F. (1990). Platelet-activating factor and related acetylated lipids as potent biologically active cellular mediators. Am. J. Physiol 259, C697–C708.

Spitznagel, T.K. (1990). Antibiotic proteins of human neutrophils. J. Clin. Invest. 86, 1381–1386.

Spitznagel, K.K. and Chi, H.-Y. (1963). Cationic proteins and antibacterial properties of infected tissues and leukocytes. Am. J. Path. 43, 697–711.

Stafforini, D.M., Prescott, S.M. and McIntyre, T.M. (1987). Human plasma platelet-activating factor acetyl hydrolase: purification and properties. J. Biol. Chem. 282, 4223–4230.

Stein, O., de Fries, A. and Katchalski, E. (1956). The effect of polyamino acids on the blood vessels of the rat. Arch. Int. Pharmacodyn. 107, 243–253.

Stewart, A.G. and Dusting, G.J. (1988). Characterization of receptors for platelet-activating factor on platelets, polymorphonuclear leukocytes and macrophages. Br. J. Pharmacol. 94, 1225–1233.

Stewart, A.G., Dubbin, P.N., Harris, T. and Dusting, G.J. (1990). Platelet-activating factor may act as a second messenger in the release of eicosanoids and superoxide anion from leukocytes and endothelial cells. Proc. Natl Acad. Sci. USA 87, 3215–3219.

Stjerschantz, J. (1984). The leukotrienes. Med. Biol. 62, 215–230.

Stoeckle, M.Y. and Barker, K.A. (1990). Two burgeoning families of platelet factor 4-related proteins: mediators of the inflammatory response. N. Biol, 2, 313–323.

Strieter, R.M., Kunkel, S.L., Showell, H.J., Remick, D.G., Phan, S.H., Ward, P.A. and Mark, R.M. (1989a). Endothelial cell gene expression of a neutrophil chemotactic factor by TNFα, LPS and IL-1β. Science 243, 1467–1469.

Strieter, R.M., Phan, S.H., Showell, H.J., Remick, D.G., Lynch, J.P., Genord, M., Raiford, C., Eskandari, M., Marks, R.M. and Kunkel, S.L. (1989b). Monokine-induced neutrophil chemotactic factor gene expression in human fibroblasts. J. Biol. Chem. 264, 10621–10626.

Sturk, A., Schaap, M.C.L., Prins, A., Wouter ten Cate, J. and Van den Bosh, H. (1989). Synthesis of platelet-activating factor by human blood platelets and leukocytes. Evidence against selective utilization of cellular ether-linked phospholipids. Biochim. Biophys. Acta 993, 148–156.

Sunnergren, K.P., Fairman, R.P., Deblois, G.G. and Glanser, F.L. (1987). Effects of protamine, heparinase and hyaluronidase on endothelial permeability and surface charge. J. Appl. Physiol. 63, 1987–1992.

Territo, M.C., Ganz, T., Selsted, M.E. and Lehrer, R. (1989). Monocyte-chemotactic activity of defensins from human neutrophils. J. Clin. Invest. 84, 2017–2020.

Tiku, K., Tiku, M.L. and Skosey, J.L. (1986). Interleukin 1 production by human polymorphonuclear neutrophils. J. Immunol. 136, 3677–3685.

Triggiani, M., Hubbard, W.C. and Chilton, F.H. (1990). Synthesis of 1-acyl-2-acetyl-sn-glycero-3-phosphocholine by an enriched preparation of the human lung mast cell. J. Immunol. 144, 4773–4780.

Triggiani, M., D'Souza, D.M. and Chilton, F.H. (1991a). Metabolism of 1-acyl-2-acetyl-sn-glycero-3-phosphocholine in the human neutrophil. J. Biol. Chem. 266, 6928–6935.

Triggiani, M., Goldman, D.W. and Chilton, F.H. (1991b). Biological effects of 1-acyl-2-acetyl-sn-glycero-3-phosphocholine in the human neutrophil. Biochim. Biophys. Acta 1084, 41–47.

Tufano, M.A., Tetta, C., Biancone, L., Ioro, E.L., Basoni, A., Giovane, A. and Camussi, G. (1992). Salmonella typhimurium porins stimulate platelet-activating factor synthesis by human polymorphonuclear neutrophils. J. Immunol. 149, 1023–1030.

Valone, F. and Goetzl, E.J. (1983). Specific binding by human polymorphonuclear leukocytes of the immunological mediator 1-O-hexadacyl/octadecyl-2-acetyl-sn-glycero-3-phosphorylcholine. J. Immunol. 48, 141–149.

Van Damme, J., Opdenaker, J., Simpson, R.J., Rubira, M.R., Cayphas, S., Vink, A., Billiau, A. and Snick, J.F. (1987). Identification of the human 26-kD protein, interferon-beta 2 (IFN-beta2), as a B cell hybridoma/plasmacytoma growth factor induced by interleukin 1 and tumor necrosis factor. J. Exp. Med. 165, 914–919.

Vehaskari, V.M., Chang, C.T.C., Steven, J.K. and Robson, A.M. (1984). The effects of polycations on vascular permeability in the rat: a proposed role for charge sites. J. Clin. Invest. 73, 1053–1061.

Vercellotti, G.M., Yin, H.Q., Gustafson, K.S., Nelson, R.D. and Jacob, J.S. (1988). Platelet-activating factor primes neutrophil responses to agonists: role in promoting neutrophil-mediated endothelium damage. Blood 71, 1100–1107.

Vercellotti, G.M., Moldow, C.F., Wickham, N.W., and Jacob,

H.S. (1990). Endothelial cell platelet-activating factor primes neutrophil responses: amplification of endothelial activation by neutrophil products. J. Lipid Mediators 2, 523–530.

Wakabayashi, G., Gelfand, J.A., Burke, J.F., Thompson, R.C. and Dinarello, C.A. (1991). A specific receptor antagonist for interleukin 1 prevents Escherichia coli-induced shock in rabbits. FASEB J. 5, 338–343.

Waksman, Y., Golde, D.W., Savion, N. and Fabian, I. (1990). Granulocyte–macrophage colony-stimulating factor enhances cationic antimicrobial protein synthesis by human neutrophils. J. Immunol. 144, 3437–3443.

Warner, S.J.C., Auger, K.R. and Libby, P. (1987). Interleukin-1 induces interleukin-1. II. Recombinant human interleukin 1 induces interleukin 1 production by adult human vascular endothelial cells. J. Immunol. 139, 1911–1917.

Wedmore, C.V. and Williams, T.J. (1981). Control of vascular permeability by polymorphonuclear leukocytes in inflammation. Nature 289, 646–650.

Weintraub, S.T., Ludwig, J.C., Mott, G.E., McManus, L.M., Lear, C. and Pinckard, R.N. (1985). Fast atom bombardment-mass spectrometric identification of molecular species of platelet-activating factor produced by stimulated human polymorphonuclear leukocytes. Biochem. Biophys. Res. Comm. 129, 868–876.

Weisbart, R.H. and Golde, D.W. (1989). Physiology of granulocyte and macrophage colony-stimulating factors. Hematol. Oncol. Clinics N. Am, 3, 401–409.

Weissman, G., Zurier, R.B., Spieler, P.J. and Goldstein, I.M. (1971). Mechanisms of lysosomal enzyme release from leukocytes exposed to immune complexes and other particles. J. Exp. Med. 134, 149S–165S.

Willis, A.L. and Smith, J.B. (1981). Some perspectives on platelets and prostaglandins. Prog. Lipid Res. 20, 387–406.

Wilson, T. and Treisman, R. (1988). Removal of poly(A) and consequent degradation of c-fos mRNA facilitated by 3′ AU-rich sequences. Nature 336, 396–399.

Wolfe, L.S. (1982). Eicosanoids, prostaglandins, thromboxanes, leukotrienes and other derivatives of carbon-20 unsaturated fatty acids. J. Neurochem. 38, 1–14.

Wolfe, S.D. and Cerami, A. (1989). Macrophage inflammatory proteins 1 and 2: members of a novel superfamily of cytokines. FASEB J. 3, 2565–2573.

Worthen, G.S., Seccombe, J.F., Guthrie, K.L. and Johnston, R.B. (1988). The priming of neutrophils by lipopolysaccharide for production of intracellular platelet-activating factor. Potential role in mediation of enhanced superoxide secretion. J. Immunol. 140, 3553–3559.

Xie, W., Robertson, D.L. and Simmons, D.L. (1992). Mitogen-inducible prostaglandin G/H synthase: a new target for nonsteroidal antiinflammatory drugs. Drug Dev. Res. 25, 249–265.

Yamoto, K., el-Hajjaoui, Z. and Koeffler, H.P. (1989). Regulation of levels of IL-1 mRNA in human fibroblasts. J. Cell. Physiol. 139, 610–616.

Ye, R.D., Prossnitz, E.R., Zou, A.M. and Cochrane, G.G. (1991). Characterization of a human cDNA that encodes a functional receptor for platelet activating factor. Biochem. Biophys. Res. Comm. 180, 105–111.

Yoshimura, T., Matsushima, K., Tanaka, S., Robinson, E.A., Appella, E., Oppenheim, J.J. and Leonard, E.J. (1987). Purification of a human monocyte-derived neutrophil chemotactic factor that has peptide sequence similarity to other host defense cytokines. Proc. Natl Acad. Sci. USA 84, 9233–9237.

Zhou, W., Javors, M.A. and Olson, M.S. (1992). Platelet-activating factor as an intercellular signal in neutrophil-dependent platelet activation. J. Immunol. 149, 1763–1769.

Zimmerman, G.A., McIntyre, T.M., Mehra, M. and Prescott, J.M. (1990). Endothelial cell-associated platelet-activating factor: a novel mechanism for signaling intracellular adhesion. J. Cell Biol. 110, 529–540.

Note Added in Proof

Recent studies have shown that neutrophils synthesize and release macrophage inflammatory protein 1α in response to LPS, and that the production of MIP-1α accounts for a substantial percentage of the monocyte chemotactic activity present in stimulated neutrophil supernatants (Kasama et al. 1993). Upregulation of MIP-1α mRNA expression was also observed. In that study, incubation of neutrophils with GM-CSF failed to induce MIP-1α gene expression. Studies in our laboratory (SRM) have shown that, in addition to MIP-1α, MIP-1β gene expression is also upregulated in neutrophils (Hachicha, M., Rathanaswami, P. and McColl, S.R., in preparation). In our hands, TNFα is a potent inducer of both MIP-1α and β gene expression, and unlike the study of Kasama et al., we have found that GM-CSF is also an effective agonist.

Clearly, in light of these new findings, the role of neutrophils in the inflammatory response must again be reconsidered since in vitro experiments show that MIP-1α and β are chemoattractants for different CD4$^+$ and CD8$^+$ lymphocyte subsets (Taub et al., 1993; Schall et al., 1993). Moreover, MIP-1α is chemotactic for B lymphocytes. These properties, combined with the observation that MIP-1α and β are chemotactic for monocytes, would imply that stimulated human neutrophils produce chemokines that are capable of directing the recruitment of all of the major mononuclear components of the immune system.

References

Kasama, T., Streiter, R.M., Standiford, T.J., Burdick, M.D. and Kunkel, S.L. (1993). Expression and regulation of human neutrophil-derived macrophage inflammatory protein-1α. J. Exp. Med. 178, 63–72.

Schall, T.J., Bacon, K. Camp, R.D.R., Kaspari, J.W. and Goeddel, D.V. (1993). Human macrophage inflammatory protein (MIP-1α) and MIP-1β chemokines attract distinct populations of lymphocytes. J. Exp. Med. 177, 1821–1826.

Taub, D.D., Conlon, K., Lloyd, A.R., Oppenheim, J.J. and Kelvin, D.J. (1993). Preferential migration of CD4$^+$ and CD8$^+$ T cells in response to MIP-1α and MIP-1β. Science 260, 355–358.

6. Molecular Biology of Human Neutrophil Chemotactic Receptors

Craig Gerard and Norma P. Gerard

1. Introduction

The basic mission of the neutrophil is host defence, as shown by the problems encountered in patients with neutropenia or chronic granulomatous disease. The mature neutrophil has a brief life span, measured in hours, following discharge from the bone marrow (see Chapter 2). During that time, circulating neutrophils can sense signals in the environment directing them to a site which is frequently extravascular. The summoned neutrophil secondarily responds to increased concentrations of signal by discharging lysosomal enzymes and producing activated species of oxygen and nitric oxide. The cell may also engulf particulate matter. The ultimate goal of this activity is to clear the host of foreign material. Inappropriate generation of chemotactic signals in the absence of exogenous pathogens can also lead to injury to the host, as in autoimmune diseases. Thus, the vectorial summoning of circulating neutrophils (chemotaxis) by environmental signals (chemotactic factors) can be viewed as a problem in sensation and signal transduction.

The past 2 years have witnessed multiple breakthroughs regarding the chemotactic receptors present on human polymorphonuclear leucocytes. The molecular cloning of cDNAs encoding the binding sites for formyl peptides, C5a anaphylatoxin, PAF and several members of the IL-8/NAP-1 (chemokine) family establishes G-protein-coupled receptors containing seven transmembrane segments as the paradigm for sensory processing by neutrophils. The linkage of chemotactic receptors to visual and olfactory receptors will be viewed below. In this chapter we will summarize the current understanding of the chemotactic receptors and describe the ongoing work which seeks to link biochemical structure with function. With regard to work performed before receptor cloning was accomplished, there are literally several thousand references dealing with the biology and/or pharmacology of the chemotactic factors and their receptors. In order to present a more detailed view on the receptors themselves, we will forego review of this literature, with the exception of selected key references.

2. Selected Events Leading to Receptor Cloning

In the mid- to late 1970s, the biological descriptions of chemotactic factors (Shin *et al.*, 1968; Ward and Newman, 1969; Ward, 1976) logically proceeded to pharmacological characterization of their cognate binding sites on PMN leucocytes. The first significant characterizations were for the putative "bacterial factor" which was mimicked by N-formylated hydrophobic oligopeptides

Immunopharmacology of Neutrophils
ISBN 0–12–339250–0

(Schiffmann et al., 1975; Showell et al., 1976). Curiously, the original test peptide, FMLP, is among the most potent ligands found, and was subsequently isolated from bacterial cultures (Marasco et al., 1984). Binding studies with radiolabelled ligand revealed an easily measurable, saturable, specific binding site which correlated in affinity with agonist potency (Aswanikumar et al., 1977; Williams et al., 1977; Schiffmann et al., 1978).

Shortly thereafter, binding of human C5a anaphylatoxin to a PMN receptor was demonstrated (Chenoweth and Hugli, 1978). In both cases, the leucocyte receptors displayed ligand affinity in the nanomolar range, and the number of receptor sites per cell was relatively abundant at ~100 000 sites per cell. In the case of the formyl peptide, two receptor classes were distinguished based on Scatchard analyses, differing in affinity by about one order of magnitude (Mackin et al., 1982). The C5a receptor appeared to exist in a single high affinity state (Chenoweth and Hugli, 1978).

Between 1980 and 1990 several additional neutrophil chemotactic ligands were chemically characterized, including the lipoxygenase product of arachidonic acid, LTB$_4$ and the ether lipid, PAF (Blank et al., 1979; Demopoulous et al., 1979; Camp et al., 1982). The lipid mediators, in contrast to the peptides, have corresponding receptors that are much less abundant. The most recent addition to the characterized chemotactic factors are the chemokines typified by IL-8/NAP-1 (Schmid and Weissmann, 1987; Schroder et al., 1987; Walz et al., 1987; Yoshimura et al., 1987).

In the case of all the above ligands, the development of a sensitive and specific receptor assay was the most critical first step towards chemically characterizing the receptor. The crosslinking of radiolabelled ligands for formal peptides and C5a established that the major binding component in each case appeared to be a single polypeptide chain (Huey and Hugli, 1985; Johnson and Chenoweth, 1985a; Marasco et al., 1985; Rollins and Springer, 1985). A detailed study of the ligand-crosslinked formyl peptide receptor provided chemical evidence that the core binding unit was a discrete single chain polypeptide. Papain treatment of the receptor did not abolish radioligand binding, but removed the N-glycanase substrate(s) indicating that the N-linked oligosaccharides were not essential (Malech et al., 1985). These data suggested that the binding domain was different from the glycosylated domain, a point which will be discussed further below.

Pharmacological studies by a number of investigators established that the chemotactic receptors were coupled to pertussis-toxin sensitive substrates in the neutrophil (Snyderman et al., 1984; Feltner et al., 1986; Jesaitis et al., 1988; Polakis et al., 1988). Advances in the understanding of the rhodopsin visual system and the adrenergic receptor led to the concept of GTP-binding proteins as transducing amplifiers between membrane receptors and effector systems. Solubilization and partial purification of the formyl peptide and C5a receptors suggested that the high affinity receptor complex contained associated pertussis toxin-sensitive G-proteins (Polakis et al., 1988; Rollins et al., 1988, 1991; Siciliano et al., 1990). Further purification of the chemotactic receptors was hampered by the instability of the partially purified receptors, the small quantities of receptor present (~1 nmol/1 × 10^9 neutrophils), and lack of synthetic ligands which could be useful for affinity chromatography.

The development of expression cloning strategies in the mid-1980s was the pivotal technological breakthrough in the field of receptor biology (Wong et al., 1985; Aruffo and Seed, 1987). Using this approach, the necessary conditions for molecular cloning of a receptor are: (1) a dependable specific binding assay and radioligand of high specific activity; (2) a single gene product encoding the receptor; and (3) a source of high-quality mRNA for the construction of a cDNA expression library. A second expression methodology relies on microinjected Xenopus laevis oocytes translating RNA transcribed from plasmid libraries separated in pools of 500–1000 clones (Hediger et al., 1987). Expression in oocytes precludes accurate binding studies due to the relatively trivial amount of protein synthesized per egg, but sensitive assays involving ligand-dependent signal transduction may be employed. More traditional cloning strategies require either amino-acid sequence data (requiring pure protein in some quantity) or antisera to the receptor.

The studies described above clearly demonstrate that sensitive binding assays were available for the chemotaxins. In the case of formyl peptide and C5a, a single molecular species appeared to bind ligand. As far as a high-quality source of RNA for library construction is concerned, neutrophils are relatively poor in mRNA and what little there is can often be isolated in a degraded form despite experienced hands. Several human myeloid cell lines were characterized which expressed chemotactic receptors following in vitro differentiation, notably U937 human lymphoma cells (Chenoweth and Soderberg, 1985) and human leukaemia HL-60 cells (Harris and Ralph, 1985). Since chemotactic responsiveness appeared following manipulation of the culture, it suggested that the mRNA encoding these receptors was newly transcribed, or possessed a longer half-life than prior to differentiation. Other mechanisms, however, including translational control, cryptic receptors or post-translational processing are also possible. The demonstration that FMLP, C5a and PAF responses could be detected by calcium fluxes in microinjected Xenopus oocytes proved that cultured myeloid cells contained receptor-encoding mRNA (Murphy and McDermott, 1991).

3.   The Formyl Peptide Receptor

The first clone for the human PMN formyl peptide

receptor was reported in May 1990 (Boulay *et al.*, 1990a). Boulay and co-workers first synthesized a novel formyl peptide reporter ligand based on previous work in Vignais' laboratory with hydrophilic peptides derived from the ADP/ATP transporter. The concept was to create a chimeric molecule. High polarity and a tyrosyl residue for iodination to high specific activity were provided by a dodecapeptide which was coupled by a C-terminal cysteine sulphydryl group to the epsilon amino-group of lysine on *N*-formyl-Met-Leu-Phe-Lys. This chimeric ligand, FMLPK-pep12, elicited superoxide anion formation with a four-fold lower ED_{50} than parent FMLPK. The high polarity of FMLPK-pep12 decreased non-specific binding compared with unmodified formyl peptide, which is typically dissolved in non-aqueous solvents and can associate non-specifically with membranes. This ligand, labelled to high specific activity with ^{125}I, was separated from free iodine by gel filtration (also more difficult with parent *n*-formyl derivatives by virtue of their low molecular weight) and was 1500–2000 dpm/fmol. A cDNA library constructed in the mammalian cell expression vector pCDM8 was transfected as plasmid from pools of 500 clones into COS cells. The pool containing clone FMLP-R98 bound nine-fold more iodinated peptide than other pools, which averaged 1800 ± 300 dpm. The eventual isolation of the pure clone from this pool allowed expression studies revealing biphasic Scatchard plots with high (0.5–1.0 nM) and low (5–10 nM) binding affinities.

Sequence analysis of the cloned FMLPK-pep12 binding protein revealed that it contained seven hydrophobic segments similar to rhodopsin-type receptors (Dohlman *et al.*, 1991). In many ways, this paper threw the first light on what was to become a major conceptual advance in the chemotactic receptor field. At this time, a variety of receptors for neurotransmitters and neuropeptides were shown to be homologous to rhodopsin, and to couple pharmacologically to G-proteins (Birnbaumer and Brown, 1990).

This initial study did not report on the signalling potential of the cloned formyl peptide receptor, nor did it provide characterization of RNA expression, or genomic analysis. Data on some of these issues were addressed by a subsequent report from this laboratory (Boulay *et al.*, 1990b). In this work, allelic variants were described for Val 101 and Glu 396 in clone R-26, replacing leucyl and alanyl residues, respectively, which were described in the original R-98 clone. It is possible that differences in the isoelectric point of the receptor relate to these polymorphisms. No differences in ligand binding were detected between these isoforms. Additional differences were detected in the 5′ and 3′ flanking regions, including a 16 bp deletion in clone R-98 at position -39. Clone R-98 also contained an additional 661 bp of 3′-untranslated sequence containing Alu repeat elements but no polyadenylation signal. Recent reports from the laboratories of Wetsel and Perez indicate

that these findings are explained by a single intron in the 5′-flanking region which undergoes alternative splicing, and by alternative polyadenylation patterns in the 3′ UTR (Perez *et al.*, 1992, personal communication; Wetsel, 1992, personal communication). More details on the chemotactic receptor genes will be addressed later in this review.

The transfected receptor was shown to endocytose rhodamine-labelled formyl peptide in COS cells. RNA blot analysis revealed strongly hybridizing signals at 1.6–1.7 kb and weaker signals at 2.3 and 3.1 kb. The genomic DNA analysis revealed multiple hybridizing bands with full length probe. Since the probe used did not contain restriction sites for the digesting enzyme, either multiple related genes or introns could explain these findings. Thus in two important papers, Boulay and co-workers opened the field for formyl peptide receptor biochemistry.

The subsequent appearance of several papers confirmed the initial reports by measuring signal transduction to homologous receptors (Murphy and McDermott, 1991; Prossnitz *et al.*, 1991; Didsbury *et al.*, 1992). Working in the oocyte system, Murphy and McDermott demonstrated that the formyl peptide receptor permitted ligand-dependent calcium currents in oocytes, but only in the presence of a ~ 3.5 kb "complementary factor". Microinjection of cRNA enoding the receptor alone was not enough to produce a calcium flux upon stimulation with ligand. The "complementary factor" was not the G-protein alpha subunit $G_{i\alpha 1, 2}$ or $_3$. This accessory factor was also not unique to HL-60 cells, as it was found in liver but not brain or spleen. The lack of "complementary factor" in spleen is curious because this organ contains myeloid cells which respond to formyl peptides. That this factor might be a "housekeeping gene" is suggested by the data collected by Prossnitz *et al.* (1991) and Didsbury *et al.* (1992), since their studies demonstrated signal transduction mediated by the receptor cDNA alone in mammalian cells.

The structure of the formyl peptide receptor is shown in Figure 6.1. When modelled as a seven-transmembrane segment receptor, by analogy with the adrenergic receptors and rhodopsin for which orientation has been probed (Dohlman *et al.*, 1991), the amino-terminal region is extracellular and seven transmembrane segments create three extracellular and three cytoplasmic loops with a carboxy-terminal segment in the cytoplasm. Glycosylation consensus sequences are present twice in the amino-terminal extracellular peptide. When this structure is taken together with the data of Malech *et al.* (1985), it appears that the amino-terminal region may be removed with papain without affecting FMLP binding to the receptor. These data suggest that the binding site for the hydrophobic oligopeptide may be present in the pocket created by the circular alignment of the seven transmembrane segments. Data supporting a model where the receptor forms a pore was obtained by Sklar

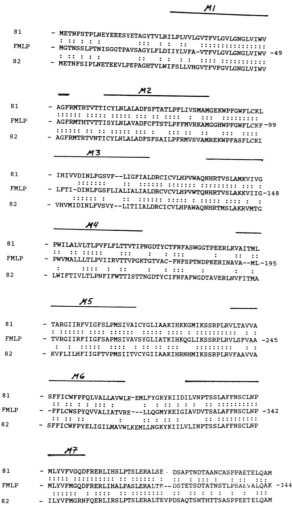

Figure 6.1 Deduced protein sequences for the FPR family. FMLP refers to the FPR, which binds bacterial chemotactic peptides and induces leucocyte activation. Clones 81 (FPRH1) and 82 (FPRH2) are orphan receptors isolated by homology with the FMLP receptor. The seven predicted membrane-spanning domains are indicated by bars over the sequence.

and colleagues (1990). A progressively longer series of N-formylated oligopeptides containing a C-terminal fluorescein group displayed quenching through five amino acids. When hexapeptides or larger were bound to the receptor, the C-terminal fluorescent group was no longer quenched. These data are consistent with a model where a receptor pore binds formyl peptide with the formyl group deepest into the plane of the membrane, and a length of five amino acids for the pore's "depth".

At present, mutagenesis data and interspecies comparisons of the formyl peptide receptor are being analysed in several laboratories. Preliminary reports from Bokoch's group suggest that the critical site for interaction of the receptor and G-protein may be contained in a segment of

the C-terminal peptide which can be competitively analysed using synthetic peptides (Schreiber, 1992, personal communication). Additional studies will likely find that for the oligopeptides, the transmembrane helices are critical for binding and signal transduction, as is the case for the adrenergic receptor and visual opsins. An interesting approach currently being explored employs the formyl peptide receptor homologues, FPRH1 and FPRH2 (Lu *et al.*, 1992; Murphy *et al.*, 1992; Ye *et al.*, 1992). As described above, studies by Boulay *et al.* (1990a) suggested that introns or related molecules are needed to explain the Southern analyses of genomic DNA using formyl peptide receptor probes. Screening of HL-60 cDNA libraries identified one homologue (Murphy *et al.*, 1992; Ye *et al.*, 1992), while screening of human genomic DNA libraries yielded both (Lu *et al.*, 1992). The sum of these studies is that there are at least two other genes with a high degree of sequence identity with the formyl peptide receptor. Neither FPRH1, with 66% identity, nor FPRH2, with 56% identity, bind formylated oligopeptides. These two homologues (Figure 6.1) are located close to the FPR on chromosome 19 at the q13.3/13.4 interface, along with the C5a receptor (see Section 5). Therefore, the orphan receptor homologies to FPR may have evolved to perform a similar function. Perhaps all three receptors evolved to recognize distinct bacterial products. Notwithstanding, the high degree of structural identity allows the construction of chimeric receptors between the FPR, FPRH1 and FPRH2 which may be useful in defining binding and signal transduction sites.

This has been exploited previously for the adrenergic receptor subtypes. Ye *et al.* (1992) demonstrated calcium transients transduced in fibroblasts stably transfected with FPRH1 in response to FMLP at micromolar concentrations. We have recently confirmed this transduction by measuring production of inositol phosphates in response to micromolar FMLP in transfected COS cells (N.P. Gerard, unpublished data).

4. The Platelet-activating Factor Receptor

Soon after structural characterization by several groups in 1980 (Blank *et al.*, 1979; Demopoulos *et al.*, 1979), the perceived importance of this lipid mediator in a host of pathophysiological situations led to questions regarding its mechanism of action. Additionally, the search for compounds which could antagonize PAF was joined. Several excellent reviews exist covering these developments (Hanahan, 1986; Prescott *et al.*, 1990; Snyder, 1990). With respect to the antagonists, many compounds including natural products, structural analogues and synthetic organic molecules have been described (Shen *et al.*, 1985; Casals-Stenzel *et al.*, 1987). Unlike the case observed with adrenergic receptors, where particular biological responses are differentially antagonized and define receptor subtypes, no striking differences emerge with PAF receptor antagonists in multiple bioassay systems. However, some pharmacological differences do occur (Hwang, 1988), raising the possibility for PAF receptor subtypes.

The first report of a PAF receptor cDNA appeared in January 1991 (Honda et al., 1991). Honda and colleagues screened the Xenopus oocyte expression system for chloride current with pools of cRNA from a guinea-pig lung library, identifying and cloning a single molecular species which conferred PAF-dependent responses. The isolated receptor conceptually encodes a 342 amino-acid protein with seven hydrophobic segments, characteristic of members of the rhodopsin family. In multiple guinea-pig tissues, Northern analysis demonstrated several molecular species hybridizing with the lung cDNA probe at 2.2, 3.0 and 4.0 kb. Sucrose gradient-fractionated RNAs suggested that the 3.0 kb species was responsible for the signal transduction observed in injected oocytes. The nature of the other hybridizing transcripts, as subtypes or closely related molecules, was not determined. This structure was the first reported for any lipid mediator, and opened the way for characterizing the human homologue(s). Within months, human homologues were reported from several groups, including ours (Ye et al., 1991; Kunz et al., 1992). The structures reported from human neutrophils, HL-60 and U-937 cells were identical, and are presented along with the guinea-pig sequence in Figure 6.2. The orientation of the PAF receptor was established through the construction of a Flag-sequence-bearing epitope (Kunz et al., 1992). Attachment of the sequence MYKDDDDK to the N-terminus of the human receptor did not markedly diminish cell surface binding to transfected COS cells. The epitope was shown to exist extracellularly in transfected cells by binding monoclonal antibody, thus the N-terminus of the PAF receptor is extracellular (Figure 6.3). Topologies for other seven-transmembrane segment receptors have only previously been determined for rhodopsin and the beta receptor (Bayramashuili et al., 1984; Dohlman et al., 1987). Sequence analysis of the human receptor reveals it to be the first lacking an N-linked glycosylation site in the amino-terminal region. The reason for this is unclear at present, however, other G-protein-coupled receptors can clearly bind and transduce signals normally when mutated to remove the glycosylation site (Rands et al., 1990).

Alignment of the deduced amino-acid sequences reveals ~ 83% sequence identity between the human and guinea-pig molecules. Conserved amino acids also include 10 unique cysteine residues in the putative transmembrane regions. Since thiol titrants were shown to block PAF binding to its receptor (Ng and Wong, 1988), perhaps these cysteines form part of the ligand binding site. Additional unique features of the PAF receptor include absence of the canonical DRY sequence at the C-terminus of the third hydrophobic segment, replaced with NRF in the PAF receptor, and the presence of an aspartic acid in the middle of the seventh transmembrane segment. The primary structure of the TXA$_2$ receptor (Hirata et al., 1991) is almost 50% identical to the PAF receptor at the nucleotide level, however, when translated, the identity is less than 22%. Since the degree of sequence identity between adrenergic receptors, dopaminergic receptors and tachykinin receptors among

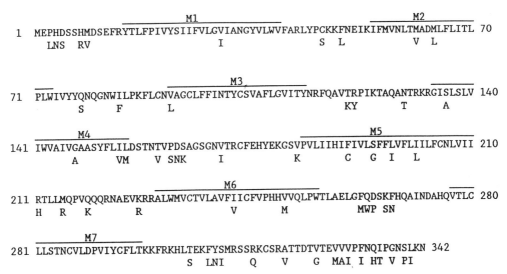

Figure 6.2 Comparison of human and guinea-pig PAF receptor protein sequences. The 342 amino-acid sequence is shown with the non-identical residues found in the guinea pig indicated. The seven predicted membrane-spanning domains are indicated by bars over the sequence.

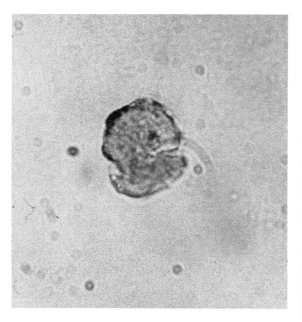

Figure 6.3 Immunohistochemical staining of the human PAF receptor transfected in COS cells. COS cells transfected with the PAF-Flag/pCDM8 plasmid were stained with M5 anti-Flag monoclonal antibody, followed by biotinylated anti-mouse IgG and avidin–biotin horseradish peroxidase. Antibody staining of the PAF receptor is localized to the perimeter of the cell, characteristic of a cell surface epitope.

species is typically higher than this, the issue of PAF-receptor subtypes arises. The human PAF receptor hybridizes with a unique mRNA at 3.7–4 kb in multiple tissue and cell types (Murphy et al., 1990), unlike the guinea pig where multiple hybridizing transcripts are seen (Honda et al., 1991). A single simple hybridization pattern was observed on Southern analysis (Kunz et al., 1992), predicting a single gene in man. This gene has been found to map to chromosome 1 and like many other members of the rhodopsin family is intronless (Seyfried et al., 1992). At the molecular hybridization level, while multiple receptor subtypes may exist in the guinea pig, the human transcript appears to be the product of a single gene. Pharmacological differences among tissues or cell types may reflect different high affinity states produced by receptor coupling with unique G-proteins.

Biological and pharmacological analyses of the cloned human PAF receptor are consistent with coupling to G-proteins (Nakamura et al., 1991), thus the isolated transfected molecule appears to satisfy all the characteristics predicted from previous studies. The chloride current in microinjected oocytes was inhibitable by GTPγS, and ligand-dependent metabolites of phosphatidyl inositol are observed in COS cells transfected with the human receptor cDNA. The antagonism by

WEB2086 in transfected cells is also specific for both the human and guinea-pig PAF receptors, and the affinity constants are within range of those previously reported (Kunz et al., 1992). Binding analysis using membranes from transfected COS cells (Nakamura et al., 1991) appears to be much more difficult than binding to intact cells (Kunz et al., 1992), since the membrane fraction displays 70–80% non-specific binding while the whole cell monolayer assay yields non-specific binding of less than 15%. The previously noted homologous desensitization properties of the PAF receptor were evident both in the oocyte and the COS cell systems. In the case of COS cells, preincubation with increasing concentrations of PAF at 4°C for 20 min led to a dose-dependent inhibition of subsequent binding of 2 nM radiolabelled ligand (Kunz et al., 1992). Whether the loss of surface binding was due to phosphorylation, uncoupling from G-protein, or internalization of the receptor is not known at present. Preliminary data using the PAF-Flag receptor construct suggest that the antigenic sites are preserved on the surface, while the specific binding is decreased by 70% arguing against internalization or sequestration.

An interesting phenomenon was noted when the whole cell binding assay was performed at 4°C versus 22°C or 37°C. In a receptor-dependent fashion, the mass of radiolabel accumulated over a 1 h incubation with ligand was 10–20-fold greater at elevated temperature. These data suggest that at physiological temperature the PAF receptor can ferry ligand intracellularly and recycle to the surface to bind additional ligand. On whole neutrophils, "loading" of cells with PAF or other phospholipids can occur in a fashion independent of the receptor by a pathway which is up-regulated in activated cells (Bratton et al., 1992). In the case of COS cells, however, the magnitude of the receptor independent uptake of ligand is relatively small compared to that obtained in receptor-bearing cells (Gerard and Gerard, 1994).

Are there additional PAF receptors yet to be cloned? Based on the evidence gathered to date with the human molecule, such candidates will have to be significantly divergent at the primary structure level given the Southern analysis described above and isolation of a single genomic clone. Since there is no intron in the coding sequence, the possibility for alternative processing such as is seen with the dopamine receptor is unlikely (Monsma et al., 1989; Van Tol et al., 1992). There may be additional molecules, however, which bind ether lipids with high avidity. The antitumour effects of ether lipid analogues of PAF are not satisfactorily explained at present, but do not seem to require the PAF receptor (Berdel et al., 1987). Perhaps the target of these compounds is a second distinct PAF receptor.

5. The C5a Receptor

The C5a receptor was first cloned using an "orphan

receptor" strategy which recognized the homologies among seven transmembrane segment receptors. Work by late 1989 clearly established that a wide variety of signalling molecules were pharmacologically coupled to G-proteins. Studies reported in 1989 by Parmentier and colleagues demonstrated that degenerate PCR oligo-deoxynucleotide primers based on the known sequences of a few diverse receptors coupled to G-proteins could be used to generate probes from genomic DNA (Libert et al., 1989; Parmentier et al., 1989). These PCR probes could then be used to identify candidate transcripts. For example, the TSH receptor transcript would be expected to be present specifically in thyroid tissues. Although the approach is quite labour intensive, a number of clones have subsequently been identified including those for

```
        10        20        30        40        50        60        70
         *         *         *         *         *         *         *
AGGGGGAGCCCAGGAGACCAGAACATGAACTCCTTCAATTATACCACCCCTGATTATGGGCACTATGATG
                         MetAsnSerPheAsnTyrThrThrProAspTyrGlyHisTyrAsp>

        80        90       100       110       120       130       140
         *         *         *         *         *         *         *
ACAAGGATACCCTGGACCTCAACACCCCTGTGGATAAAACTTCTAACACGCTGCGTGTTCCAGACATCCT
AspLysAspThrLeuAspLeuAsnThrProValAspLysThrSerAsnThrLeuArgValProAspIleLeu>

       150       160       170       180       190       200       210
         *         *         *         *         *         *         *
GGCCTTGGTCATCTTTGCAGTCGTCTTCCTGGTGGGAGTGCTGGGCAATGCCCTGGTGGTCTGGGTGACG
AlaLeuValIlePheAlaValValPheLeuValGlyValLeuGlyAsnAlaLeuValValTrpValThr>

       220       230       240       250       260       270       280
         *         *         *         *         *         *         *
GCATTCGAGGCCAAGCGGACCATCAATGCCATCTGGTTCCTCAACTTGGCGGTAGCCGACTTCCTCTCCT
AlaPheGluAlaLysArgThrIleAsnAlaIleTrpPheLeuAsnLeuAlaValAlaAspPheLeuSer>

       290       300       310       320       330       340       350
         *         *         *         *         *         *         *
GCCTGGCGCTGCCCATCTTGTTCACGTCCATTGTACAGCATCACCACTGGCCCTTTGGCGGGGCCGGCTG
CysLeuAlaLeuProIleLeuPheThrSerIleValGlnHisHisHisTrpProPheGlyGlyAlaAlaCys>

       360       370       380       390       400       410       420
         *         *         *         *         *         *         *
CAGCATCCTGCCCTCCCTCATCCTGCTCAACATGTACGGCCAGCATCCTGCTCCTGGCCACCATCAGCGCC
SerIleLeuProSerLeuIleLeuLeuAsnMetTyrAlaSerIleLeuLeuAlaThrIleSerAla>

       430       440       450       460       470       480       490
         *         *         *         *         *         *         *
GACCGCTTTCTGCTGGTGTTTAAACCCATCTGGTGCCAGAACTTCCGAGGGGCCGGCTTGGCCTGGATCG
AspArgPheLeuLeuValPheLysProIleTrpCysGlnAsnPheArgGlyAlaGlyLeuAlaTrpIle>

       500       510       520       530       540       550       560
         *         *         *         *         *         *         *
CCTGTGCCGTGGCTTGGGGTTTAGCCCTGCTGCTGACCATACCCTCCTTCCTGTACCGGGTGGTCCGGGA
AlaCysAlaValAlaTrpGlyLeuAlaLeuLeuLeuThrIleProSerPheLeuTyrArgValValArgGlu>

       570       580       590       600       610       620       630
         *         *         *         *         *         *         *
GGAGTACTTTCCACCAAAGGTGTTGTGTGGCGTGGACTACAGCCACGACAAACGGCGGGAGCGAGCCGTG
GluTyrPheProProLysValLeuCysGlyValAspTyrSerHisAspLysArgArgGluArgAlaVal>

       640       650       660       670       680       690       700
         *         *         *         *         *         *         *
GCCATCGTCCGGCTGGTCCTGGGCTTCCTGTGGCCTCTACTCACGCTCACGATTTGTTACACTTTCATCC
AlaIleValArgLeuValLeuGlyPheLeuTrpProLeuLeuThrLeuThrIleCysTyrThrPheIle>

       710       720       730       740       750       760       770
         *         *         *         *         *         *         *
TGCTCCGGACGTGGAGCCGCAGGGCCACGCGGTCCACCAAGACACTCAAGGTGGTGGTGGCAGTGGTGGC
LeuLeuArgThrTrpSerArgArgAlaThrArgSerThrLysThrLeuLysValValValAlaValValAla>

       780       790       800       810       820       830       840
         *         *         *         *         *         *         *
CAGTTTCTTTATCTTCTGGTTGCCCTACCAGGTGACGGGGATAATGATGTCCTTCCTGGAGCCATCGTCA
SerPhePheIlePheTrpLeuProTyrGlnValThrGlyIleMetMetSerPheLeuGluProSerSer>

       850       860       870       880       890       900       910
         *         *         *         *         *         *         *
CCCACCTTCCTGCTGCTGAATAAGCTGGACTCCCTGTGTGTGTCCTTTGCCTACATCAACTGCTGCATCA
ProThrPheLeuLeuLeuAsnLysLeuAspSerLeuCysValSerPheAlaTyrIleAsnCysCysIle>

       920       930       940       950       960       970       980
         *         *         *         *         *         *         *
ACCCCATCATCTACGTGGTGGCCGGCCAGGGCTTCCAGGGCCGACTGCGGAAATCCCTCCCCAGCCTCCT
AsnProIleIleTyrValValAlaGlyGlnGlyPheGlnGlyArgLeuArgLysSerLeuProSerLeuLeu>

       990      1000      1010      1020      1030      1040      1050
         *         *         *         *         *         *         *
CCGGAACGTGTTGACTGAAGAGTCCGTGGTTAGGGAGAGCAAGTCATTCACGCGGCTCCACAGTGGACACT
ArgAsnValLeuThrGluGluSerValValArgGluSerLysSerPheThrArgSerThrValAspThr>

      1060      1070      1080      1090      1100      1110      1120
         *         *         *         *         *         *         *
ATGGCCCAGAAGACCCAGGCAGTGTAGGCGACAGCCTCATGGGCCACTGTGGCCCGATGTCCCCTTCCTT
MetAlaGlnLysThrGlnAlaVal***>
```

```
      1130      1140      1150      1160      1170      1180      1190
         *         *         *         *         *         *         *
CCCGGCCATTCTCCCTCTTGTTTTCACTTCACTTTTCGTGGGATGGTGTTACCTTAGCTAACTAACTCTC

      1200      1210      1220      1230      1240      1250      1260
         *         *         *         *         *         *         *
CTCCATGTTGCCTGTCTTTCCCAGACTTGTCCCTCCTTTTCCAGCGGGACTCTTCTCATCCTTCCTCATT

      1270      1280      1290      1300      1310      1320      1330
         *         *         *         *         *         *         *
TGCCAAGGTGAACACTTCCTTCTAGGGAGCACCCTCCCACCCCCCACCCCCCCCCACACACCATCTTTCCA

      1340      1350      1360      1370      1380      1390      1400
         *         *         *         *         *         *         *
TCCCAGGCTTTTGAAAAACAAACAGAAACCCGTGTATCTGGGATATTTCCATATGGCAATAGGTGTGAAC

      1410      1420      1430      1440      1450      1460      1470
         *         *         *         *         *         *         *
AGGGAACTCAGAATACAGACAAGTAGAAAGATTCTCGCTTAAAAAAATGTATTTATTTTATGGCAAGTTG

      1480      1490      1500      1510      1520      1530      1540
         *         *         *         *         *         *         *
GAAAATATGTAACTGGAATCTCAAAAGTTCTTTGGGACAAAACAGAAGTCCATGGAGTTATCTAAGCTCT

      1550      1560      1570      1580      1590      1600      1610
         *         *         *         *         *         *         *
TGTAAGTGAGTTAATTTAAAAAAGAAAATTAGGCTGAGAGCAGTGGCTCACGCCTGTAATCCCAGAACTT

      1620      1630      1640      1650      1660      1670      1680
         *         *         *         *         *         *         *
TGGGAGGCTAAGGTGGGTGGATCACCTGAGGTCAAGAGTTCCAGACCAGGCTGGCCAGCATGGTGAAACC

      1690      1700      1710      1720      1730      1740      1750
         *         *         *         *         *         *         *
CCGTCTGTACTAAAAATACAAAAAATTAACTGGGCATGGTAGTGGGTGCCTGTAATCCCAGCTACTTGGG

      1760      1770      1780      1790      1800      1810      1820
         *         *         *         *         *         *         *
AGGCTGAGGTGGGAGAATTGCTCGAACCTTGGAGGTGGAGGTTGTGGTGAGCCATGATCGCACCACTGCA

      1830      1840      1850      1860      1870      1880      1890
         *         *         *         *         *         *         *
CTCTAGCCTGGGTGACCGAGGGAGGCTCTGTCTCAAAAGCAAAGCAAAAACAAAAACAAAAACACCTAAA

      1900      1910      1920      1930      1940      1950      1960
         *         *         *         *         *         *         *
AAACCTGCAGTTTTGTTTGTACTTTGTTTTTAAATTATGCTTTCTATTTTGAGATCATTGCAAACTCAAC

      1970      1980      1990      2000      2010      2020      2030
         *         *         *         *         *         *         *
ACAATTGTAAGTAATGATACAGAGGGATCTTGTGTACCCTTCACCCAGCCTCCCCCAATGGCAACATCTT

      2040      2050      2060      2070      2080      2090      2100
         *         *         *         *         *         *         *
GCAAAACTACAATGTAGTCTCATAACCAGGATATTGACATTGATACAGTGAAGATACAGGACATTCTCAT

      2110      2120      2130      2140      2150      2160      2170
         *         *         *         *         *         *         *
CACCACAGGGATCCCCAGGATGCCCACTTCCCTCCACCCCCACACCCCAGCCGTGTCCCTAACCCCTGGC

      2180      2190      2200      2210      2220      2230      2240
         *         *         *         *         *         *         *
AACCAGGAATCCACTCTCCATTTCTATAATGTTGTCATTTCAAGAATGTTATTCAATGGAATCATATAGT

      2250      2260      2270      2280      2290      2300      2310
         *         *         *         *         *         *         *
ATGTAACCTGTTTTGAGCTTAAAAAAAAAAGTATACATGACTTTAATGAGGAAAATAAAAATGAATATTG

      2320
         *
AAAAAAAAAACTTTAGAG
```

Figure 6.4 Nucleotide and deduced protein sequence of the human PMN C5a receptor.

adenosine A1 and A2 receptors (Maenhaut et al., 1990; Libert et al., 1991). A crucial assumption for the success of this approach is an intronless gene structure in the region of the probe. This assumption is generally valid in seven-transmembrane segment receptors, with the notable exception of the human tachykinin receptor genes (for substance P and neurokinin A), which we showed to have a five-exon structure (Gerard et al., 1990, 1991). A variation on this approach is to prepare cDNA from polyA+ selected RNA derived from the tissue of interest and then perform PCR, which subverts the intron problem. We rejected this approach for cloning the C5a receptor because the primer selection clearly biases the PCR yield. However, analysis of available sequences at that time (less than 20 receptors were cloned) revealed that the longest, least degenerate structure occurred in the seventh transmembrane domain including the sequence NPXXY, where X is a hydrophobic amino acid.

As previously mentioned, differentiated human myeloid cell lines, HL-60 and U-937, express C5a and FPRs. Therefore, a plus–minus strategy could be envisaged where candidate clones could be screened. Using this approach, an abundant "orphan receptor" with novel sequence was identified in March 1990. This clone hybridized to transcripts in concordance with the expression of C5a receptors was undetectable in undifferentiated HL-60 and U937 cells, and was closely related structurally to the FPR, with some cytoplasmic and membrane-spanning regions being more than 50% identical. Expression of this receptor in COS cells conferred binding of radiolabelled C5a, and affected polyphosphoinositol metabolism (Gerard and Gerard, 1991). The sequence of the clone NPIIY-18 (C5a receptor) is shown in Figure 6.4. Independently, the laboratory of Boulay and co-workers also identified a C5a receptor by expression cloning using the same library they used to isolate the first formyl peptide receptor. The two clones are identical in the deduced coding sequence (Boulay *et al.*, 1991; Gerard and Gerard, 1991).

The genomic organization of the C5a receptor is unusual in that the first exon encodes the 5'-untranslated region and the initiating methionyl residue, while the second exon contains the receptor, otherwise intronless. The 5'-flanking region contains a number of regulatory sequences, including several AP-1 sites, but does not contain CREB/cAMP sites. This is interesting since dibutyryl cAMP is a potent differentiating agent in myeloid cell lines leading to expression of the C5aR. Myeloid specific promoter activity of the C5aR 5'-flanking sequence is detectable in the myeloid rat basophilic leukaemia RBL-1 line, but is seen as a suppressor of gene transcription in non-myeloid lines (Gerard *et al.*, 1992). In the case of both the C5a and formyl peptide receptors, a single large intron is present (Gerard *et al.*, 1992; Perez *et al.*, 1992), apparently dividing the regulatory sequences by 5–10 kb away from the coding sequences. The genes for the FPR, C5a receptor and the two FPRHs are located on human chromosome 19 at the q13.3/13.4 interface (Figure 6.5) (Gerard *et al.*, 1992).

The nature of the binding site for the C5a receptor has been approached through site-directed mutagenesis, limited proteolysis and the formation of chimeric receptors. Preliminarily to beginning the mutagenesis studies, we elected to characterize a second species of C5a receptor. Previous investigators clearly demonstrated a specific binding site for C5a on murine myeloid cell lines using human C5a as the ligand (Goodman *et al.*, 1982), and the affinity of the mouse receptor for the human ligand was almost the same as in the homotypic system. Thus the comparison of human and mouse structures was expected to reveal some interspecies variations in sequence which did not affect binding.

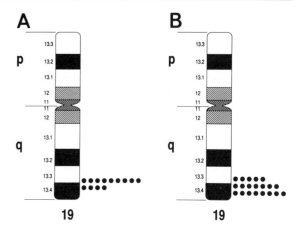

Figure 6.5 (A) Idiogram showing the distribution of signals for C5aR on both chromatids of chromosome 19. (B) Idiogram of the distribution of signals for FPR, FPRH1 and FPRH2 on both chromatids of chromosome 19.

As seen in Figure 6.6, the alignment of the mouse and human structures for the C5a receptor in a topological display demonstrates that the extracellular regions are the most divergent (65%) while the transmembrane segments and selected cytoplasmic sequences are highly conserved (over 70% identical). This diversity in the putative extracellular (binding) domain is at present the highest seen among 115 G-protein coupled receptors for which two species are compared. For comparison, the ten most divergent pairs are noted (Table 6.1). Interestingly, the

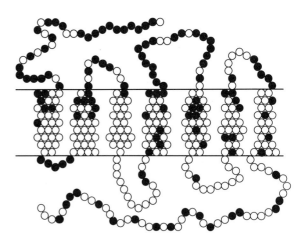

Figure 6.6 Schematic comparison of the mouse and human receptors. Residues conserved between species are depicted in open circles, while divergent positions are filled circles. The amino terminal and extracellular sequences are at the top of the figure and the carboxyl terminus is at the bottom. The majority of sequence divergence (55 of 79 residues) is extracellular. Transmembrane segments M1–M7 and cytoplasmic loops 2 and 3 display high sequence identities, along with the proximal C-terminal region.

Table 6.1   Comparison of divergent and conserved receptors. Comparison of percentage sequence identities for G-protein receptors among species indicates human and mouse C5a receptors are most divergent.

Human C5aR – mouse C5aR	65.3%
Human calcitonin R – Pig calcitonin R	69.5%
Xenopus D2 dopamine R – mouse D2 dopamine R	71.7%
Human IL-8R – rabbit IL-8R	72.8%
Human bradykinin BK2AI – rabbit B2 bradykinin receptor	74.6%
Bovine angiotensin 1R – human angiotensin-1R	95.3%
Rat NK1 – mouse NK1	98.8%
Mouse M1 AchR – rat M1 AchR	98.9%
Sheep NPY R – bovine NPY R	99.2%
Mouse D2 dopamine R – rat D2 dopamine R	100%

IL-8 receptors from human and rabbit also show a high degree of diversity. The highly cationic C5a molecule is known to bind receptors with an ionic component, since concentrations of sodium chloride above 0.25 M can inhibit binding. As noted in the original publication, this feature was consistent with an acidic N-terminal domain seen in the receptor (Gerard and Gerard, 1991; Gerard et al., 1992). In comparing the mouse and human sequences, it is clear that this feature is conserved. As might be expected, also conserved are two cysteine residues in the first and second extracellular loops which form a disulphide in opsin-type receptors (Dohlman et al., 1991). An unusual pentapeptide in the third extracellular loop (ProSerSerProThr) is also conserved. The positioning of two prolyl residues in this small (12 amino acid) loop between the sixth and seventh membrane spanning segments suggested a structural feature to this loop which may be important in ligand binding.

Using the mouse sequence as a starting point, oligonucleotide-directed mutagenesis studies targeted a number of residues spaced throughout the human C5a receptor. The mutant receptors were tagged with a Flag monoclonal epitope in the N-terminus so as to enable detection of expression in the case of non-binding mutants. A number of these mutations were associated with loss or diminution of ligand binding; mutation of one, two and three aspartyl residues from the N-terminus was associated with a progressive loss of binding (N. P. Gerard and C. Gerard, in preparation). The extracellular cysteine residues (Cys 109 and Cys 188) cannot be changed to serine while maintaining ligand binding. Surprisingly, of the six cysteine residues present in the hydrophobic membrane spanning segments, five of them can be mutagenized to serine with no change in receptor activity. One cysteinyl residue at 221 in the fourth membrane spanning segment is essential for high affinity C5a binding. The structure of the third extracellular loop is critical since change of Pro-270 to Leu or change of

Leu-277 to Pro diminishes or extinguishes binding. Prolines in the transmembrane domains are of variable importance and clearly form structural "pockets" as they do in the adrenergic receptors. Canonical aspartate residues in the second transmembrane segment and at the C-terminus of the third segment were both predicted to be essential based on earlier work with other receptors. While Asp 132 behaved as expected, Asp 82 mutated to Asn affected neither binding nor signal transduction. In the case of the LH and TSH receptors, this invariant Asp is critical for signal transduction (Ji and Ji, 1991b). These data are important because they reveal that the mechanisms for binding and signal transduction are divergent while the overall paradigm of G-protein coupling is preserved.

We were unable in this preliminary survey to generate mutants which uncoupled binding from signal transduction, although mutations in the third intracellular loop and C-terminal deletion mutants confirm these sites as important for G-protein coupling. Work by Springer's group have demonstrated that a protease in snake venom can cleave the C5a receptor in the extracellular domain in a limited fashion, resulting in abrogation of binding of the intact anaphylatoxin (M. Springer, personal communication). Chimeric C5a/FPRs made by Perez and colleagues reveal similar information as we determined from mutagenesis, specifically in regard to the role of the amino terminus (H. D. Perez and C. Gerard, unpublished).

A model for the C5a receptor was first envisaged by work done in Hugli's laboratory in the late 1970s and early 1980s (Chenoweth and Hugli, 1980; Hugli, 1981). In this model, the 69-residue disulphide-linked core of C5a was termed the "binding domain" and the C-terminal pentapeptide MQLGR was termed the "activating domain." Subsequent site-directed mutagenesis of C5a and chemical modification studies with the natural factor suggested multiple points of interaction of the ligand with its receptor (Gerard et al., 1985; Johnson and Chenoweth, 1985b; Mollison et al., 1989). In light of the present preliminary analysis of the C5a receptor, we propose that the extracellular segments perform the function of recognizing the bulk of the C5a molecule and presenting the C-terminal pentapeptide to a pore created by the seven transmembrane segments. Work remains to be done in this area to validate these concepts, much of which should rely on the important studies with C5a agonist synthetic peptides described now by several groups (Kwai et al., 1991; Ember et al., 1992). The original model and the present representation for the C5a receptor system is presented in Figure 6.7.

6.   *The Interleukin-8/NAP-1 Receptor*

The cellular receptors for members of the IL-8 gene family were soon found, following the discovery of their

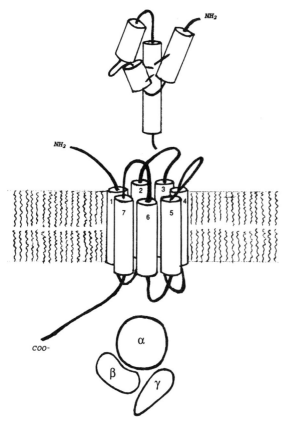

Figure 6.7 Model of the C5a ligand receptor system. The receptor is depicted as a circular structure in the membrane, as suggested by studies on other seven-transmembrane segment receptors. The C5a molecule docks with the receptor via the COOH-terminus and subtle high-affinity interactions, with the extracellular segments and amino terminal acidic segment while interaction of the receptor with a heterotrimeric Gi protein consisting of α,β and γ subunits forms a high-affinity binding complex.

neutrophils using a long oligonucleotide patterned after the adrenergic receptors. When cRNA from their clone, called F3R, was injected into *Xenopus* oocytes, a calcium transient was reportedly observed only in the presence of formyl peptide. Membranes from these oocytes were shown specifically to bind iodinated formyl peptide and displacement by unlabelled ligand yielded a nanomolar K_d for binding. The Northern analysis of the putative rabbit FMLP receptor was absolutely unique to neutrophils; notably absent in lung RNA samples. Surprisingly, the deduced protein sequence for the rabbit receptor was < 30% identical to the isolated human clone (Boulay *et al.*, 1990a). This degree of difference has not been observed for any other cross-species pair or among receptor subtypes of any members of the G-protein

(a)

```
           10        20        30        40        50        60        70
            *         *         *         *         *         *         *
CCTGGCCGGTGCTTCAGTTAGATCAAACCATTGCTGAAACTGAAGAGGACATGTCAAATATTACAGATCC
                                                     MetSerAsnIleThrAspPro>

           80        90       100       110       120       130       140
            *         *         *         *         *         *         *
ACAGATGTGGGATTTTGATGATCTAAATTTCACTGGCATGCCACCTGCAGATGAAGATTACAGCCCCTGT
GlnMetTrpAspPheAspAspLeuAsnPheThrGlyMetProProAlaAspGluAspTyrSerProCys>

          150       160       170       180       190       200       210
            *         *         *         *         *         *         *
ATGCTAGAAACTGAGACACTCAACAAGTATGTTGTGATCATCGCCTATGCCCTAGTGTTCCTGCTAGGCTCA
MetLeuGluThrGluThrLeuAsnLysTyrValValIleIleAlaTyrAlaLeuValPheLeuLeuSer>

          220       230       240       250       260       270       280
            *         *         *         *         *         *         *
TGCTGGGAAACTCCCTGGTGATGCTGGTCATCTTATACAGCAGGGTCGGCCGCTCCGTCACTGATGTCTA
LeuLeuGlyAsnSerLeuValMetLeuValIleLeuTyrSerArgValGlyArgSerValThrAspValTyr>

          290       300       310       320       330       340       350
            *         *         *         *         *         *         *
CCTGCTGAACCTGGCCTTGGCCGACCTACTCTTTGCCCTGACCTTGCCCATCTGGGCCGCCTCCAAGGTG
LeuLeuAsnLeuAlaLeuAlaAspLeuLeuPheAlaLeuThrLeuProIleTrpAlaAlaSerLysVal>

          360       370       380       390       400       410       420
            *         *         *         *         *         *         *
AATGGCTGGATTTTTGGCACATTCCTGTGCAAGGTGGTCTCACTCCTGAAGGAAGTCAACTTCTACAGTG
AsnGlyTrpIlePheGlyThrPheLeuCysLysValValSerLeuLeuLysGluValAsnPheTyrSer>

          430       440       450       460       470       480       490
            *         *         *         *         *         *         *
GCATCCTGCTCGTTGGCCTGCATCAGTGTGGACCGTTACCTGGCCATTGTCCATGCCACACGCACACTGAC
GlyIleLeuLeuLeuValGlyLeuHisGlnCysIleSerValAspArgTyrLeuAlaIleValHisAlaThrArgThrLeuThr>

          500       510       520       530       540       550       560
            *         *         *         *         *         *         *
CCAGAAGCGTCACTTGGTCAAGTTTGTTTGTCTTGGCTGCTGGGGACTGTCTATGAATCTGTCCCTGCCC
GlnLysArgHisLeuValLysPheValCysLeuGlyCysTrpGlyLeuSerMetAsnLeuSerLeuPro>

          570       580       590       600       610       620       630
            *         *         *         *         *         *         *
TTCTTCCTTTTCCGCCAGGCTTACCATCCAAACAATTCCAGTCCAGTTTGCTATGAGGTCCTGGGAAATG
PhePheLeuPheArgGlnAlaTyrHisProAsnAsnSerSerProValCysTyrGluValLeuGlyAsn>

          640       650       660       670       680       690       700
            *         *         *         *         *         *         *
ACACAGCAAAATGGCGGATGGTGTTGCGGATCCTGCCTCACACCTTTGGGCTTCATCGTGCCGCTGTTTGT
AspThrAlaLysTrpArgMetValLeuArgIleLeuProHisThrPheGlyPheIleValProLeuPheVal>

          710       720       730       740       750       760       770
            *         *         *         *         *         *         *
CATGCTGTTCTGCTATGGATTCACCCTGCGTACACTGTTTAAGGCCCACATGGGGCAGAAGCACCGAGCC
MetLeuPheCysTyrGlyPheThrLeuArgThrLeuPheLysAlaHisMetGlyGlnLysHisArgAla>

          780       790       800       810       820       830       840
            *         *         *         *         *         *         *
ATGAGGGTCATCTTTGCTGTCGTCCTCATCTTCCTGCTTTTGCTGGCTGGCCTACAACCTGGTCCTGCTGG
MetArgValIlePheAlaValValLeuIlePheLeuLeuLeuCysTrpLeuProTyrAsnLeuValLeuLeu>

          850       860       870       880       890       900       910
            *         *         *         *         *         *         *
CAGACACCCTCATGAGGACCCAGGTGATCCAGGAGACCTGTGAGCGCCGCAACAACATCGGCCGGGCCCT
AlaAspThrLeuMetArgThrGlnValIleGlnGluThrCysGluArgArgAsnAsnIleGlyArgAlaLeu>

          920       930       940       950       960       970       980
            *         *         *         *         *         *         *
GGATGCCACTGAGATTCTGGGGATTTCTCCATAGCTGCCTCAACCCCATCATCTACGCCTTCATCGGCCAG
AspAlaThrGluIleLeuGlyIlePheLeuHisSerCysLeuAsnProIleIleTyrAlaPheIleGlyGln>

          990      1000      1010      1020      1030      1040      1050
            *         *         *         *         *         *         *
AATTTTCGCCATGGATTCCTCAAGATCCTGGCTATGCATGGCCTGGTCAGCAAGGAGTTCTTGGCACGTC
AsnPheArgHisGlyPheLeuLysIleLeuAlaMetHisGlyLeuValSerLysGluPheLeuAlaArg>

         1060      1070      1080      1090      1100      1110      1120
            *         *         *         *         *         *         *
ATCGTGTTACCTCCTACACTTCTTCGTCTGTCAATGTCTCTTCCAACCTCTGAAAACCATCGATGAAGGA
HisArgValThrSerTyrThrSerSerSerValAsnValSerSerAsnLeu***>
```

ligands. Characterization of the binding of radiolabelled NAP-1 or IL-8 was reported in 1990–91 by several groups (Grob *et al.*, 1990; Beckmann *et al.*, 1991). Data concerning this receptor are somewhat complicated from the start because the ligand series is more heterogeneous. The careful studies of Clark-Lewis *et al.* (1991) indicated that IL-8/NAP–1 can bind two classes of receptors on neutrophils, while the related molecules NAP-2 and MGSA/Gro can only interact with a single class of receptors (Cheng *et al.*, 1992). These forecasts are now known to be accurate.

Ironically, the IL-8 receptor was already cloned in 1990 but was not recognized as such. The cloning of the human FPR by Boulay and colleagues (1990a) was followed 6 months later by the publication of a clone that was billed as the rabbit FMLP receptor (Thomas *et al.*, 1990). While Boulay used a direct expression strategy, Thomas *et al.* cloned an orphan receptor from rabbit

```
        1130      1140      1150      1160      1170      1180      1190
ATATCTCTTCTCAGAAGGAAAGAATAACCAACACCCTGAGGTTGTGTGTGGAAGGTGATCTGGCTCTGGA

        1200      1210      1220      1230      1240      1250      1260
CAGGCACTATCTGGGTTTTGGGGGGACGCTATAGGATGTGGGGAAGTTAGGAACTGGTGTCTTCAGGGGC

        1270      1280      1290      1300      1310      1320      1330
CACACCAACCTTCTGAGGAGCTGTTGAGGTACCTCCAAGGACCGGCCTTTGCACCTCCATGGAAACGAAG

        1340      1350      1360      1370      1380      1390      1400
CACCATCATTCCCGTTGAACGTCACATCTTTAACCCACTAACTGGCTAATTAGCATGGCCACATCTGAGC

        1410      1420      1430      1440      1450      1460      1470
CCCGAATCTGACATTAGATGAGAGAACAGGGCTGAAGCTGTGTCCTCATGAGGGCTGGATGCTCTCGTTG

        1480      1490      1500      1510      1520      1530      1540
ACCCTCACAGGAGCATCTCCTCAACTCTGAGTGTTAAGCGTTGAGCCACCAAGCTGGTGGCTCTGTGTGC

        1550      1560      1570      1580      1590      1600      1610
TCTGATCCGAGCTCAGGGGGGTGGTTTTCCCATCTCAGGTGTGTTGCAGTGTCTGCTGGAGACATTGAGG

        1620      1630      1640      1650      1660      1670      1680
CAGGCACTGCCAAAACATCAACCTGCCAGCTGGCCTTGTGAGGAGCTGGAAACACATGTTCCCCTTGGGG

        1690      1700      1710      1720      1730      1740      1750
GTGGTGGATGAACAAAGAGAAAGAGGGTTTGGAAGCCAGATCTATGCCACAAGAACCCCCTTTACCCCCA

        1760      1770      1780      1790      1800      1810      1820
TGACCAACATCGCAGACACATGTGCTGGCCACCTGCTGAGCCCCAAGTGGAACGAGACAAGCAGCCCTTA

        1830      1840      1850      1860      1870      1880      1890
GCCCTTCCCCTCTGCAGCTTCCAGGCTGGCGTGCAGCATCAGCATCCCTAGAAAGCCATGTGTCAGCCACC

        1900      1910      1920      1930
AGTCCATTGGGCAGGCAGATGTTCCTAATAAAGCTTCTGTTCC
```

```
        850       860       870       880       890       900       910
GGCAGACACCCTCATGAGGACCCAGGTGATCCAGGAGACCTGTGAGCGCCGCAATCACATCGACCGGGCT
AlaAspThrLeuMetArgThrGlnValIleGlnGluThrCysGluArgArgAsnHisIleAspArgAla>

        920       930       940       950       960       970       980
CTGGATGCCACCGAGATTCTGGGCATCCTTCACAGCTGCCTCAACCCCCTCATCTACGCCTTCATTGGCC
LeuAspAlaThrGluIleLeuGlyIleLeuHisSerCysLeuAsnProLeuIleTyrAlaPheIleGly>

        990       1000      1010      1020      1030      1040      1050
AGAAGTTTCGCCATGGACTCCTCAAGATTCTAGCTATACATGGCTTGATCAGCAAGGACTCCCTGCCCAA
GlnLysPheArgHisGlyLeuLeuLysIleLeuAlaIleHisGlyLeuIleSerLysAspSerLeuProLys>

        1060      1070      1080      1090      1100      1110      1120
AGACAGCAGGCCTTCCTTTGTTGGCTCTTCTTCAGGGCACACTTCCACTACTCTCTAAGACCTCCTGCCT
AspSerArgProSerPheValGlySerSerSerGlyHisThrSerThrThrThrLeu***>

        1130      1140      1150      1160      1170      1180      1190
AAGTGCAGCCCGTGGGGTTCCTCCCTTCTCTTCACAGTCACATTCCAAGCCTCATGTCCACTGGTTCTTC

        1200      1210      1220      1230      1240      1250      1260
TTGGTCTCAGTGTCAATGCAGCCCCCATTGTGGTCACAGGAAGCAGAGGAGGCCACGTTCTTACTAGTTT

        1270      1280      1290      1300      1310      1320      1330
CCCTTGCATGGTTTAGAAAGCTTGCCCTGGTGCCTCACCCCTTGCCATAATTACTATGTCATTTGCTGGA

        1340      1350      1360      1370      1380      1390      1400
GCTCTGCCCATCCTGCCCCTGAGCCCATGGCACTCTATGTTCTAAGAAGTGAAAATCTACACTCCAGTGA

        1410      1420      1430      1440      1450      1460      1470
GACAGCTCTGCATACTCATTAGGATGGCTAGTATCAAAAGAAAGAAAATCAGGCTGGCCAACGGGATGAA

        1480      1490      1500      1510
ACCCTGTCTCTACTAAAAAATACAAAAAAAAAAAAAAAAAA
```

Figure 6.8 Nucleotide and deduced amino-acid sequences of the human IL-8 receptors, (a) IL-8RA and (b) IL-8RB. IL-8RA binds to IL-8NAP1 as well as Gro/MGSA, IL-8RB binds IL-8 exclusively.

(b)

```
        10        20        30        40        50        60        70
GTCAGGATTTAAGTTTACCTCAAAAATGGAAGATTTTAACATGGAGAGTGACAGCTTTGAAGATTTCTGG
                                    MetGluSerAspSerPheGluAspPheTrp>

        80        90        100       110       120       130       140
AAAGGTGAAGATCTTAGTAATTACAGTTACAGCTCTACCCTGCCCCCTTTTCTACTAGATGCCGCCCCAT
LysGlyGluAspLeuSerAsnTyrSerTyrSerSerThrLeuProProPheLeuLeuAspAlaAlaPro>

        150       160       170       180       190       200       210
GTGAACCAGAATCCCTGGAAATCAACAAGTATTTTGTGGTCATTATCTATGCCCTGGTATTCCTGCTGAG
CysGluProGluSerLeuGluIleAsnLysTyrPheValValIleIleTyrAlaLeuValPheLeuLeuSer>

        220       230       240       250       260       270       280
CCTGCTGGGAAACTCCCTCGTGATGCTGGTCATCTTATACAGCAGGGTCGGCCGCTCCGTCACTGATGTC
LeuLeuGlyAsnSerLeuValMetLeuValIleLeuTyrSerArgValGlyArgSerValThrAspVal>

        290       300       310       320       330       340       350
TACCTGCTGAACCTAGCCTTGGCCGACCTACTCTTTGCCCTGACCTTGCCCATCTGGGCCGCCTCCAAGG
TyrLeuLeuAsnLeuAlaLeuAlaAspLeuLeuPheAlaLeuThrLeuProIleTrpAlaAlaSerLys>

        360       370       380       390       400       410       420
TGAATGGCTGGATTTTTGGCACATTCCTGTGCAAGGTGGTCTCACTCCTGAAGGAAGTCAACTTCTATAG
ValAsnGlyTrpIlePheGlyThrPheLeuCysLysValValSerLeuLeuLysGluValAsnPheTyrSer>

        430       440       450       460       470       480       490
TGGCATCCTGCTACTGGCCTGCATCAGTGTGGACCGTTACCTGGCCATTGTCCATGCCACACGCACACTG
GlyIleLeuLeuLeuAlaCysIleSerValAspArgTyrLeuAlaIleValHisAlaThrArgThrLeu>

        500       510       520       530       540       550       560
ACCCAGAAGCGCTACTTGGTCAAATTCATATGTCTCAGCATCTGGGGTCTGTCCTTGCTCCTGGCCCTGC
ThrGlnLysArgTyrLeuValLysPheIleCysLeuSerIleTrpGlyLeuSerLeuLeuLeuAlaLeu>

        570       580       590       600       610       620       630
CTGTCTTACTTTTCCGAAGGACCGTCTACTCATCCAATGTTAGCCCAGCCTGCTATGAGGACATGGGCAA
ProValLeuLeuPheArgArgThrValTyrSerSerAsnValSerProAlaCysTyrGluAspMetGlyAsn>

        640       650       660       670       680       690       700
CAATACAGCAAACTGGCGGATGCTGTTACGGATCCTGCCCCAGTCCTTTGGCTTCATCGTGCCACTGCTG
AsnThrAlaAsnTrpArgMetLeuLeuArgIleLeuProGlnSerPheGlyPheIleValProLeuLeu>

        710       720       730       740       750       760       770
ATCATGCTGTTCTGCTACGGATTCACCCTGCGTACGCTGTTTAAGGCCCACATGGGGCAGAAGCACCGGG
IleMetLeuPheCysTyrGlyPheThrLeuArgThrLeuPheLysAlaHisMetGlyGlnLysHisArg>

        780       790       800       810       820       830       840
CCATGCGGGTCATCTTTGCTGTGGTCCTCATCTTCCTGCTTTGCTGGCTGCCCTACAACCTGGTCCTGCT
AlaMetArgValIlePheAlaValValLeuIlePheLeuLeuCysTrpLeuProTyrAsnLeuValLeuLeu>
```

receptor family. Holmes and colleagues (1991) subsequently cloned a human IL-8 receptor using an expression strategy identical to that used for formyl peptide and were surprised to observe >80% sequence identity with the rabbit F3R FMLP receptor. Beckmann et al. (1991) further showed that the putative rabbit FMLP receptor did not interact with FMLP, but in fact bound IL-8 and Gro. This rabbit cDNA additionally differed from Thomas' published sequence in several locations by single or dinucleotide deletions. Murphy and Tiffany (1991) also isolated a human homologue of the rabbit F3R "FMLP receptor" and found that it did not respond to formyl peptide following injection into oocytes. It did, however, transduce a calcium signal when challenged with IL-8 and Gro. Based upon the dose–response data with oocytes, these authors (Murphy and Tiffany, 1991) suggested that their IL-8 receptor was of lower affinity than the molecule identified by Holmes et al. (1991). Subsequent reports from the Navarro laboratory corrected the sequence of F3R, in agreement with the results of Beckmann et al. (1991) and Lee et al. (1992a), and confirmed that F3R did in fact respond to IL-8 (Thomas et al., 1991). Unfortunately, no retraction of the initial error in the first rabbit FMLP receptor report has appeared, while the data are clearly irreproducible and inexplicable.

Comparison of the human sequences is shown in Figure 6.8. The two receptors (IL-8RA and IL-8RB) are nearly 80% identical, with the bulk of the sequence divergence occurring in the N-terminal region (only 28% identical) and the predicted second extracellular loop. These data suggest that the ligand binding specificity may be localized to these sites, with perhaps some participation of transmembrane segment 4. Experiments by LaRosa and colleagues using chimeric receptors suggest that the N-terminus dictates ligand specificity (LaRosa). Transfection of the IL-8RA and IL-8RB clones into 293 cells reveals that IL-8RA, the "low affinity" receptor described by Murphy and Tiffany (1991) binds IL-8 with a K_d of 1.2 nM and Gro with a K_d of 0.8 nM by direct binding. Similar data were obtained by competition binding (Lee et al., 1992b). The IL-8RB clone, described by Holmes et al. (1991), as a high affinity IL-8 receptor binds IL-8/NAP-1 with a K_d of 1.7 nM, but recognizes Gro with an extremely low affinity of 450 nM.

```
            1                                                    50
Humpafr     .......... .........   ..MEPHDSSH MDSEFRYTLF
Gpipafrec   .......... .........   ..MELNSSSR VDSEFRYTLF
Rabil8c     MEVNVWNMTD LWTWFEDEFA NAT...GMPP VEKDYSPCLV VTQTLNKYVV
Humil8ra    ....MSNITD PQMWDFDDL. NFT...GMPP ADEDYSPCML ETETLNKYVV
Humintleu8  ....MESDSF EDFWKGEDLS NYSYSSTLPP FLLDAAPCEP ESLEINKYFV
Humc5anapl  ....MNSFNY TTPDYGHYDD KDTLDLNTPV DKTSNTLRVP .D.....ILA
Musc5r      ....MNS.SF EI....NYDH YGTMDPNIPA DGIHLPKRQP GD.....VAA
Humfmlpx    .......... .........   .METNFSTPL NEYEEVSYES AGYTVLRILP
Humfmlpy    .......... .........   .METNFSIPL NETEEVLPEP AGHTVLWIFS
Humfmlp     .......... .........   .METNSSLPT NISGGTPAVS AGYLFLDIIT

            51                                                   100
Humpafr     PIVYSIIFVL GVIANGYVLW VFARLYPCKK FNEIKIFMVN LTMADMLFLI
Gpipafrec   PIVYSIIFVL GIIANGYVLW VFARLYPSKK LNEIKIFMVN LTVADLLFLI
Rabil8c     VVIYALVFLL SLLGNSLVML VIL..YSRSN RSVTDVYLLN LAMADLLFAL
Humil8ra    IIAYALVFLL SLLGNSLVML VIL...YSRVG RSVTDVYLLN LALADLLFAL
Humintleu8  VIIYALVFLL SLLGNSLVML VIL...YSRVG RSVTDVYLLN LALADLLFAL
Humc5anapl  LVIFAVVFLV GVLGNALVVW VTA..F.EAK RTINAIWFLN LAVADFLSCL
Musc5r      LIIYSVVFLV GVPGNALVVW VTA..F.EPD GPSNAIWFLN LAVADLLSCL
Humfmlpx    LVVLGVTFVL GVLGNGLVIW VAG..F.RMT RTVTTICYLN LALADFSFTA
Humfmlpy    LLVHGVTFVF GVLGNGLVIW VAG..F.RMT RTVNTICYLN LALADFSFSA
Humfmlp     YLVFVATFVL GVLGNGLVIW VAG..F.RMT HTVVTTISYLN LAVADFCFTS

            101                                                  150
Humpafr     TLPLWIVYYQ NQGNWILPKF LCNVAGCLFF INTYCSVAFL GVITYNRFQA
Gpipafrec   TLPLWIVYYS NQGNWFLPKF LCNLAGCLFF INTYCSVAFL GVITYNRFQA
Rabil8c     TMPIWAVSKE KG..WIFGTP LCKVVSLVKE VNFYSGILLL ACISVDRYLA
Humil8ra    TLPIWAASKV NG..WIFGTF LCKVVSLLKE VNFYSGILLL ACISVDRYLA
Humintleu8  TLPIWAASKV NG..WIFGTF LCKVVSLLKE VNFYSGILLL ACISVDRYLA
Humc5anapl  ALPFLFTSIV QHHHWPFGGA ACSILPSLIL LNMYASILLL ATISADRFLL
Musc5r      AMPVLFTTVL NHNYWYFDAT ACIVLPSLIL LNMYASILLL ATISADRFLL
Humfmlpx    TLPFLIVVSMA MGEKWPFGWF LCKLIHIVVD INLFGSVFLI GFIALDRCIC
Humfmlpy    ILPFRMVSVA MREKWPFASF LCKLVHVMID INLFVSVYLI TIIALDRCIC
Humfmlp     TLPFFMVRKA MGGHWPFGWF LCKFLFTIVD INLFGSVFLI ALIALDRCVC

            151                                                  200
Humpafr     VTRPIKTAQA NTRKRGISLS LVIWV..AIV GAASYFLILD STNTVPDSAG
Gpipafrec   VKYPIKTAQA TTRKRGIALS LVIWV..AIV AAASYFLVMD STNVVSNKAG
Rabil8c     IVHATRTLTQ KRH.LVKFIC LGIWALSLIL SLPFFLFRQV FSPNNSSPVC
Humil8ra    IVHATRTLTQ KRH.LVKFVC LGCWGLSMNL SLPFFLFRQA YHPNNSSPVC
Humintleu8  IVHATRTLTQ KRY.LVKFIC LSIWGLSLLL ALPVLLFRRT VYSSNVSPAC
Humc5anapl  VFKPIWCQNF RGAGLAWIAC AVAWGLALLL TIPSFLYRVV REEYFPPKVL
Musc5r      VFKPIWCQKV RGTGLAWMAC GVAWVLALLV TIPSFVYREA YKHFYSEHTV
Humfmlpx    VLHPVWAQNH RTVSLAMKVI VGPWILALVL TLPVFLFLTT VTI.PNGDTY
Humfmlpy    VLHPAWAQNH RTMSLAKRVM TGLWIFTIVL TLPNFIFWTT IST.TNGDTY
Humfmlp     VLHPVWTQNH RTVSLAKKVI IGPWVMALLL TLPVIIRVTT VPG.KTGTVA

            201                                                  250
Humpafr     SGNVTRCFEH YEKGSVPVLI IH......IF IVFSFFLVFL IILFCNLVII
Gpipafrec   SGNITRCFEH YEKGSKPVLI IH......IC IVLGFFIVFL LILFCNLVII
Rabil8c     ....YEDLGH NTAKWRMV... ....LRILP HTFGFIVPLL VMLFCYGFTL
Humil8ra    ....YEVLGN DTAKWRMV... ....LRILP HTFGFIVPLF VMLFCYGFTL
Humintleu8  ....YEDMGN NTANWRML.. ....LRILP QSFGFIVPLL IMLFCYGFTL
Humc5anapl  CGVDYSH.DK .RRER...... ..AVAIVR LLFWLPYNIL TICYTFLL
Musc5r      CGINYGG.GS FPPKEN..... ..AVAILR LMVGFVLPLL TLNICYTFLL
Humfmlpx    CTFNFASWGG TPEERLKVAI TMLTARGIIR FVIGFSLPMS IVAICYGLIA
Humfmlpy    CIFNFAFWGD TAVERLNVFI TMAKVFLILH FIIGFTVPMS IITVCYGLIA
Humfmlp     CTFNFSPWTN DPKERINAV AMLTVRGIIR FIIGFSAPMS IVAVSYGLIA

            251                                                  300
Humpafr     RTLLMQPVQQ QRNAEVKRRA LWMVCTVLAV FIICFVPHHV VQL....PWTL
Gpipafrec   HTTLLRQPVKQ QRNAEVRRRA LWMVCTVLAV FVICFVPHHM VQL...PWTL
Rabil8c     RTLFQAHMGQ ......KHRA MRVIFAVVLI FLLCWLPYNL V.LLADTLMR
Humil8ra    RTLFKAHMGQ ......KHRA MRVIFAVVLI FLLCWLPYNL V.LLADTLMR
Humintleu8  RTLFKAHMGQ ......KHRA MRVIFAVVLI FLLCWLPYNL V.LLADTLMR
Humc5anapl  LRTWSRRATR ......STKT LKVVVAVVAS FFIFWLPYQV TGIMMSFLEP
Musc5r      LRTWSRRATR ......STKT LKVVMAVVIC FFIFWLPYQV TGVMIAWLPP
Humfmlpx    AKIHKKGMIK ......SSRP LRVLTAVVAS FFICWFPYQL VALLGTVWLK
Humfmlpy    AKIHRNHMIK ......SSRP LRVFAAVVAS FFICWFPYEL IGILMAVWLK
Humfmlp     TKIHKQGLIK ......SSRP LRVLSFVAAA FFLCWSPYQV VALIATVRIR

            301                                                  350
Humpafr     AELGFQDSKF HQAINDAHQV TLCLLSTNCV LDPVIYCFLT KKFRKHLTEK
Gpipafrec   AELGMWPSSN HQAINDAHQV TLCLLSTNCV LDPVIYCFLT KKFRKHLSEK
Rabil8c     THVIQETCQR RNDIDRALDA TEILGFLHSC LNPIIYAFIG QNFRNGFLKM
Humil8ra    TQVIQETCER RNNIGRALDA TEILGFLHSC LNPIIYAFIG QNFRHGFLKI
Humintleu8  TQVIQETCER RNHIDRALDA TEILGILHSC LNPLIYAFIG QKFRHGLLKI
Humc5anapl  S...SPTFLL ..LNKLDSL CVSPAYINCC INPIIYVVAG QGFQGRLRKS
Musc5r      S...SPTLRR ..VEKLNSL CVSLAYINCC VNPIIYVMAG QGFHGRLLRS
Humfmlpx    EMLFYGKYKI ...IDILVNP TSSLAFFNSC LNPMLYVFVG QDFRERLIHS
Humfmlpy    EMLLNGKYKI ...ILVLINP TSSLAFFNSC LNPILYVFMG RNFQERLIRS
Humfmlp     E.LLQGMYKE ...IGIAVDV TSALAFFNSC LNPMLYVFMG QDFRERLIHA

            351                                        387
Humpafr     FYSMRSSRKC SRATTCDTVTE VVVPFNQIPG NSLKN..
Gpipafrec   LNIMRSSQKC SRVTTDTGTE MAIPINHTPV NPIKN..
Rabil8c     LAA...RGLI SKEFLTRHRV TSYTSSSTNV PSNL...
Humil8ra    LAM...HGLV SKEFLARHRV TSYTSSSVNV SSNL...
Humintleu8  LAI...HGLI SKDSLPKDSR PSFVGSSSGH TSTTL..
Humc5anapl  LPSLLRNVLT E.ESVVRESK SFTRSTVDTM AQKTQAV
Musc5r      LPSIIRNALS E.DSVGRDSK TFTPSTDDTS GRKSQAV
Humfmlpx    LPTSLERALS E.DSAPTND TAANCASPPA ETELQAM
Humfmlpy    LPTSLERALT EVPDSAQTSN THTTSASPPE ETELQAM
```

Figure 6.9 Comparison of the predicted amino-acid sequences of neutrophil chemotactic receptors. Aligned sequences are Humpafr, human PAF receptor; gpipafrec, guinea-pig PAF receptor; Rabil8c, rabbit IL-8 receptor; Humil8ra, human IL-8RA; Humintleu8, human IL-8RB; Humc5anapl, human C5a receptor; Musc5r, mouse C5a receptor; Humfmlpx, human FPRH1; Humfmlpy, human FPRH2; Humfmlp; human FPR. Gaps are introduced to maximize sequence identity.

These binding data were fully supported by calcium transients detected in the transfectants, demonstrating functional expression. When the transfected cell system is compared with human neutrophils, the data are also consistent. In essence, two receptors for IL-8/NAP-1 occur on human neutrophils which are ~77% identical. Both bind IL-8 with high affinity. One of the receptors (IL-8RB) binds IL-8 exclusively, while the other (IL-8RA) binds both IL-8/NAP-1 and Gro/MGSA equally well.

Questions about the multiplicity of receptors has led to characterization of their genes. Ahuja et al. (1992) determined that the IL-8 receptors clustered at human chromosome 2q34/35 along with a pseudogene. The genomic clones are intronless in their coding sequences. The gene clustering is reminiscent of the C5a/formyl peptide group. An intriguing observation in this study recognizes that the chemokines are clustered on chromosome 4q13–21, and are multiple, while the two receptors have evolved the ability to recognize multiple ligands. Perhaps the presence of a related pseudogene reflects evolutionary constraints dealt by the multiplicity of ligands and receptors. The IL-8 family of ligands are derived from multiple diverse sources, including epithelium, endothelium, tumour cells and connective tissue, as well as monocytes and platelets (reviewed in Oppenheim et al., 1991). It is clear that at the receptor binding and signal transduction level, all of the ligand diversity feeds into a final common pathway for neutrophil activation. Thus, this gives the IL-8 system the versatility that is not possible in the C5a/formyl peptide systems, which recognize complement activation, tissue autolysis or bacterial invasion. A similar level of versatility is seen in the PAF and LTB₄ systems, since these stimuli are also generated relatively non-specifically from a variety of sources.

7. Structural and Functional Analysis of the Neutrophil Chemotactic Receptors

The five receptors discussed above are presented in computed alignment in Figure 6.9. Casual inspection of the sequences discloses that the N-terminal peptide prior to the first transmembrane segment, the second extra-cellular loop, and the third intracellular loop are the sites of the largest gaps between alignments. While these data implicate these regions in ligand specificity and signal transduction, it will be necessary to perform detailed studies to ascertain the facts. Unlike the adrenergic receptor field, where decades of pharmacological study identified myriad compounds useful to probe structure: activity relationships, our tools for the study of chemotactic receptors are much more limited. Receptor subtypes do not appear to exist for the C5a and PAF receptors, while the IL-8 and FPR clearly have related structures. Interacting sites on the receptor that confer specificity to ligand subtypes may be probed by the creation of chimeric receptors, as has been preliminarily reported for the IL-8 receptor (LaRosa *et al.*, 1992). The most powerful technique available at present is site directed mutagenesis followed by transfection into appropriate host cells. This is a developing area and requires some additional work to validate the approaches, as discussed below.

There are several fundamentally different questions we would like to answer. First, what is the nature of the ligand:receptor binding site? Second, how does ligand binding initiate the biological response? Third, why do these ligands evoke different responses? In order to address these questions, the cloned receptor cDNA offers a powerful tool, but one with limitations. The trans-fection systems available at the moment include mostly established non-myeloid cells such as COS (Africa green monkey kidney) and 293 (human embryonic kidney), as well as *Xenopus*. However, these cell lines are not usual hosts for the chemotactic receptors. They may or may not contain the appropriate alpha, beta and gamma G-protein subunits. Differences exist as well in the downstream effectors of G-proteins, for example, the isotype of phospholipase C, protein kinases, or phos-phatases etc., which are activated and may ultimately determine the outcome of a particular stimulation. Didsbury and colleagues reported that TSA cells, a subline of HEK 293 cells stably transfected with the SV40 large T antigen, could co-express C5aR and FPR and that calcium transients were measurable in response to ligand (Didsbury *et al.*, 1992). Similar data cannot be

obtained in COS cells, apparently because the signal is too small. These co-expressed receptors exhibited specific heterologous desensitization when stimulated at low agonist concentrations, an effect which can also be observed in neutrophils. However, when we try to measure phosphatidyl inositol metabolites expected to coincide with such calcium signals in COS cells, we observe effects detectable by isotope tracer but not by lipid mass. Co-transfection of $G_{\alpha 16}$, a pertussis toxin-insensitive G-protein subunit found in monocytes, with the receptors, greatly facilitates measurement of inositol metabolites in these cells (Amatruda *et al.* 1993). Thus, reconstitution of the inositol signalling system triggered by these receptors appears promising.

Another potential avenue will be to transfect more appropriate host cells, for example U-937 cells, and study the expressed mutant molecules in the absence of cell differentiation. The benefit of this system is that post-receptor signalling pathways should be intact. The limitation of this system is that U-937 and HL-60 cells are very poorly transfected, and the practicality of selecting stable lines for each mutant is questionable. Therefore, preliminary screening for interesting mutants can be performed in 293 cells. The rat myeloid RBL line can also be transfected following electroporation and selection can be performed for stable lines which signal appropriately (J. Didsbury and R. Snyderman, N.P. Gerard and C. Gerard, unpublished observations).

The difficulties in transfection aside, expression of mutant receptors requires strict controls to allow inter-pretation of data. Unlike production of mutant poly-peptides in *E. coli* or baculovirus, where the mutant is produced in bulk and can be chemically characterized, overexpressed receptors are still rare. For example, a typical dish of transfected cells containing $\sim 10^7$ cells with an average expression of 20 000 sites/cell translates to picomolar quantities of receptor. Thus, the binding constants for mutants must be determined by Scatchard analyses. In the case of low affinity or "knockout" mutations one must prove that the mutation still allows surface expression of the receptor. Since such mutants are not amenable to Scatchard analysis, the number of sites/cell must be estimated by another method. Quanti-fication by radiolabelled anti-receptor antibody is accept-able, as is any other immunochemical approach, provided the cells are not permeabilized or disrupted. Mutants of the opsin receptor have been described which are not processed to the final disc membrane (Sung *et al.*, 1991). Such receptors phenotypically appear to be "knockout" or low affinity mutants; in reality, they simply are not present where they should be to function.

Antisera raised against the receptors will be useful for following their biosynthesis and processing, as well as trafficking and turnover following interaction with ligand. The state of phosphorylation of the receptors can also be followed given well-characterized antibodies. To date, no antisera have been raised against the intact receptors, although anti-peptide antisera have been tried for some.

8. Conclusion

The once-distant goal of knowing the structures for the major neutrophil chemotactic receptors has largely been achieved through expression-cloning strategies. The structures turn out to be far more interesting because the common theme of seven transmembrane segments and G-protein coupling provide a conceptual link to other sensing systems such as vision, olfaction, endocrine and neurotransmission. The broad perspective is now established, and the "i-dot and t-cross" experiments will now deepen our understanding of the mechanisms by which neutrophils respond to their environment.

9. References

Ahuja, S.K., Ozcelik, T., Milatovitch, A., Francke, U. and Murphy, P.M. (1992). Molecular evolution of the interleukin-8 receptor gene cluster. Nature Genetics 2, 31–36.

Amatruda, T.T. 3rd, Gerard, N.P., Gerard, C. and Simon, M. I. (1993). Specific interaction of chemoattractant factor receptors with G-proteins. J. Biol. Chem. 268, 10139–10144.

Aruffo, A. and Seed, B. (1987). Molecular cloning of a CD28 cDNA by a high efficiency COS cell expression system. Proc. Natl Acad. Sci. USA 84, 8573–8577.

Aswanikumar, S., Corcoran, B., Schiffman, E., Day, A.R., Freer, R.J., Showell, H.J. and Becker, E.L. (1977). Demonstration of a receptor on rabbit neutrophils for chemotactic peptides. Biochem. Biophys. Res. Comm. 74, 810–817.

Bayramashuili, D.I., Drachev, A.L., Drachev, L.A., Kaulen, A.D., Kudelin, A.B., Martynov, V.I. and Skulachev, V.P. (1984). Proteinase-treated photoreactor discs. Photoelectric activity of the partially-digested rhodopsin and membrane orientation. Eur. J. Biochem. 142, 583–590.

Beckmann, M.P., Munger, W.E., Kozlosky, C., VandenBos, T., Price, V., Lyman, S., Gerard, N.P., Gerard, C. and Cerretti, D.P. (1991). Molecular characterization of the interleukin-8 receptor. Biochem. Biophys. Res. Comm. 179, 784–789.

Berdel, W.E., Korth, R., Reichert, A., Houlihan, W.J., Bicker, U., Nomura, H., Vogler, W.R., Benveniste, J. and Rastetter, J. (1987). Lack of correlation between cytotoxicity of agonists and antagonists of platelet activating factor (paf-acether) in neoplastic cells and modulation of [^{3}H]-paf-acether binding to platelets from humans in vitro. Anticancer Res. 7, 1181–1187.

Birnbaumer, L. and Brown, A.M. (1990). G-Proteins and the mechanism of action of hormones, neurotransmitters, and autocrine and paracrine regulatory factors. Am. Rev. Respir. Dis. 141, S106–114.

Blank, M.L., Snyder, F., Byers, L.W., Brooks, B. and Muirhead, E.E. (1979). 1-Alkyl-2-acetyl-sn-glycero-3-phosphocholine, derived chemically from choline plasmalogens of beef heart, has been shown to possess powerful antihypertensive activity. Biochem. Biophys. Res. Comm. 90, 1194–1200.

Boulay, F., Tardif, M., Brouchon, L. and Vignais, P. (1990a). The human N-formylpeptide receptor. Characterization of two cDNA isolates and evidence for a new subfamily of G-protein-coupled receptors. Biochemistry 29, 11123–11133.

Boulay, F., Taridif, M. and Vignais, P. (1990b). Synthesis and use of a novel N-formyl peptide derivative to isolate a human N-formyl peptide receptor cDNA. Biochem. Biophys. Res. Comm. 168, 1103–1109.

Boulay, F., Mery, L., Tardif, M., Brouchon, L. and Vignais, P. (1991). Expression cloning of a receptor for C5a anaphylatoxin on differentiated HL-60 cells. Biochemistry 30, 2993–2999.

Bratton, D.L., Dreyer, E., Kailey, J.M., Fadok, V.A., Clay, K.L. and Henson, P.M. (1992). The mechanism of internalization of platelet-activating factor in activated human neutrophils. Enhanced transbilayer movement across the plasma membrane. J. Immunol. 148, 514–523.

Camp, R.D., Woollard, P.M., Mallet, A.I. Fincham, N.J., Ford-Hutchinson, A.W and Bray, M.A. (1982). Neutrophil aggregating and chemokinetic properties of a 5,12, 20-trihydroxy-6,8,10,14-eicosatetraenoic acid isolated from human leukocytes. Prostaglandins 23, 631–641.

Casals-Stenzel, J., Muacevic, G. and Weber, K.H. (1987). Pharmacological actions of WEB 2086, a new specific antagonist of platelet activating factor. J. Pharmacol. Exp. Ther. 241, 974–981.

Cheng, Q.C., Han, J.H., Thomas, H.G., Balentien, E. and Richmond, A. (1992). The melanoma growth stimulatory activity receptors consist of two proteins: ligand binding results in enhanced tyrosine phosphorylation. J. Immunol. 148, 451–456.

Chenoweth, D.E. and Hugli, T.E. (1978). Demonstration of specific C5a receptor on intact human polymorphonuclear leukocytes. Proc. Natl Acad. Sci. USA 75, 3943–3947.

Chenoweth, D.E. and Hugli, T.E. (1980). Human C5a and C5a analogs as probes of the neutrophil C5a receptor. Mol. Immunol. 17, 151–161.

Chenoweth, D.E. and Soderberg, C. (1985). Prog. Leukocyte Biol. 4, 439–446.

Clark-Lewis, I., Schumacher, C., Baggiolini, M., and Moser, B. (1991). Structure–activity relationships of interleukin-8 determined using chemically synthesized analogs. Critical role of NH$_2$-terminal residues and evidence for uncoupling of neutrophil chemotaxis, exocytosis, and receptor binding activities. J. Biol. Chem. 266, 23128–23134.

Demopoulos, C.A., Pinckard, R.N. and Hannahan, D.J. (1979) Platelet-activating factor. Evidence for 1-O-alkyl-acetyl-sn-glyceryl-3-phosphorylcholine as the active component (a new class of lipid chemical mediators). J. Biol. Chem. 254, 9355–9358.

Didsbury, J.R., Uhing, R.J., Tomhave, E., Gerard, C., Gerard, N. and Snyderman, R. (1992). Functional high efficiency expression of cloned leukocyte chemoattractant receptor cDNA's. FEBS Lett. 297, 275–279.

Dohlman, H.G., Bouvier, M., Benovic, J.L., Caron, M.G. and Lefkowitz, R.J. (1987). The multiple membrane spanning topography of the beta 2-adrenergic receptor. Localization of the sites of binding, glycosylation, and regulatory phosphorylation by limited proteolysis. J. Biol. Chem. 262, 14282–14288.

Dohlman, H.G., Thorner, J., Caron, M.G. and Lefkowitz, R.J. (1991). Model systems for the study of seven-transmembrane-segment receptors. Annu. Rev. Biochem. 60, 653–688.

Ember, J.A., Sanderson, S.D., Taylor, S.M., Kawahara, M. and Hugli, T.E. (1992). Biologic activity of synthetic analogues of C5a anaphylatoxin. J. Immunol. 148, 3165–3173.

Feltner, D.E., Smith, R.H. and Marasco, W.A. (1986). Characterization of the plasma membrane bound GTPase from rabbit neutrophils. I. Evidence for an Ni-like protein coupled to the formyl peptide, C5a, and leukotriene B4 chemotaxis receptors. J. Immunol. 137, 1961–1970.

Gerard, C., Showell, H.J., Hoeprich, P.D., Jr, Hugli, T.E. and Stimler, N.P. (1985). Evidence for a role of the amino-terminal region in the biological activity of the classical anaphylatoxin, porcine C5a des-Arg-74. J. Biol. Chem. 260, 2613–2616.

Gerard, N.P. and Gerard, C. (1991). The chemotactic receptor for human C5a anaphylatoxin. Nature 349, 614–617.

Gerard, N.P. and Gerard, C. (1994). Receptor-dependent internalization of platelet-activating factor (PAF). J. Immunol. (in press).

Gerard, N.P., Eddy, R.L., Jr, Shows, T.B. and Gerard, C. (1990). The human neurokinin A (Substance K) receptor. J. Biol. Chem. 265, 20455–20462.

Gerard, N.P., Garraway, L.A., Eddy, R.L., Jr, Shows, T.B., Iijima, H., Paquet, J.-L. and Gerard, C. (1991). Human substance P receptor (NK-1): organization of the gene, chromosome localization, and functional expression of cDNA clones. Biochemistry 30, 10640–10646.

Gerard, N.P., Lu, B., He, X-P, Eddy, R.L., Jr, Shows, T.B. and Gerard, C. (1992). Human chemotaxis receptor genes cluster at 19q13.3–13.4. Characterization of the human C5a receptor gene. Biochemistry 32, 1243–1250.

Goodman, M.G., Chenoweth, D.E. and Weigle, W.O. (1982). Induction of interleukin 1 secretion and enhancement of humoral immunity by binding of human C5a to macrophage surface C5a receptors. J. Exp. Med. 156, 912–917.

Grob, P.M., David, E., Warren, T.C., DeLeon R.P., Farina, P.R. and Homon, C.A. (1990). Characterization of a receptor for human monocyte-derived neutrophil chemotactic factor/interleukin-8. J. Biol. Chem. 265, 8311–8316.

Hanahan, D.J. (1986). Platelet-activating factor: a biologically active phosphoglyceride. Annu. Rev. Biochem. 55, 483–509.

Harris, P. and Ralph, P. (1985). Human leukemia models of myelomonocytic development: a review of the HL60 and U937 cell lines. J. Leuk. Biol. 407–422.

Hediger, M.A., Coady, M.J., Ikeda, T.S. and Wright, E.M. (1987). Expression cloning and cDNA sequencing to the Na⁺/glucose co-transporter. Nature 330, 379–381.

Hirata, M., Hayashi, Y., Ushikubi, F., Yokota, Y., Kageyama, R., Nakanishi, S. and Narumiyai, S. (1991). Cloning and expression of cDNA for a human thromboxane A2 receptor. Nature 349, 617–620.

Holmes, W.E., Lee, J., Kuang, W.J., Rice, G.C. and Wood, W.I. (1991). Structure and functional expression of a human interleukin-8 receptor. Science 253, 1278–1280.

Honda, Z., Nakamura, M., Miki, I., Minami, M., Watanabe, T., Seyama, Y., Okado, H., Toh, H., Ito, K., Miyamoto, T. and Shimizu, T. (1991). Cloning by functional expression of platelet-activating factor receptor from guinea-pig lung. Nature 349, 342–346.

Huey, R. and Hugli, T.E. (1985). Characterization of a C5a receptor on human polymorphonuclear leukocytes. J. Immunol. 135, 2063–2068.

Hugli, T.E. (1981). The structural basis for anaphylatoxin and chemotactic functions of C3a, C4a, and C5a. Crit. Rev. Immunol. 1, 321–366.

Hwang, S.B. (1988). Identificaton of a second putative receptor of platelet-activating factor from human polymorphonuclear leukocytes. J. Biol. Chem. 263, 3225–3233.

Jesaitis, A.J., Bokoch, G.M., Tolley, J.O. and Allen, R.A. (1988). Lateral segregation of neutrophil chemotactic receptors into actin- and fodrin-rich plasma membrane microdomains depleted in guanyl nucleotide regulatory proteins. J. Cell Biol. 107, 921–928.

Ji, I.H. and Ji, T.H. (1991a). Human choriogonadotropin binds to a lutropin receptor with essentially no N-terminal extension and stimulates cAMP synthesis. J. Biol. Chem. 266, 13076–13079.

Ji, I. and Ji, T.H. (1991b). Asp383 in the second transmembrane domain of the lutropin receptor is important for high affinity hormone binding and cAMP production. J. Biol. Chem. 266, 14953–14957.

Johnson, R.J. and Chenoweth, D.E. (1985a). Labeling the granulocyte C5a receptor with a unique photoreactive probe. J. Biol. Chem. 260, 7161–7164.

Johnson, R.J. and Chenoweth, D.E. (1985b). Structure and function of human C5a anaphylatoxin. Selective modification of tyrosine 23 alters biological activity but not antigenicity. J. Biol. Chem. 260, 10339–10345.

Kunz, D., Gerard, N.P. and Gerard, C. (1992). The human leukocyte platelet-activating factor receptor. J. Biol. Chem. 267, 9101–9106.

Kwai, M., Quincy, D.A., Lane, B., Mollison, K.W., Luly, J. and Carter, G.W. (1991). Identificaton and synthesis of a receptor binding site of human anaphylatoxin C5a. J. Med. Chem. 31, 2068–2071.

LaRosa, G.J., Thomas, K.M., Kaufmann, M.E., Mark, R., White, M., Taylor, L., Gray, G., Witt, D., and Navarro, J. (1992). Amino terminus of the interleukin-8 receptor is a major determinant of receptor subtype specificity. J. Biol. Chem. 267, 25402–25406.

Lee, J., Kuang, W.J., Rice, G.C. and Wood, W.I. (1992a). Characterization of complementary DNA clones encoding the rabbit IL-8 receptor. J. Immunol. 148, 1261–1264.

Lee, J., Horuk, R., Rice, G.C., Bennett, G.L., Camerato, T. and Wood, W.I. (1992b). Characterization of two high affinity human interleukin-8 receptors. J. Biol. Chem. 267, 16283–16287.

Libert, F., Parmentier, M., Lefort, A., Dinsart, C., Van Sande, J., Maenhaut, C., Simons, M.J., Dumont, J.E. and Vassart, G. (1989). Selective amplification and cloning of four new members of the G protein-coupled receptor family. Science 244, 569–572.

Libert, F., Schiffman, S.N., Lefort, A., Parmentier, M., Gerard, C., Dumont, J.E., Vanderhaegen, J.J. and Vassart, G. (1991). The orphan receptor cDNA RDC7 encodes an A1 adenosine receptor. EMBO J. 10, 1677–1682.

Lu, B., Gerard, N.P., Eddy, R.L., Jr, Shows, T.B. and Gerard, C. (1992). Mapping of genes for the human C5a receptor (C5aR), human FMLP receptor (FPR), and two FMLP receptor homologue orphan receptors (FPRH1, FPRH2) to chromosome 19. Genomics 13, 437–440.

Mackin, W.M., Huang, C.K. and Becker, E.L. (1982). The formylpeptide chemotactic receptor on rabbit peritoneal neutrophils. I. Evidence for two binding sites with different affinities. J. Immunol. 129, 1608–1611.

Maenhaut, C., Van Sande, J., Libert, F., Abramowicz, M., Parmentier, M., Vanderhaegen, J.J., Dumont, J.E., Vassart, G. and Schiffman, S. (1990). RDC8 codes for an adenosine A2 receptor with physiological constitutive activity. Biochem. Biophys. Res. Comm. 173, 1169–1178.

Malech, H.L., Gardner, J.P., Heiman, D.F., and Rosenzweig, S.A. (1985). Asparagine-linked oligosaccharides on formyl peptide chemotactic receptors of human phagocytic cells. J. Biol. Chem. 260, 2509–2514.

Marasco, W.A., Phan, S.H., Krutzsch, H., Showell, H.J., Feltner, D.E., Nairn, R., Becker, E.L. and Ward, P.A. (1984). Purification and identification of formyl-methionyl-leucyl-phenylalanine as the major peptide neutrophil chemotactic factor produced by Escherichia coli. J. Biol. Chem. 259, 5430–5439.

Marasco, W.A., Becker, K.M., Feltner, D.E., Brown, C.S., Ward, P.A. and Nairn, R. (1985). Covalent affinity labelling, detergent solubilization, and fluid-phase characterization of the rabbit neutrophil formyl peptide chemotaxis receptor. Biochemistry 24, 2227–2236.

Mollison, K.W., Mandecki, W., Zuiderweg, E.R., Fayer, A., Krause, R.A., Conway, R.G., Miller, L. Edalji, R.P., Shallcross, M.A. Lane, B., Fox, J.L., Green, J. and Carter, G.W. (1989). Identification of receptor-binding residues in the inflammatory complement protein C5a by site-directed mutagenesis. Proc. Natl Acad. Sci. USA 86, 292–296.

Monsma, F.J., Jr, McVittie, L.D., Gerfen, C.R., Mahan, L.C. and Sibley, D.R. (1989). Multiple D2 dopamine receptors produced by alternative RNA splicing. Nature 342, 926–929.

Murphy, P.M. and McDermott, D. (1991). Functional expression of the human formyl peptide receptor in Xenopus oocytes requires a complementary human factor. J. Biol. Chem. 266, 12560–12567.

Murphy, P.M. and Tiffany, H.L. (1991). Cloning of complementary DNA encoding a functional human interleukin-8 receptor. Science 253, 1280–1283.

Murphy, P.M., Gallin, E.K. and Tiffany, H.L. (1990). Characterization of human phagocytic cell receptors for C5a and platelet activating factor expressed in Xenopus oocytes. J. Immunol. 145, 2227–2234.

Murphy, P.M., Ozcelik, T., Kenney, R.T., Tiffany, H.L., McDermott, D. and Francke, U. (1992). A structural homologue of the N-formyl peptide receptor. Characterization and chromosome mapping of a peptide chemoattractant receptor family. J. Biol. Chem. 267, 7637–7643.

Nakamura, M., Honda, Z., Izumi, T., Sakanaka, H., Minami, M., Bito, H., Seyama, Y., Matsumoto, T., Noma, M. and Shimizu, J. (1991). Molecular cloning and expression of platelet-activating factor receptor from human leukocytes. J. Biol. Chem. 266, 20400–20405.

Ng, D.S. and Wong, K. (1988). Effect of sulfhydryl reagents on PAF binding to human neutrophils and platelets. Eur. J. Pharmacol. 154, 47–52.

Oppenheim, J.J., Zachariae, C.O., Mukaida, N. and Matsushima, K. (1991). Properties of the novel proinflammatory supergene "intercrine" cytokine family. Annu. Rev. Immunol. 9, 617–648.

Parmentier, M., Libert, F., Maenhaut, C., Lefort, A., Gerard, C., Perret, J., Van Sande, J., Dumont, J.E. and Vassart, G. (1989). Molecular cloning of the thyrotropin receptor. Science 246, 1620–1622.

Perez, H.D., Holmes, R., Kelly, E., McClary, J., Chou, Q. and Andrews, W.H. (1992). Cloning of the gene coding for a human receptor for formylpeptides: characterization of a promoter region and evidence for polymorphic expression. Biochemistry 31, 11595–11599.

Polakis, P.G., Uhing, R.J. and Snyderman, R. (1988). The formylpeptide chemoattractant receptor copurifies with a GTP-binding protein containing a distinct 40-kDa pertussis toxin substrate. J. Biol. Chem. 263, 4969–4976.

Prescott, S.M., Zimmerman, G.A. and McIntyre, T.M. (1990). Platelet-activating factor. J. Biol. Chem. 265, 17381–17384.

Prossnitz, E.R., Quehenberger, O., Cochrane, C.G. and Ye, R.D. (1991). Transmembrane signalling by the N-formyl peptide receptor in stably transfected fibroblasts. Biochem. Biophys. Res. Comm. 179, 471–476.

Rands, E., Candelore, M.R., Cheung, A.H., Hill, W.S., Strader, C.D. and Dixon, R.A. (1990). Mutational analysis of beta-adrenergic receptor glycosylation. J. Biol. Chem. 265, 10759–10764.

Rollins, T.E. and Springer, M.S. (1985). Identification of the polymorphonuclear leukocyte C5a receptor. J. Biol. Chem. 260, 7157–7160.

Rollins, T.E., Siciliano, S. and Springer, M.S. (1988). Solubilization of the functional C5a receptor from human polymorphonuclear leukocytes. J. Biol. Chem. 263, 520–526.

Rollins, T.E., Siciliano, S., Kobayashi, S., Cianciarulo, D.N., Bonilla-Argudo, V., Collier, K. and Springer, M.S. (1991). Purification of the active C5a receptor from human polymorphonuclear leukocytes as a receptor-gi complex. Proc. Natl Acad. Sci. USA 88, 971–975.

Schiffman, E., Corcoran, B.A. and Wahl, S.M. (1975). N-Formylmethionyl peptides as chemoattractants for leucocytes. Proc. Natl Acad Sci. USA 72, 1059–1062.

Schiffman, E., Corcoran, B.A. and Aswanikumar, S. (1978). In "Leukocyte Chemotaxis" (eds J.I. Gallin and P.G. Quire), pp. 97–111. Raven Press, New York.

Schmid, J. and Weissmann, C. (1987). Induction of mRNA for a serine protease and a β-thromboglobulin-like protein in mitogen-stimulated human leukocytes. J. Immunol. 139, 250.

Schroder, J.-M., Mrowietz, U., Morita, E. and Christophers, E. (1987). Purification and partial biochemical characterization of a human monocyte-derived, neutrophil-activating peptide that lacks interleukin 1 activity. J. Immunol. 139, 3474.

Seyfried, L.E., Schweikert, V.L., Godiska, R. and Gray, P.W. (1992). The human PAF receptor gene (PTAFR) contains no introns and maps to chromosome 1. Genomics 13, 832.

Shen, T.Y., Hwang, S.B., Chang, M.N., Doebber, T.W., Lam, M.H., Wu, M.S., Wang, X., Han, G.Q and Li, R.Z. (1985). Characterization of a platelet-activating factor receptor antagonist isolated from haifenteng (Piper futokadsura): specific inhibition of in vitro and in vivo platelet-activating factor-induced effects. Proc. Natl Acad. Sci. USA 82, 672–676.

Shin, H.S., Snyderman, R., Friedman, E., Mellors, A. and Mayer, M.M. (1968). Chemotactic and anaphylatoxic fragment cleaved from the fifth component of guinea pig complement. Science 162, 361–363.

Showell, H.J., Freer, R.J., Zigmond, S.H., Schiffman, E., Aswanikumar, S., Corcoran, B. and Becker, E.L. (1976). The structure–activity relations of synthetic peptides as chemotactic factors and inducers of lysosomal secretion for neutrophils. J. Exp. Med. 143, 1154–1169.

Siciliano, S.J., Rollins, T.E. and Springer, M.S. (1990). Interaction between the C5a receptor and Gi in both the membrane-bound and detergent-solubilized states. J. Biol. Chem. 265, 19568–19574.

Sklar, L.A., Fay, S.P., Seligmann, B.E., Freer, R.J., Muthukumaraswamy, N. and Mueller, H. (1990) Fluorescence analysis of the size of a binding pocket of a peptide receptor at natural abundance. Biochemistry 29, 313–316.

Snyder, F. (1990). Platelet-activating factor and related acetylated lipids as potent biologically active cellular mediators. Am. J. Physiol. 259, C697–708.

Snyderman, R., Pike, M.C., Edge, S. and Lane, B. (1984). A chemoattractant receptor on macrophages exists in two affinity states regulated by guanine nucleotides. J. Cell Biol. 98, 444–448.

Sung, C.H., Schneider, B.G., Agarwal, N., Papermaster, D.S. and Nathans, J. (1991). Functional heterogeneity of mutant rhodopsins responsible for autosomal dominant retinitis pigmentosa. Proc. Natl Acad. Sci. USA 88, 8840–8844.

Thomas, K.M., Taylor, L. and Navarro, J. (1990). Molecular cloning of the fMet-Leu-Phe receptor from neutrophils. J. Biol. Chem. 265, 20061–20064.

Thomas, K.M., Taylor, L. and Navarro, J. (1991). The interleukin-8 receptor is encoded by a neutrophil-specific cDNA clone, F3R. J. Biol. Chem. 266, 14839–14841.

Van Tol, H.H., Wu, C.M., Guan, H.C., Ohara, K., Bunzoq, J.R., Civelli, O., Kennedy, J., Seeman, P., Niznik, H.B. and Jovanovic, V. (1992). Multiple dopamine D4 receptor variants in the human population. Nature 358, 149–152.

Walz, A., Peveri, P., Aschauer, H. and Baggiolini, M. (1987). Purification and amino acid sequencing of NAF, a novel neutrophil-activating factor produced by monocytes. Biochem. Biophys. Res. Comm. 149, 755.

Ward, P.A. (1976). Biological aspects of leukotactic factors. J. Allergy Clin. Immunol. 58, 224–228.

Ward, P.A. and Newman, L.J. (1969). A neutrophil chemotactic factor from human C5. J. Immunol. 102, 93–99.

Williams, L.T., Snyderman, R., Pike, M.C. and Lefkowitz, R.J. (1977). Specific receptor sites for chemotactic peptides on human polymorphonuclear leukocytes. Proc. Natl Acad. Sci. USA 74, 1204–1208.

Wong, G., Witek, J.S., Temple, P.A., Wilkens, K.M., Leary, A.C., Luxenberg, D.P., Jones, S.S., Brown, E.L., Kay, R.M., Orr, E.C., Shoemaker, C., Golde, D.W., Kaufman, R.J., Hewick, R.M., Wang, E.A. and Clark, S.C. (1985). Human GM-CSF: molecular cloning of the complementary DNA and purification of the natural and recombinant proteins. Science 228, 810.

Ye, R.D., Prossnitz, E.R., Zou, A.H. and Cochrane, C.G. (1991). Characterization of a human cDNA that encodes a functional receptor for a platelet activating factor. Biochem. Biophys. Res. Comm. 180, 105–111.

Ye, R.D., Cavanagh, SL., Quehenberger, O., Prossnitz, E.R. and Cochrane, C.G. (1992). Isolation of a cDNA that encodes a novel granulocyte N-formyl peptide receptor. Biochem. Biophys. Res. Comm. 184, 582–589.

Yoshimura, T., Natsushima, K., Oppenheim, J.J. and Leonard, E.J. (1987). Neutrophil chemotactic factor produced by lipopolysaccharide (LPS)-stimulated human blood mononuclear leukocytes: partial characterization and separation from interleukin 1 (IL-1). J. Immunol. 139, 788–793.

7. Neutrophil Adhesion Receptors

A.J. Wardlaw and G.M. Walsh

1. Introduction

Neutrophil-mediated defence mechanisms are an important part of the host response to bacterial and parasite infection. For neutrophils to carry out this role they need to be able to migrate rapidly from the vascular bed into the extracellular tissue, and then interact with the extracellular matrix and other cells in the tissue such as epithelial cells and fibroblasts. Finally neutrophils need to be able to recognize and phagocytose bacteria and other foreign bodies which threaten the host. These functions are crucially dependent on the ability of the neutrophil to adhere to other cells as well as extracellular matrix proteins. This adhesion process is part of a widespread biological phenomenon which involves all aspects of cellular function from embryogenesis and maintenance of tissue integrity through to wound healing and thrombogenesis. Cellular adhesion is mediated through interaction between adhesion receptors on the surface of cells and their counter-structures (ligands) on other cells or matrix proteins. Over the last 10 years there has been a considerable advance in our knowledge of the receptors involved and an understanding of the role that they play in individual cellular functions. The importance of adhesion in leucocyte function has opened up the exciting possibility that inhibition of adhesion-dependent functions by blocking adhesion receptor interactions may be an effective therapeutic approach in a number of inflammatory-based diseases. This is particularly true of the neutrophil which is increasingly seen to play an important tissue damaging role in a number of conditions as diverse as septic shock, ARDS and myocardial infarction.

Immunopharmacology of Neutrophils
ISBN 0–12–339250–0

In the first part of this review the structure and expression of the numerous adhesion molecules will be described, with emphasis on those with importance for neutrophil function. Secondly the *in vitro* studies that have defined the role of these receptors in neutrophil function will be summarized. Lastly the *in vivo* studies that have suggested a use for antiadhesion strategies in the treatment of human disease will be outlined. A detailed discussion of the involvement of adhesion molecules in neutrophil accumulation in tissues will be found in Chapter 10.

2. Structure and Expression of Neutrophil Adhesion Receptors

There are three main families of molecules important in neutrophil adhesion. These families are defined according to structural criteria with considerable homology between family members in both nucleotide and amino-acid sequence. The three families are the selectins, the integrins and members of the immunoglobulin gene superfamily (Table 7.1). A fourth family of adhesion receptors, the cadherins, are important in maintaining the integrity of endothelial and epithelial tissue but have not been shown to have a role in leucocyte function (Takeichi, 1990).

2.1 THE SELECTINS

Three members of this family have so far been characterized. Before being designated "selectins" (derived from "lectin" and "select" which share the same Latin origin meaning to separate by picking out) each member of the family had a number of alternative names which made the terminology confusing (Bevilacqua *et al.*, 1991). Expression of E-selectin (formerly called ELAM-1) is confined to vascular endothelium. P-selectin (GMP-140, PADGEM, CD62) is expressed on platelets and endothelial cells and L-selectin (MEL-14, gp90^{mel}, Leu 8, LECAM-1, LAM-1, LEC-CAM-1) is expressed on

leucocytes. All three members of the family are type 1 (i.e. the N-terminus is extracellular) membrane proteins with a hydrophobic transmembrane domain and a cytoplasmic domain. The extracellular region is characterized by an N-terminal domain homologous to various calcium-dependent (C type) animal lectins (Drickamer, 1988; McEver, 1991). Related lectins include the low-affinity IgE receptor CD23 and the asialoglycoprotein receptor. The lectin domain is joined to a domain related to epithelial growth factor (EGF-like domain) followed by a variable number of repeat domains related to the complement regulatory proteins such as DAF and CR1 and CR2 (Figure 7.1). The presence of a lectin binding domain, suggesting that the counter-structure recognized by selectins is carbohydrate in nature, was consistent with the longstanding observation that the adhesion function of the selectins, particularly L-selectin could be blocked by sugars such as mannose which bind certain animal lectins (Stoolman *et al.*, 1984).

2.1.1 E-Selectin

E-Selectin was initially characterized by mAbs raised against IL-1 and TNF-stimulated HUVEC which blocked neutrophil adhesion (Pober *et al.*, 1986a; Bevilacqua *et al.*, 1987). It had been shown that neutrophils bound more avidly to HUVEC stimulated with these cytokines than to unstimulated HUVEC and a mAb, H18/7, was generated which blocked this enhanced adhesion. This antibody precipitated a single chain polypeptide of 115 kD which was termed ELAM-1. Treatment with *N*-glycosidase to remove N-linked sugars revealed a peptide backbone of 78 kD. Although E-selectin was originally thought only to mediate neutrophil adhesion (Bevilacqua *et al.*, 1987; Dobrina *et al.*, 1989), it has now been shown that eosinophils (Kyan-Aung *et al.*, 1991), monocytes (Carlos *et al.*, 1991), NK cells (Ohmori *et al.*, 1989) and a subpopulation of skin-homing T cells (Graber *et al.*, 1990; Shimuzu *et al.*, 1991; Berg *et al.*, 1991; Picker *et al.*, 1991a) which express a receptor termed CLA, can all recognize E-selectin.

The cDNA for E-selectin was obtained by expression cloning using RNA from HUVEC treated with IL-1 for

Table 7.1   Endothelial adhesion receptors and their counter receptors on leucocytes

Endothelium	Gene family	Counter-receptor	Gene family	Leucocyte
ICAM-1	Ig	LFA-1 + Mac-1	Integrin	All leucocytes
ICAM-2	Ig	LFA-1	Integrin	All leucocytes
VCAM-1	Ig	VLA-4	Integrin	EO + LO + MO + BO
PECAM	Ig	PECAM + ?	Proteoglycans	All leucocytes
E-Selectin	Selectin	SLe^x	Carbohydrate	All leucocytes
P-Selectin	Selectin	SLe^x	Carbohydrate	All leucocytes
SLe^x? (Glycam-1)	Carbohydrate	L-Selectin	Selectin	All leucocytes

LO, lymphocyte; MO, monocyte, BO, basophil

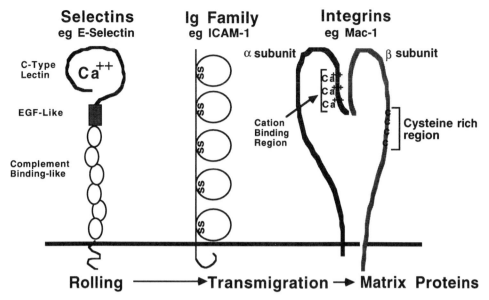

Figure 7.1 Schematic outline of the structure of the three major supergene families of receptors involved in neutrophil adhesion.

2.5 h (Bevilacqua *et al.* 1989). The E-selectin cDNA was 3.85 kb and consisted of a 116 base 5'-untranslated region, a continuous open reading frame of 1830 bases and a relatively long 3'-untranslated region of 1898 bases. The 3'-untranslated region encodes eight repeats of the sequences ATTTA found in cDNAs encoding various transiently expressed molecules suggesting this sequence is associated with unstable mRNAs. This would be consistent with the kinetics of expression of E-selectin RNA in endothelial cells after cytokine stimulation. Whereas unstimulated HUVEC express no E-selectin mRNA, after continuous stimulation of HUVEC with IL-1, a single 3.9 kb transcript appears within 1 h which is maximal after 2–4 h and has disappeared by 24 h. This mirrors the expression of E-selectin on HUVEC *in vitro* which is maximal at 4 h and virtually gone by 24 h (Bevilacqua *et al.*, 1987). The primary structure of E-selectin consists of an N-terminal domain of 120 amino acids, a 34 aa EGF-like domain and six tandem repetitive motifs of 60 aa related to complement binding proteins with six cysteines within each repeat. The lectin and EGF-like domain share considerable homology with the respective domains in L-selectin. Southern blotting of chromosomal DNA for E-selectin suggested that it is a single copy gene. It is located on chromosome 1 and is geographically closely related to the genes for both L-selectin and P-selectin as well as serum coagulation factor 5 (Watson *et al.*, 1990). Genes encoding several of the complement binding proteins have also been localized to the long arm of chromosome 1. The chromosomal localization of mouse selectins appears to be very similar suggesting that the selectin family arose through multiple gene duplication before genetic divergence of mouse and human.

2.1.2 P-Selectin

P-Selectin is an integral membrane protein found in the α-granules of human platelets (Hsu-Lin *et al.*, 1984) and the Weibel-Palade bodies of human endothelial cells (McEver *et al.*, 1989; Bonfanti *et al.*, 1989). Activation of these cells with heparin, thrombin or oxygen radicals results in the rapid translocation of P-selectin to the cell surface within minutes (Hattori *et al.*, 1989; Toothill *et al.*, 1990; Patel *et al.*, 1991). The exact function of P-selectin *in vivo* has not been well defined (see Chapter 10), however, it can mediate adhesion of neutrophils and other leucocytes to appropriately stimulated vascular endothelium (Geng *et al.*, 1990), as well as platelet adhesion to neutrophils and monocytes (Larsen *et al.*, 1990). In contrast to neutrophil adhesion via the leucocyte integrins, activation of neutrophils does not appear to be a requirement for adhesion via P-selectin (Moore *et al.*, 1991). P-Selectin is a cysteine-rich N-linked glycosylated protein with a SDS–PAGE-defined molecular weight of 140 000 kD and a protein backbone of 126 400 kD. The cDNA for P-selectin has a 5'-untranslated region of 38 bp followed by an open reading frame of 2490 bp coding for a protein of 830 amino acids (Johnston *et al.*, 1989). The mature protein without the signal peptide has a predicted 789 aa. The 3'-untranslated sequence is 64 bp. The lectin domain is 118 aa, the EGF-like domain 40 amino acids. P-selectin has 9 complement regulatory protein domains each of 62 amino acids. The cytoplasmic domain is 35 amino acids. Some cDNA clones isolated predicted a soluble form of P-selectin without a transmembrane region. Soluble P-selectin, isolated from plasma, bound to the same neutrophil receptor as the membrane-bound form (Dunlop *et al.*, 1992). Fluid-phase P-selectin was anti-inflammatory and down-regulated CD18-dependent neutrophil adhesion and respiratory burst. Thus, its presence in plasma may be important in preventing inadvertent activation of neutrophils in the circulation. Northern analysis of P-selectin RNA demonstrated that expression of P-selectin RNA was restricted to megakaryocytes and endothelial cells. Southern analysis suggested that a single gene encodes P-selectin.

2.1.3 L-Selectin

Peripheral blood lymphocyte circulation is spatially deter-mined by "homing receptors" on the lymphocyte mem-brane reacting with counter-structures called "addressins" on specialized endothelial cells termed HEVs within lymphoreticular tissue (Butcher, 1986, 1990; Yednock and Rosen, 1989). At least three different patterns of lymphocyte recirculation have been deter-mined, one to peripheral lymph nodes, one to Peyers patches in the gut and one to the lung (Butcher *et al.*, 1980; Chin *et al.*, 1984, 1986; Jalkanan *et al.*, 1986; Yednock and Rosen, 1989). A mAb against mouse lymphocytes termed Mel-14 inhibited binding of lymphocytes to HEVs from peripheral lymph nodes and recognized the peripheral lymph node lymphocyte homing receptor (Gallatin *et al.*, 1983). The Mel-14 antigen (gp90^{MEL}) has now been shown to be the mouse form of L-selectin (Bowen *et al.*, 1989). Although originally described as a lymphocyte homing receptor, L-selectin is expressed on all leucocytes including neutrophils and is likely to play an important role in neutrophil migration into tissues (Jutila *et al.*, 1989; Kishimoto *et al.*, 1991; Smith *et al.*, 1991; Watson *et al.*, 1991). An interesting feature of L-selectin expression on neutrophils is down-regulation after stimulation with chemotactic peptides such as FMLP (Kishimoto *et al.*, 1990). This is mediated by proteolytic cleavage and shedding of a 100 kD fragment (5 kD shorter than the cell-associated protein). However, cell activation also increases binding of PPME (a ligand for L-selectin) by increasing affinity, despite a reduction in expression of L-selectin (Yednock *et al.*, 1987; Imai *et al.*, 1990). Regulation of L-selectin function on neutrophils is there-fore complex. The cDNA for L-selectin encodes an open reading frame of 372 aa with a molecular mass of 42.2 kD with 26 cysteine residues and eight potential glyco-sylation sites (Bowen *et al.*, 1989; Camerini *et al.*, 1989; Siegelman and Weissman, 1989; Tedder *et al.*, 1989). Like the earlier reported mouse cDNA (Lasky *et al.*, 1989; Siegelman *et al.*, 1989) human L-selectin had the three-domain structure characteristic of the selectins. The

lectin-binding domain was lysine rich suggesting that charge may be important in ligand binding. L-selectin has two complement regulatory protein domains which in mouse, but not human, are identical. There was 83% sequences conservation in the lectin and EGF domains suggesting an important structural role for these regions in L-selectin function between mouse and human with 79–63% conservation in the complement regulatory repeats which include a region of potential importance to the function of both L-selectin and E-selectin (Jutila *et al.*, 1992).

2.1.4 Selectin Ligands

Early observations of lymphocyte homing suggested that the selectins may recognize a carbohydrate determinant. Thus the binding of lymphocytes to peripheral lymph node HEVs, which is now known to be mediated primarily by L-selectin, was inhibited by high concen-trations of charged saccharides such as PPME, a mannose phosphate polysaccharide complex derived from yeast, as well as mannose-6-phosphate. In addition, pretreatment of the endothelium with neuraminidase abolished binding suggesting that the carbohydrate involved was sialylated. This was supported by the cDNA cloning of the selectins which revealed the shared C-type lectin domain at the N-terminus. A number of papers have been published, mainly concerning E-selectin, which suggest that a major component of the carbohydrate moiety recognized by the selectins is SLe^x (Lowe *et al.*, 1990; Phillips *et al.*, 1990; Walz *et al.*, 1990; Springer and Lasky, 1991). Leucocytes which bind E-selectin express high amounts of both SLe^x and Le^x and neutro-phils are rich in both molecules (Fukuda *et al.*, 1984; Symington *et al.*, 1985). Monoclonal antibodies against SLe^x inhibited binding of neutrophils and a variety of cell lines to E-selectin expressing endothelial cells, as well as purified E-selectin. A variant of HL60 cells which did not express SLe^x bound very poorly to HUVEC in an E-selectin-dependent adhesion assay, whereas HL60 cells which expressed a normal amount of SLe^x bound very well. Transfection of COS cells and CHO cells with an $\alpha(1,3)$fucosyltransferase cDNA which caused expression of SLe^x and Le^x on the cell surface resulted in these cells becoming adhesive for TNF-stimulated HUVEC in an E-selectin-dependent manner. A highly purified glycolipid fraction of neutrophils which bound to E-selectin-transfected COS cells was found to have a structure similar to SLe^x except the fucose was linked to the penultimate rather than the ultimate *N*-acetyl glucosamine. This structure is identical to CD65, although expression of CD65 did not correlate with E-selectin binding capacity.

Despite these conclusive experiments more work needs to be done to characterize the ligand for E-selectin com-pletely. For example, the ligand appears to differ between cells. A monoclonal antibody which recognizes a non-SLe^x carbohydrate determinant ligand for E-selectin on neutrophils does not bind to NK cells. The CLA antigen on a subpopulation of skin-homing T lymphocytes which is the ligand on these cells for E-selectin is immunologically distinct from the SLe^x structure on neutrophils, although neuraminidase treatment of CLA$^+$ T cells but not CLA$^-$ T cells uncovered the expression of Le^x (CD15) structures (Berg et al., 1991). The mAb which recognizes CLA also recognizes SLe^x on neutrophils. It is therefore likely that the CLA antigen is a modified form of SLe^x. SLe^x is attached to a range of glycolipids and glycoproteins on leucocytes and the importance of the backbone structure containing the SLe^x has not been determined. Treatment of neutrophils with trypsin abolished specific P-selectin binding indicating that the predominant ligand for P-selectin is on surface glycoproteins rather than glycolipids (Moore et al., 1991). It is not clear whether the EGF domain and CPR domains are simply acting as spacers or whether they confer specificity to the interactions between the selectins and their ligands. However, studies with mAb raised against the various structural domains of E-selectin have demonstrated the importance of the lectin domain in cell binding and that the EGF-like domain is important in maintaining its conformation (Pigott et al., 1991). Antibodies against the mouse or human L-selectin EGF domain block lymphocyte adhesion to HEV but have little effect on carbohydrate binding. Recently it has been shown that neutrophil L-selectin is a potential counter-receptor for E-selectin, however, most L-selectin positive lymphocytes bind poorly, if at all, to E-selectin (Picker et al., 1991b).

The ligand specificities of P-selectin have been less clearly characterized. One study demonstrated that mAb to CD15, a carbohydrate antigen that includes the Le^x structure, inhibited binding of neutrophils and monocytes to P-selectin (Larsen et al., 1990). However, this inhibition was incomplete and another mAb against CD15 used in a subsequent report failed to inhibit binding (Moore et al., 1991). In addition, cells expressing Le^x failed to bind P-selectin and neuraminidase treatment of myeloid cells abolished platelet adhesion to these cells, which is a P-selectin-dependent phenomenon (Corral et al., 1990). Transfection of CHO cells with an $\alpha(1-3/4)$ fucosyltransferase which caused the cells to express SLe^x as well as other related carbohydrate structures conferred binding of the CHO cells to purified P-selectin (Zhou et al., 1991). Neuraminidase

treatment of the CHO cell (so converting SLe^x to Le^x) abolished the ability of the transfected CHO cells to bind P-selectin. However, the affinity of binding of P-selectin to SLe^x-like structures is dependent on other as yet undetermined factors. Thus, transfected CHO cells express much higher levels of SLe^x than HL60 cells but bind to P-selectin with a much lower affinity. Although P-selectin appears to recognize similar carbohydrate structures to E-selectin, the binding patterns are not identical. For example, HT-29 cells express SLe^x determinants and bind avidly to E-selectin but do not bind to P-selectin (Zhou et al., 1991). P-Selectin binds to oligosaccharide ligands in a Ca^{2+}-dependent manner. Studies using purified P-selectin have demonstrated two high affinity binding sites for Ca^{2+}. Occupancy of these sites alters the conformation of the protein exposing an epitope in the lectin domain which appears important for neutrophil recognition (Geng et al., 1991).

Further insights into the nature of the counter-structures that bind the selectins have come from studies using a modified form of L-selectin consisting of a chimeric molecule (LEC-IgG) containing the extracellular domain of mouse L-selectin and the hinge CH2 and CH3 regions of human IgG. This reagent was able to stain lymph node HEV (L-selectin is a lymphocyte-homing receptor for peripheral lymph nodes) and block lymphocyte attachment to HEV in vitro (Watson et al., 1990). Using LEC-IgG as the basis for an immunaffinity column, Imai et al. (1991) precipitated a 50 kD and a 90 kD component from a detergent lysate of lymph nodes that had been metabolically labelled with [^{35}S]-sulphate or [^{3}H]fucose. Purification and subsequent cDNA cloning of the 50 kD component has revealed a novel mucin-like glycoprotein with a serine/threonine-rich protein core that is likely to function as a scaffold for the extensive O-linked sialylated carbohydrate groups that bind to the lectin domain of L-selectin (Lasky et al., 1992). Expression of this molecule, which the authors have termed GlyCAM-1, was preferential for peripheral lymph node HEV consistent with it being a peripheral lymph node addressin.

In conclusion, the selectins appear to recognize one or more members of a family of $\alpha(2-3)$sialylated, $\alpha(1-3)$fucosylated lactosaminoglycans that can be expressed on both myeloid and non-myeloid cells (Figure 7.2). Subtle differences in the structure of the carbohydrate

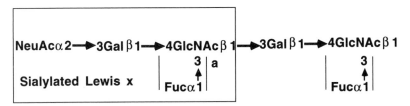

Figure 7.2 Structure of the carbohydrate moieties of the selectin ligands with the SLe^x structure in the boxed area.

moieties, or the protein or lipid on which they are expressed, may be responsible for the differing affinities and specificities of the different selectins for their ligand, as reflected in distinct, selectin-dependent, functional responses between leucocytes. The expression of differing SLe^x-like molecules may be controlled by differing expression of a family of fucosyl transferases such as the recently described $\alpha(1–3)$fucosyltransferase expressed only in myeloid cells.

2.2 INTEGRINS

Integrins are a superfamily of α, β, heterodimeric, type 1 transmembrane glycoproteins, non-covalently expressed on the cell surface. They were termed integrins because they were perceived as forming a bridge between an extracellular ligand, particularly proteins of the extracellular matrix, and the intracellular cytoskeletal proteins such as actin, talin and vinculin (Hynes, 1987, 1992). One of the earliest integrins to be characterized was the major platelet receptor gp IIb–IIIa, a heterodimeric protein through which platelets adhere to fibrinogen, von-Willebrand factor, fibronectin and vitronectin. The use of mAbs to block cellular interactions with matrix proteins led to the characterization of a related yet distinct set of receptors which bound vitronectin, fibronectin and laminin. All these matrix proteins contain an Arg-Gly-Asp (RGD) sequence which was shown to be important for ligand binding. Independent from work on platelets and matrix protein receptors was the observation that a number of adhesion related events on leucocytes was mediated by two groups of receptors with an α/β heterodimeric structure. One group of receptors, subsequently termed the leucocyte integrins, were important in leucocyte adhesion to endothelium, T-cell proliferation and cytotoxic T-cell killing. The second group were termed the VLA proteins because the first two identified, i.e. VLA-1 and VLA-2, appear very late after lymphocyte activation. Full characterization of these receptors resulted in a classification based on complementarity at the nucleotide and amino-acid level. Three subfamilies of integrins were defined based on a common β chain combining with a number of α chains: the $\beta1$ integrin family which consisted of a single β chain (CD29) combining with six α chains (CD49a–f, $\alpha_{1–6}/\beta1$) to form the VLA family; the $\beta2$ integrin family or leucocyte integrins (CD11a–c/CD18 or LFA-1, Mac-1, p 150,95 or $\alpha_L/\beta2$, $\alpha_M/\beta2$, $\alpha_X/\beta2$; and the $\beta3$ family or cytoadhesins (gpIIb/IIIa or CD41/CD61; vitronectin receptor or $\alpha_v\beta3$ or CD51/CD61) of which gpIIb-IIIa is the most abundant platelet receptor playing a crucial role in platelet aggregation. Since that original classification it has become apparent that the association between α and β chains is not as restricted as once thought. In addition a number of new α and β chains have been characterized giving the integrin family another level of complexity (Figure 7.3). To date only

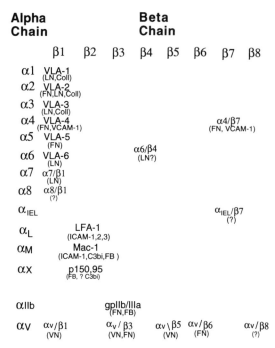

Figure 7.3 Outline of the members of the integrin superfamily with their ligands (in brackets). FN, fibronectin; FB, fibrinogen; VN, vitronectin; LN, laminin; Coll, collagen.

the leucocyte integrins have been shown to be expressed by neutrophils although other integrin-like molecules on neutrophils have been described.

2.2.1 Leucocyte Integrins

Mac-1 (also known as Mo-1, OKM-1 and CR3) was first defined by mAbs as a marker for myeloid cells (Springer et al., 1979). LFA-1 was identified by screening mAbs that blocked killing by cytotoxic T lymphocytes of tumour cells (Davignon et al., 1981a, 1981b). It became apparent that these two receptors shared a similar structure, with a high molecular weight α chain and a common β chain. Characterization of the third member of the family p150,95 followed shortly (Schwarting et al., 1985; Miller et al., 1986). Expression of the leucocyte integrins is restricted to cells of the immune system with LFA-1 expressed by virtually all leucocytes (Krensky et al., 1983) and Mac-1 expressed by myeloid cells, large granular lymphocytes and a subset of B cells (Arnaout and Colten), 1984). p150,95 is expressed on macrophages and is a marker for hairy cell leukaemia. It is only weakly expressed on neutrophils and has been designated CR4 (Myones et al., 1988). The importance of the leucocyte integrins was underlined by the realization that a rare autosomal recessive immunodeficiency disorder termed LAD was caused by lack of expression of the three members of the $\beta2$ integrins by all leucocytes (Anderson and Springer, 1987). This disease is characterized by life-threatening septicaemia, indolent superficial infections which fail to respond to antibiotics and, commonly, death in early infancy. Neutrophils from LAD patients exhibit a marked *in vitro* defect in adhesion-related functions such as chemotaxis and phagocytosis. Biopsies from infected wounds revealed large numbers of neutrophils in the vasculature but very few in the tissue, thus emphasizing the important role of cell trans-migration in the integrity of the immune response and the importance of the leucocyte integrins in mediating that migratory event. This fascinating disease will be discussed in more detail in the next section.

The complete primary structures of the α subunits of LFA-1 (Larson *et al.*, 1989), Mac-1 (Arnaout *et al.*, 1988; Corbi *et al.*, 1988a) and p150,95 (Corbi *et al.*, 1987) have been determined. The subunits have a molecular weight of 180, 170 and 150 kD, respectively which after deglycosylation are reduced to 149, 137 and 132 kD. The common β subunit has a molecular weight of 95 kD (78 kD deglycosylated). The α subunits of all leucocyte integrins are synthesized as lower molecular weight precursors which contain high mannose N-linked oligosaccharides. These are processed to complex-type N-linked oligosaccharides after α/β chain association in the Golgi. If this association does not occur the α chain is degraded and is not expressed (Corbi *et al.*, 1988a; Larson *et al.* 1989).

cDNA cloning of the β chain revealed a deduced sequence of 769 amino acids with an N-terminal extra-cellular domain of 677 amino acids with six potential N-glycosylation sites, a 23 amino acid transmembrane domain and a 46 amino acid cytoplasmic domain (Kishimoto *et al.*, 1987a; Law *et al.*, 1987). There was a high cysteine content (7.4%) which was concentrated in a cysteine rich (20%) region of 186 amino acids giving the subunit a rigid tertiary structure. There was general homology with the β1 and β3 integrin subunits (37–45% shared identity) with particularly high homology in the cytoplasmic domain, the transmembrane domain and a region of 241 amino acids in the extracellular domain (64%). Cross-linking studies of RGD peptide binding to gp IIb-IIIa suggests that this latter region is important in ligand binding (D'Souza *et al.*, 1988). In addition, in several LAD patients the mutation in the β chain responsible for the disease is located in this region suggesting that it is important for α/β association. All 56 cysteine residues are conserved between the three family members. The genes for the α subunits of LFA-1, CR3 and p150,95 have been located to the short arm of chromosome 16 between bands p11 and p13.1 (Corbi *et al.*, 1988b), while the gene for the β2 chain is located to chromosome band 21q/22.3 on chromosome 21 (Marlin *et al.*, 1986).

The α subunit cDNAs revealed deduced primary structures, characterized by long extracellular domains (approximately 1000 amino acids) and short cytoplasmic domains (19–53 amino acids). An important feature of all three α chains are three homologous repeats that have putative cation-binding sites which are similar to the "EF-hand loop" found in other calcium-binding proteins such as calmodulin. These sites may account for the magnesium dependency of leucocyte integrin-dependent adhesion. Mac-1 and p150,95 α chains share 63% identity with each other but only 35% identity with the LFA-1 α subunit. The α subunits of the integrin super-family share 25–63% amino-acid identity. There are certain shared features within the superfamily which suggest an evolutionary grouping of the α chains (Figure 7.4). Thus a number of α chains, such as those of VLA-5, VLA-3, $\alpha_v/\beta3$ and $\alpha_{IIb}/\beta3$, share a sequence in the C-terminal end of the extracellular domain which is post-translationally cleaved with resulting fragments bridged by a disulphide bond. VLA-4 has a unique cleavage site in the centre of the extracellular domain to give approximately equal sized fragments (Hemler, 1990). The leucocyte integrins do not have a cleavage site but do have a 200 amino acid region which is present in VLA-2 but none of the other α chains. This region has been termed the I domain for inserted or interactive domain. A similar domain appears in a number of other proteins including collagen, various collagen-binding proteins such as cartilage matrix proteins and von Willebrand factor and the complement factors B and C2. The collagen-binding nature of several I domain-containing proteins including VLA-2 suggests that this

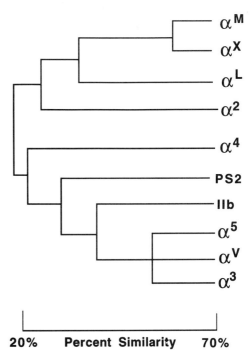

20%   Percent Similarity   70%

Figure 7.4 Evolutionary development of the integrin superfamily based on structural homology (after Hemler, 1990).

region may be involved in collagen recognition, although the leucocyte integrins have not been shown to bind collagen.

The expression of the leucocyte integrins on neutrophils has been extensively studied. Both LFA-1 and Mac-1 are well expressed by resting neutrophils, whereas expression of p150,95 is low (Anderson et al., 1986). LFA-1 expression is not greatly changed on neutrophil activation. A striking feature of Mac-1 on neutrophils in vitro is the rapid and marked increase in expression after cell activation by inflammatory mediators. After de novo synthesis, neutrophil Mac-1 is stored in intracellular pools within the peroxidase-negative granules (Bainton et al., 1987; Miller et al., 1987; see Chapter 4). This pool can be rapidly mobilized in response to stimulus with a number of chemoattractants including FMLP, C5a, LTB$_4$ (Fearon and Collins, 1983; Arnaout and Colten, 1984; Berger et al., 1984), PAF (Shalit et al., 1988) and GM-CSF (Buckle and Hogg, 1989). Granule exocytosis and Mac-1 mobilization and expression appear to be controlled by distinct signal-transduction pathways (Brown et al., 1991). Up-regulation of Mac-1 is a sensitive marker of neutrophil activation to the extent that it is readily induced by neutrophil separation techniques unless special precautions are taken. The functional role of this up-regulation of expression is uncertain. The function of Mac-1 is dependent on cell activation (Smith et al., 1989) and it was thought that the increased expression was an integral part of this process. However, there is evidence that the newly expressed receptors are functionally inactive (Buyon et al., 1988; Phillips et al., 1988; Vedder and Harlan, 1988; Nourshargh et al., 1989; Schleiffenbaum et al., 1989). It appears more likely that receptor activation is due to a conformational change in constitutively expressed receptors as has been well established for LFA-1 and a number of other integrins (Chatila et al., 1989; Dustin and Springer, 1989; Dransfield, 1991). This activation step is possibly mediated by a recently described lipid factor generated during neutrophil priming with inflammatory mediators (Hermanowski-Vosatka et al., 1992) and may involve changes in calcium flux (Graham and Brown, 1991). However, neither rapid rises in intracellular calcium nor specific granule fusion with the plasma membrane were required for neutrophil migration across resting or cytokine-activated endothelium (Kuijpers et al., 1992). The concept of a conformational change in the receptor leading to its functional activation has been supported by mAbs which recognize only the activated form of the receptor or induce its activation (Altieri and Edgington, 1988; Dransfield and Hogg, 1989). Binding activity may also be enhanced by receptor clustering (Detmers et al., 1988).

2.2.2   Integrin Counter-receptors

A number of ligands or counter-receptors for the leucocyte integrins have been described. LFA-1 was shown to bind to a member of the immunoglobulin gene superfamily called ICAM-1. Since then two other ICAM-like molecules which bind LFA-1 have been described (ICAM-2, ICAM-3) and ICAM-1 has been shown to bind Mac-1, although with a lower affinity than LFA-1. These receptors will be discussed in more detail in the next section.

Mac-1 appears to have an extensive range of binding activities. It binds the "inactivated" opsonic C3b (iC3b) component (Beller et al., 1982). Binding of iC3b does not depend on neutrophil activation but is increased by activation. Although iC3b contains an RGD sequence binding is not dependent on this region. Neutrophils can also bind fibrinogen (Altieri et al., 1988; Wright et al., 1988) and Leishmania gp63 (Russell and Wright, 1988) through Mac-1. These proteins also have RGD sequences although Mac-1 binding to these proteins does not appear to be RGD-dependent. Another binding site on Mac-1 is "lectin-like" and binds to various ligands such as unopsonized rabbit erythrocytes, bakers yeast particles and its capsule extract zymosan. In addition, Mac-1 is responsible for neutrophil binding to unstimulated vascular endothelium, plastic and glass surfaces, and neutrophil aggregation (Anderson et al., 1986; Wallis et al., 1986). The ligands for these binding activities have not been clearly defined. The adhesive function of Mac-1 appears to involve binding sites distinct from that involved in soluble ligand binding and adhesion as these functions are blocked by different mAbs (Anderson et al., 1986; Dana et al., 1986). Antibodies to Mac-1 also block Fc receptor-mediated phagocytosis, suggesting that the two molecules may be in close proximity (Brown et al., 1988).

2.3   IMMUNOGLOBULIN FAMILY MEMBERS AND THEIR LIGANDS

2.3.1   Intercellular Adhesion Molecule-1 (ICAM-1, CD54)

It was observed that homotypic aggregation of lymphoid cells was mediated through LFA-1, binding to a counterstructure distinct from itself (Rothlein et al., 1986). mAbs were raised against EBV-transformed B cells from a patient with LAD, which therefore did not express LFA-1. This panel of mAbs were screened for their ability to inhibit LFA-1-dependent homotypic aggregation. One mAb (RR1/1) was characterized which inhibited this function (Rothlein and Springer, 1986). It defined a 76–114 kD heavily glycosylated single-chain transmembrane receptor with a peptide backbone of 55 kD, the variable molecular weight being due to different degrees of glycosylation of its eight potential, N-linked glycosylation sites (Dustin et al., 1986; Rothlein et al., 1986). A number of approaches including binding between purified ICAM-1 and LFA-1 conclusively demonstrated that ICAM-1 was a receptor for LFA-1 (Marlin and Springer, 1987). cDNA cloning of ICAM-1 revealed that it was a member of the immunoglobulin gene superfamily, and was thus the first demonstration of an interaction between members of the integrin and immunoglobulin gene families (Dustin *et al.*, 1988b; Simmons *et al.*, 1988; Staunton *et al.*, 1988). ICAM-1 contains five Ig-like domains, with homology to the N-CAM and MAG, another neural adhesion protein. As well as binding LFA-1 and Mac-1 (Dustin and Springer, 1988; Smith *et al.*, 1989; Diamond *et al.*, 1990), ICAM-1 is also a receptor for *Plasmodium falciparum* (Berendt *et al.*, 1989) and the major group of rhinovirus (Greve *et al.*, 1989; Staunton *et al.*, 1989b; Tomassini *et al.*, 1989). A soluble form of ICAM-1 lacking the transmembrane and cytoplasmic domains binds the human rhinovirus inhibiting infection (Marlin *et al.*, 1990). LFA-1, rhinovirus and *Plasmodium falciparum* bind to distinct regions of the first two amino-terminal domains of ICAM-1, with the first domain being of particular importance (Staunton *et al.*, 1990), whereas Mac-1 binds to the third amino-terminal domain (Diamond *et al.*, 1991). As a result there is a difference in the pattern of mAb inhibition of ICAM-1/β2 integrin interactions. For example, mAb RR1/1 inhibits LFA-1/ICAM-1 interactions but not Mac-1/ICAM-1 interactions whereas mAb R6.5 inhibits both. cDNA clones of ICAM-1 predicted a soluble form of the receptor and soluble forms have been detected in serum in both health and disease with some evidence to suggest that there is an increase in serum levels of soluble ICAM-1 in certain inflammatory conditions (Seth *et al.*, 1991). ICAM-1 is a widely expressed molecule being found on vascular endothelium, leucocytes, dendritic cells, fibroblasts and epithelial cells (Rothlein *et al.*, 1986; Dustin *et al.*, 1988a; Makgoba *et al.*, 1988; Vogetseder *et al.*, 1989; Weetman *et al.*, 1989). In contrast to the integrins, its function appears to be regulated by increased expression rather than a conformational change of constitutively expressed molecules. Expression is increased on most cell types by a number of cytokines including IL-1, TNF and IFN-γ with some specificity between cytokine and cell type (Dustin *et al.*, 1986; Pober *et al.*, 1986b). For example, keratinocyte ICAM-1 is induced by IFN-γ and less well by TNF whereas IFN-γ, TNF and LPS are all good inducers of ICAM-1 on fibroblasts. Increased expression *in vitro* is protein synthesis dependent, detectable after about 4 h and maximal by 24 h. ICAM-1 has been implicated in a large number of cellular functions including leucocyte migration, lymphocyte homing, CTL and large granular lymphocyte cytotoxicity, antigen presentation and thymocyte maturation.

Functional studies with lymphocyte cell lines suggested that LFA-1 had ligands other than ICAM-1. Two other ICAMs have been characterized. ICAM-2 is a 60 000 kD single-chain transmembrane receptor with a peptide backbone of 31 kD. Like ICAM-1, ICAM-2 is a member of the immunoglobulin superfamily with two Ig-like domains which are most homologous (35%) to the two amino-terminal domains of ICAM-1. ICAM-2 is constitutively expressed on vascular endothelial cells and expression is not increased by cytokine activation (Staunton *et al.*, 1989a). It is also expressed on lymphocytes and monocytes but there is very little on neutrophils (de Fougerolles *et al.*, 1991). ICAM-3 is a highly glycosylated protein of 124 kD which is well expressed on all leucocytes including neutrophils but not endothelial cells (de Fougerolles and Springer 1992; Fawcett *et al.*,1992; Vazeux *et al.*, 1992). In assays of adhesion of resting lymphocytes to purified LFA-1, ICAM-3 appeared to have the greatest role (compared with ICAM-1 and 2) in modulating lymphocyte function. A role for ICAM-2 and ICAM-3 in neutrophil function has not yet been determined.

2.3.2 Vascular Cell Adhesion Molecule-1 (VCAM-1)

Functional studies with lymphocytic cell lines had demonstrated an adhesion pathway independent of the leucocyte β2 integrins and ICAM-1 (Dustin and Springer, 1988). The endothelial receptor responsible for this pathway was attributed to a 110 kD protein initially termed INCAM-110 (Rice and Bevilacqua 1989; Rice *et al.*, 1990). The name VCAM-1 was ascribed to a molecule characterized by an elegant functional expression cloning technique (Osborn *et al.*, 1989). A cDNA library made from mRNA from cytokine-activated HUVECs was transiently expressed in COS cells. Ramos cells, which had been shown to use this leucocyte β2 integrin-independent pathway preferentially, were added to the transfected COS cells and plasmid DNA recovered from the COS cells which bound Ramos cells. After several rounds of purification a full length cDNA was obtained which encoded a transmembrane receptor termed VCAM-1. Subsequently VCAM-1 was shown to bind to VLA-4 on the surface of the Ramos cells (Elices *et al.*, 1990). This pathway has subsequently been shown to be important in monocyte, lymphocyte, eosinophil and basophil adhesion to HUVEC (Campanero *et al.*, 1990; Schwartz *et al.*, 1990; Bochner *et al.*, 1991; Dobrina *et al.*, 1991; Walsh *et al.*, 1991; Weller *et al.*, 1991). However, neutrophils do not express VLA-4 (Hemler *et al.*, 1984; Hemler, 1988) and cannot bind to VCAM-1.

2.3.3 PECAM-1

Another member of the immunoglobulin family involved in adhesion is PECAM-1 (CD31) (Albelda *et al.*, 1991). PECAM is structurally most closely related to ICAM-1 and VCAM-1. As well as being constitutively expressed on platelets and endothelial cells it is expressed by granulocytes, monocytes and lymphocytes. In culture it accumulates at endothelial cell–cell borders and it has been suggested that it is involved in regulation of endothelial growth. It appears to bind to itself as well as proteoglycans. It has not as yet been shown to play a role in neutrophil adhesion or migration.

2.4   OTHER ADHESION AND RELATED NEUTROPHIL RECEPTORS

2.4.1   Extracellular Matrix Receptors

Not all receptors for extracellular matrix proteins are integrins. CD44, as well as being a lymphocyte homing receptor, has been shown to recognize hyaluronate (Aruffo et al., 1990; Miyake et al., 1990). CD44 was originally described as a lymphocyte homing receptor for mucosal and peripheral lymph node HEV which was defined by a mAb termed Hermes. CD44 is an acidic, sulphated transmembrane protein with a molecular weight of 90 kD that contains both O- and N-linked sugars. It has a C-terminal cytoplasmic region, a 23 aa hydrophobic transmembrane region and a 248 aa extracellular domain with a distal region that is homologous to tandem repeat domains of the cartilage link and proteoglycan core proteins (Stamenkovic et al., 1989). CD44 is expressed on lymphocytes, granulocytes, epithelial cells and fibroblasts with many different isoforms due to alternative splicing of up to 10 exons as well as extensive post-translational modifications including glycosylation and addition of chondroitin sulphate. The extent to which it plays a role in neutrophil function has not been determined.

2.4.2   Fcγ Receptors

Fcγ receptors are important in a number of neutrophil effector functions including degranulation, the respiratory burst, clearance of immune complexes, ADCC and phagocytosis. Three types of Fcγ receptor have been identified on human leucocytes (Fanger et al., 1989; Unkeless, 1989). FcγRI (CD64) is a 72 kD high-affinity receptor which is constitutively expressed on monocytes and induced on both eosinophils and neutrophils by culture in IFNγ. FcγRII (CD32) is a 40 kD lower affinity receptor which is highly expressed by neutrophils and is also expressed by a number of cell types including monocytes, eosinophils, platelets and B cells. FcγRIII (CD16) is also a low affinity receptor of 50–70 kD which is constitutively expressed by neutrophils and NK cells and is induced by IFNγ on monocytes and eosinophils. Neutrophils highly express CD16 and the difference in CD16 expression by neutrophils and unstimulated eosinophils can be utilized to purify eosinophils using immunoselection (Hartnell et al., 1990; Hansel et al., 1991). All three receptors are members of the immunoglobulin superfamily and have highly homologous extracellular domains (Stuart et al., 1987; Allen and Seed, 1988; Simmons and Seed, 1988; Kinet, 1989).

Two isoforms of CD16 encoded by two distinct genes have been identified (Ravetch and Perussia, 1989: Scallon et al., 1989). CD16-1 is expressed by neutrophils and is anchored to the membrane by a phosphatidylinositol glycan anchor. This receptor is shed from neutrophils on stimulation with FMLP and can be detected in human plasma (Huizinga et al., 1988). CD16-2 is expressed by NK cells and is a transmembrane protein with a cytoplasmic region and a hydrophobic sequence which anchors it within the membrane. Surface expression of CD16-2 is dependent on co-expression of the γ chain of the high affinity FcεRI receptor or the ζ chain of CD3 (Hibbs et al., 1989; Kurosaki and Ravetch, 1989; Lanier et al., 1991). This additional chain is also essential for signal transduction by CD16-2. Signal transduction through CD16 and CD32 is, unlike the FMLP-induced pathway, pertussis toxin insensitive (Brennan et al., 1991; Reibman et al., 1991; Walker et al., 1991). CD16-1 promotes the binding of immune complexes, particularly small ones, by neutrophils and mediates degranulation whereas CD32, in addition to these functions, is essential for respiratory burst and phagocytosis (Tosi and Berger, 1988; Kimberly et al., 1990). There is some evidence that CD16 co-operates with CD32 to facilitate cell activation (Salmon et al., 1991). Although highly expressed, CD16 expression can be increased by stimulation of neutrophils by IFNγ and GM-CSF (Buckle and Hogg, 1989).

2.5   IN VIVO EXPRESSION OF ADHESION RECEPTORS

The in vivo expression of adhesion receptors in many diseases remains to be clarified. Much attention has been focused on the possibility that up-regulation of endothelial adhesion receptors in vivo, particularly ICAM-1 and E-selectin, as a result of locally released cytokines, is responsible for migration of inflammatory cells into tissue with differential recruitment potentially owing to differential expression of leucocyte-specific receptors. For example, expression of E-selectin expression in vivo has been observed at sites of acute inflammation (Cotran et al., 1986; Goerdt et al., 1987; Munro et al., 1989). VCAM-1, which is selectively up-regulated in vitro by IL-4 (Masinovsky et al., 1990; Thornhill et al., 1990), may be responsible for the characteristic selective accumulation of eosinophils and mononuclear cells, without increased numbers of neutrophils, in allergic inflammation. In some tissues, such as the skin, in vivo expression appears to mirror in vitro findings. For example, Kyan-Aung et al. (1991) examined skin biopsies, 6 h after challenge with antigen or saline, for expression of E-selectin or ICAM-1 using an alkaline phosphatase immunostaining technique. Levels of both E-selectin and ICAM-1 were increased in biopsies taken from sites challenged with antigen. Furthermore, a prominent eosinophil infiltrate was observed in the biopsies from those sites challenged with antigen. Mononuclear cell and neutrophil infiltration were also observed, but in smaller numbers (Kyan Aung *et al.*, 1991).

This work was supported by a similar study of allergic reactions in the skin (Leung *et al.*, 1991). In addition to demonstrating increased E-selectin expression concurrently with an inflammatory cell infiltrate, these workers observed the same E-selectin increases in atopic skin cultured *in vitro* and challenged with allergen suggesting that resident cells in the skin, rather than infiltrating leucocytes, appeared to be the source of the cytokines that mediated the endothelial activation. Similarly, marked expression of both ICAM-1, VCAM-1 and E-selectin has been described in synovial tissues from patients with rheumatoid and osteoarthritis (Koch *et al.*, 1991). In this study there was no control group so it is difficult to ascertain the extent to which expression was increased compared with normal synovium. These studies suggest an important role for E-selectin and ICAM-1 in inflammation in the skin and joints. In addition, increased ICAM-1 expression has been detected in alcoholic and viral hepatitis (Burra *et al.*, 1990; Volpes *et al.*, 1990), and in liver and renal graft rejection (Adams *et al.*, 1989; Faull and Russ, 1989). ICAM-1 is widely expressed and increased expression in tissue can be due to infiltration with monocytes and lymphocytes or increased expression on endothelial cells, epithelial cells, fibroblasts and dendritic cells. In other tissues such as those of the upper and lower airways, there is marked constitutive expression of ICAM-1 and E-selectin in normal individuals with little if any increase in diseases such as asthma and allergic rhinitis (Bentley *et al.*, 1993). This may be due to the chronic stimulation of the airway mucosa by air pollutants. ICAM-1 expression was, however, increased on the epithelium of steady-state asthmatics compared with normal controls.

Increased expression of ICAM-2, in addition to ICAM-1 and VCAM-1, was observed in malignant lymphoma lymph nodes compared with non-malignant ones (Renkonen *et al.*, 1992). The observation that ICAM-2 expression was upregulated *in vivo* was interesting, as *in vitro* cytokine-treated endothelial cells do not demonstrate enhanced expression of ICAM-2 (Staunton *et al.*, 1989; de Fougerolles *et al.*, 1991; Nortamo *et al.*, 1991). In baboons subjected to *E. coli*-induced septic shock, E-selectin expression was observed in the capillaries, venules, small veins, arterioles, and arteries of the lungs, liver and kidneys. In contrast, animals subjected to traumatic/hypovolaemic shock had minimal E-selectin expression emphasizing the importance of circulating cytokines in septic shock (Redl *et al.*, 1991). In general, therefore, endothelial adhesion receptors, particularly ICAM-1 and E-selectin, are highly expressed in a range of inflammatory conditions with patterns of expression consistent with *in vitro* studies. However, the paucity of kinetic studies, the lack in some cases of proper

controls and the intense staining in some tissues in normal individuals make it difficult to assess from histochemical studies the extent to which modulation of endothelial adhesion receptors control the flux of leucocytes across the vascular endothelium in inflammatory states.

Integrins are widely expressed and their expression is less obviously regulated by inflammatory stimuli than VCAM-1, E-selectin or ICAM-1. Immunohistochemical studies have therefore not generally revealed any marked differences between normal and inflammatory tissue other than that due to increased leucocyte infiltration, although some differences have been detected in malignant lung tissue (Damjanovich *et al.*, 1992).

3. Adhesion Receptors and Neutrophil Function

Having described the various families of receptors involved in neutrophil adhesion we will now outline the role they may play in neutrophil function. The fundamental importance of the leucocyte integrins to proper functioning of neutrophils has been highlighted by our understanding of an immunodeficiency disease, LAD. Although rare, this disease has cast many insights into the role of adhesion receptors in leucocyte function and we will therefore describe it in some detail.

3.1 LEUCOCYTE ADHESION DEFICIENCY

3.1.1 Clinical Features

In the late 1970s a group of children were described with a severe immunodeficiency disease related to defects in neutrophil mobility and phagocytosis (Hayward *et al.*, 1979). About 60 patients with the disease have now been described worldwide. Clinically the disease is characterized by recurrent necrotic and indolent infections of the soft tissues usually involving the skin, mucous membranes and gastrointestinal tract. Superficial infections are resistant to antimicrobial therapy and invade both locally and systemically, resulting in life-threatening septicaemia or severe cellulitis (Anderson *et al.*, 1985; Anderson and Springer, 1987). Gingivitis and recurrent otitis media are common and there is often a history of delayed umbilical cord separation. Deep-seated granulomatous infections seen in defects in intracellular killing by neutrophils have not been observed in LAD patients. In addition, susceptibility to viral infections is not a prominent feature. There are two clinical phenotypes. A severe phenotype with death in early infancy and a moderate phenotype in which patients often survive into adulthood. The clinical phenotype correlates with expression of the leucocyte integrins. In the severe form expression is absent whereas in the moderate phenotype up to 10% of normal expression is observed. Despite a marked peripheral blood granulocytosis, which is a consistent feature of the disease even in the absence of active infection, biopsies of infected lesions reveal a virtual absence of granulocytes in the extracellular tissue and neutrophils fail to migrate into Rebuck skin windows. Leucocyte transfusion results in the migration of donor neutrophils into the tissue. There is a less profound effect on mononuclear cells and eosinophils which can be seen in the inflammatory infiltrates presumably because they can use the VLA-4/VCAM-1 pathway to transmigrate across the vascular endothelium.

3.1.2 Inheritance

Family studies have demonstrated that LAD is an autosomal recessive disease, although there was a suggestion of X-linked inheritance in one family. Family members who are clinically unaffected may have 50% of normal expression of the leucocyte integrins. Affected families often give a history of consanguinous marriages, and male and female incidence is equal.

3.1.3 The Molecular Basis of LAD

In 1980, Crowley et al. reported that LAD patients had a defect in neutrophil adhesion and that this was associated with loss of a major cell surface protein with a molecular weight of 110 000. It was subsequently shown that the defect was associated with lack of expression of any member of the leucocyte integrins. Several lines of evidence have indicated that the defect in LAD is in the common β chain. No patient with loss of expression of just one member of the family has been described. In mouse/human lymphocyte hybrids it was possible to recover expression of the human α subunit of LFA-1 in combination with the mouse β subunit; however recovery of the human β subunit in combination with the mouse α subunit was seen in healthy but not patient cells (Marlin et al., 1986). Biosynthetic studies of the α subunit of LFA-1 in patient EBV-transformed B cells demonstrated that apparently normal synthesis of the LFA-1 α subunit occurred in LAD patients, but that it failed to be processed to the mature form and was degraded without being expressed (Springer et al., 1984). Studies using a rabbit antiserum against the β subunit to undertake biosynthetic labelling studies and a β subunit cDNA probe demonstrated heterogeneity in the pattern of β subunit abnormality (Kishimoto et al., 1987b). Five patterns of abnormality were found: (1) absent β subunit mRNA and protein precursor; (2) low levels of β subunit mRNA and protein precursor; (3) an aberrantly large β subunit precursor probably due to an extra glycosylation site; (4) an aberrantly small precursor; and (5) a grossly normal precursor. Similar findings were reported by a second group (Dimanche-Boitrel et al., 1988). Final confirmation that defects in the β subunit were responsible for the disease was obtained by studies that analysed

the abnormalities at a nucleotide level and by recovery of expression by transfection of a normal β subunit gene. Thus, Hibbs and colleagues (1990) were able to stably transfect a normal β subunit gene into EBV-transformed B cells from patients with LAD with variable patterns of abnormality, including patients with normal β subunit mRNA expression and a normal-looking protein precursor. Transfection of the normal gene rescued expression of LFA-1 in the cells and resulted in a return of leucocyte integrin-dependent functions including homotypic aggregation and the ability to bind to ICAM-1-coated plates.

Studies investigating the defect in the β subunit at the nucleotide level revealed a number of abnormalities. In the family with a small protein precursor mentioned above, there was a base pair substitution in the consensus splicing site that resulted in aberrant splicing and the excision in 95% of the mRNA of a 90 bp exon. The 5% of normal mRNA in this group of patients allowed some leucocyte integrin expression and resulted in a moderate clinical phenotype (Kishimoto et al., 1989). In two patients with a grossly normal β subunit mRNA and protein precursor there were distinct, single base-pair defects resulting in a non-conservative amino-acid substitution in the highly conserved region of the β subunit which, in the gpIIb-IIIa receptor is involved in binding of RGD oligopeptides (Wardlaw et al., 1990). Several other mutations have been localized to this site emphasizing the importance of this region to α/β association. In addition, mutations in the cysteine-rich region of the β subunit, and frameshift and initiation codon mutations have been described (Arnaout et al., 1990; Nelson et al., 1992; Sligh et al., 1992).

3.2   NEUTROPHIL ADHESION RECEPTORS AND THE VASCULAR ENDOTHELIUM

The sequence of events resulting in the extravasation of leucocytes in response to inflammatory stimuli can be summarized as follows. Inflammatory substances generated at the site of inflammation activate the circulating leucocyte and adjacent endothelium. Activation results in changes in adhesion receptor expression and/or affinity/conformation, the net result being one or both of these cells becoming more adhesive. Over a hundred years ago, Cohnheim (1889) described that, within minutes of injury to the adjacent tissue, leucocytes first marginate and then begin to interact with the vessel wall by rolling along the endothelium. The number of rolling cells increases dramatically as the inflammatory reaction proceeds (Atherton and Born, 1972, 1973) and this appears to be an important step in the accumulation of cells at inflammatory sites (Fiebig et al., 1991). The endothelium becomes paved with leucocytes and the rolling decreases in velocity until the cells come to a dead stop (Cohnheim, 1889). They then migrate along the endothelium, become flattened and insert a pseudopod between the junction of two endothelial cells (Marchesi, 1961). The leucocytes then undergo diapedesis and finally make their way through the extracellular matrix to the site of the inflammatory reaction. Variations in the kinetics of emigration and accumulation of different types of leucocytes may be explained, at least in part, by the selective effects of diverse inflammatory mediators and/or differences in expression or configuration of leucocyte/endothelial cell adhesion molecules and their ligands.

An array of receptors can mediate neutrophil adhesion to endothelium. Thus, in static *in vitro* assays of neutrophil adhesion to unstimulated endothelial cells, there is a low background adhesion which is markedly increased by activation of the neutrophils with mediators such as PAF and FMLP (Tonnesen *et al.*, 1984; O'Flaherty *et al.*, 1985; McIntyre *et al.*, 1986; Garcia *et al.*, 1988; Lo *et al.*, 1989). This increase in adhesion is primarily dependent on Mac-1 on the neutrophil binding to constitutively expressed ICAM-1 and possibly another, as yet unidentified, ligand. Stimulation of the endothelium with thrombin or histamine for 5–10 min results in enhanced neutrophil adhesion which is transient and primarily dependent on P-selectin (Zimmerman *et al.*, 1985; Geng *et al.*, 1990; Toothill *et al.*, 1990). Stimulation of the endothelium with cytokines such as IL-1 and TNF-α for between 4 and 24 h results in markedly increased neutrophil adhesion as well as transmigration which is due to LFA-1 and Mac-1 on the neutrophil binding to ICAM-1 and ICAM-2 on the endothelium and E-selectin on the endothelium binding to its SLe^x ligand on the neutrophil (Bevilacqua *et al.*, 1985; Gamble *et al.*, 1985; Pohlman *et al.*, 1986; Schleimer and Rutledge, 1986; Smith *et al.*, 1988, 1989; Furie and McHugh, 1989; Moser *et al.*, 1989). ICAM-1 interaction with the CD11/CD18 complex on neutrophils appeared primarily responsible for transmigration (Smith *et al.*, 1989). One study demonstrated that blocking mAb to the $\beta2$ integrin and E-selectin each inhibited IL-1-enhanced migration of neutrophils across endothelial monolayers by over 90% (Luscinskas *et al.*, 1991). However Furie *et al.* (1992) demonstrated that E-selectin only appeared to operate in transmigration of neutrophils when endothelial monolayers were stimulated with low concentrations of IL-1, higher amounts of IL-1 resulted in a mainly $\beta2$-dependent pathways.

What role do these receptors play *in vivo*? The observation that loss of expression of the leucocyte integrins as seen in LAD patients was sufficient to prevent neutrophil extravasation raised questions about the importance of other receptors in neutrophil migration. However, it is now appreciated that the sequential events described above which lead to neutrophil extravasation are the result of distinct patterns of receptor interactions which are crucially dependent on the physiological flow rates seen in the postcapillary venules (Ley *et al.*, 1991; Von

Adrian *et al.*, 1991). The first step, which occurs under the high sheer stress conditions normally present in the venule, involves neutrophil adherence via the selectins. Selectins bind to their ligands in a reversible manner with rapid on/off rates which results in the rolling movement described above (Williams, 1991). Under these high flow rates integrin/Ig family receptor interactions do not occur. With the neutrophil arrested in the vessel through a selectin-dependent mechanism, inflammatory mediators can activate the neutrophil which then binds more firmly to the endothelium via integrin/Ig family receptors. This mainly irreversible binding results in flattening and transmigration of the neutrophil through the endothelium (Figure 7.5) (Smith *et al.*, 1991). These events were illustrated in an elegant study by Lawrence and Springer (1991). Purified P-selectin and ICAM-1 were inserted into artificial lipid bilayers either alone or in combination. Neutrophil adhesion to these molecules was then observed in a chamber which allowed the effects of different flow rates to be assessed. Neutrophils were observed to "roll" on bilayers containing P-selectin at physiological flow rates similar to those found in post-capillary venules. In contrast, resting or activated neutrophil adhesion to bilayers containing only ICAM-1 did not occur at these rates. However, addition of a chemoattractant to activate LFA-1 and Mac-1 resulted in the rapid arrest and subsequent flattening of neutrophils rolling on bilayers containing both P-selectin and ICAM-1. The mechanism of neutrophil activation in these circumstances is not entirely clear. Soluble neutrophil-activating mediators released into the vessel lumen would be rapidly diluted. One possible mechanism would be the presentation of neutrophil chemoattractants by the endothelium. Thus, endothelial-associated PAF generated by thrombin or histamine has been shown to activate neutrophils, as determined by Ca^{2+} flux and increased expression of Mac-1, during P-selectin binding in what has been termed a "juxtacrine" form of stimulation (Zimmerman *et al.*, 1990). Alternatively, neutrophil adhesion to plastic surfaces coated with purified E-selectin resulted in increased expression and activation of $\beta2$ integrins suggesting that the ligand for E-selectin on neutrophils can act as a signalling receptor.

A number of observations remain only partly explained. For example, IL-8, which generally activates neutrophils, inhibited enhanced neutrophil adhesion to cytokine-activated endothelial monolayers by an as yet undetermined mechanism (Gimbrone *et al.*, 1989). The role of L-selectin is still not entirely clear. Although clearly able to mediate neutrophil adhesion to endothelium, activation of neutrophils results in shedding of L-selectin which is a potentially down-regulatory adhesion mechanism (Kishimoto *et al.*, 1990). However, although activation results in a reduced number of L-selectin receptors on neutrophils those remaining appear to have increased affinity for its

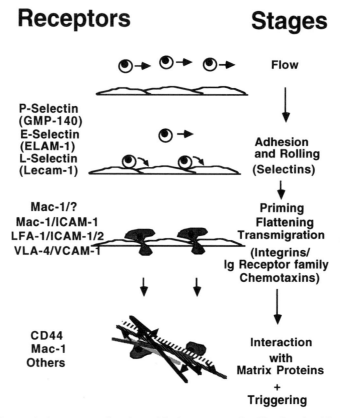

Receptors   **Stages**

Flow

P-Selectin
(GMP-140)
E-Selectin
(ELAM-1)
L-Selectin
(Lecam-1)

Adhesion
and Rolling
(Selectins)

Mac-1/?
Mac-1/ICAM-1
LFA-1/ICAM-1/2
VLA-4/VCAM-1

Priming
Flattening
Transmigration
(Integrins/
Ig Receptor family
Chemotaxins)

CD44
Mac-1
Others

Interaction
with
Matrix Proteins
+
Triggering

Figure 7.5 Stages in leucocyte migration with the receptor families involved in each stage.

endothelial ligand. In summary, neutrophils do not normally adhere to vascular endothelium. An inflammatory insult results in neutrophil adherence to endothelium initially via selectins, possibly P-selectin and L-selectin in the initial stages with E-selectin more prominent after a few hours. If the neutrophils rolling along the endothelium come into contact with an inflammatory mediator such as PAF, their $\beta2$ integrins will be activated and bind to ICAM-1 or other ligands on the endothelium which will result in a firmer adhesion and transmigration.

3.3 NEUTROPHIL ADHESION RECEPTORS AND THE EXTRACELLULAR MATRIX

It is increasingly clear that interactions between integrins and matrix proteins have a far more profound effect on cellular function than merely mediating cell attachment. Adhesion of cells to matrix proteins has been shown to result in: tyrosine phosphorylation; cytoplasmic alkalinization in platelets, fibroblasts, lymphocytes and endothelial cells; activation of lymphocytes; differentiation of myoblasts and keratinocytes; and activation of leucocyte secretion (Schubert, 1992). Adhesion of

monocytes to fibronectin resulted in the generation of GM-CSF (Thorens *et al.*, 1987), while adhesion to collagen resulted in secretion of TNF-α (Eierman *et al.*, 1989) suggesting the possibility of linkage between different integrin receptors and transcription of specific genes. Adhesion of neutrophils to a number of matrix proteins acted as a co-stimulus for induction of the respiratory burst (Nathan *et al.*, 1989). Neutrophils were much more effective at killing *Staphylococcus aureus* when adhering to a variety of matrix proteins compared with adhesion to albumin (Hermann *et al.*, 1990). Neutrophils will bind to fibrinogen via Mac-1 (Altieri *et al.*, 1988). Fibrinogen contains a ligand for Mac-1 in the C-terminus of the γ chain and neutrophils stimulated with phorbol esters will adhere to fibrinogen-coated, but not albumin-coated, surfaces in a Mac-1-dependent fashion. In contrast, TNF-stimulated neutrophils adhered to fibrinogen via p150,95 which recognizes a Gly-Pro-Arg sequence in the N-terminal domain of the α chain of fibrinogen (Loike *et al.*, 1991). Mac-1 affinity for fibrinogen is enhanced by the substitution of Mn^{2+} for Ca^{2+} and Mg^{2+} ions (Altieri, 1991). This effect appears to be due to insertion of Mn^{2+} into the divalent cation binding site of Mac-1 (Gailit and Ruoslahti, 1988). Neutrophils were thought not to express any members of the $\beta1$ integrin family due to their low surface density.

However, there are reports of expression of VLA-5 as well as a $\beta 1$ integrin that recognized laminin. Adhesion to laminin by activated neutrophils has a $\beta 2$-dependent component. However, with neutrophils from LAD patients or in the presence of an anti-$\beta 2$ mAb, stimulated neutrophil adhesion to laminin appeared to be mediated by VLA-6 (Bohnsack et al., 1990; Bohnsack, 1991). Neutrophil adhesion to fibronectin was enhanced in the presence of Mn^{2+}. This increased adhesion was inhibited by mAb to VLA-5 and also by a synthetic peptide, GRGDSP. The contribution of VLA-5 could only be detected when the $\beta 2$ pathway was blocked by mAb or $\beta 2$-deficient neutrophils were used and was more transient than $\beta 2$-dependent adhesion (Bohnsack and Zhou, 1992). It is apparent therefore that Mn^{2+} induces increased neutrophil adherence through its effect on at least two integrin receptors, i.e. Mac-1 and VLA-5. Earlier reports suggested that the fibronectin receptor on neutrophils was related to the $\beta 3$ integrins (Brown and Goodwin, 1988), however, this receptor activity has not yet been fully characterized. Interestingly, stimulation of neutrophils did not lead to up-regulation of VLA-5, although VLA-5 shares an internal PMN compartment (the adhesome) with Mac-1 whose expression is up-regulated following stimulation (Singer et al., 1989). This work requires confirmation in view of the apparent variability in $\beta 1$ receptor expression by neutrophils with some groups able to detect expression and others finding expression to be absent (Hemler, 1988) together with the tendency of platelets, which do express VLA-5 and VLA-6, to adhere to neutrophils in vitro. Although neutrophils do not appear to express any $\beta 3$ integrins it has been shown that macrophages recognize apoptotic neutrophils through their vitronectin receptor (Savill et al., 1990).

4. Adhesion Receptors as Targets for Therapy

One of the most exciting aspects of our increased understanding of the receptors involved in leucocyte adhesion is the potential for using strategies that block adhesion receptor interactions to treat disease. In addition, this provides in vivo evidence for a role for these receptors in leucocyte function. For a full discussion, see Chapter 10. To date, most studies have used mAbs directed against a variety of adhesion receptors with most information being gained on the role of CD18 receptors and ICAM-1. A popular model has been that of reperfusion injury as a model for myocardial infarctions and related vascular diseases. Vedder and co-workers (1990) have used a rabbit model in which the rabbit ear is amputated and reattached after a period of about 4–6 h. Without treatment the ear became completely necrotic within 7 days. Antibodies against CD18, ICAM-1 and L-selectin were all able to considerably ameliorate this process if given within 1 h of reattachment. A number of studies have used reperfusion injury to the myocardium as a model. In the dog, anti-$\beta 2$ mAb given intravenously diminished the size of myocardial damage suggesting a possible role in the treatment of acute myocardial infarction (Simpson et al., 1988). This has been confirmed by other workers in other animals. Similarly, in a rabbit model of hypovolaemic shock, anti-$\beta 2$ mAb resulted in decreased mortality (Vedder et al., 1988). A crucial aspect of these studies is the timing of the antiadhesion therapy for a requirement to give the antibody well before the injury would limit any clinical use. At the moment the evidence is mixed but in most studies in which the antibody was given post-reperfusion the therapy was ineffective.

Another area in which antiadhesion therapy may be of use is transplantation. In renal transplants in baboons anti-ICAM-1 antibodies considerably enhanced graft survival (Cosimi et al., 1990). Phases I/II open trials of renal transplantation in humans using a mouse monoclonal anti-ICAM-1 antibody have also been encouraging and double-blind controlled trials are now under way. One group has demonstrated indefinite survival of cardiac allografts in completely incompatible strains of mice. Interestingly, simultaneous infusion of both anti-LFA-1 and ICAM-1 mAbs was required for the effect, infusion of either mAb alone was insufficient to prolong graft survival (Isobe et al., 1992). Furthermore, anti-$\beta 2$ mAbs have been used successfully in preventing graft versus host reactions and the rejection of non-HLA-matched bone marrow transplants (Fischer et al., 1986). Although anti-ICAM-1 has been shown to inhibit transplant rejection in primate renal allografts (Cosimi et al., 1990), ICAM-1 is also important in the interaction between antigen presenting cells and antigen-specific T cells (reviewed in Springer, 1990) and this may explain the efficacy of these mAbs in this situation. To date, there are few reported studies in which mAbs to P-selectin, ICAM-2 or VCAM-1 have inhibited the adhesion or extravasation of leucocytes in vivo (see Chapter 10). This is in contrast to studies showing that mAbs to $\beta 2$ (Arfors et al., 1987; Nourshargh et al., 1989) or L-selectin inhibited neutrophil accumulation in vivo (Price et al., 1987; Jutila et al., 1989). In a recent study, the relationship between E-selectin expression and neutrophil influx in acute and late-phase airway obstruction was assessed using a primate model of extrinsic asthma. In antigen-sensitive animals, a single inhalation exposure induced expression of E-selectin on the vascular endothelium within 6 h of challenge. This expression correlated with the influx of neutrophils into the lungs and the onset of late-phase airway obstruction. Infusion of a mAb to E-selectin blocked both the neutrophil influx and the late-phase reaction. A mAb to ICAM-1 had no effect in this system nor were significant numbers of eosinophils observed. Thus, in primates at least, the elicited late-phase response appeared due to an E-selectin-dependent influx of neutrophils (Gundel *et al.*, 1991). A different response was observed in animals subjected to repeated allergen challenge. In these circumstances eosinophil rather than neutrophil influx was the predominant feature. Influx of eosinophils correlated with the development of bronchial hyper-responsiveness and both of these events were inhibited by an antibody against ICAM-1 but not E-selectin (Wegner *et al.*, 1990). This illustrates the effects of subtle differences in inflammatory stimulus and the resultant differences in the pattern of adhesion receptor expression.

In a rat model of neutrophil-mediated lung injury, pretreatment with an anti-E-selectin mAb gave a 70% reduction in neutrophil numbers in glycogen-induced peritoneal exudates. Furthermore, vascular damage associated with induction of IgG immune complex deposition and subsequent neutrophil infiltration was inhibited by prophylactic mAb treatment. Increased expression of E-selectin was observed in the animals with immune complex deposition in their lungs indicating an important role for this molecule in the associated neutrophil influx and subsequent damage (Mulligan *et al.*, 1991).

It seems that the relative importance of various adhesion receptors in neutrophil-mediated disease is crucially dependent on the precise details of the experiment, in particular, the species used and type of injury being studied. In addition, the timing of the antibody infusion and other factors such as the temperature at which the experiment is carried out are important variables.

5. Conclusions

In no area of cell biology over the last 10 years has there been a greater advance in our understanding of the basic mechanisms involved than in the field of adhesion. In particular, there has been a detailed characterization of the mechanisms that lead to leucocyte extravasation from the vasculature and the adhesion events involved in leucocyte effector function. What has emerged is a picture of considerable complexity with several families of adhesion receptors interacting to form a concerted pattern of events which control leucocyte migration both in health and during inflammatory events. Already it is becoming clear that blockage of any one of these pathways can inhibit leucocyte, and particularly neutrophil migration, into tissues with a therapeutic potential for a wide range of acute and chronic diseases. Much remains to be done, in particular, unravelling the dominant receptor interactions in different diseases so that receptor blockade can be tailored to the inflammatory condition. In this way it may be possible to inhibit an adhesion-mediated event without resulting in potentially damaging immune suppression. The future nonetheless looks bright with adhesion-related therapy offering major advances for treatment in the 21st century.

6. References

Adams, D.H., Hubscher, S.G., Shaw, J., Rothlein, R. and Neuberger, J.M. (1989). Intercellular adhesion molecule 1 on liver allografts during rejection. Lancet ii. 1122–1125.

Albelda, S.M., Mullen, W.A., Buck, C.A. and Newman, P.J. (1991). Molecular and cellular properties of PECAM-1 (endo CAM/CD31): a novel vascular cell–cell adhesion molecule. J. Cell Biol. 114, 1059–1068.

Allen, J. and Seed, B. (1988). Isolation and expression of functional high affinity Fc receptor complementary cDNAs. Science 243, 378–381.

Altieri, D.C. (1991). Occupancy of CD11b/CD18 (Mac-1) divalent ion binding site(s) induces leukocyte adhesion. J. Immunol. 147, 1891–1898.

Altieri, D.C. and Edgington, T.S. (1988). A monoclonal antibody reacting with distinct adhesion molecules defines a transition in the functional state of the receptor CD11b/CD18 (Mac-1). J. Immunol. 141, 2656–2660.

Altieri, D.C., Bader R., Mannucci, P.M. and Edgington, T.S. (1988). Oligospecificity of the cellular adhesion receptor Mac-1 encompasses an inducible recognition specificity for fibrinogen. J. Cell. Biol. 107, 1893–1900.

Anderson, D.C. and Springer T.A. (1987). Leukocyte adhesion deficiency: an inherited defect in the Mac-1, LFA-1 and p150,95 glycoproteins. Ann. Rev. Med. 38, 175–194.

Anderson, D.C., Schmalsteig F.C., Finegold, M.J., Hughes, B.J., Rothlein, R., Miller, L.J., Kohl, S., Tosi, M.F., Jacobs R.L., Waldrop, T.C., Goldman, A.S., Shearer, W.T. and Springer, T.A. (1985). The severe and moderate phenotypes of heritable Mac-1, LFA-1 deficiency: their quantitative definition and relation to leukocyte dysfunction and clinical features. J. Infect. Dis. 152, 668–689.

Anderson, D.C., Miller, L.J., Schmalsteig F.C., Rothlein, R. and Springer, T.A. (1986). Contributions of the Mac-1 glycoprotein family to adherence-dependent granulocytic functions: structure–function assessments employing sub-unit specific monoclonal antibodies. J. Immunol. 137, 15–27.

Arfors, K.E., Lundberg, C., Lindbonn, L., Lundberg K., Beatty, P.G. and Harlan, J.M. (1987). A monoclonal antibody to the membrane glycoprotein complex CD18 inhibits polymorphonuclear leukocyte accumulation and plasma leakage *in vivo*. Blood 69, 338–340.

Arnaout, M.A. and Colten, H.R. (1984). Complement C3 receptors: structure and function. Mol. Immunol. 21, 1191–1199.

Arnaout, M.A., Gupta, S.K., Pierce, M.W. and Tenen, D.G. (1988). Amino acid sequence of the alpha subunit of human leukocyte adhesion receptor Mo1 (complement receptor type 3). J. Cell Biol. 106, 2153–2918.

Arnaout, M.A., Dana, N., Gupta, S.K., Tenen D.G. and Fathallah, D.M. (1990). Point mutations impairing cell surface expression of the common β subunit (CD18) in a patient with leukocyte adhesion molecule (Leu-CAM) deficiency. J. Clin. Invest. 85, 977–981.

Arrufo, A., Stamenkovic, I., Melnick, M., Underhill, C.B. and Seed, B. (1990). CD44 is the principal cell surface receptor for hyaluronate. Cell 61, 1303–1313.

Atherton, A. and Born, G.V.R. (1972). Quantitative investigation of the adhesiveness of circulating polymorphonuclear neutrophils to blood vessel walls. J. Physiol. 222, 447–474.

Atherton, A. and Born, G.V.R. (1973). Relationship between the velocity of rolling granulocytes and that of the blood flow in venules. J. Physiol. 233, 157–165.

Bainton, D.F., Miller, L.J., Kishimoto, T.K. and Springer, T.A. (1987). Leukocyte adhesion receptors are stored in peroxidase-negative granules of human neutrophils. J. Exp. Med. 166, 1641–1653.

Beller, D.I., Springer, T.A. and Schreiber, R.D. (1982). Anti-Mac-1 selectively inhibits the mouse and human type three complement receptor. J. Exp. Med. 156, 1000–1009.

Bentley, A.M., Robinson, D.S., Menz, G., Storz, C., Durham S.R., Cromwell, O., Kay, A.B. and Wardlaw, A.J. (1992). Expression of the endothelial and leukocyte adhesion molecules ICAM-1, E-selectin and VCAM-1 in the bronchial mucosa in steady state and allergen induced asthma. J. All. Clin. Immunol. (in press).

Berendt, A.R. Simmons, D.L., Tansy, J., Newbold, C.I. and Marsh, K. (1989). Intercellular adhesion molecule-1 is an endothelial cell adhesion receptor for Plasmodium falciparum. Nature 341, 57–59.

Berg, E.L., Yoshino, T., Rott, L., Robinson, M.K., Warnock, R.A., Kishimoto, T.K., Picker, L.J. and Butcher, E.C. (1991). The cutaneous lymphocyte antigen is a skin lymphocyte homing receptor for the vascular lectin endothelial cell-leukocyte adhesion molecule-1. J. Exp. Med. 174, 1461–1566.

Berger, M., O'Shea, J., Cross, A.S., Folks, T.M., Chused, T.M., Brown E.J and Frank M.M. (1984). Human neutrophils increase expression of C3bi as well as C3b receptors upon activation. J. Clin. Invest. 74, 1566–1571.

Bevilacqua, M.P., Pober, J.S., Wheeler, M.E., Cotran, R.S. and Gimbrone, A. (1985). Interleukin-1 acts on cultured human vascular endothelium to increase the adhesion of polymorphonuclear leukocytes, monocytes, and related leukocyte cell lines. J. Clin. Invest. 76, 2003–2011.

Bevilacqua, M.P., Pober, J.S., Mendrick, D.L., Cotran, R.S. and Gimbrone, M.A. (1987). Identification of an inducible endothelial-leukocyte adhesion molecule, ELAM-1. Proc. Natl Acad. Sci. USA 84, 9238–9242.

Bevilacqua, M.P., Stengelin, S., Gimbrone, M.A. and Seed, B. (1989). Endothelial leukocyte adhesion molecule-1. An inducible receptor for neutrophils related to complement regulatory proteins and lectins. Science 243, 1160–1165.

Bevilacqua, M., Butcher E., Furie, B., Gallatin, M., Gimbrone, M., Harlan, J., Kishimoto, K., Lasky, L., McEver, R., Paulson, J., Rosen, S., Seed, B., Siegelman, M., Springer, T., Strolman, L., Tedder, T., Varki, A., Wagner, D., Weissman, I. and Zimmerman, G. (1991). Selectins: a family of adhesion receptors. Cell 67, 233.

Bochner, B.S., Luskinas, F.W., Gimbrone, M.A., Newman W., Sterbinsky, A., Derse-Anthony, C.P., Klunk, D. and Schleimer, R.P. (1991). Adhesion of human basophils, eosinophils and neutrophils to interleukin-1-activated human vascular endothelial cells: contributions of endothelial cell adhesion molecules. J. Exp. Med. 173, 1553–1556.

Bonfanti, R., Furie, B.C., Furie, B. and Wagner, D.D. (1989).

PADGEM (GMP-140) is a component of Weibel-Palade bodies of human endothelial cells. Blood 73, 1109–1112.

Bohnsack, J.F. (1991). VLA-6 is present on human neutrophils and mediates neutrophil adherence to laminin. Blood 79, 1545–1552.

Bohnsack, J.F and Zhou, X.N. (1992). Divalent cation substitution reveals CD18- and very late antigen-dependent pathways that mediate human neutrophil adherence to fibronectin. J. Immunol. 149, 1340–1347.

Bohnsack, J.F., Akiyama, S.K., Damsky, C.H., Knape, W.A. and Zimmerman, G.A. (1990). Human neutrophil adherence to laminin in vitro. J. Exp. Med. 171, 1221–1237.

Bowen, B.R., Nguyen, T. and Lasky, L.A. (1989). Characterisation of human homologue of the murine peripheral lymph node homing receptor. J. Cell. Biol. 109, 421–427.

Brennan, P.J., Zigmond, S.H., Schreiber, A.D., Smith E.R. and Southwick, F.S. (1991). Binding of IgG containing immune complexes to human neutrophil FcγRII and FcγRIII induces actin polymerization by a pertussis toxin-insensitive transduction pathway. J. Immunol. 146, 4282–4288.

Brown, E.J. and Goodwin, J.L. (1988). Fibronectin receptors of phagocytes. J. Exp. Med. 167, 777–793.

Brown, E.J., Bohnsack, J.F. and Gresham, H.D. (1988). Mechanism of inhibition of immunoglobulin G-mediated phagocytosis by monoclonal antibodies that recognize the Mac-1 antigen. J. Clin. Invest. 81, 365–375.

Brown, G.E., Reed, E.B. and Lanser, M.E. (1991). Neutrophil CR3 expression and specific granule exocytosis are controlled by different signal transduction pathways. J. Immunol. 147, 965–971.

Buckle, A.M. and Hogg, N. (1989). The effect of IFN-gamma and colony-stimulating factors on the expression of neutrophil cell membrane receptors. J. Immunol. 143, 2295–2301.

Burra P., Hubscher, S.C., Shaw, J. Elias, C. and Adams, D.H. (1990). Is the ICAM-1/IFA-1 pathway of leukocyte adhesion involved in the hepatocyte damage of alcoholic hepatitis? Hepatology 12, 394 (abstract).

Butcher, E. (1986). The regulation of lymphocyte traffic. Curr. Top. Microbio. Immunol. 128, 85–122.

Butcher, E.C. (1990). Cellular and molecular mechanisms that direct lymphocyte traffic. Am. J. Pathol. 136, 3–12.

Butcher, E., Scollay, R. and Weissman, I. (1980). Organ specificity of lymphocyte migration: mediation by highly sensitive lymphocye interaction with organ-specific determinants on high endothelial venules. Eur. J. Immunol. 10, 556–561.

Buyon, J.P., Abramson, S.B., Phillips, M.R., Slade, S.G., Ross, G.D., Weissmann, G. and Winchester, R.J. (1988). Dissociation between increased surface expression of gp165/95 and homotypic neutrophil aggregation. J. Immunol. 140, 3156–3160.

Camerini, D., James, S.P., Stamenkovic, J. and Seed, B. (1989). Leu-8/TQ-1 is the human equivalent of the MEL-14 lymph node homing receptor. Nature (Lond.) 342, 78–82.

Campanero, M.R., Puliod, R., Ursa, M.A., Rodriguez-Moya, M., de Landazuri, M.O. and Sanchez-Madrid, F. (1990). An alternative leukocyte adhesion mechanism, LFA-1/ICAM-1 independent, triggered through the human VLA-4 integrin. J. Cell Biol. 110, 2157–2165.

Carlos, T., Kovach, N., Schwartz, B., Rosa,M., Newman, B., Wayner, E., Benjamin, C., Osborn, L., Lobb, R. and Harlan, J. (1991). Human monocytes bind to cytokine-induced adhesive ligands on cultured human endothelial cells: endothelial-leukocyte adhesion molecule-1 and vascular cell adhesion molecule-1. Blood 77, 2266–2271.

Chatila, T.A., GehaR.S. and Arnaout, M.A. (1989). Constitutive and stimulus-induced phosphorylation of CD11/18 leukocyte adhesion molecules. J. Cell Biol. 109, 3435–3444.

Chin, Y., Rasmussen, J., Cakiroglu, A. and Woodruff, J. (1984). Lymphocyte recognition of lymph node high endothelium. VI. Evidence of distinct structures mediating binding to high endothelial cells of lymph nodes and Peyer's patches. J. Immunol. 133, 2961–2965.

Chin Y., Rasmussen R., Woodruff J. and Easton T.A. (1986). Monoclonal anti-HEBFpp antibody with specificity for lymphocyte surface molecules mediating adhesion to Peyer's patch high endothelium of the rat. J. Immunol. 136, 2556–2561.

Cohnheim, J. (1889). Lectures on General Pathology: A Handbook for Practioners and Students. The New Sydenham Society, London.

Corbi, A.L., Miller, L.J., O'Connor, K., Larson, R.S. and Springer, T.A. (1987). cDNA cloning and complete primary structure of the alpha subunit of a leukocyte adhesion glycoprotein, p 150,95. EMBO J. 6, 4023–4028.

Corbi, A.L., Kishimoto, T.K., Miller, L.J. and Springer, T.A. (1988a). The human leukocyte adhesion glycoprotein Mac-1 (Complement receptor type 3, CD11b) alpha subunit. Cloning, primary structure, and relation to the integrins, von Willebrand factor and factor B. J. Biol. Chem. 263, 12403–12411.

Corbi, A.L., Larson, R.S., Kishimoto, T.K., Springer, T.A. and Morton C.C. (1988b). Chromosomal location of the genes encoding the leukocyte adhesion receptors LFA-1, Mac-1 and p150,95: identification of a gene cluster involved in cell adhesion. J. Exp. Med. 176, 1597–1607.

Corral, L., Singer, M.S., Matcher, B.A. and Rosen, S.D. (1990). Requirement for sialic add on neutrophils in a GMP-140 (PADGEM) mediated adhesive interaction with activated platelets. Biochem. Biophys. Res. Commun. 172, 1349–1356.

Cosimi, A.B., Conti, D., Delmonico, F.L., Preffer, F.I., Wee, S.-L., Rothlein, R., Faanes, R. and Colvin R.B. (1990). In vivo effects of monoclonal antibody to ICAM-1 (CD54) in nonhuman primates with renal allografts. J. Immunol. 144, 4604–4612.

Cotran, R.S., Gimbrone, M.A., Jr, Bevilacqua, M.P., Mendrick, D.L. and Pober, J.S. (1986). Induction and detection of a human endothelial activation antigen in vivo. J. Exp. Med. 164, 661–666.

Crowley, C.A., Curnette, J.T., Rosin, R.E., Andre-Schwartz, J., Gallin, J.L. et al. (1980). An inherited abnormality of neutrophil adhesion: its genetic transmission and its association with a missing protein. N. Engl. J. Med. 302, 1163–1168.

Damjanovich, L., Abelda, S.M., Mette, S.A. and Buck, C.A. (1992). Distribution of integrin cell adhesion receptors in normal and malignant lung tissue. Am. J. Respir. Cell Mol. Biol. 6, 197–206.

Dana, N., Styrt, B., Griffin, J., Todd, R.F., III, Klempner, M. and Amaout, M.A. (1986). Two functional domains in the phagocyte membrane glycoprotein Mol identified with monoclonal antibodies. J. Immunol. 137, 3259–3263.

Davignon, D., Martz, E., Reynolds, T., Kurzinger, K. and Springer, T.A. (1981a). Monoclonal antibody to a novel lymphocyte function-associated antigen (LFA-1): mechanism of blocking of T lymphocyte-mediated killing and effects on other T and B lymphocyte functions. J. Immunol. 127, 590–595.

Davignon, D., Martz, E., Reynolds, T., Kurzinger, K. and Springer, T.A. (1981b). Lymphocyte function-associated antigen 1 (LFA-1): a surface antigen distinct from Lyt–2,3 that participates in T lymphocytc-mediated killing. Proc. Natl Acad. Sci. 78, 4535–4539.

de Fougerolles, A.R. and Springer, T.A. (1992). Intercellular adhesion molecule 3, a third adhesion counter receptor for lymphocyte function-associated molecule-1 on resting lymphocytes. J. Exp. Med. 175, 185–190.

de Fougerolles, A.R., Stacker, S.A., Schwartting, R. and Springer, T.A. (1991). Characterisation of ICAM-2 and evidence for a third counter-receptor for LFA-1. J. Exp. Med. 174, 253–267.

Detmers, P.A., Wright, S.D., Olsen, E., Kimball, B. and Cohn, Z.A. (1988). Aggregation of complement receptors on human neutrophils in the absence of ligand. J. Cell Biol. 105, 1137–1145.

Diamond, M.S., Staunton, D.E., de Fougerolles, A.R., Stacker, S.A., Garcia-Aguilar, J., Hibbs, M.L. and Springer, T.A. (1990). ICAM-1 (CD54): a counter-receptor for Mac-1 (CD11b/CD18). J. Cell Biol. 111, 3129–3139.

Diamond, M.S., Staunton, D.E., Marlin, S.D. and Springer, T.A. (1991). Binding of the integrin Mac-1 (CD11b/CD18) to the third immunoglobulin-like domains of ICAM-1 (CD54) and its regulation by glycosylation. Cell 65, 961–971.

Dimanche-Boitrel, M.T., Guyot, A., De Saint-Basile, G., Fischer, A., Griscelli, C. and Lisowska-Grospierre, B. (1988). Heterogeneity in the molecular defect leading to the leukocyte adhesion deficiency. Eur. J. Immunol. 18, 1575–1579.

Dobrina A., Schwartz, B.R., Carlos, T.M., Ochs, H.D., Beatty, P.G. and Harlan, J.M. (1989). CD11/CD18-independent neutrophil adherence to inducible endothelial-leucocyte adhesion molecules (ELAM-l) in vitro. Immunol. 67, 502–508.

Dobrina, A., Menegazzi., R., Carlos, T.M., Nardon, E., Cramer, R., Zacchi, T., Ryan, J.M. and Patriarca, P. (1991). Mechanisms of eosinophil adherence to cultured vascular endothelial cells: Eosinophils bind to the cytokine-induced endothelial ligand vascular cell adhesion molecule-1 via the very late activation antigen-4 integrin receptor. J. Clin. Invest. 88, 20–26.

Dransfield, I. (1991). Regulation of leukocyte integrin function. In "Integrins and ICAM-1 in Immune Responses". (ed. N. Hogg) Chemical Immunology, Vol. 50. Karger, Basel.

Dransfield, I. and Hogg, N. (1989). Regulated expression of a Mg^{2+} binding epitope on leukocyte integrin alpha subunits EMBO J. 12, 3759–3765.

Drickamer, K. (1988). Two distinct classes of carbohydrate recognition domains in animal lectins. J. Biol. Chem. 263, 9557–9560.

D'Souza, S.E., Ginsburg, M.H., Burke, T.A., Lam, S.C.T. and Plow, E.F. (1988). Localization of a ARG-GLY-ASP recognition site within an integrin adhesion receptor. Science 242, 91–93.

Dunlop, L.C., Skinner, M.P., Bendall, L.J., Favaloro, E.J., Castaldi, P.A., Gorman, J.J., Gamble, J.R., Vadas, M.A. and Berndt, M.C. (1992). Characterization of GMP-140 (P-selectin) as a circulating plasma protein. J. Exp. Med. 175, 1147–1150.

Dustin, M.L. and Springer, T.A. (1988). Lymphocyte function associated antigen-1 (LFA-1) interaction with intercellular adhesion molecule-1 (ICAM-1) is one of at least three mechanisms for lymphocyte adhesion to cultured endothelial cells. J. Cell Biol. 107, 321–331.

Dustin, M.L. and Springer, T.A. (1989). T cell receptor cross-linking transiently stimulates adhesiveness through LFA-1. Nature 341, 619–624.

Dustin, M.L., Rothlein, R., Bhan, A.K., Dinarello, C.A. and Springer, T.A. (1986). Induction by IL-1 and interferon-gamma: tissue distribution, biochemistry and function of natural adherence molecule (ICAM-1). J. Immunol. 137, 245–254.

Dustin, M.L., Singer, K.H., Tuck, D.T. and Springer, T.A. (1988a). Adhesion of T lymphoblasts to epidermal keratinocytes is regulated by interferon gamma and is mediated by intercellular adhesion molecule-1 (ICAM-1). J. Exp. Med. 167, 1323–1340.

Dustin, M.L., Staunton, D.E. and Springer, T.A. (1988b). Supergene families meet in the immune system. Immunol. Today 9, 213–215.

Eierman, D.F., Johnson, C.E. and Haskill, J.S. (1989). Human monocyte inflammatory mediator gene expression is selectively regulated by adherence substrates. J. Immunol. 142, 1970–1976.

Elices, M.J., Osborn, L., Takada, Y., Carouse, C., Luhowskyj, S., Hemler, M.E. and Lobb, R.R. (1990). VCAM-1 on activated endothelium interacts with the leukocyte integrin VLA 4 at a binding site distinct from the VLA 4/fibronectin binding site. Cell 60, 577–584.

Fanger, M.W., Shen, L., Graziano, R.F. and Guyre, P.M. (1989). Cytotoxicity mediated by human Fc receptors for IgG. Immunol. Today 10, 92–99.

Faull, R.J. and Russ G.R. (1989). Tubular expression of intercellular adhesion molecule-1 during renal allograft rejection. Transplantation 48, 226–230.

Fawcett, J., Holness, C.L.L., Needham, L.A., Turley, H., Gaffer, K.C., Mason, D.Y. and Simmons, D.C. (1992). Molecular cloning of ICAM-3, a third ligand for LFA-1 constitutively expressed on resting leukocytes. Nature (Lond.) 360, 481–484.

Fearon, D.T. and Collins, L.A. (1983). Increased expression of C3b receptors on polymorphonuclear leukocytes induced by chemotactic factors and by purification procedures. J. Immunol. 130, 370–375.

Fiebig, E., Ley, K. and Arfors, K.E. (1991). Rapid leucocyte accumulation by "spontaneous" rolling and adhesion in the exteriorized rabbit mesentery. Int. J. Microcirc. Clin. Exp. 10, 127–144.

Fischer, A., Blanche, S., Veber, F., LeDeist, F., Gerota I., Lopez, M., Durandy, A. and Griscelli, C. (1986). In "Recent Advances in Bone Marrow Transplantation" (ed. R.P. Gale) A.R. Liss, New York.

Fukuda, M., Spooncer, E.S., Oates, J.E., Dell, A. and Klock, J.C. (1984). Structure of sialyated fucosyl lactoaminoglycan isolated from human granulocytes. J. Biol. Chem. 259, 10925–10935.

Furie, M.B. and McHugh, D.D. (1989). Migration of neutrophils across endothelial monolayers is stimulated by treatment of the monolayer with interleukin-1 or tumor necrosis factor-alpha. J. Immunol. 143, 3309–3317.

Furie, M.B., Burns, M.J., Tancinco, M.C., Benjamin, C.D. and Lobb, R.R. (1992). E-Selectin (endothelial-leukocyte adhesion molecule-1) is not required for the migration of neutrophils across IL-1-stimulated endothelium in vitro. J. Immunol. 148, 2395–2404.

Gailit, J. and Ruoslahti, E. (1988). Regulation of the fibronectin receptor affinity by divalent cations. J. Biol. Chem. 263, 12927–12932.

Gallatin, W.M., Weismann, I.L. and Butcher, E.C. (1983). A cell surface molecule involved in organ-specific homing of lymphocytes. Nature (Lond.) 303, 30–34.

Gamble, J.R., Harlan, J.M., Klebanoff, S.J., Lopez, A.F. and Vadas, M.A. (1985). Stimulation of the adherence of neutrophils to umbilical vein endothelium by human recombinant tumor necrosis factor. Proc. Natl Acad. Sci. USA 82, 8667–8674.

Garcia, J.G.N., Azghani, A., Callahan, K.S. and Johnson, A.R. (1988). Effect of platelet activating factor on leukocyte-endothelial cell interactions. Thromb. Res. 51, 83.

Geng, J.G., Bevilacqua, M.P., Moore, K.L., McIntyre, T.M., Prescott, S.M., Kim, J.M., Bliss, G.A., Zimmerman, G.A. and McEver, R.P. (1990). Rapid neutrophil adhesion to activated endothelium mediated by GMP-140. Nature (Lond.) 343, 757–759.

Geng, J.G., Moore, K.L., Johnson, A.E. and McEver, R.P. (1991). Neutrophil recognition requires a $Ca^{(2+)}$-induced conformational change in the lectin domain of GMP-140. J. Biol. Chem. 266, 22313–22318.

Gimbrone, M.A., Jr, Obin, M.S., Brock, A.F., Luis, E.A., Hass, P.E., Hebert, C.A., Yip, Y.K., Leung, D.W., Lowe, D.G., Kohr, W.J., Darbonne, W.C., Bechtol, K.B. and Baker, J.B. (1989). Endothelial interleukin-8: a novel inhibitor of leukocyte endothelial interactions. Science 246, 1601–1603.

Goerdt, S., Zwaldo, G., Schlegel, R., Hagemeier, H.H. and Sorg, C. (1987). Characterisation of endothelial activation antigen present in vivo only in acute inflammatory tissues. Exp. Cell Biol. 55, 117–126.

Graber, N., Gopak, T.V., Wilson, D., Beall, L.D., Polte, T. and Newman, W. (1990). T cells bind to cytokine-activated endothelial cells via a novel, inducible sialoglycoprotein and endothelial leukocyte adhesion molecule-1. J. Immunol. 145, 819–830.

Graham I.L. and Brown, E.J. (1991). Extracellular calcium results in a conformational change in Mac-1 (CD11b/CD18) on neutrophils. Differentiation of adhesion and phagocytosis functions on Mac-1. J. Immunol. 146, 685–691.

Greve J.M., Davies, G., Meyer, A.M., Forte, C.P., Yost, S.C., Marlow, C.W., Kamarck, M.E. and McClelland, A. (1989). A major human rhinovirus receptor is ICAM-1. Cell 56, 839–847.

Gundel, R.H., Wegner, C.D., Torcellini, C.A., Clarke C.C., Haynes N., Rothlein R., Smith C.W. and Letts L.G. (1991). Endothelial leukocyte adhesion molecule-1 mediates antigen-induced acute airway inflammation and late phase obstruction in monkeys. J. Clin. Invest. 88, 1407–1411.

Hansel, T.T., de Vries, J.M., Iff, T., Rihs, S., Wandzilak M., Betz, S., Blaser, K. and Walker, C. (1991). An improved immunomagnetic procedure for the isolation of highly purified human blood eosinophils. J. Immunol. Meth. 145, 105–110.

Harlen, J.M., Killen, P.D., Senecal, F.M., Schwartz, B.R., Yee, E.K., Taylor, R.F., Beatty, P.G., Price, T.H. and Ochs,

H.D. (1985). The role of neutrophil membrane glycoprotein Gp-150 in neutrophil adhesion to endothelium in vitro. Blood 66, 167–178.

Hartnell, A., Moqbel, R., Walsh, G.M., Bradley, B. and Kay, A.B. (1990). Fcγ and CD11/CD18 receptor expression on normal human density and low density human eosinophils. Immunology 69, 264–270.

Hattori, R., Hamilton, K.K., Fugate, R.D., McEver, R.D. and Sims, P.J. (1989). Stimulated secretion of endothelial von Willebrand factor is accompanied by rapid redistribution to the cell surface of the intracellular granule membrane protein GMP-140. J. Biol. Chem. 264, 7768–7771.

Hayward A.R., Leonard, J., Wood, C.B.S., Harvey, B.A.M., Greenwood M.C. and Soothill, J.F. (1979). Delayed separation of the umbilical cord, widespread infections and defective neutrophil mobility. Lancet 1, 1099–1101.

Hemmer, M.E. (1988). Adhesive protein receptors on haemopoietic cells. Immunol. Today 9, 109–113.

Hemler, M.E. (1990). VLA proteins in the integrin family. Structures, functions and their role on leukocytes. Ann. Rev. Immunol. 8, 365–400.

Hemler, M.E., Sanchez-Madrid, F., Flotte, T.J., Krensky, A.M., Burakoff, S.J., Bhan, A.K., Springer, T.A. and Strominger, J.L. (1984). Glycoproteins of 210,000 and 130,000 molecular weight on activated T cells: cell distribution and antigenic relation to components on resting cells and T cell lines. J. Immunol. 132, 3011–3018.

Hermann, M., Jaconi, M.E.E., Dahlgren, C., Waldvogel, F.A., Stendahl, O. and Law, D.P. (1990). Neutrophil bactericidal activity against Staphylococcus aureus adherent on biological surfaces. J. Clin. Invest. 86, 942–951.

Hermanowski-Vosatka, A., Van Strijp, J.A., Swiggard, W.J. and Wright, S.D. (1992). Integrin modulating factor-1; a lipid that alters the function of leukocyte integrins. Cell 68, 341–352.

Hibbs, M.L., Selveraj, P., Carpen, O., Springer, T.A., Kuster, H., Jouvin, M.H.E. and Kinet, J.P. (1989). Mechanisms, for regulating expression of membrane isoforms for FcγRIII. Science 246, 1608–1611.

Hibbs, M.L., Wardlaw, A.J., Stacker, S.A., Anderson, D.C., Lee, A., Roberts, T.M. and Springer, T.A. (1990). Transfection of cells from patients with leukocyte adhesion deficiency with an integrin β subunit (CD18) restores lymphocyte function-associated antigen-1 expression and function. J. Clin. Invest. 85, 674–681.

Hsu-Lin, S.C., Berman, C.L., Furie, B.C., August, D. and Furie, B. (1984). A platelet membrane protein expressed during platelet activation. J. Biol. Chem. 259, 9121–9126.

Huizinga, T.W.J., Van der Schoot, C.E., Jost, C., Klassen, R., Kleijer, M., Kr. von dem Borne, A.E.G., Roos, D. and Tetteroo, (1988). The PI-linked receptor FcRIII is released on stimulation of neutrophils. Nature (Lond.) 333, 667–669.

Hynes, R.O. (1987). Integrins: a family of cell surface receptors. Cell 48, 549–554.

Hynes, R.O. (1992). Integrins: versatility, modulation and signalling in cell adhesion. Cell 69, 11–25.

Imai, Y., True, D.D., Singer, M.S. and Rosen, S.D. (1990). Direct demonstration of the lectin activity of gp90MEL-14, a lymphocyte homing receptor. J. Cell Biol. 111, 1225–1232.

Imai, Y., Singer, M., Fennie, C., Lasky, L. and Rosen, S.D. (1991). Identification of a carbohydrate-based endothelial ligand for a lymphocyte homing receptor. J Cell Biol. 113, 1213–1221.

Isobe, M., Yagita, H., Okumura, K. and Ihara, A. (1992). Specific acceptance of cardiac allograft after treatment with antibodies to ICAM-1 and LFA-1. Science 255, 1125–1127.

Jalkanen, S., Steere, A., Fox, E. and Butcher, E. (1986). A distinct endothelial cell recognition system that controls traffic into inflamed synovium. Science 233, 556–558.

Johnston, G.I., Cook, G.R. and McEver, R.P. (1989). Cloning of GMP-140, a granule membrane protein of platelets and endothelium; sequence similarity to proteins involved in cell adhesion and inflammation. Cell 56, 1033–1044.

Jutila, M.A., Rott, L., Berg, E.L. and Butcher, E.C. (1989). Function and regulation of the neutrophil MEL-14 antigen in vivo: comparison with LFA-l and MAC-1. J. Immunol. 143, 3318–3324.

Jutila, M.A., Watts, G., Walcheck, B. and Kansas, G.S. (1992). Characterisation of a functionally important and evolutionarily well conserved epitope mapped to the short consensus repeats of E-selectin and L-selectin. J. Exp. Med. 175, 1565–1573.

Kimberly, R.P., Ahlstrom, J.W., Click, M.E. and Edberg, J.C. (1990). The glycosyl phosphatidylinositol-linked FcγRIII$_{PMN}$ mediates transmembrane signalling events distinct from RCγRII. J. Exp. Med. 171, 1239–1255.

Kinet, J.P. (1989). Antibody–cell interactions Fc receptors. Cell 57, 351–354.

Kishimoto, T.K., O'Connor, K., Lee, A., Roberts, T.M. and Springer, T.A. (1987a). Cloning of the beta subunit of the leukocyte adhesion proteins: homology to an extracellular matrix receptor defines a novel supergene family. Cell 48, 681–690.

Kishimoto, T.K., Hollander, N., Roberts, T.M., Anderson, D.C. and Springer, T.A. (1987b). Heterogenous mutations in the beta subunit common to the LFA-1, Mac-1 and p150,95 glycoproteins cause leukocyte adhesion deficiency. Cell 50, 193–202.

Kishimoto, T.K., O'Connor, K. and Springer, T.A. (1989). Leukocyte adhesion deficiency. Aberrant splicing of a conserved integrin sequence causes a moderate deficiency phenotype. J. Biol. Chem. 264, 3588–3595.

Kishimoto, T.K., Jutila, M.A. and Butcher, E.C. (1990). Identification of a human peripheral lymph node homing receptor: a rapidly down-regulated adhesion molecule. Proc. Natl Acad. Sci. USA 87, 2244–2248.

Kishimoto, T.K., Warnock, R.A., Jutila, M.A., Butcher, E.C., Lane, C., Anderson, D.C. and Smith, C.W. (1991). Antibodies against human neutrophil LECAM-l(LAM-1/Leu8/DREG-56 antigen) and endothelial adhesion molecule-1 inhibit a common CD18-independent adhesion pathway in vitro. Blood 78, 805–811.

Koch, A.E., Burrows, J.C., Haines, K.G., Carlos, T.M., Harlan., J.M., Joseph, S. and Leibovich, S. (1991). Immunolocalisation of endothelial and leukocyte adhesion molecules in human rheumatoid and osteoarthritic synovial tissues. Lab. Invest. 64, 313–320.

Krensky, A.M., Sanchez-Madrid, F., Robbins, E., Nagy, J., Springer, T.A. and Burakoff, S.J. (1983). The functional significance, distribution and structure of LFA-1, LFA-2 and LFA-3: cell surface antigens associated with CTL-target interactions. J. Immunol. 131, 611–616.

Kuijpers, T.W., Hoogerwerf, M. and Roos, D. (1992). Neutrophil migration across monolayers of resting or cytokine-activated endothelial cells. J. Immunol. 148, 72–77.

Kurosaki, T. and Ravetch, J.V. (1989). A single amino acid in the glycosyl phosphatidylinositol attachment domain determines the membrane topology of FcγRIII. Nature 342, 805–807.

Kyan-Aung, U., Haskard, D.O., Poston, R.N., Thornhill, M.H. and Lee, T.H. (1991). Endothelial leukocyte adhesion molecule-1 and intercellular adhesion molecule-1 mediate adhesion of eosinophils to endothelial cells *in vitro* and are expressed by endothelium in allergic cutaneous inflammation *in vivo*. J. Immunol. 146, 521–528.

Lanier, L.L., Yu, G. and Phillips, (1991). Analysis of FcγRIII (CD16) membrane expression and association with CD3-zeta and FcεRI-γ by site-directed mutation. J. Immunol. 146, 1571–1576.

Larsen, E., Palabrica, T., Sajer, S., Gilbert, G.E., Wagner, D.D., Furie, B.C. and Furie, B. (1990). PADGEM-dependent adhesion of platelets to monocytes and neutrophils is mediated by a lineage-specific carbohydrate, LNF III (CD15). Cell 63, 467–474.

Larson, R.S., Corbi, A.L., Berman, L. and Springer, T.A. (1989). Primary structure of the LFA-1 alpha subunit. An integrin with an embedded domain defining a protein superfamily. J. Cell Biol. 108, 703–712.

Lasky, L.A., Singer, M.S., Yednock, T.A., Dowbenko, D., Fennie, C., Rodriguez, H., Nguyen, T., Stachel, S. and Rosen, S.D. (1989). Cloning of a lymphocyte homing receptor reveals a lectin domain. Cell 56, 1045–1055.

Lasky, L.A., Singer, M.S., Dowbenko, D., Imai, Y., Henzel, W.J., Grimley C., Fennie, C., Gillett, C., Watson, S.R. and Rosen, S.D. (1992). An endothelial ligand for L-selectin is a novel mucin-like molecule. Cell 69, 927–938.

Law, S.K.A., Gagnon, J., Hildreth, J.E.K., Wells, C.E., Willis, A.C. and Wong, A.J. (1987). The primary structure of the beta subunit of the cell surface adhesion glycoproteins LFA-1, CR3 and p150,95 and its relationship to the fibronectin receptor. EMBO J. 6, 915–919.

Lawrence, M.B. and Springer, T.A. (1991). Leukocytes roll on a selectin at physiologic flow rates: distinction from and prerequisite for adhesion through integrins. Cell 65, 859–873.

Ley, K., Gaehtgens, P., Fennie, C., Singer, M.S., Lasky, L.A. and Rosen, S.D. (1991). Lectin-like cell adhesion molecule 1 mediates leukocyte rolling in mesenteric venules in vivo. Blood 77, 2553–2555.

Leung, D.Y.M., Pober, J.S. and Cotran, R.S. (1991). Expression of endothelial-leukocyte adhesion molecule-1 (ELAM-1) in elicited late phase allergic reactions. J. Clin. Invest. 87, 1805–1809.

Lo, S.K., Detmers, P.A., Levin, S.M. and Wright, S.D. (1989). Transient adhesion of neutrophils to endothelium. J. Exp. Med. 169, 1779–1793.

Loike, J.D., Sodeik, B., Cao, L., Leucona, S., Weitz, J.I., Detmers, P.A., Wright, S.D. and Silverstein, S.C. (1991). CD11c/CD18 on neutrophils recognizes a domain at the N terminus of the A alpha chain or fibrinogen. Proc. Natl Acad. Sci. USA 88, 1044–1048.

Lowe, J.B., Stoolman, L.M., Nair, R.P., Larsen, R.D., Berhend, T.L. and Marks, R.M. (1990). ELAM-1-dependent cell adhesion to vascular endothelium determined by a transfected human fucosyl transferase cDNA. Cell 63, 475–484.

Luscinskas, F.W., Cybulsky, M.I., Kiely, J.M., Peckins, C.S., Davis, V.M. and Gimbrone, J.R. (1991). Cytokine-activated human endothelial monolayers support enhanced neutrophil transmigration via a mechanism involving both endothelial-leukocyte adhesion molecule-1 and intercellular adhesion molecule-1. J. Immunol. 146, 1617–1625.

Makgoba, M.W., Sanders, M.E., Ginther, G.E. *et al.* (1988). ICAM-1 a ligand for LFA-1-dependent adhesion of B, T, and myeloid cells. Nature (Lond.) 331, 86–88.

Marchesi, V.T. (1961). The site of leukocyte emigration during inflammation. Q. J. Exp. Physiol. 46, 115–133.

Marlin, S.D. and Springer, T.A. (1987). Purified intercellular adhesion molecule-1 (ICAM-1) is a ligand for lymphocyte function-associated antigen 1 (LFA-1). Cell 51, 813–819.

Marlin, S.D., Morton, C.C., Anderson, D.C. and Springer, T.A. (1986). Definition of the genetic defect and chromosomal mapping of a and β subunits of the lymphocyte function-associated antigen-1 (LFA-1) by complementation in hybrid cells. J. Exp. Med. 164, 855–867.

Marlin, S.D., Staunton, D.E.. Springer, T.A., Stratowa, C., Sommergruber, W. and Merluzzi, V. (1990). A soluble form of intercellular adhesion molecule-1 inhibits rhinovirus infection. Nature (Lond.) 344, 70–72.

Masinovsky B., Urdal, D. and Gallatin, W.M. (1990). IL-4 acts synergistically with IL-1 to promote lymphocyte adhesion to microvascular endothelium by induction of vascular cell adhesion molecule-1. J. Immunol. 145, 2886–2895.

McEver, R.P. (1991). Selectins: novel receptors that mediate leukocyte adhesion during inflammation. Thromb. Haemostasis 65, 223–228.

McEver, R.P., Beckstead, J.H., Moore, K.L., Marshall-Carlson, L. and Bainton, D.F. (1989). GMP-140, a platelet alpha-granule membrane protein is also synthesised by vascular endothelial cells and is localised in the Weibel–Palade bodies. J. Clin. Invest. 84, 92–99.

McIntyre, T.M., Zimmerman, G.A. and Prescott, S.M. (1986). Leukotrienes C4 and D4 stimulate endothelial cells to synthesize platelet activating factor and bind neutrophils. Proc. Natl Acad. Sci. USA 83, 2204.

Miller, L.J., Schwarting, R. and Springer, T.A. (1986). J. Immunol, 137, 2891–2900.

Miller, L.J., Bainton, D.F., Borregaard, N. and Springer, T.A. (1987). Stimulated mobilisation of monocyte Mac-1 and p150,95 adhesion proteins from an intracellular vascular compartment to the cell surface. J. Clin. Invest. 80, 535–544.

Miyake, K. Underhill, C.B., Lesley, J. and Kincade, P.W. (1990). Hyaluronate can function as a cell adhesion molecule and CD44 participates in hyaluronate recognition. J. Exp. Med. 172, 69–75.

Moser, R., Schleiffenbaum, B., Groscurth, P. and Fehr, J. (1989). Interleukin-1 and tumor necrosis factor stimulate human vascular endothelial cells to promote transendothelial neutrophil passage. J. Clin. Invest. 83, 444–455.

Moore, K.L., Varki, A. and McEver, R.P. (1991). GMP-140 binds to a glycoprotein receptor on human neutrophils: Evidence for a lectin-like interaction. J. Cell Biol. 112, 491–499.

Mulligan, M.S., Varani, J., Dame, M.K., Lane, C.L., Smith, C.W., Anderson, D.C. and Ward, P.A. (1991). Role of endothelial leukocyte adhesion molecule-1 (ELAM-1) in neutrophil-mediated lung injury in rats. J. Clin. Invest. 88, 1396–1406.

Munro J.M., Pober, J.S. and Cotran, R.S. (1989). Tumour necrosis factor and interferon-gamma induce distinct patterns of endothelial activation and associated leukocyte accumulation in the skin of *Pabio anubis*. Am. J. Pathol. 153, 121–133.

Myones, B.L., Daizell, J.G., Hogg, N. and Ross, G.D. (1988). Neutrophil and monocyte cell surface p150,95 has iC3b-receptor (CR4) activity resembling CR3. J. Clin. Invest. 82, 640–651.

Nathan, C., Srimal, S., Farber, C. Sanderz, E., Kabbash, L., Asch, A., Gailit, J. and Wright, S.D. (1989). Cytokine-induced respiratory burst of human neutrophils: dependence on extracellular matrix proteins and CD11/CD18 integrins. J. Cell Biol. 109, 1341–1349.

Nelson C., Rabb, H. and Arnaout, M.A. (1992). Genetic cause of leukocyte adhesion deficiency. J. Biol. Chem. 267, 3351–3357.

Nortamo, P., Rui, L., Renkonen, R., Timonen, T., Preito, J., Pataroyo, M. and Gahmberg, C.G. (1991). The expression of human intercellular adhesion molecule-2 is refractory to inflammatory cytokines. Eur. J. Immunol. 21, 2629–2632.

Nourshargh, S., Rampart, M., Hellewell, P.G., Jose, P.J., Harlan, J.M., Edwards, A.J. and Williams, T.J. (1989). Accumulation of ^{111}In-neutrophils in rabbit skin in allergic and non-allergic inflammatory reactions in vivo. J. Immunol. 142, 3193–3198.

Ohmori, K., Yoneda, T., Ishihara, G., Shigeta, K., Hirashima, K., Kanai, M., Itai, S., Sasaoki, T., Arii, S., Anita, H. and Kannagi, R. (1989). Sialyl SSEA-1 antigen as a carbohydrate marker of human natural killer cells and immature lymphoid cells. Blood 74, 255–261.

Osborn, L., Hession, C., Tizard, R., Vassallo, C., Luhowskyj, S., ChiRosso, G. and Lobb, R. (1989). Direct expression cloning of vascular adhesion molecule 1, a cytokine induced endothelial protein that binds to lymphocytes. Cell 59, 1203–1211.

Patel, D.K., Zimmermann, G.A., Prescott, S.M., McEver, R.P. and McIntyre, T.M. (1991). Oxygen radicals induce human endothelial cells to express GMP-140 and bind neutrophils. J. Cell Biol. 112, 749–759.

Phillips, M.L., Nudelman, E., Gaeta, F.C.A., Perez, M., Singhal, A.K., Hakomori, S.I. and Paulson, J.C. (1990). ELAM-1 mediates cell adhesion by recognition of a carbohydrate ligand, sial-le[x]. Science 250, 1130–1132.

Phillips, M.R., Buyon, J.P., Winchester, R., Weissmann, G. and Abramson, S.B. (1988). Upregulation of the iC3b receptor (CR3) is neither necessary nor sufficient to promote neutrophil aggregation. J. Clin. Invest. 82, 495–501.

Picker, L.J., Kishimoto, T.K., Smith, C.W., Warnock, R.A. and Butcher, E.C. (1991a). ELAM-1 is an adhesion molecule for skin-homing T cells. Nature, (Lond.) 349, 796–798.

Picker, L.J., Warnock, R.A., Burns, A.R., Doerschuk, C.M., Berg, E.L and Butcher, E.C. (1991b). The neutrophil selectin LECAM-1 presents carbohydrate ligands to the vascular selectins ELAM-1 and GMP-140. Cell 66, 921–933.

Pigott, R., Needham, L.A., Edwards, R.M., Walker, C. and Powers, C. (1991). Structural and functional studies of the endothelial activation antigen endothelial adhesion molecule-1 using a panel of monoclonal antibodies. J. Immunol. 147, 130–135.

Pober, J.S., Bevilacqua, M.P., Mendrick, D.L., Lapierre, L.A.

Fiers, W. and Gimbrone, M.A. Jr (1986a). Two distinct monokines, interleukin-1 and tumor necrosis factor each independently induce biosynthesis and transient expression of the same antigen on the surface of cultured human vascular endothelial cells. J. Immunol. 136, 1680–1687.

Pober, J.S., Gimbrone, M.A., Jr Lapierre, L.A., Mendrick, D.L., Fiers, W., Rothlein, R. and Springer, T.A. (1986b). Overlapping patterns of activation by human endothelial cells by interleukin-1, tumor necrosis factor and immune interferon. J. Immunol. 137, 1893–1896.

Pohlman, T.H., Stanness, K.A., Beatty, P.G., Ochs, H.D. and Harlan, J.M. (1986). An endothelial cell surface factor(s) induced in vitro by lipopolysaccharide, interleukin-1 and tumor necrosis factor-alpha increases neutrophil adherence by a CDw 18-dependent mechanism. J. Immunol. 136, 4548–4553.

Price, T.H., Beatty, P.G. and Corpus, S.R. (1987). *In vivo* inhibition of neutrophil function in the rabbit using monoclonal antibody to CD18. J. Immunol. 139, 4174–4177.

Ravetch, J.V. and Perussia, B. (1989). Alternative membrane forms of FcγRIII (CD16) on human natural killer cells and neutrophils. J. Exp. Med. 170, 481–497.

Redl, H., Dinges, H.P., Buurman, W.A., Van der Linden, C.J., Pober, J.S., Cotran, R.S. and Schlag, G. (1991). Expression of endothelial leukocyte adhesion molecule-1 in septic but not traumatic/hypovolemic shock in the baboon. Am. J. Pathol. 139, 461–466.

Reibman, J., Haines, K.A., Gude, A. and Weissman, G. (1991). Differences in signal transduction between Fcγ receptors (FcγRII FcγRIII) and FMLP receptors in neutrophils. J. Immunol. 146, 988–996.

Renkonen, R., Paavonen, T., Nortamo, P. and Gahmberg, C.G. (1992). Expression of endothelial molecules *in vivo*; increased endothelial ICAM-2 expression in lymphoid malignancies Am. J. Pathol. 140, 763–767.

Rice, G.E. and Bevilacqua, M.P. (1989). An inducible endothelial cell surface glycoprotein mediates melanoma adhesion. Science 246, 1303–1374.

Rice, G.E., Munro, J.M. and Bevilacqua, M.P. (1990). Inducible cell adhesion molecule-110 (INCAM-110) is an endothelial receptor for lymphocytes. II. A CD11/CD18-independent adhesion mechanism. J. Exp. Med. 171, 1369–1374.

Rothlein, R. and Springer, T.A. (1986). The requirement for lymphocyte function-associated antigen 1 in homotypic leukocyte adhesion stimulated by phorbol ester. J. Exp. Med. 163, 1132–1149.

Rothlein R., Dustin, M.L., Martin, S.D. and Springer, T.A. (1986). A human inter-cellular adhesion molecule (ICAM-1) distinct from LFA-1. J. Immunol. 137, 1270–1274.

Russell, D.G. and Wright, S.D. (1988). Complement receptor type 3 (CR3) binds to an arg-gly-asp containing region of the major surface glycoprotein, gp63, of *Leishmania promastigotes*. J. Exp. Med. 168, 279–292.

Salmon, J.E., Brogle, N.L., Edberg, J.C. and Kimberly, R.P. (1991). Fcγ receptor III induces actin polymerisation in human neutrophils and primes phagocytosis mediated by Fcγ receptor II. J. Immunol, 146, 997–1004.

Savill, J., Dransfield, I., Hogg, N. and Haslett, C. (1990). Vitronectin receptor-mediated phagocytosis of cells undergoing apoptosis. Nature (Lond.) 343, 170–173.

Scallon, B.J., Scigliano, E., Freedman, V.H., Miedel. M.C., Pan, Y.C.E., Unkeless, J.C. and Kochan, J.P. (1989). A human immunoglobulin G receptor exists in both polypeptide-anchored and phosphatidylinositol-anchored forms. Proc. Natl Acad. Sci. USA 86, 5079–5083.

Schleiffenbaum, B., Moser, R., Patarroyo, M. and Fehr, J. (1989). The cell surface glycoprotein Mac-1 (CD11b/CD18) mediates neutrophil adhesion and modulates degranulation independently of its quantitative cell surface expression. J. Immunol. 142, 3537–3545.

Schwarting, R., Stein, H. and Wang, C.Y. (1985). Blood 65, 974–983.

Schwartz, B.R., Wayner, E.A., Carlos, T.M., Ochs, H.D. and Harlan, J.M. (1990). Identification of surface proteins mediating adherence of CD11/18-deficient lymphoblastoid cells to cultured endothelium. J. Clin. Invest. 85, 2019–2022.

Schleimer, R.P. and Rutledge, B.K. (1986). Cultured human vascular endothelial cells acquire adhesiveness for neutrophils after stimulation with interleukin-1, endotoxin and tumor promoting phorbol diester. J. Immunol. 136, 649–654.

Schubert, D. (1992). Collaborative interactions between growth factors and the extracellular matrix. Trends Cell Biol. 2, 63.

Seth, R., Raymond, F.D. and Makgoba, M.W. (1991). Circulating ICAM-1 isoforms: diagnostic prospects for inflammatory and immune disorders. Lancet 338, 83–84.

Shalit, M., von Allmen, C., Atkins, P.C. and Zweiman, B. (1988). Platelet activating factor increases expression of complement receptors on human neutrophils. J. Leuk. Biol. 44, 212–217.

Shimuzu, Y., Newman, W., Gopal, T.V., Hogan, K.J., Graber, N., Dawson-Beall, L., van Seventer, G.A. and Shaw, S. (1991). Four molecular pathways of T cell adhesion to endothelial cells: roles of LFA-1, VCAM-1 and ELAM-1 and changes in pathway hierarchy under different activation conditions. J. Cell Biol. 113, 1203–1212.

Siegelman, M.H. and Wiessman, I.L. (1989). Human homologue of mouse lymph node homing receptor: evolutionary conservation at tandem cell interaction domains. Proc. Natl Acad. Sci. USA 86, 5562–5566.

Siegelman, M.H., van de Rijn, M. and Wiessman, I.L. (1989). Mouse lymph node homing receptor cDNA encodes a glycoprotein revealing tandem interaction domains. Science 243, 1165–1172.

Simmons, D. and Seed, B. (1988). The Fcγ receptor of natural killer cells is a phospholipid-linked membrane protein. Nature (Lond.) 333, 568–570.

Simmons, D., Makgoba, M.W. and Seed, B. (1988). ICAM, an adhesion ligand of LFA-1, is homologous to the neural cell adhesion molecule NCAM. Nature (Lond.) 331, 624–627.

Simpson, P.J., Todd, R.F., III, Fantone, J.C., Mickelson, J.K., Griffin, J.D., Lucchesi, B.R., Adams, M.D., Hoff, P., Lee, K. and Rogers, C.E. (1988). Reduction of experimental canine myocardial reperfusion injury by a monoclonal antibody (anti-Mol, anti-CD11b) that inhibits leukocyte adhesion. J. Clin. Invest. 81, 624–629.

Singer, I.I., Scott, S., Kawka, W. and Kazazis, D.M. (1989). Adesomes; specific granules containing receptors for laminin, C3bi/fibrinogen, fibronectin and vitronectin in human polymorphonuclear leukocytes and monocytes. J. Cell Biol. 109, 3169–3182.

Sligh, J.E., Hurwitz, M.Y., Zhu, C., Anderson, D.C. and Beaudet, A.L. (1992). An initiation codon mutation in CD18 in association with the moderate phenotype of leukocyte adhesion deficiency. J. Biol. Chem. 267, 714–718.

Smith, C.W., Rothlein, R., Hughes, B.J., Mariscalco, M.M., Rudloff, H.E., Schmalstieg, F.C. and Anderson, D.C. (1988). Recognition of an endothelial determinant for CD18-dependent human neutrophil adherence and transendothelial migration. J. Clin. Invest. 82, 1746–1756.

Smith, C.W., Marlin, S.D., Rothlein, R., Toman, C. and Anderson, D.C. (1989). Cooperative interactions of LFA-1 and Mac-1 with intercellular adhesion molecule-1 in facilitating adherence and transendothelial migration of human neutrophils in vitro. J. Clin. Invest. 83, 2008–2017.

Smith, C.W., Kishimoto, T.K., Abbass, O., Hughes, B.J., Rothlein, R., McIntyre, L.V., Butcher, E. and Anderson, D.C. (1991). Chemotactic factors regulate lectin adhesion molecule-1 (LECAM-1)-dependent neutrophil adhesion to cytokine-stimulated endothelial cells in vitro. J Clin. Invest. 87, 609–618.

Springer T.A. (1990). Adhesion receptors of the immune system. Nature (Lond.) 346, 425–434.

Springer, T.A. and Lasky, L.A. (1991). Sticky sugars for selectins. Nature (Lond.) 349, 196–197.

Springer, T.A. Galfre, G., Secher, D.S. and Milstein, C. (1979). Eur. J. Immunol. 9, 310–316.

Springer, T.A., Thompson, W.S., Miller, L.J., Schmalstieg, F.C. and Anderson, D.C. (1984). Inherited deficiency of the MAC-1, LFA-1, p150,95 glycoprotein family and its molecular basis. J. Exp. Med. 160, 1901–1980.

Stamenkovic, I., Amiot, M., Pasando, M. and Seed, B. (1989). A lymphocyte molecule implicated in lymph nods homing is a member of the cartilage link protein family. Cell 56, 1057–1062.

Staunton, D.E., Marlin, S.D., Stratowa, C., Dustin, M.L. and Springer, T.A. (1988). Primary structure of intercellular adhesion molecule 1 (ICAM-1) demonstrates interaction between members of the immunoglobulin and integrin supergene families. Cell 52, 925–933.

Staunton, D.E. Dustin, M.L. and Springer, T.A. (1989a). Functional cloning of ICAM-2, a cell adhesion ligand for LFA-1 homologous to ICAM-1. Nature (Lond.) 339, 61–64.

Staunton, D.E., Merluzzi, V.J., Rothlein, R., Barton, R., Marlin, S.D. and Springer, T.A. (1989b). A cell adhesion molecule, ICAM-1, is the major surface receptor for rhinoviruses. Cell 56, 849–853.

Staunton., D.E., Dustin, M.L., Erickson, H.P. and Springer, T.A. (1990). The arrangement of the immunoglobulin-like domains of ICAM-1 and the binding sites for LFA-1 and rhinovirus. Cell 61, 243–254.

Stoolman, L.M., Tenforde, T.S. and Rosen, S.D. (1984). Phosphomannosyl receptors may participate in the adhesive interactions between lymphocytes and high endothelial venules. J. Cell Biol. 99, 1535–1540.

Stuart, S.G., Trounstine, M.L., Vaux, D.J.T., Koch, T., Martens, C.L., Mellman, I. and Moore, K.W. (1987). Isolation and expression of cDNA clones encoding a human receptor for IgG(FcγRII). J. Exp. Med. 166, 1668–1684.

Symington, F.W., Hedges, D.L. and Hakomori, S.I. (1985). Glycolipid antigens of human polymorphonuclear neutrophils and the inducible HL-60 myeloid leukaemia line. J. Immunol. 134, 2498–2506.

Takeichi, M. (1990). Cadherins: a molecular family important in selective cell-cell adhesion Annu. Rev. Biochem. 59, 237–252.

Tedder, T.F., Issacs, T., Ernst, G., Demetri, G., Alder, G. and Disteche, C. (1989). Isolation and chromosomal localisation of cDNAs encoding a novel human lymphocyte cell surface molecule, LAM-1: homology with the mouse lymphocyte homing receptor and other human adhesion molecules. J. Exp. Med. 170, 123–133.

Thorens, B., Mermod, J.J. and Vassalli, P. (1987). Phagocytosis and inflammatory stimuli induce GM-CSF mRNA in macrophages through post-transcriptional regulation. Cell 48, 671–679.

Thornhill, M.H. and Haskard, D.O. (1990). IL-4 regulates endothelial cell activation by IL-1, tumor necrosis factor of IFN-gamma. J. Immunol. 145, 865–872.

Thornhill, M.H., Kyan-Aung, U. and Haskard, D.O. (1990). IL-4 increases human endothelial cell adhesiveness for T cells but not neutrophils. J. Immunol. 144, 3060–3065.

Tomassini,J.E., Graham, D., DeWitt, C.M., Lineberger, D.W., Rodkey, J.A., and Colonno, R.J. (1989). cDNA cloning reveals that the major group rhinovirus receptor on HeLa cells is intercellular adhesion molecule 1. Proc. Natl Acad. Sci. USA 86, 4907–4911.

Tonnesen, M.G., Smedly, L.A. and Henson, P.M. (1984). Neutrophil-endothelial cell interactions. Modulation of neutrophil adhesiveness induced by complement fragments C5a and C5a des Arg and formylmethionyl-leucyl-phenylalanine in vitro. J. Clin. Invest. 74, 1581–1592.

Tosi, M.F. and Berger, M. (1988). Functional differences between the 40 kDa and 50–70 kDa IgG Fc receptors on human neutrophils revealed by elastase treatment and anti-receptor antibodies. J.Immunol. 146, 2097–2103.

Toothill, V.J., van Mourik, J.A., Niewenhuis. H.K., Metzelaar, M.J. and Pearson, J.D. (1990). Characterization of the enhanced adhesion of neutrophil leukocytes to thrombin-stimulated endothelial cells. J. Immunol. 145, 283–291.

Unkeless, J.C. (1989). Function and heterogeneity of human Fc receptors for immunoglobulin G. J. Clin. Invest. 83, 355–361.

Vazeux, R., Hoffman, P.A., Tomiton, J.K., Dickinson, E.S., Jarman, R.L., St. John, T. and Gallatin, W.M. (1992). Cloning and characterization of a new intercellular adhesion molecule ICAM-R. Nature (Lond.) 360, 485–488.

Vedder, N.B. and Harlan, J.M. (1988). Increased surface expression of CD11b/CD18 (Mac-1) is not required for stimulated neutrophil adherence to cultured endothelium. J. Clin. Invest. 81, 676–682.

Vedder N.B., Winn, R.K., Rice, C.L., Chi, E.Y., Arfors, K.E. and Harlan, J.M. (1988). A monoclonal antibody to the adherence-promoting leukocyte glycoprotein, CD18, reduces organ injury and improves survival from hemorrhagic shock and resuscitation in rabbits. J. Clin. Invest. 81, 939–944.

Vedder, N.B., Winn, R.K., Rice, C.L., Chi, E.Y., Arfors, K.E. and Harlan, J.M. (1990). Inhibition of leukocyte adherence by anti-CD18 monoclonal antibody attenuates reperfusion injury in the rabbit ear. Proc. Natl Acad. Sci. USA 87, 2643–2646.

Vogetseder, W., Feichtinger, H., Schultz., T.F. et al. (1989). Expression of 7F7-antigen, a human adhesion molecule identical to intercellular adhesion molecule-1 human carcinoma and their stromal fibroblasts. Int. J. Cancer 43, 768–773.

Volpes, R., Van Den Oord, J.J. and Desmet, V.J. (1990). Immunohistochemical study of adhesion molecules in liver inflammation. Hematology 12, 59–65.

Von Adrian, U., Chambers, J.D., McEvoy, L.M., Bargatze, R.F., Arfors, K.E. and Butcher, E.C. (1991). Two-step model of leukocyte-endothelial cell interaction in inflammation. Proc. Natl Acad. Sci. USA 88, 7538–7542.

Walker, B.A.M., Hagnelocker, B.E., Stubbs, E.B. Jr., Sandborg, R.R., Agranoff, B.W. and Ward, P.A. (1991). Signal transduction events and FcγR engagement in human neutrophils stimulated with immune complexes. J. Immunol. 146, 735–741.

Wallis, W.J., Hickstein, D.D., Schwartz, B.R., June, C.H., Ochs, H.D., Beatty, P.G., Klebanoff, S.J. and Harlan, J.M. (1986). Monoclonal antibody-defined functional epitopes on the adhesion-promoting glycoprotein complex (CDw18) of human neutrophils. Blood 67, 1007–1013.

Walsh, G.M., Mermod, J.J., Hartnell, A., Kay, A.B. and Wardlaw, A.J. (1991). Human eosinophil, but not neutrophil, adherence to IL-1 stimulated HUVEC is α4β1 (VLA-4) dependent. J. Immunol. 146, 3419–3423.

Walz, G.A., Aruffo, A., Kolanus, W., Bevilacqua, M. and Seed, B. (1990). Recognition by ELAM-1 of the sial-le^x. Science 250, 1132–1135.

Wardlaw, A.J., Hibbs, M.L., Stacker, S.A. and Springer, T.A. (1990). Distinct mutations in two patients with leukocyte adhesion deficiency and their functional correlates. J. Exp. Med. 172, 335–345.

Watson, S., Imai, Y., Fennie, C., Geoffroy, J.S., Rosen, S.D. and Lasky, L.A (1990). A homing receptor IgG chimera as a probe for adhesive ligands of lymph node high endothelial venules. J. Cell Biol. 110, 2221–2229.

Watson, S., Fennie, C., and Lasky, L.A. (1991). Neutrophil influx into an inflammatory site inhibited by a soluble homing receptor-IgG chimaera. Nature (Lond.) 349, 164–167.

Weetman, A.P., Cohen, S., Mategoba, M.W. and Borysiewicz, L.K. (1989). Expression of an intercellular adhesion molecule-1, ICAM-1, by human thyroid cells. J. Endocrinol. 122, 185–191.

Wegner, C.D., Gundel, R.H., Reilly, P., Haynes, N., Letts, G.L. and Rothlein, R. (1990). Intercellular adhesion molecule-1 (ICAM-1) in the pathogenesis of asthma. Science 247, 456–459.

Weller, P.F., Rand, T.H., Goetzl, S.E., Chi-Rosso, G. and Lobb, R.R. (1991). Human eosinophil adherence to vascular endothelium mediated by binding to vascular cell adhesion molecule-1 and endothelial molecule-1. Proc. Natl Acad. Sci. USA 88, 7430–7433.

Williams, A.F. (1991). Out of equilibrium, Nature (Lond.) 352, 473–474.

Wright, S.D., Weitz, J.I., Huang, A.J., Levin, S.M., Silverstein S.C. and Loike, J.D. (1988). Complement receptor three (CD11b/CD18) of human polymorphonuclear leukocytes recognises fibrinogen. Proc. Natl Acad. Sci. USA 85, 7734–7738.

Yednock, T.A, and Rosen, S.D. (1989). Lymphocyte homing. Adv. Immunol. 44, 313–378.

Yednock, T.A., Butcher, E.C., Stoolman, L.M. and Rosen, S.D. (1987). Receptors involved in lymphocyte homing: relationship between a carbohydrate-binding receptor and the MEL-14 antigen. J. Cell Biol. 104–725.

Zhou, Q., Moore., L.K., Smith, D.F., Varki, A., McEver, R.P. and Cummings, R.D. (1991). The selectin GMP-140 binds to sialyated fucosylated lactosaminoglycans on both myeloid and nonmyeloid cells. J. Cell. Biol. 115, 557–614.

Zimmerman, G.A., McIntyre, T.M. and Prescott, S.M. (1985). Thrombin stimulates the adherence of neutrophils to human endothelial cells in vitro. J. Clin. Invest. 76, 2235–2246.

Zimmerman, G.A., McIntyre, T.M., Mehra, M. and Prescott, S.M. (1990). Endothelial cell-associated platelet activating factor: a novel mechanism for signalling cell adhesion. J. Cell Biol. 110, 529–540.

8. Receptor-mediated Signal Transduction Pathways in Neutrophils: Regulatory Mechanisms that Control Phospholipases C, D and A₂

Shamshad Cockcroft

1. Introduction

Cell surface receptors provide the link between the extracellular milieu and the intracellular environment. Receptors bind to their cognate ligands on the external face of the plasma membrane and this interaction sets into motion a cascade of biochemical events which control the intracellular machinery of the cell. Transmembrane signalling is the key mechanism by which intracellular events can be controlled with precision. The

Immunopharmacology of Neutrophils
ISBN 0–12–339250–0

Copyright © 1994 Academic Press Limited
All rights of reproduction in any form reserved.

neutrophil responds to external stimulation in a variety of ways including chemotaxis, phagocytosis, degranulation, respiratory burst, aggregation and many of these functional events are triggered in an ordered manner. The transmembrane signalling pathways provide "second messengers" released in the cell interior, and they in turn can initiate subsequent biochemical reactions such as phosphorylation and dephosphorylation of proteins. Second messengers are generally derived from enzymatic reactions which are regulated by the activated receptor. The use of catalytic reactions allows the initial signal to be greatly amplified when relayed through the signalling cascade.

Many of the receptors for soluble agonists present on neutrophils have been cloned (see Chapter 6). These are the FMLP receptor (Boulay *et al.*, 1990), C5a receptor (Gerard and Gerard, 1991), IL-8 receptor (Thomas *et al.*, 1991) and the PAF receptor (Honda *et al.*, 1991) and they all belong to the superfamily of G protein-linked receptors (Strosberg, 1991). In the neutrophil, many of these G protein-linked receptors stimulate the activation of three phospholipases PLC, PLD and PLA$_2$ (Figure 8.1). It is now generally accepted that the phosphoinositide-specific PLC can be coupled to the receptor via a G protein, G$_p$ (Cockcroft, 1987). The mechanism of how cell-surface stimulation leads to the activation of PLD and PLA$_2$ has yet to be firmly established. Substantial evidence has now emerged suggesting that these reactions are also regulated by G proteins.

In addition to the G protein-coupled receptors, there are also receptors for the components of complement C3b/bi, receptors for lectins (responding to Con A) and the Fc domain of IgG (FcγR) (see Chapter 7). All these receptors also stimulate the three phospholipases, PLC, PLD and PLA$_2$, although many of them do not belong to the superfamily of G protein-coupled receptors (Ravtech and Kinet, 1991). Three antigenically, biochemically and functionally distinct Fc receptors for IgG (FcγRI, FcγRII and FcγRIII) have been identified on neutrophils (Ravtech and Kinet, 1991). FcγRI (CD64) is a high-affinity receptor and can bind monomeric IgG whilst FcγRII (CD32) and FcγRIII (CD16) are low-affinity receptors. Current evidence indicates that the Fc receptors activate PLC by a different mechanism compared to G protein-coupled receptors. In common with the IgE receptor and the T-cell antigen receptor, Fcγ receptors appear to use tyrosine kinase-mediated signalling pathways involving phosphorylation of specific isoforms of PLC (Cockcroft and Thomas, 1992; Rhee and Choi, 1992). Fcγ receptors also stimulate PLD and PLA$_2$ but the mechanism of activation is incompletely understood (Della Bianca *et al.*, 1991).

PLC, PLA$_2$ and PLD have the potential to deliver intracellular signals that can be integrated to yield the terminal physiological response of the cell. In the case of the neutrophil, the physiological end point includes adherence, aggregation, chemotaxis, exocytosis of secretory granules as well as the activation of the NADPH oxidase (respiratory burst). How does activation of these three phospholipases result in triggering the various neutrophil functions? The FMLP receptor also stimulates the rapid activation of phosphatidylinositol-3-kinase (Stephens *et al.*, 1991) and tyrosine phosphorylation (Huang *et al.*, 1988; Gomez-Cambronero *et al.*, 1991). It is not clear whether these reactions are downstream events occurring subsequent to the activation of the phospholipases or whether they are triggered by separate intracellular regulatory pathways. Figure 8.2 depicts the various pathways that may potentially control many of the different end responses of the neutrophil. Multiple second messengers are generated within seconds of receptor stimulation and these "effectors" can either converge or diverge to trigger the individual functional responses in the neutrophil. The function of many of the individual second messengers has been extensively studied by controlling their endogenous production or by externally adding them into permeabilized cell preparations. From such functional studies, the role of the individual second messengers is beginning to be understood.

The potential second messengers that are derived from the activation of the three phospholipases are summarized in Figure 8.2 Activation of the PI-PLC pathway causes the generation of two products, IP$_3$, which mobilizes intracellular Ca^{2+} and DAG which activates PKC. Activation of PLD increases the membrane concentration of phosphatidate, which may act as a second messenger in its own right, or it may be further metabolized to generate DAG. Activation of PLA$_2$ leads to the release of arachidonate and this also may have a dual function. It can act as a second messenger or it can be a substrate for the synthesis of eicosanoids.

Much evidence has accrued to indicate that the activation of functional responses is dependent not just on Ca^{2+} but also on other second messengers. This has been demonstrated by using a variety of approaches. From studies in permeabilized neutrophils or HL60 cells, it has been shown that secretion requires at least two separate G protein-regulated pathways (Barrowman *et al.*, 1986; Stutchfield and Cockcroft, 1988; Cockcroft,

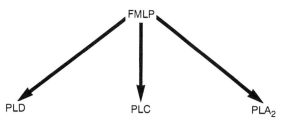

Figure 8.1 Three phospholipases triggered by the FMLP receptor in neutrophils. PLD, phospholipase D; PLC, phosphoinositide-specific phospholipase C; PLA$_2$, phospholipase A$_2$.

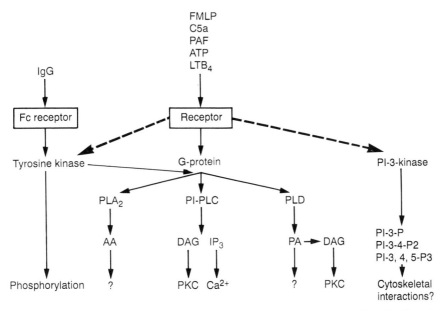

Figure 8.2 Multiple second messengers derived from signalling pathways triggered by the G-protein-coupled receptors and Fc receptors. Rapid activation of three phospholipases as well as the activation of tyrosine phosphorylation and phosphatidylinositol-3-kinase are known to be regulated by occupied receptors. The products of the individual reactions which function as second messengers are indicated as well as the downstream events that they regulate.

1991). Using 17-hydroxywortmannin as an inhibitor of receptor-mediated neutrophil responses, evidence for two transduction sequences initiated by receptor agonists was obtained for the induction of the respiratory burst (Dewald *et al.*, 1988). Clearly, functional responses such as secretion or the respiratory burst are under complex regulatory control rather than under a single second messenger.

The presence of multiple signalling pathways invoked by a single ligand can be interpreted differently. It may reflect a built-in redundancy in the signalling molecules. It can be shown that different combinations of second messengers can trigger functional responses (Stutchfield and Cockcroft, 1988). Another feature to consider is that the individual second messengers allow functional responses to be triggered at thresholds which can be modulated by the presence of second signals. For example, an increment in Ca^{2+} sets the system to a receptive state, but does not actually trigger a response. A small change in a second parameter, e.g. an increase in DAG or PA, then is sufficient for the system to pass a threshold such that a physiological response can now occur. The use of multiple signalling pathways permits a sophisticated means of controlling output and the responsiveness of the cells can be fine-tuned.

1.1 MEMBRANE PHOSPHOLIPIDS AS A SOURCE OF SECOND MESSENGERS

The main substrates for the different phospholipases as

well as PI-3-kinase are phospholipids resident in the membrane. The biological membrane is organized as a bilayer consisting of several phospholipids mainly phosphatidylcholine, phosphatidylethanolamine, phosphatidylserine, phosphatidylinositol and sphingomyelin. The lipid composition of the membrane will influence the ability of the individual phospholipases to hydrolyse its specific substrate. In general, when enzyme activity is monitored *in vitro*, the substrate is presented either as lipid vesicles comprising a single lipid or with a defined lipid composition very often in the presence of detergents. *In vivo*, of course, the phospholipases (PLs) will be presented with their substrate in the membrane. Thus caution must be exercised when comparisons are made between *in vitro* assays for PLs where the substrate is presented in a non-bilayer form and *in vivo* studies where the substrate is provided in a biological membrane. Enzyme regulation by other molecules or by protein phosphorylation may not manifest itself *in vitro* but may do so when the enzyme is studied using a biological membrane. For example, in cells there is enough PLC activity present to hydrolyse all the inositol lipid within seconds and yet the enzyme, because it is unable to get access to its substrate, is essentially inactive. Cell surface stimulation clearly brings about a change in the enzyme or the membrane such that the enzyme is now able to "see" its substrate in the membrane.

The main substrate(s) for PLC and PI-3-kinase are the inositol-containing lipids. The fatty-acid composition of the inositol lipids in many cells including human neutrophils show a consistent pattern whereby the sn-1 position normally contains stearic acid (C_{18}) and the sn-2 position contains arachidonic acid ($C_{20:4}$) (Cockcroft and Allan, 1984). Two kinases are responsible for phosphorylating PI to generate PI(4,5)P$_2$, the primary substrate for both PLC and PI-3-kinase. The inositol lipids only comprise 5–8% of the total phospholipids. In comparison PC, the substrate for both PLD and PLA$_2$, accounts for 40% of the total phospholipid pool (Cockcroft, 1984). The sn-1 position of PC can be either acyl-linked or alkyl-linked whereas the sn-2 position is invariably acyl-linked. In neutrophils, alkyl-PC (1-O-alkyl-PC) accounts for up to 40% of the total PC pool, the remainder being diacyl-PC (Billah et $al.$, 1986) and both are substrates for PLD and PLA$_2$. 1-O-Alkyl-PC is the source for PAF, a product made by neutrophils in substantial amounts on cell-surface stimulation.

2. Phosphoinositide-specific Phospholipase C

A plasma-membrane localized Ca^{2+}-activated PLC was first demonstrated in neutrophils in 1984 (Cockcroft et $al.$, 1984) and subsequently shown that this activity could be regulated by a G-protein (designated G$_p$) (Cockcroft and Gomperts, 1985). Since then much work has followed to establish the role of an intermediary G protein that couples receptors to phospholipase C. Many of the receptors on phagocytic cells have been recently cloned and it is clear that receptors for FMLP (Boulay et $al.$, 1990; Thomas et $al.$, 1990), C5a (Rollins et $al.$, 1991; Gerard and Gerard, 1991), PAF (Honda et $al.$, 1991) and IL-8 (Thomas et $al.$, 1991; Murphy and Tiffany, 1991) all belong to the superfamily of G protein-coupled receptors (Strosberg, 1991). Other G protein-coupled receptors that are present on neutrophils are LTB$_4$ receptors (Lew et $al.$, 1987; Omann et $al.$, 1987; McLeish et $al.$, 1989) and a novel puringeric receptor(s) whose pharmacological characteristics are distinct in comparison to previously characterized purinergic receptors (Kuhns et $al.$, 1988; Ward et $al.$, 1988; Seifert et $al.$, 1989a, 1989b; Cockcroft and Stutchfield, 1989a, 1989b; Stutchfield and Cockcroft, 1990; Merritt and Moores, 1991).

A common feature among the G protein-linked receptors is that they span the cell membrane seven times, forming three extracellular and three intracellular loops and a cytoplasmic carboxy-terminal tail. Although most of the G protein-coupled receptors in neutrophils stimulate the same intracellular signalling pathways in most cases, the third cytoplasmic loop and the carboxy-terminal tail display extensive variability in length and sequence, which has led to the proposal that these parts of the receptor are responsible for the selective inter-action with the various regulatory G proteins (Cotecchia

et $al.$, 1990; Lechleiter et $al.$, 1990; Liggett et $al.$, 1991). Clearly the sequence dictates that the receptor–G protein interaction will be different for individual receptors. Already evidence supporting this notion has been presented for the FMLP and the LTB$_4$ receptor in HL60 cells (McLeish et $al.$, 1989; Schepers et $al.$, 1992).

In general, there is little evidence to suggest that isoforms of the C5a or PAF receptor exist, indicating that the multiple PLs stimulated by these receptors arise from the activation of a single receptor (Gerard and Gerard, 1991; Honda et $al.$, 1991). Although two cDNA clones have been identified for the human FMLP receptor, they represent allelic variations of the same gene (Boulay et $al.$, 1990). The FMLP receptor from rabbit neutrophils has also been cloned and this showed only 28% homology with the human FMLP receptor (Thomas et $al.$, 1990). More recent studies by the same workers now indicate that the clone from the rabbit neutrophils in fact encodes the IL-8 receptor (Thomas et $al.$, 1991). When the human FMLP receptor was functionally expressed in $Xenopus$ oocytes, a requirement for a complementary factor was identified which was found to be present in undifferentiated and differentiated HL60 cells as well as in liver cells (Murphy and McDermott, 1991). In contrast, functional expression of the single-chain FMLP receptor into mouse fibroblasts was sufficient in mediating ligand-induced early transmembrane signalling events (Prossnitz et $al.$, 1991). Identification of the factor required for expression in $Xenopus$ oocytes may provide valuable clues for understanding how many components comprise the signalling pathway that FMLP regulates.

Initial studies to demonstrate that PLC was regulated by a G protein were done in membrane preparations. It was anticipated that an effector system that is linked to receptors is likely to be present at the plasma membrane, in analogy to the adenylate cyclase system. [Adenylate cyclase is a transmembrane glycoprotein (Bakalyar and Reed, 1990)]. Indeed in 1984, a polyphosphoinositide-specific PLC was identified in membranes that was activated by millimolar levels of Ca^{2+} (Cockcroft et $al.$, 1984). The endogenous polyphosphoinositides served as substrate and on addition of 500 μM Ca^{2+}, 40–60% of the preformed polyphosphoinositides were hydrolysed to diacylglycerol and the corresponding inositol phosphates.

Since the resting level of Ca^{2+} in cells is normally 100 nM and since this level of Ca^{2+} was ineffective at stimulating PLC activity, this preparation served as a testing ground for other controlling pathways. GTP-γ-S proved to be an effective stimulator of the membrane-bound PLC (Cockcroft and Gomperts, 1985). Within a few years many studies were published establishing that membranes from different cell types contained both a GTP-γ-S activated as well a GTP-dependent receptor-activated PLC see (Cockcroft, 1987, for review).

The basic characteristics of this PLC activation in neutrophils/HL60 cells can be summarized as follows.

(1) GTP analogues show a particular potency (GTP-γ-S > GppNHp > GppCH2p) characteristic of G-protein activation (Cockcroft and Stutchfield, 1988a; Stutchfield and Cockcroft, 1988).

(2) Fluoride in the presence of aluminium stimulates the enzyme (Cockcroft and Stutchfield, 1988a; Geny *et al.*, 1988; Randriamampita and Trautmann, 1990).

(3) Activation via a G protein is dependent on Ca^{2+} in the resting physiological range (i.e. 100 nM); increasing Ca^{2+} to the stimulatory range (i.e. 1–10 μM) potentiates this activation (Cockcroft, 1986a; Smith *et al.*, 1986; Anthes *et al.*, 1987; Cockcroft and Stutchfield, 1988a; Cowen *et al.*, 1990b).

(4) Ligand activation is dependent on GTP (Smith *et al.*, 1985, 1986; Kikuchi *et al.*, 1986, 1987; Anthes *et al.*, 1987; Cowen *et al.*, 1990a, 1990b; Stutchfield and Cockcroft, 1991). In the majority of studies FMLP has been used as the ligand.

(5) Stimulation by some ligands such as FMLP, PAF, LTB4, C5a, ATP, UTP, etc. is blocked by pertussis toxin pretreatment (Becker *et al.*, 1985; Brandt *et al.*, 1985; Goldman *et al.*, 1985; Krause *et al.*, 1985; Okajima *et al.*, 1985; Cockcroft and Stutchfield, 1988a). In some cases inhibition is partial (Cowen *et al.*, 1990a; Brunkhorst *et al.*, 1991) implying a role for pertussis toxin-insensitive G proteins as well.

All the above statements are generally applicable to most cell types examined with minor variations but statement (5) is restricted to only a small range of cell types (Cockcroft and Stutchfield, 1988b). In a large proportion of cell types the G protein regulating the PLC is *not* sensitive to pertussis toxin pretreatment (Cockcroft and Thomas, 1992). In neutrophils and HL60 cells, the pertussis toxin sensitivity is an important indicator as to the nature of the G protein involved in coupling the activated receptor to PLC. It narrows the field to the G_i family, the only pertussis toxin-sensitive G proteins so far identified in these cells. Indeed G_{i1} is not present either; thus it is either G_{i2} or G_{i3} (Uhing *et al.*, 1987; Goldsmith *et al.*, 1988; Gierschik *et al.*, 1989). The nature of the pertussis-insensitive G-proteins regulating PLC is not known in neutrophils but it is likely to involve members of the G_q family which regulate the PLC-β1 isoform (Amatruda *et al.*, 1991; Shenker *et al.*, 1991; Smrcka *et al.*, 1991; Taylor *et al.*, 1991).

2.1 G PROTEINS IDENTIFIED IN NEUTROPHIL/HL60 CELLS

Both heterotrimeric G proteins (composed of $\alpha\beta\gamma$) as well as monomeric GTP-binding proteins with molecular masses ranging from 20–26 kD have been found in phagocytic cells. Table 8.1 provides a summary of the GTP-binding proteins that have been identified so far in

Table 8.1 GTP-binding proteins identified in neutrophils/HL60 cells

Protein	Description	Reference
Heterotrimeric G proteins		
G_{i2}	Major substrate for pertussis toxin	Uhing *et al.* (1987), Falloon *et al.* (1986), Offermans *et al.* (1990)
G_{i3}	Substrate for pertussis toxin	Uhing *et al.* (1987), Goldsmith *et al.* (1988)
G_{16}/G_{15}	Specifically expressed in haematopoietic cells	Amatruda *et al.* (1991), Wilkie *et al.* (1991)
G_q/G_{11}	Ubiquitous	Mitchell *et al.* (1991), Pang and Sternweis (1989), Strathmann and Simon (1990)
G_{12}/G_{13}	Ubiquitous	Strathmann and Simon (1991)
G_s	Substrate for cholera toxin	Bokoch (1987)
Small GTP binding proteins – the *ras* superfamily		
Ras family		
Ras		Philips *et al.* (1991)
Rap1A	Also known as Krev1/*smg*21	Bokoch and Quilliam (1990), Quilliam *et al.* (1991), Quinn *et al.* (1992)
Rap1/2	Translocates from granules to plasma membranes	Maridonneau-Parini and de Gunzburg (1992)
Rho family		
Rho	Substrate for botulinum toxin	Quilliam *et al.* (1989)
G22K	Major substrate for botulinum toxin	Quilliam *et al.* (1989), Bokoch *et al.* (1988)
Rac1/2	Substrate for botulinum C3 toxin	Didsbury *et al.* (1989)

In neutrophils, as many as 10–15 different low molecular weight proteins have been identified in secretory granule membranes as well as plasma membranes (Dexter *et al.*, 1990; Philips *et al.*, 1991). The identity of many of these proteins remains to be confirmed by specific antibodies.

neutrophils/HL60 cells. (HL60 is a promyelocytic cell line which can be differentiated to either macrophage-like or a neutrophil-like cell depending on the inducing agent. It is widely used as a model for neutrophils.) Of the heterotrimeric G proteins, the G_i family is represented by only two of its members, G_{i2} and G_{i3}, the two main pertussis-toxin substrates in these cells (Falloon et al., 1986; Murphy et al., 1987; Uhing et al., 1987; Goldsmith et al., 1988, Offermans et al., 1990). G_o is known to be absent (Murphy et al., 1987). Two new families of G proteins (G_q and G_{12} family) have been recently identified by cloning (Simon et al., 1991) and of these new families, a member of the G_q family (G_{16}) is specifically expressed in haematopoietic cells (Amatruda et al., 1991). The level of G_{16} is decreased when HL60 cells are induced to differentiate towards a neutrophil-like cell. The restricted expression of this G protein suggests that it may regulate cell-type specific signalling pathways, which are not inhibited by pertussis toxin. (G_{16} is not a substrate for pertussis toxin because it lacks the cysteine residue required for this modification.) In contrast to G_{16}, G_{i2} and G_{i3} levels increase when HL60 cells differentiate into a mature form (Falloon et al., 1986).

There are at least 25 distinct low molecular mass GTP-binding proteins in eukaryotic cells (Hall, 1990; Grand and Owen, 1991). These proteins are collectively referred to as belonging to the *ras* superfamily which are classified into three distinct subgroups, the *ras*, *rho* and *rab* families. The function of the *ras* and *rho* family is not clear (although there is much speculation) whilst many members of the *rab* family are clearly involved in vesicular traffic in the endocytic and exocytic pathway (Balch, 1990). In neutrophils, members of both the *ras* and *rho* families have been unambiguously identified (see Table 8.1). Rap1A, a *ras*-related protein, is a substrate for cAMP-dependent protein kinase in human neutrophils and may play a role in mediating the inhibitory effects of cAMP-elevating agents upon receptor-mediated cell activation (Quilliam et al., 1991). Both the secretory granules and the plasma membrane contain specific subsets of some of these G proteins (Dexter et al., 1990; Philips et al., 1991). Both Rac1 and Rac2 have recently been identified to be one of the three components required for the activation of the NADPH oxidase in a reconstitution system (Abo et al., 1991; Knaus et al., 1991). Since the NADPH oxidase has a specific role in phagocytic cells, this would imply that the small GTP-binding proteins may serve particular functions in individual cell types. Rac1 and Rac2 expression increases when HL60 cells are differentiated towards neutrophils (Didsbury et al., 1989) and indeed Rac2 appears to be restricted to cells of myeloid origin.

2.2 IDENTITY OF G PROTEINS THAT COUPLE RECEPTORS TO PLC

Two lines of evidence indicate that G_{i2}/G_{i3} are the two potential candidates for being G_p in these cells. The major pertussis toxin substrate in neutrophils and HL60 cells is a 40 kD protein identified immunologically as G_{i2} and is predominantly localized at the plasma membrane (Gierschik et al., 1986, 1987; Murphy et al., 1987; Uhing et al., 1987). The predominant G protein which is associated with the FMLP receptor was found to be G_{i2}. A more interesting approach to demonstrate this association was to use the ability of cholera toxin to ADP-ribosylate G_{i2} and G_{i3} but only in the presence of the agonist FMLP (Gierschik and Jacobs, 1987; Gierschik et al., 1989). This was used as evidence that the FMLP receptor specifically interacted with these two G proteins. The G_i family, transducin and G_s, have an arginine residue (at position-174 on transducin) which is subject to modification by cholera toxin. However, it appears that cholera toxin cannot access this site for ADP-ribosylation in G_i. If the G protein is activated by the ligand in the absence of GTP or GTP-γ-S, then the toxin gains access to the amino acid on the G protein and ADP-ribosylates it. This technique of receptor-dependent modification of a G protein permits the identification of which G protein associates with the receptor (Verghese et al., 1986; Gierschik and Jacobs, 1987). The use of a photoreactive GTP analogue provides further evidence that not only the FMLP receptor but also receptors for C5a and LTB$_4$ appear to interact with G_{i2} (Offermans et al., 1990).

Whilst the identity of the G protein(s) that are associated with the FMLP receptor is well-substantiated, that does not establish which G protein is responsible for activating PLC. It is generally assumed that G_{i2}/G_{i3} must be the candidate for activating the effector, PLC. As discussed later, it appears that PLD and PLA$_2$ (discussed in Sections 3 and 4) are also activated via a G protein by FMLP, and therefore assigning the right G protein to its target effector system may prove to be more difficult than originally thought.

Because the G protein is a substrate for pertussis toxin, an approach taken by Kikuchi et al. (1986) was to prepare membranes from pertussis toxin-pretreated cells and then add back individual G proteins to restore FMLP-stimulated PLC activation. (Pertussis toxin pretreatment ADP-ribosylates a cysteine residue four amino acids from the C-terminus present in some G proteins and this interrupts the activation of the G proteins by their receptors.) Exogenous G proteins prepared from rat brain (G_i and G_o) were tested for their ability to reconstitute the FMLP-stimulated PLC response. (The G_i preparation used was a mixture of G_{i1}, G_{i2} and G_{i3} as revealed by subsequent studies.) Both G_o and G_i were equipotent in restoring responsiveness. Because the stimulation by FMLP in membranes is small in comparison to intact or permeabilized cells, this approach may be more useful to apply in reconstitution systems employing exogenous phospholipases (see later). The availability of recombinant G proteins may allow the problem of purity to be circumvented as it is inevitable that purified G proteins from tissues may subsequently be proven to be contaminated by unknown G proteins.

Both G_i and G_o were equipotent in reconstituting the FMLP response in HL60 cells. It is now understood that HL60 cells/neutrophils lack G_o (Murphy *et al.*, 1987). But G_o has been reported to couple to PLC when stimulated with muscarinic receptors in brain and clearly has the potential to interact with PLC (Kroll *et al.*, 1991; Padrell *et al.*, 1991). In the light of these results with reconstitution experiments using purified G proteins, it becomes increasingly important to analyse the interaction of G proteins and their effectors in their natural plasma membrane environment as well. Also, the ratio of the individual G proteins to specific receptors and effectors may dictate which receptor and effector interacts with which G protein. The assignment of specific G proteins to specific effectors is especially highlighted with the observation that G_s, generally known to activate adenylate cyclase, can also activate PLC via the β-adrenergic receptor in turkey erythrocytes (Rooney *et al.*, 1991). G proteins can indeed be promiscuous (Asano *et al.*, 1984; Cerione *et al.*, 1985).

2.3 PLC REGULATION IN MEMBRANES VERSUS PERMEABILIZED CELLS

Two observations suggested that the studies on the regulation of PLC activity by receptors and G proteins in membrane preparations did not represent the complete picture. PLC activation by receptors or directly via G proteins in membrane preparations is small (Smith *et al.*, 1985; Kikuchi *et al.*, 1986, 1987; Smith *et al.*, 1986). The availability of permeabilized cell preparations made it possible to study PLC regulation by receptors and G proteins in an environment where the cytosolic components were still present (Stutchfield and Cockcroft, 1988). It appears that PLC activation in membrane preparations only represents a small fraction of the response that could be observed in permeabilized cell preparations (Cockcroft and Stutchfield, 1988a; Stutchfield and Cockcroft, 1991). The percentage of the inositol lipid hydrolysed in permeabilized cells is 10-fold greater than the response in membranes when PLC is activated by GTP-γ-S. However, the characteristics for membrane preparations and permeabilized preparations are remarkably similar otherwise, i.e. Ca^{2+} requirement and GTP-γ-S-dependence, etc. An identical picture is observed when receptor-mediated PLC activation is analysed. For example, FMLP-mediated PLC activation is 10 times better preserved in permeabilized cells in comparison to membrane preparations (Stutchfield and Cockcroft, 1991). To fully appreciate these results, it is necessary to digress a little to appreciate the problems of quantifying stimulation of PLC activity using the endogenous substrate.

In neutrophils or HL60 cells it has not been possible to show that exogenously added substrate can be hydrolysed by receptor/G-protein-activated PLC. Therefore, the majority of studies concerning the activation of PLC by G protein have been done using the endogenous substrate present in the membranes. To label the inositol-containing lipids, the cells are generally preincubated with [^{3}H]inositol. At least three inositol-containing lipids, PI, PI-4-P and PI-4,5-P_2, are found in the plasma membrane. The concentration of the phosphorylated derivatives of PI is controlled by two lipid kinases, PI kinase and PI-4-kinase (Cockcroft, 1986b; Pike and Arndt, 1988; Geny *et al.*, 1991), and as PIP_2 gets degraded by PLC, the pool is replenished by the kinases from PI *in situ*. Thus the substrate concentration cannot be controlled effectively when biological membranes are used. Even if the substrate concentration could be calculated minute by minute, concentration in the conventional sense is not a meaningful concept, since a biological membrane is essentially two dimensional. A more meaningful approach would be to quantify the amount of moles per unit area. This is technically difficult to achieve.

Therefore, how does one quantify the activity of the PLC under this situation. The substrate concentration is continually changing as more and more PI becomes phosphorylated but only when the equilibrium is altered by degradation of substrate by PLC. An approach that can be taken is to express the product formed (i.e. the total inositol phosphates) as a function of all three inositol lipids (PI + PIP + PIP_2). The drawback with this approach is that there may be separate pools of inositol lipids that are not available to the PLC. For example, inositol lipids are present in Golgi, lysosomes and secretory granules, where the function of the lipid may be quite different. Nonetheless, if the cells are prelabelled to equilibrium (only possible for HL60 cells but not neutrophils), then expressing the formation of labelled product as a function of the total inositol lipids does provide an approximate measure for comparing membrane preparations with permeabilized cells. Using this approach, it has been demonstrated that the amount of inositol lipids hydrolysed due to receptor- or G-protein-activation is 10-fold greater in permeabilized cells compared to membrane preparations (Cockcroft and Stutchfield, 1988a; Stutchfield and Cockcroft, 1991).

2.4 CA^{2+} DEPENDENCE OF PLC ACTIVATION

It is sufficiently clear that both activation of PLC by receptors or G proteins requires the presence of nanomolar levels of Ca^{2+}. Moreover, Ca^{2+}, when present at micromolar levels, *potentiates* the receptor-mediated stimulation of PLC (see Figure 8.7). Does Ca^{2+} alone stimulate PLC activation?

Early studies in membrane preparations had clearly indicated that Ca^{2+} in the micromolar range was ineffective at PLC activation (Cockcroft *et al.*, 1984; Cockcroft, 1986a). In contrast, when one examines the Ca^{2+} requirement for PLC activation in permeabilized HL60 cells, the results show that Ca^{2+} in the micromolar range is effective at stimulating PLC (Stutchfield and Cockcroft, 1988; Geny *et al.*, 1988). All the studies in permeabilized cells were done in the presence of MgATP, but the membrane studies were done in the absence of MgATP. It is, therefore, likely that the response to Ca^{2+}, observed in the presence of ATP, can be explained as an activation of PLC by the ATP receptor present on these cells (Dubyak *et al.*, 1988, Cockcroft and Stutchfield, 1989a, 1989b; Cowen *et al.*, 1990a; Merritt and Moores, 1991). Indeed, ATP (as well as UTP and ATP-γ-S) will stimulate PLC in the micromolar range when GTP is available in HL60 membranes (Cowen *et al.*, 1990b) This response is clearly receptor mediated. The presence of ATP receptors may complicate the interpretation of many of the studies where MgATP is routinely added for intracellular requirements.

2.5 ENZYMOLOGY OF PLC

From functional studies it is clear that a membrane-associated PLC is present, i.e. membranes are able to hydrolyse the endogenous polyphosphoinositides. The enzyme activity present in membranes does not discriminate between PIP and PIP$_2$ in that both are effectively hydrolysed (Cockcroft *et al.*, 1984; Cockcroft and Gomperts, 1985; Cockcroft, 1986a). In contrast, PI does not get hydrolysed at all.

Since the late 1970s much effort had gone into purifying PLC and studying the isolated enzyme *in vitro* (see Rhee *et al.*, 1989; Kritz *et al.*, 1990; Meldrum *et al.*, 1991; Rhee, 1991; Rhee and Choi, 1992; Cockcroft and Thomas, 1992, for recent reviews). The majority of PLC activity has been found to be localized in the cytosol with some activity in the membrane. The membrane activity can be stripped by using high ionic strength buffers indicating that PLC is not an integral membrane protein. Table 8.2 summarizes our current knowledge regarding PLC isozymes studied in a variety of tissues. PLCs fall into at least three families: PLC-γ(150 kD), β(148 kD) and δ(85 kD). These enzymes are separate gene products. Within each family there are subtypes; two members of the γ family have been identified, PLC-γ1 and PLC-γ2, the β family has three members, β1, β2 and β3, as does the δ family, δ1, δ2 and δ3.

Figure 8.3 compares the linear sequence of the cloned members of the PLC β, γ and δ families. Also included is the PLC sequence from *Drosophila* which shows strong sequence homology to the PLC-β family. What emerges is that there are only two regions of homology shared by the three families, designated X and Y. The X and Y regions comprise 150 and 240 amino acids, respectively

Table 8.2   Classification of PLC isozymes characterized from different tissues

Name	Size (kD)	Source (Reference)
β family		
β1	150–154	Brain (Katan *et al.*, 1988)
β2	134	HL60 cDNA (Kritz *et al.*, 1990)
β3	—	Fibroblast cDNA (Kritz *et al.*, 1990)
γ family		
γ1	145	Brain (Suh *et al.*, 1988)
γ2	146	HL60 (Emori *et al.*, 1989)
δ family		
δ1	85	Brain (Homma *et al.*, 1988)
δ2	85	Brain (Meldrum *et al.*, 1989)
δ3	84	Fibroblast cDNA (Kritz *et al.*, 1990)
δ or ε family ???		
ε	85	Brain (Thomas *et al.*, 1991)
ε	88	Brain (Rebecchi and Rosen, 1987)
ε	87	Liver (Fukui *et al.*, 1988)
α family		
α	70	Liver (Takenawa and Nagai, 1981)
α	65	Seminal vesicular gland (Hofmann and Majerus, 1982)
α	70	Thymocyte (Wang *et al.*, 1986)
α	62	Uterus (Bennett and Crooke, 1987)
α	61	Platelet (Banno *et al.*, 1988)

This is a representative selection of the PLC isozymes. For a more complete list, see Rhee and Choi (1992) and Cockcroft and Thomas (1992).

(Rhee *et al.*, 1991). The two domains are about 60% and 40% identical, respectively. These regions might constitute, separately or jointly, the catalytic domain. The PLC-γ isoform has been found to contain the *src* homology domains, SH2 and SH3. These domains govern protein–protein interactions; SH2 domain targets the molecule to tyrosine phosphorylated sequences present in other proteins (e.g. PDGF receptor) and the SH3 domain targets it to cytoskeletal components. These domains are found in a large number of unrelated proteins such as GAP, PI-3-kinase, tyrosine phosphatases and kinases (see Koch *et al.*, 1991, for review).

There are probably two other families whose sequences are not yet available, the PLC-α and PLC-ε. The presence of PLC-α is deduced from purification of PLCs having a molecular weight in the range of 60–70 kD, present in a wide variety of tissues including platelets, liver, etc. (Table 8.2). The presence of the PLC-ε family on the other hand is based on the knowledge that cytosols from several tissues contain a 85 kD PLC which is distinct from the δ family in terms of biochemical characteristics (Rebecchi and Rosen, 1987; Fukui *et al.*, 1988: Homma *et al.*, 1988; Thomas *et al.*, 1991). The main biochemical characteristic that distinguishes PLC-ε from PLC-δ family is the substrate specificity for the enzyme in an *in vitro* assay. Generally speaking, all the PLCs so far identified can use PI, PIP or PIP$_2$ when presented in an *in vitro*

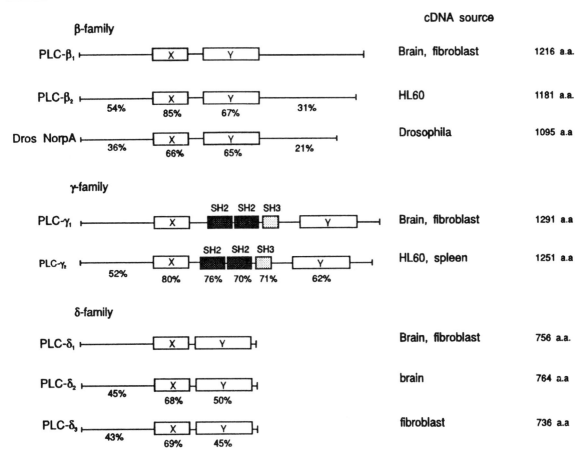

Figure 8.3 Linear representation of the members of the PLC-β, γ and δ families. Percentages reflect the degree of sequence identity within each PLC family. a.a., amino acids.

assay. PLC-ε appears not to utilize PI under most conditions, i.e. varying pH, Ca^{2+}, and including detergents.

Our knowledge of which PLC isozymes are present in phagocytic cells is limited but it is clear that both the β (β2) and γ (γ2) family are present in these cells based on cDNA analysis (Kritz et al., 1990). At the protein level, PLC-γ2 has been purified to homogeneity from spleen and its biochemical properties studied (Homma et al., 1990). That the HL60 or neutrophil cytosol contains inositol lipid hydrolysing activity is clear as assessed biochemically (Camps et al., 1990; Thomas et al., 1991). At least two peaks of PLC activity were found in differentiated HL60 cells (Camps et al., 1992). In an in vitro assay in the presence of detergents and 1 mM Ca^{2+}, one of these activities was specifically activated by βγ subunits of G proteins. Whether this activation is physiologically relevant is not clear because of the conditions of the assay. More importantly, βγ subunits of transducin were more potent than those prepared from bovine brain. In human neutrophils, we have also identified two peaks of PLC activity when the cytosol was fractionated on heparin sepharose (our unpublished observations).

The activity in the cytosol appears to be stimulated by GTP-γ-S in the absence of membranes only when the concentration of the protein is sufficiently high. The effect of GTP-γ-S was attributed to the activation of a soluble GTP-binding protein which relieved an inhibitory constraint from the PLC (Camps et al., 1990). This interpretation has to be accepted with caution since G proteins are generally tethered to membranes. Other studies have also demonstrated that a cytosolic PLC from platelets, brain and thymocytes could be activated by guanine nucleotides (Banno et al., 1986; Deckmyn et al., 1986; Baldassare et al., 1988). Baldassare et al. (1988) identified a 29 kD GTP-binding protein. On the other hand, it has been demonstrated that, in a different assay system, platelet-soluble PLC activity is non-specifically stimulated by several nucleotides (Rock and Jackowski, 1987; Sommermeyer et al., 1989). In a recent study, the GTP-γ-S-binding activity associated with the platelet cytosolic PLC was purified and was identified as an actin/gelsolin (1:1) complex (Banno et al., 1992). The obvious lesson to learn from here is that all effects of GTP-γ-S are not always mediated by G proteins. Clearly further studies need to be done to establish a role for soluble G proteins.

What is the role of these cytosolic enzymes in cell signalling? This question can now be answered with some confidence. The cytosolic PLCs are critical in cell signalling (Thomas *et al.*, 1991). They are recruited by the G protein from the cytosol. An approach that addressed this question specifically was to allow the endogenous cytosolic PLCs to exit from the cell after permeabilization with a cytolysin, streptolysin O, that makes lesions in the plasma membrane of 15 nm dimensions (Thomas *et al.*, 1991). Loss of enzymes such as lactate dehydrogenase occurs within 5 min after permeabilization is initiated (Stutchfield and Cockcroft, 1988). When PLC activation by GTP-γ-S is assessed at different times after permeabilization, the response to GTP-γ-S decays as the permeabilization interval is increased. The general idea was to allow the endogenous PLC to leak out of the cells and the time-course of this leakage should coincide with the loss of GTP-γ-S stimulated PLC. activity. The correspondence between these parameters is not exact. The exit of PLC from the cells is slower than the decay of GTP-γ-S-stimulated PLC. This is not surprising since it is likely that leakage of PLC measures all the isoforms of PLC whilst only some isoforms will be coupled to G proteins. A good example is the PLC-γ family which is regulated by tyrosine phosphorylation and not by G proteins (Ullrich and Schlessinger, 1990; Rhee, 1991).

2.6   WHICH PLC ISOFORMS ARE G-PROTEIN REGULATED?

The cytosol of cells contains PLC isoforms of which two isoforms have been identified to be G-protein-regulated. PLC-β1 has been shown to reconstitute in an *in vitro* assay with a purified G protein, G_q (Smrcka *et al.*, 1991; Taylor and Exton, 1991; Taylor *et al.*, 1991). Moreover, *in vivo*, endogenous G proteins from HL60 cells are also able to recruit exogenously added PLC-β1 (Thomas *et al.*, 1991). The G_q family of G proteins was identified both by protein purification as well as by cDNA analysis. The G_q family of G proteins was originally purified by Sternweis and his colleagues (Pang and Sternweis, 1989) and shown to reconstitute with an enriched preparation of PLC-β1 (Smrcka *et al.*, 1991) using an *in vitro* assay method. The partial amino-acid sequence was identical to that encoded by a cDNA designated α_q (Strathmann *et al.*, 1989; Strathmann and Simon, 1990; Simon *et al.*, 1991).

The G_q family comprises at least five G proteins, G_q, G_{11}, G_{14}, G_{15} and G_{16} (Simon *et al.*, 1991). G_q and G_{11}, which are 88% identical, are both capable of activating PLC (Blank *et al.*, 1991; Taylor and Exton, 1991; Wu *et al.*, 1992). These two G proteins are ubiquitously expressed (Strathmann *et al.*, 1989; Wilkie *et al.*, 1991; Mitchell *et al.*, 1991) and can selectively activate PLC-β1 but not PLC-γ1 or PLC-δ1 (Taylor *et al.*, 1991). More

recently, it was shown that α_q subunit (purified from a βγ-affinity gel) stimulates PLC-β1 but not PLC-β2 (Rhee and Choi, 1992). G_{14}, G_{15} and G_{16} are expressed in a tissue-restricted fashion and of these G proteins, G_{15} and G_{16} are specifically expressed in cells of the haematopoietic lineage (Amatruda *et al.*, 1991; Wilkie *et al.*, 1991) together with PLC-β2 (Kritz *et al.*, 1990). Not surprisingly, it was found that $G\alpha_{16}$ (and less effectively, $G\alpha_q$, $G\alpha_{11}$, $G\alpha_{14}$) when expressed in COS-7 cells was most effective in reconstituting with PLC-β2 (Rhee and Choi, 1992). Since in HL60 cells, G_{16} is specifically expressed as is PLC-β2, it follows that the pertussis toxin-insensitive response observed in neutrophils and HL60 cells may be a result of G_{16} regulating PLC-β2.

The receptors that interact with G_{16} in these cells have yet to be identified. The ATP receptor is one possible candidate. That different members of the G_q family activate PLC-β isoforms selectively provides ample room for subtle differences in activation characteristics. The mix and match approach of G proteins and PLCs provides a system which is extremely versatile, and can be easily tailored to the requirement of any particular cell.

In addition to the PLC-β family, a second PLC (designated PLC-ε) is also recruited by G-proteins in undifferentiated as well as differentiated HL60 cells (Thomas *et al.*, 1991). PLC-ε was identified in the following way. Rat brain cytosol was fractionated on heparin sepharose and three major peaks of PLC were observed. Peaks II and III were identified as containing PLC-γ1 and PLC-β1 + PLC-δ1 respectively by western blotting. The activity in Peak I was found to contain PLC of 86 kD. Of the three peaks of activity, Peak I was found to be activated in the presence of GTP-γ-S or FMLP when added back to HL60 cell "ghosts" (where the endogenous PLCs had been removed during pre-permeabilization). The nature of the G-proteins that interact with the PLC has yet to be identified. Also, it remains to be established whether PLC-ε type PLC is present in neutrophils and HL60 cells.

The cytosolic enzymes are clearly involved in signalling and therefore the recruitment of these enzymes by the activated G-protein residing in the membrane is of some interest. Mechanisms for recruiting molecules from the cytosol on receptor activation is known to occur after stimulation in a number of situations, and the elements that control interactions of cytoplasmic signalling proteins in some cases have been identified to be the SH2 and SH3 domains (*src* homology domains) (Koch *et al.*, 1991). The PDGF receptor when activated recruits a number of proteins including PLC-γ1, PI-3-kinase, $p21^{ras}$ GTPase-activating protein (GAP) and Src and Src-like tyrosine kinases (Ullrich and Schlessinger, 1990). This association is dependent on the presence of a Src homology region SH2. The SH2 domain is a sequence of ~ 100 amino acids and it is implicated in regulating protein–protein interactions. SH2 domains regulate protein–protein interactions by recognizing peptide sequences that encompass tyrosine phosphorylated sites.

Thus tyrosine phosphorylation of the PDGF receptor acts as a switch to induce high-affinity SH2 binding. Most of the SH2-containing proteins also possess a distinct motif of ~ 45 amino acids termed the SH3 domain. SH3-like sequences have been identified in a variety of proteins that comprise or associate with the cytoskeleton and membrane (Rodaway et al., 1990). SH2 and SH3 domains are not obligate partners and some proteins only contain SH3 domains. These include two neutrophil NADPH oxidase-associated proteins, p47 and p67 (Rodaway et al., 1990).

It is now apparent that PLA2 is also recruited to the membrane due to the presence of a Ca^{2+}-dependent translocation domain also found to be present in PKC, GAP and PLC-γ1 (Clark et al., 1991). Clearly, the SH2 domain and Ca^{2+}-dependent translocation domain hold the key to recruiting PLC-γ1 from the cytosol by the activated PDGF receptor. The docking protein that recognizes the presence of the Ca^{2+}-dependent translocation domain in PLC-γ1 or GAP is not yet known. Although the precise mechanism for recruiting PLCs by G proteins is not yet known, it could be envisaged that the activated G protein exposes a domain that can bind PLC-β or ε with high affinity. Although PLC-β, a G-protein-regulated PLC, has not been identified to contain either a Ca^{2+}-dependent translocation domain or an SH2 or SH3 domain, a possible mechanism for recruitment to the membrane may yet depend on Ca^{2+}. PLC-δ apparently has a single EF-hand Ca^{2+}-binding motif which may be involved in some form of Ca^{2+}-dependent regulation (Bairoch and Cox, 1990).

2.7 MEMBRANE-ASSOCIATED PHOSPHOLIPASE C

As indicated earlier, many of the PLs have been purified from the cytosol but since membrane preparations are responsive to GTP-γ-S- or Ca^{2+}-mediated stimulation of PLC, this makes it clear that there is a tightly associated membrane activity in many cells including neutrophils. The only PLC isoform that has been identified so far that is associated with membranes is PLC-β1. Membranes from brain contain PLC-β1 that is indistinguishable from its cytosolic counterpart. From the amino-acid sequence there is no indication of any regions that may be involved in membrane interactions. Since HL60 cells do contain a representative of the PLC-β family (PLC-β2) (Kritz et al., 1990), it would suggest that this enzyme may be responsible for the responses observed in membrane preparations. The observation that PLC-β can be tightly associated with membranes could be used to discover whether interaction with another protein is responsible for its membrane attachment. Does immunoprecipitation of PLC-β from membranes pull out an associated protein? The availability of PLC-β antibodies will certainly provide the tools for addressing these questions shortly.

If PLC-β2 is the isoform that is present in HL60 cell membranes as suggested above, then clearly the β isoform may be responsible for the stimulation observed by GTP-γ-S or FMLP in HL60 membranes. Since the FMLP response in membranes can be inhibited by pertussis toxin treatment, this would imply that PLC-β can couple to both pertussis toxin-sensitive and pertussis toxin-insensitive G proteins, i.e. G_q as well as the $G_{i/o}$ family. Identification of the PLCs in neutrophil membranes will help in addressing this issue.

2.8 ADDITIVITY OF PLC ACTIVATION BY DIFFERENT AGONISTS

An interesting observation pertains to the ability of different agonists on HL60 cells to stimulate PLC in an additive fashion (Stutchfield and Cockcroft, 1991). The response to FMLP and ATP in intact cells is additive at all concentrations of both agonists. Such additivity is also observed when permeabilized HL60 cells are stimulated with FMLP and GTP-γ-S either in the presence or absence of MgATP. GTP-γ-S should activate all the endogenous G proteins, and therefore, addition of an agonist (i.e. FMLP) should not provide a further stimulation. In the absence of MgATP, the stimulation by GTP-γ-S is small and that is not due to lack of the substrate, PIP2, since a further addition of FMLP stimulates a robust stimulation. This result indicates that the G protein coupled to the FMLP receptor cannot be activated by GTP-γ-S directly. This could arise if G proteins associated with receptors are present in a precoupled state in the membrane.

Such additivity could also arise if GTP-γ-S and FMLP stimulated different G proteins and also if they activated different isoforms of PLC. In the neutrophil/HL60, it is clear that both pertussis toxin-sensitive and -insensitive G proteins are coupled to PLC. In the case of PLCs, two isoforms have been shown to be regulated in a G-protein-dependent manner in HL60 cells (Thomas et al., 1991). There are other examples where distinct receptor-types can stimulate phosphoinositide hydrolysis in an additive manner (Ashkenazi et al., 1989; Raymond et al., 1991). This was shown to be due to distinct G proteins selectively coupling to different receptors in the same cell.

2.9 ACTIVATION OF G PROTEIN BY NUCLEOSIDE DIPHOSPHATE KINASE?

The accepted dogma, supported by abundant evidence, is that G proteins are activated by exchange of bound GDP for GTP, a reaction catalysed by the occupied receptor (Birnbaumer et al., 1990). An alternative means of activating G proteins is, theoretically, phosphorylation of bound GDP to GTP directly by NDP kinases with no intermediate exchange event. Evidence that the small GTP-binding proteins may be regulated by these means has been presented (Ohtsuki and Yokoyama, 1987;

Jakobs and Wieland, 1989; Randazzo *et al.*, 1991; Teng *et al.*, 1991). HL60 membranes also appear to exhibit NDP kinase activity (Seifert *et al.*, 1988). This has been demonstrated by incubating HL60 membranes with ATP-γ-S which leads to thiophosphorylation of the bound form of endogenous GDP to GTP-γ-S. Further studies will need to be done to clarify which pools of GDP serve as phosphate acceptors, i.e. little G proteins or the heterotrimeric G proteins. It is interesting to note that in permeabilized HL60 cells, activation of PLC by FMLP is not dependent on addition of exogenous GTP; the presence of ATP appears to be sufficient. The addition of micromolar levels of GTP appears to activate PLC independently of the FMLP response (Stutchfield and Cockcroft, 1991). This result supports the (heretical) concept that heterotrimeric G proteins can be regulated by either exchange or by phosphorylation of bound GDP by NDP kinase.

2.10 REGULATION OF PLC-γ FAMILY BY TYROSINE PHOSPHORYLATION

The regulation of PLC-γ family by tyrosine phosphorylation has been reviewed recently (Rhee, 1991). The first indication that tyrosine phosphorylation may regulate PLC activity came from the published sequence of PLC-γ1 (Stahl *et al.*, 1988). The predicted amino-acid sequence for the PLC derived from complementary DNA cloning revealed that it possessed regions homologous to the products of various tyrosine kinase-related oncogenes (*yes, src, fgr, abl, fps, fes, tck* and *crk*) (Mayer *et al.*, 1988; Stahl *et al.*, 1988; Suh *et al.*, 1988). The next significant finding was the demonstration that PLC-γ1 was a substrate for receptor protein-tyrosine kinases. Both EGF and PDGF receptors, when activated, could phosphorylate PLC-γ1 on tyrosine and serine residues both *in vivo* and *in vitro* (Margolis *et al.*, 1989; Meisenhelder *et al.*, 1989; Nishibe *et al.*, 1989; Wahl *et al.*, 1989). By virtue of being phosphorylated on tyrosine residues, phosphotyrosine antibodies could immunoprecipitate PLC-γ1 from EGF-activated A-431 cells (Wahl *et al.*, 1988). A physical association of PLC-γ1 with the PDGF and EGF receptor could also be demonstrated (Kumjian *et al.*, 1989, Nishibe *et al.*, 1990).

Four sites of tyrosine phosphorylation in PLC-γ1 have been identified. Purified EGF receptor phosphorylates tyrosine residues 771, 783, 1254 and to a lesser extent, tyrosine 472 (Kim *et al.*, 1990; Wahl *et al.*, 1990). The major sites of phosphorylation by EGF and PDGF receptors *in vivo* and *in vitro* appear to be identical (Meisenhelder *et al.*, 1989). Tyr-771 is adjacent to regions of PLC-γ1 that contain high homology to the non-catalytic, amino-terminal region of the *src* tyrosine kinase. Tyr-1254 lies near the carboxyl terminus of the PLC molecule. By site-directed mutagenesis, it was established that Tyr-783 and Tyr-1254 were essential for PLC-γ1 activation (Kim *et al.*, 1991). However, mutation at residues 771, 783 and 1254 does not change the catalytic activity of PLC-γ1 measured *in vitro* (Kim *et al.*, 1991).

PLC-γ2 appears to be present in abundance in haematopoietic cells (Emori *et al.*, 1989; Banno *et al.*,

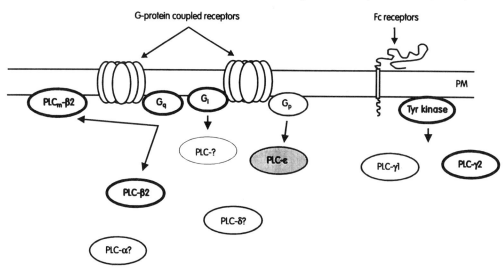

Figure 8.4 Differential regulation of PLC isoforms by G-protein-coupled receptors and Fc receptors.
G-protein-coupled receptors interact with specific G proteins to stimulate different isozymes of PLC. G_p denotes any G protein that activates a PLC (a functional definition). G_q and G_i denote defined G-protein families which are known to interact with either specific receptors (e.g. FMLP) or with specific PLC isoforms (e.g. PLC-β2). Fc receptors stimulate the PLC-γ1 and γ2 isoforms of PLC by interacting with a soluble tyrosine kinase of the *src* family. The molecular entities that are enclosed in heavy type are known to be present in neutrophils/HL60 cells. The other entities are possibilities that have to be substantiated. PLC-ε (shaded) indicates that this enzyme has been shown to reconstitute in HL60 cells.

SH3 domains as well as equivalents of tyrosine residues 771 and 783 of PLC-γ1 but not tyrosine residue 1254. Nonetheless, PLC-γ2 appears to be regulated in a similar manner to PLC-γ1. *In vivo*, PDGF stimulates tyrosine phosphorylation of PLC-γ2 when overexpressed in rat-2 cells (Sultzman *et al.*, 1991) or in NIH 3T3 fibroblasts (Totzke *et al.*, 1992). Although the PDGF receptor can phosphorylate PLC-γ2, it is unlikely to be the natural regulator of this enzyme. PDGF receptors are normally not found in haematopoietic cells where PLC-γ2 is specifically expressed. However, there are several candidate receptors that are either intrinsic tyrosine kinases or can activate *src*-related soluble tyrosine kinases expressed in haematopoietic cells whose activation could be linked to PLC-γ2 activation.

Cross-linking of Fc receptors for IgG (FcγRs) on neutrophils mediated by immune complexes, or opsonized antigen activates a multitude of biological functions, such as phagocytosis, degranulation and respiratory burst. Cross-linking of the FcγRI and FcγRII results in a rapid tyrosine phosphorylation of PLC-γ1 (Liao *et al.*, 1992). Because amino-acid sequence data indicate that FcγRI and FcγRII are not intrinsic tyrosine kinases, these receptors must be functionally coupled to soluble tyrosine kinases. As discussed above, human neutrophils do not contain PLC-γ1 in substantial amounts and therefore it is expected that PLC-γ2 may be the relevant PLC isoform that is regulated by the FcγRI and FcγRII in neutrophils. In U937 cells, a monocytic cell-line, it has been shown that PLC-γ1 is regulated by FcγRI and FcγRII (Liao *et al.*, 1992).

Figure 8.4 summarizes the mechanisms involved in the differential regulation of phospholipases by G-protein-coupled receptors and by Fc receptors in neutrophils/HL60 cells. The Fc receptors regulate soluble tyrosine kinase activity and this in turn phosphorylates the PLC-γ family, -γ1 and -γ2, depending on the availability of the specific isoform present in the cells. In neutrophils, the major isoform is expected to be PLC-γ2 but this has to be rigorously established. On the other hand, the G-protein-coupled receptors appear to activate G proteins possibly belonging to the G_i family as well as the G_q family. G_p is defined functionally as the G proteins that regulate PLC. G_p, is shown to activate an 86 kD PLC (PLC-ε) purified from brain cytosol. It remains to be established whether such an enzyme is actually present in neutrophils/HL60 cells. PLC-ε can also be activated by FMLP. The specific isoform of PLC regulated by the G_i family is not yet established. On the other hand, PLC-β2 isoform is expected to be regulated by a member of the G_q family, possibly G_{16}. Also shown in Figure 8.4 is the possible localization of the enzymes. Only PLC-β2 is expected to be present at the plasma membrane. Clearly a more detailed picture is beginning to emerge regarding the regulation of PLCs in these cells.

3. PHOSPHOLIPASE D

Phospholipase D catalyses the hydrolytic cleavage of the terminal phosphate diester bond of phosphatidylcholine with the formation of phosphatidic acid and the water-soluble headgroup, choline. PLD-catalysed hydrolysis might theoretically occur by cleavage of the P–O or C–O bond (see Figure 8.5). In an elegant study by Holbrook *et al.* (1991) evidence has now been presented that the reaction mechanism involves cleavage of the P–O bond. Using [^{18}O] water, ^{18}OH from H_2O is incorporated into PA, rather than into the headgroup. Also shown in Figure 8.5 is the ability of PLD to transfer the phosphatidyl portion of the PC molecule to ethanol. In this case, the product that is formed is the unusual lipid, phosphatidylethanol. This lipid is generally absent in cells. It is relatively stable in comparison to PA.

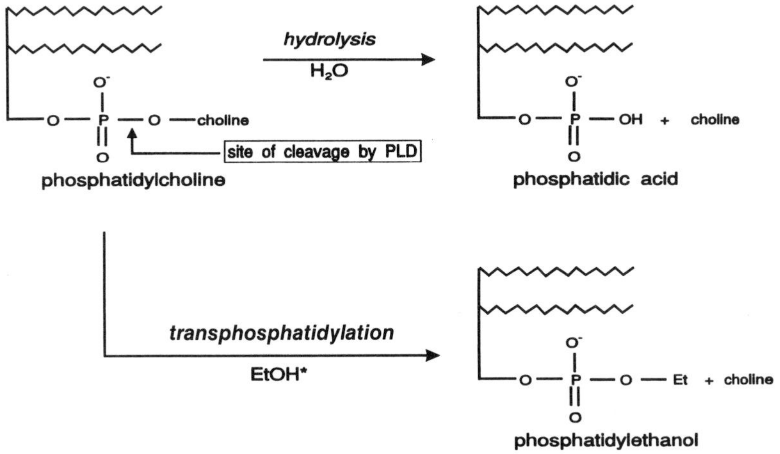

Figure 8.5 Hydrolysis of phosphatidylcholine by PLD action in the presence or absence of ethanol. PLD cleaves the -P–O- bond to release phosphatidate and choline. In the presence of ethanol, the phosphatidyl headgroup is transferred preferentially to the enthanol (rather than water) forming the unique lipid, phosphatidylethanol. *Other short chain alcohols can substitute for ethanol.

PLD was originally discovered in plants, where it is present in large amounts, and is also present in bacteria and fungi (Heller, 1978). The first indication that PLD may be present in mammalian tissues came from studies by Kanfer and his colleagues, and their interest in the enzyme was focused on the release of choline from PC as a source for acetylcholine synthesis (Chalifour and Kanfer, 1980; Hattori and Kanfer, 1984, 1985). The brain is unable to synthesize choline and is therefore dependent on recycling choline for acetylcholine synthesis.

Recent attention on PLD was engendered by the discovery of FMLP-stimulated activation in human neutrophils (Cockcroft, 1984). The evidence for PLD activation was derived from the observation that FMLP stimulated a rise in PA levels that was *not* derived by phosphorylation of diacylglycerol but was derived directly from a phospholipid. The initial product of PLC hydrolysis is DAG and this is rapidly converted to PA by DAG kinase-dependent phosphorylation with MgATP (Cockcroft *et al.*, 1980). Thus, in principal, in ^{32}P-labelled cells where the ATP pool is labelled to equilibrium, any new PA synthesized by the PLC route would have the same specific activity as ATP. Since the specific activity of ATP can be easily determined, changes in the radioactivity in PA could be used for converting the increase in radioactivity in PA into actual changes in mass. In such an experiment, where the specific activity of the PA and ATP were both measured, it was found that the specific activity of PA actually declined whilst the mass of PA increased sharply from 1.7 nmol to 10.7 nmol/10^8 human neutrophils within 20 s. The sharp decrease in specific activity could only occur if the bulk of the PA was derived directly from a preformed phospholipid, and not by phosphorylation with ATP; the only explanation for this PA was a product of PLD action (Cockcroft, 1984.)

The source of the PA was unidentified but, since a decline in phosphatidylinositol was also apparent, it was suggested that this phospholipid was the source of the PA (Cockcroft, 1984). (It is now clear that part of the decline in PI is accounted for by PLA$_2$-mediated hydrolysis.) The fatty-acid composition of the newly synthesized PA does not resemble that of inositol phospholipids implying another source for the PA; the fatty-acid composition resembles phosphatidylcholine closely (Cockcroft and Allan, 1984).

The stimulation of PA formation by FMLP is rapid. The increase in PA is only sustained for 20 s after which the level of PA declines slowly. At the peak of PA formation, 9 nmol of PA are produced/10^8 cells and this corresponds to a net hydrolysis of 2.8% of the total PC pool. There is a slow but steady conversion of the PA into diacylglycerol such that by 2 min nearly a third of the PA is metabolized. The enzyme, phosphatidate phosphohydrolase, is responsible for this conversion (Billah *et al.*, 1989a). DAG production shows a lag of 10 s and peak increases are observed at 5 min (Honeycutt and Niedel, 1986).

The initial rate of PA formation in intact neutrophils is calculated to be 27 nmol/min per 10^8 human neutrophils. This rate should be compared with the *in vitro* activity measured in various tissues including brain and HL60 cells. The specific activity of the brain homogenate is 8 pmol/min per mg protein (Taki and Kanfer, 1979; Kobayashi and Kanfer, 1991) and similar values were obtained for HL60 cells. Since 10^8 human neutrophils is equivalent to 6 mg of protein approximately, the activity observed *in receptor-stimulated cells* is approximately 4.5 nmol/min per mg protein. This activity is 500-fold greater than that observed in an *in vitro* assay. It is possible that the low specific activity of the enzyme observed in an *in vitro* assay is due to inappropriate assay conditions or to the presence of inhibitory factors. Attempts at purifying the particulate brain enzyme over the last decade have proved to be difficult and at best a 240-fold purification has been reported (Taki and Kanfer, 1979). PLD has also been identified in the cytosol of eosinophils, lung and brain (Kater *et al.*, 1976; Wang *et al.*, 1991) and purification from this source may prove to be easier. However, the reported specific activities are still much less than expected compared to the rates observed in intact cells.

Since the original discovery of receptor-mediated formation of PA in neutrophils (Cockcroft, 1984), the number of cell types where agonist-mediated activation of PLD has been demonstrated has increased dramatically (see Billah and Anthes, 1990; Exton, 1990; Shukla and Halenda, 1991; Liscovitch, 1991, for recent reviews). Not only do G-protein-coupled receptors such as muscarinic cholinergic receptors (Martinson *et al.*, 1989; Qian and Drewes, 1989; Pepitoni *et al.*, 1991. Sandmann *et al.*, 1991), angiotensin II receptors (Bocckino *et al.*, 1987; Lassegue *et al.*, 1991), bradykinin receptors (Martin and Michaelis, 1988) and ATP receptors (Bocckino *ey al.*, 1987; Martin and Michaelis, 1989), but also receptors that are tyrosine kinases (e.g. EGF and PDGF) (Bocckino *et al.*, 1987; Ben-Av and Liscovitch, 1989) stimulate PLD in intact cells. What is interesting about the cell types listed above is that the same agonists are also activators of PLC in those cell types (Shukla and Halenda, 1991). Moreover, in many of the cell types listed above, both the phorbol ester, PMA and the calcium ionophores are activators of PLD.

Of all the cell types, studies of PLD activation in intact neutrophils/HL60 cells have grown apace (Cockcroft, 1984; Pai *et al.*, 1988a; Agwu *et al.*, 1989; Billah *et al.*, 1989b; Bonser *et al.*, 1989, 1991; Randall *et al.*, 1990; Reinhold *et al.*, 1990; Kanaho *et al.*, 1991a, 1991b). Several techniques are currently in use for measuring PLD activation in intact cells, and many of them rely on prelabelling of the phospholipid with radiolabelled precursors and measuring product formation. Most of these studies do not provide any indication of the underlying mass changes. However, these techniques are simple to use and large numbers of samples can be processed.

3.1 SUBSTRATES FOR PLD

In the initial studies on PLD activation it was suggested that PI was a substrate for PLD. More recently, Balsinde *et al.* (1988a, 1989) have observed the presence of a cytosolic PI-specific PLD in human neutrophils. The specific activity of the enzyme was 0.65 nmol/min per mg protein and was stimulated two-fold by sodium deoxycholate. The enzyme required Ca^{2+} for activity. In the subsequent work by Billah and his colleagues, the cells were prelabelled only in the phosphatidylcholine pool and therefore the question of substrate specificity has not been formally addressed. [³H]Alkyl-lyso-PC was added to the cells and this readily enters the cells and is acylated rapidly into membrane-associated [³H]alkyl-PC (Pai *et al.*, 1988b). It is clear that [³H]alkyl-PC can be hydrolysed to form phosphatidate or phosphatidylethanol (if ethanol was also present). Transphosphatidylation in which the phosphatidyl group of the phospholipid is transferred to appropriate nucleophiles such as ethanol is a unique feature of PLD (Yang *et al.*, 1967; Benthin *et al.*, 1985). This is illustrated in Figure 8.5.

In human neutrophils, PC is equally distributed between ether- and ester-linkage at the *sn*-1 position (Agwu *et al.*, 1989). Both forms of PC appear to be degraded by PLD (Agwu *et al.*, 1989; Billah *et al.*, 1989a). More interestingly, the products (PA and PEt) show a similar distribution of ether- and ester-linkages to PC but not PE or PI. Thus, this forms the main basis for stating that the main substrate for PLD is PC. Clearly, the PC specificity for FMLP-stimulated PLD is determined not by the composition of the *sn*-1 bonds but by the nature of the phospholipid base. PLD activities from other sources including brain also prefer endogenous PC as substrate.

In some cell types, PC has been shown to be hydrolysed by a pathway to generate DAG and phosphorylcholine (Exton, 1990; Choudhury *et al.*, 1991). In neutrophils there is no evidence that PC can be metabolized by this route during FMLP-mediated stimulation (Truett *et al.*, 1989). However, the possibility that other agonists may activate a PC-specific PLC cannot be excluded.

3.2 ENZYMOLOGY OF PLD

PLD activity (assayed with an exogenous substrate in the presence or absence of detergents, etc.) has been found to be associated with either membranes (Chalifour and Kanfer, 1980; Martin, 1988; Chalifa *et al.*, 1990) or cytosol (Kater *et al.*, 1976; Wang *et al.*, 1991). As discussed before, attempts at purifying the membrane-associated PLD activity or the cytosolic PLD has been disappointing (Kater *et al.*, 1976; Kanoh *et al.*, 1991). In HL60 membranes the activity of PLD appears to be dependent on the presence of cytosolic components (Anthes *et al.*, 1991; Olson *et al.*, 1991). The reported specific activities from both cytosolic and membrane-

associated activities from brain are in the range of 16 pmol/min/mg protein (Kanoh *et al.*, 1991; Wang *et al.*, 1991), much lower than that observed in intact cells stimulated with FMLP which is 4.5 nmol/min/mg protein.

Although both membranes and cytosol contain PLD activity, it has been claimed that the bulk of the activity resides in the cytosol (Wang *et al.*, 1991). By gel filtration, the apparent molecular mass of the peaks of activity observed in the cytosol were found to have an apparent mass of 30 kD and 80 kD. It was suggested that the specific activities represented a single enzyme entity with varying extents of aggregation (Wang *et al.*, 1991). Clearly, the purification of the enzyme will be much simpler if the above is true.

Another approach to assessing the requirement for cytosolic components required for PLD is to study its regulation in permeabilized cells. Both electropermeabilization and streptolysin O-mediated permeabilization have been studied. Streptolysin O induces large lesions in the plasma membrane (15 nm) allowing the exit of cytosolic enzymes including LDH and PLC in a time-dependent manner (Stutchfield and Cockcroft, 1988; Thomas *et al.*, 1991). When GTP-γ-S is added to the permeabilized cells, PLD activation can be easily measured. However, the response to GTP-γ-S is diminished if the cells are permeabilized first and GTP-γ-S is added 30 min later (Xie and Dubyak, 1991; Geny and Cockcroft, 1992). A residual component of the response does remain after 30 min, i.e. after extensive loss of cytosolic components. This would suggest that a component of the response is very tightly associated with the membranes. This component is probably akin to the GTP-γ-S-stimulated PLD activity that has been demonstrated in membrane fractions in platelets (Van Der Meulen and Haslam, 1990), NIH 3T3 cells (Kiss and Anderson, 1990), liver (Hurst *et al.*, 1990) as well as cerebral cortex (Qian *et al.*, 1990).

Another approach to illustrate that cytosolic components are required for PLD activation is to reconstitute membranes with cytosol. Membrane fractions when combined with cytosol have been shown to reconstitute the GTP-γ-S-stimulated PLD activity (Anthes *et al.*, 1991; Olson *et al.*, 1991). Therefore, it is clear that the membrane system does not contain all the components and that cytosolic factors are recruited in a Ca^{2+} and/or G-protein-dependent manner and that these factors play a major role in obtaining the full PLD response (Geny and Cockcroft, 1992).

3.3 PHOSPHATIDATE PHOSPHOHYDROLASE

As early as 1985, two separate routes for the production of DAG could be recognized in the neutrophil (Cockcroft *et al.*, 1985). An early phase of DAG production was derived from the hydrolysis of PIP_2 by PLC and a second late phase derived from PA, which itself was generated by PLD action. DAG production is biphasic, the early phase occurs without a detectable lag, whilst the second phase has a lag of 20 s (Cockcroft et al., 1985, Billah et al., 1989a). The lag can be accounted for by the enzyme phosphatidate phosphohydrolase, to act on PA. A distinct isoform of phosphatidate phosphohydrolase that is localized in plasma membranes has been identified (Jamal et al., 1991; Aridor-Piterman et al., 1992) indicating that these reactions must be occurring at the plasma membrane. Propranolol has been widely used to inhibit this enzyme (Billah et al., 1989a) and at 250 μM, it causes the virtual inhibition of DAG accumulation stimulated by FMLP (Billah et al., 1989a), C5a (Mullman et al., 1990a) and PMA (Mullman et al., 1990b).

3.4 REGULATION OF PLD

From studies in intact cells it is clear that FMLP (Cockcroft, 1984; Pai et al., 1988a, 1988b; Billah et al., 1989a), C5a (Mullman et al., 1990a), ATP (Xie et al., 1991), PAF (Reinhold et al., 1990; Kanaho et al., 1991b), LTB$_4$ (Reinhold et al., 1990), C3b/bi and IgG-opsonized yeast particles (Bonser et al., 1991; Della Bianca et al., 1991) are all able to stimulate PLD activation as do Ca^{2+} ionophores (Cockcroft, 1984; Billah et al., 1989b; Della Bianca et al., 1991), PMA (Mullman et al., 1990b) and fluoride (English and Taylor, 1991; English et al., 1991). From studies in permeabilized cells, it is also clear that guanine nucleotides are potent activators of PLD (Xie and Dubyak, 1991; Geny and Cockcroft, 1992).

Activation of the PLD by GTP-γ-S in permeabilized cells can occur to a limited extent at 10 nM Ca^{2+} but is greatly enhanced in the presence of micromolar levels of Ca^{2+} (Xie and Dubyak, 1991; Geny and Cockcroft, 1992). This enhancement by Ca^{2+} suggests that this pathway may be strongly influenced by a prior activation of the PLC pathway. Activation of PLD by GTP-γ-S in permeabilized cells is potentiated by the presence of 1 mM MgATP (Xie and Dubyak, 1991; Geny and Cockcroft, 1992). Such a potentiation by MgATP has also been reported in neural-derived NG108-15 cells (Liscovitch and Eli, 1991). The mechanism of this potentiation is not clear but products of the PLC pathway can be excluded as well as an effect of ATP on its cell-surface receptor (Xie and Dubyak, 1991; Geny and Cockcroft, 1992).

Although PMA does stimulate PLD, it cannot totally substitute for GTP-γ-S in permeabilized cells. Indeed the effects of GTP-γ-S and PMA are synergistic (Geny and Cockcroft, 1992). It is now clear that one of the pathways stimulated by GTP-γ-S or FMLP is tyrosine phosphorylation (Kraft and Berkow, 1987; Huang et al., 1988; Gomez-Cambronero et al., 1991; Kusunoki et al., 1992; Uings et al., 1992). Tyrosine kinase inhibitors (e.g. erbstatin) are inhibitors of FMLP-, PAF- and LTB$_4$- but not PMA-induced activation of PLD in intact

neutrophils (Uings et al., 1992). Moreover, the phosphotyrosine phosphatase inhibitor, pervanadate, also increases tyrosine phosphorylation as well as PLD activation (Uings et al., 1992). These results suggest that tyrosine kinases may be responsible for PLD activation.

3.4.1 Synergistic Activation of PLD by Ca, PKC and G Proteins

As mentioned above, PLD can be activated by guanine nucleotides (Olson et al., 1991; Xie and Dubyak, 1991; Geny and Cockcroft, 1992). Since addition of guanine nucleotides into permeabilized HL60 cells also leads to a stimulation of phosphoinositide-specific PLC (Stutchfield and Cockcroft, 1988), it is of importance to establish whether PLD activation by guanine nucleotides is a consequence of a primary stimulation of PLC or whether the two events are independently activated. Three separate components of PLD regulation can be discerned: a direct G-protein activation, a PKC-mediated activation and a Ca^{2+}-triggered activation. When all the pathways are stimulated simultaneously, then synergistic activation of PLD occurs (Geny and Cockcroft, 1992).

The main evidence that supports the conclusion that GTP-γ-S, PKC and Ca^{2+} may directly regulate PLD can be summarized (Xie and Dubyak, 1991; Geny and Cockcroft, 1992) as follows.

(1) In metabolically inhibited cells, conditions in which PLC activation is virtually abolished, it is still possible to stimulate PLD activation with GTP-γ-S. This response is approximately 30% of the maximal response observed with GTP-γ-S in the presence of MgATP.

(2) Evidence for PKC-mediated activation of PLD is clearly illustrated by the observation that PMA is able to stimulate PLD activation but only in the presence of MgATP. This response is much slower in comparison to that observed with GTP-γ-S.

(3) Ca^{2+} alone in the micromolar range is able to stimulate PLD.

Although multiple regulation of PLD activity occurs, these pathways are interactive and synergize to provide the full activation of PLD. Pretreatment of intact cells with PMA prior to permeabilization with streptolysin O, reveals that GTP-γ-S requires less Ca^{2+} to activate PLD. In other words, PMA and therefore presumably PKC phosphorylates PLD (most likely) and that phosphorylation decreases the Ca^{2+} requirement for GTP-γ-S-stimulated PLD activation. PKC-mediated phosphorylation cannot totally explain the enhancement observed with MgATP discussed above since PMA pretreatment does not substitute for the enhancing effects of MgATP (Geny and Cockcroft, 1992). For this reason, it is likely that a separate event such as tyrosine phosphorylation may be of importance in the regulation of PLD. Clearly, the purification and availability of purified enzymes will allow the regulatory pathways to be elucidated.

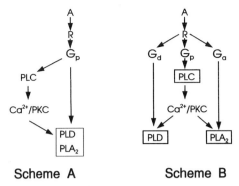

Figure 8.6 Two alternative schemes summarizing the regulatory pathways that control PLC, PLD and PLA₂ activation. In Scheme A, it is envisaged that a single G protein regulates all three phospholipases, and in Scheme B activation of the three phospholipases is controlled by three different G proteins. The primary event in both cases is PLC activation and the subsequent increase in cytosol Ca²⁺ and PKC activity in turn triggers PLD and PLA₂ downstream. Alternatively, the G protein(s) can also directly activate PLD and PLA₂. Synergistic activation of the downstream phospholipases can also occur owing to the simultaneous activation of a G protein, and an increase in Ca²⁺ and PKC activity. Gₚ, Gₐ and G_d are the G protein(s) that regulate PLC, PLA₂ and PLD, respectively. A, agonist; R, receptor.

GTP-γ-S will interact with the G protein regulating PLC in permeabilized cells as well as the G protein regulating PLD. The simultaneous activation of multiple components leads to a response which is greater than the response seen if each pathway is activated alone. A scheme that summarizes the regulatory pathways leading to PLD activation is presented in Figure 8.6. Two pathways for PLD activation can be identified – a direct G-protein regulated pathway and a Ca²⁺/PKC regulated pathway. This model encapsulates much of the available information we have about regulation of PLD in other cell types including neutrophils. These are *possible* regulatory pathways. What is not known for certain is which mechanism regulates the stimulation of PLD by receptors in *intact cells*. The stimulation of PLD by the receptor may be exclusively via the G protein. Such a possibility is suggested by the knowledge that putative inhibitors of the PKC pathway are not inhibitory to receptor-mediated PLD activation (Reinhold *et al.*, 1990).

3.4.2 Inhibition by cAMP

Agents which elevate cellular cAMP are known to inhibit certain aspects of human neutrophil activation such as secretion or the respiratory burst by receptor-linked agonists, e.g. FMLP (De Togni *et al.*, 1984; Mueller *et al.*, 1991). However, cAMP has little or no effect on FMLP-stimulated PLC activation in neutrophils (De Togni *et al.*, 1984) while it does inhibit FMLP-mediated

PLD activation (Agwu *et al.*, 1991; Tyagi *et al.*, 1991). Both the G protein and the PLD are potential targets. PMA-induced activation of PLD in not inhibited by cAMP (Agwu *et al.*, 1991; Tyagi *et al.*, 1991), but it is still possible that phosphorylation of PLD may inhibit the interaction of PLD with its G protein.

Activation of PLD by FMLP is short lived. This may be due to the rise in cAMP which is observed when neutrophils are activated by FMLP (Iannone *et al.*, 1989). The rise in cAMP is mediated by adenosine which is produced endogenously on cell activation (Iannone *et al.*, 1989). Adenosine is known to activate AC and cause an increase in cAMP levels. If adenosine is indeed responsible for the short-lived activation of PLD by FMLP in neutrophils, this could easily be tested by the addition of adenosine deaminase to remove any adenosine; preliminary studies have indicated that functional responses can be potentiated by the addition of this enzyme (Iannone *et al.*, 1989). This implies that the extent of PLD activation can directly affect the physiological output of the cell.

3.5 PHYSIOLOGICAL ROLE OF PLD

The physiological significance of PLD activation in cells is not apparent but its role is likely to be related to providing an intracellular signal for cell activation. This signal is most likely to be PA. In human neutrophils the mass of PA increases to a maximal value within 20 s from a basal level of 1.7 nmol/10^8 cells to 10.7 nmol (Cockcroft, 1984; Cockcroft and Allan, 1984). The time course for PA formation coincides with the time course of secretion from intact human neutrophils stimulated by FMLP. Abrogation of PA production by adding ethanol or butanol to intact cells leads to inhibition of exocytosis in many cell types: examples include secretion from mast cells (Gruchalla *et al.*, 1990; Lin *et al.*, 1991), platelets (Benistant and Rubin, 1990), neutrophils (Kanaho *et al.*, 1991b; Yuli *et al.*, 1982) and differentiated HL60 cells (Xie *et al.*, 1991). Moreover, generation of endogenous PA by adding exogenous PLD also stimulates physiological responses in many cell types including insulin release from islets (Metz and Dunlop, 1990) and aldosterone secretion from adrenal glomerulosa cells (Bollag *et al.*, 1990). It seems likely that PA plays a role as a second messenger and the identification of this function would aid in our understanding of cellular activation. One possibility that has been recently suggested is that PA may activate a protein kinase (Bocckino *et al.*, 1991).

Activation of NADPH oxidase by FMLP can be selectively inhibited by wortmannin as does PLD activation. Such a relationship implies that PLD-derived PA may be a necessary second messenger for activating the respiratory burst and exocytosis, but not for aggregation or adherence since the latter two responses are not affected by wortmannin (Reinhold *et al.*, 1990).

4. Phospholipase A_2 – Liberation of Arachidonic Acid

Many cell types, particularly neutrophils, release arachidonic acid specifically from their phospholipids on cell stimulation. Although the main function of AA is as a precursor for the biosynthesis of potent extracellular mediators, particularly prostaglandins and leukotrienes (collectively referred to as eicosanoids), it may also have a role to play as an intracellular second messenger. Despite the central function of intracellular PLA_2 in inflammatory processes, the identity of the enzyme responsible for AA release has only been recently characterized.

It is only in the last couple of years that serious attempts have been made at identifying the intracellular enzyme(s). Previous studies on PLA_2 had focused on the large class of closely related secretory phospholipases A_2 that are prevalent in digestive organs (e.g. pancreatic, snake venoms, and secretory granules of neutrophils and platelets) (Davidson and Dennis, 1990; Wright et al., 1990). Characteristic of their extracellular location, these secretory phospholipases A_2 contain seven disulphide bonds (Davidson and Dennis, 1990; Wery et al., 1991). This is of particular significance since the secretory phospholipases A_2 would be inactivated if they came into contact with the reducing environment of the cytosol. Moreover, the secretory phospholipases A_2 do not demonstrate any selectivity among the fatty acids in the sn-2 position of phospholipids. This lack of preference for phospholipids containing AA in the sn-2 position is noteworthy because it has been demonstrated that there is a PLA_2 activity that selectively cleaves arachidonyl PC to initiate eicosanoid and PAF production concomitantly in differentiated HL60 cells (Suga et al., 1990).

Many ligands that couple to GTP-binding proteins or activate tyrosine kinases have been shown to stimulate PLA_2 activation (Margolis et al., 1988; Kajiyama et al., 1989; Axelrod, 1990; Narasimhan et al., 1990). Interestingly, many of the ligands that stimulate PLA_2 are also Ca^{2+}-mobilizing ligands. Where is the receptor-activated PLA_2 localized? It is unlikely that PLA_2 located within a secretory granule could be directly affected by phosphorylation or by changes in cytosolic calcium concentrations. Therefore, a cytosolic form of PLA_2 is a likely candidate to interact with the diverse regulatory systems that stimulate the release of AA and lyso-PAF.

PLA_2 has been identified in the cytosol of U937 (Diez and Mong, 1990; Clark et al., 1990a, 1991; Kramer et al., 1991), RAW 264.7 cells (Channon and Leslie, 1990; Leslie, 1991), rat brain (Yoshihara and Watanabe, 1990), kidney (Gronich et al., 1990) and platelets (Kim et al., 1991; Takayama et al., 1991). The molecular weight of the enzyme has been reported to be in the range of 90–110 kD by SDS-gel electrophoresis in most cases. The cDNA clone encoding for the U937 enzyme

has been isolated and from the amino-acid sequence, it is clear that it shares no homology with the secreted forms of PLA_2. Moreover, there is no evidence (as yet) to suggest that cytosolic PLA_2 belongs to a larger multigene family as is the case for PLC and PKC. The enzyme selectively hydrolyses arachidonic acid when a natural membrane is used as the source of substrate (Clark et al., 1991).

The most interesting feature of the cytosolic PLA_2 so far identified is its ability to associate with membranes when the Ca^{2+} concentration is increased above 300 nM (Channon and Leslie, 1990; Diez and Mong, 1990; Yoshihara and Watanabe, 1990). The ability of the enzyme to translocate to membranes in a Ca^{2+}-dependent manner appears to be due to a domain 45 amino acids long that delineates a Ca^{2+}-dependent phospholipid-binding motif. This motif is also present in PKC, GAP and PLC-γ1 (Clark et al., 1991). The biochemical features of this 110 kD PLA_2 strongly suggests that this enzyme may be the target for the hormonally stimulated PLA_2 activity responsible for mobilizing arachidonic acid in many cell types including neutrophils (Clark et al., 1990; Kramer et al., 1991).

As part of its arsenal required for the elimination of bacterial invaders, PLA_2 is also present in secretory granules of neutrophils. This granule-associated PLA_2 belongs to the Group II phospholipases A_2 having a molecular weight of 14 kD (Wright et al., 1990). Stimulated neutrophils also secrete PLA_2 during degranulation in response to chemotactic as well as phagocytic stimuli (Traynor and Authi, 1981; Balsinde et al., 1988b). PLA_2 activity has been studied in fractionated neutrophils by Balsinde et al. (1988b) and they report the presence of a neutral PLA_2 in a plasma membrane fraction. No evidence for a cytosolic activity was found in contrast to the study by Alonso et al. (1986). The presence of the 110 kD PLA_2 in U937 cells, brain, kidney, macrophage cell line RAW 264.7 and platelets would strongly suggest that this enzyme is ubiquitous, and is therefore likely to also be present in neutrophils/HL60 cells.

4.1 SUBSTRATES FOR PHOSPHOLIPASE A_2

The major stores of arachidonic acid in mammalian cells are esterified at the sn-2 position of glycerophospholipids (Chilton and Murphy, 1986; Chilton, 1991). PLA_2 directly cleaves AA from the sn-2 position of the phospholipid releasing the corresponding lyso-phospholipid. In neutrophils, the predominant pools of endogenous arachidonate are distributed between PE (60%), PC (18%) and PI (18%). In contrast to the endogenous distribution of arachidonate, when cells are labelled with exogenous [^{3}H]arachidonate, the label is distributed primarily between PI (30%), PC (13%), PE (2%) and triglycerides (55%) (Chilton, 1991). Since the majority of studies concerning PLA$_2$ activation has been done in cells which have been prelabelled with radioactive arachidonate, the relative contribution by the different phospholipids is not known, for certain, for a receptor-directed agonist. Studies with labelled cells indicate that PC and PI are two sources. The formation of glycerophosphoinositol has been used to establish that PI is also a substrate for PLA$_2$ (Cockcroft and Stutchfield, 1989a; Nielson et al., 1991). Glycerophosphoinositol is derived from lyso-PI, the initial product of PLA$_2$-mediated hydrolysis of PI. Since PE is poorly labelled, it is not possible to exclude that as a potential source. The main conclusion to be drawn from these observations is that the enzyme does not appear to be specific for the phospholipid headgroup and that the specificity resides in cleaving AA.

4.2 REGULATION OF PHOSPHOLIPASE A$_2$

From studies in intact neutrophils, FMLP-mediated release of AA occurs within seconds and is sensitive to inhibition by pertussis toxin pretreatment (Okajima and Ui, 1984; Wynkoop et al., 1986; Tao et al., 1989). Early studies had indicated that Ca^{2+}/DAG may be the main regulators of PLA$_2$ (Volpi et al., 1985; Billah and Siegel, 1987), both products of the PLC pathway. More recent evidence suggests that enzyme activation may be under G-protein control in neutrophils and differentiated HL60 cells (Nakashima et al., 1988; Cockcroft, 1991; Cockcroft et al., 1991; Nielson et al., 1991) as in many other cell-types (Axelrod, 1990; Cockcroft et al., 1991).

The main evidence which indicates that FMLP may stimulate the release of AA in a G-protein-dependent manner can be summarized as below.

(1) GTP analogues, GTP-γ-S, GppNHp and GppCH$_2$p are potent activators of PLA$_2$ in permeabilized neutrophils and HL60 cells (Cockcroft, 1991; Cockcroft et al., 1991; Nielson et al., 1991).

(2) Fluoride, an activator of G-proteins, also stimulates AA release in intact or permeabilized cells (Bokoch and Gilman, 1984; Nakashima et al., 1988; Cockcroft et al., 1991).

(3) Synergistic activation of PLA$_2$ is observed when FMLP and GTP-γ-S are added together (Nakashima et al., 1988; Cockcroft, 1991).

Because GTP analogues and fluoride are potent activators of PLC in permeabilized cells (Geny et al., 1988; Stutchfield and Cockcroft, 1988), products of the PLC pathway will also be generated. It is therefore essential to establish that the activation of PLA$_2$ by GTP-γ-S is not a consequence of a rise in Ca^{2+} mediated by IP$_3$ and DAG-mediated PKC activation. Of course, in studies with permeabilized cells, Ca^{2+} is usually buffered with EGTA, and this would buffer any changes in Ca^{2+}. However, DAG would be effective at stimulating PKC. Since MgATP is generally required for both protein and

lipid phosphorylation, conditions where the activation of PLC is suppressed is easily achieved by ATP removal. In the absence of MgATP, it is still possible to observe PLA$_2$ activation by FMLP and GTP-γ-S in human neutrophils as well as in differentiated HL60 cells (Cockcroft, 1991; Nielson et al., 1991).

The G protein responsible for coupling the FMLP receptor to PLA$_2$ has yet to be identified. Despite the observation that pertussis toxin pretreatment is inhibitory to the release of AA by FMLP, ATP, etc. in intact cells, it does not necessarily follow that the G protein is pertussis toxin-sensitive. The activation of PLA$_2$ is dependent on the rise in [Ca^{2+}]$_i$ and this occurs via PLC, which may be coupled to the receptor by a pertussis toxin-sensitive G protein. Assays utilizing purified PLA$_2$ and G proteins will have to be done to establish the nature of the G protein. Alternatively, reconstitution with purified PLA$_2$ in native membranes where the endogenous G proteins are still present will be another way of addressing this question. What is emerging from studies in other cell types where PLA$_2$ has been shown to be regulated by a G protein (see Table 8.3) is that PLA$_2$ activation appears to be pertussis toxin-sensitive in many instances, but not necessarily PLC. This would imply that the G$_i$/G$_o$ family as well as another G-protein family which is pertussis toxin-insensitive must be involved in regulating PLA$_2$.

An interesting observation about the studies in permeabilized cells is the dependence on Ca^{2+} for GTP-γ-S- as well as FMLP-stimulated PLA$_2$ activity (Nakashima et al., 1988; Cockcroft, 1991; Nielson et al., 1991). For PLA$_2$ to obtain access to its substrate, the enzyme has to translocate from the cytosol to the membranes. This translocation is dependent on Ca^{2+} concentration. Between 300 nM and 10 μM Ca^{2+} is required for translocation (Clark et al., 1991). Activation by G proteins may be secondary to this translocation. Ca^{2+} per se is only a weak activator of PLA$_2$ in permeabilized cells. In the presence of FMLP, AA release is stimulated providing that Ca^{2+} is also present between 1 and 10 μM. In the combined presence of GTP-γ-S and FMLP, a significant release of AA is observed when Ca^{2+} is present at 1 μM.

That Ca^{2+} alone cannot be the trigger for PLA$_2$ activation in neutrophils was already expected from previous studies in intact cells (Cockcroft and Stutchfield, 1989a). Under conditions where [Ca^{2+}]$_i$ is elevated with a physiological stimulus (e.g. ATP or UTP), AA release is not always observed (Cockcroft and Stutchfield, 1989a; Tao et al., 1989). The neutrophil has a novel purinergic receptor which responds to ATP, ATP-γ-S, UTP and inosine triphosphate (ITP) (Cockcroft and Stutchfield, 1989a). Although all four of these agonists can cause a rise in cytosol Ca^{2+} to an equal extent, the ability of the individual nucleotides to stimulate PLA$_2$ is variable. Comparison between FMLP and ATP is even more interesting. Despite a similar rise in cytosol Ca^{2+} induced by either agonist, PLA$_2$ activation is markedly different.

Table 8.3   Systems where it has been shown that phospholipase A$_2$ can be regulated by a G protein

Cell type	Agonist	Reference
Mast cells	GTP-γ-S	Churcher et al. (1990)
RBL cells	GTP-γ-S antigen	Narasimhan et al. (1990)
Neutrophils	GTP-γ-S	Nakashima et al. (1988)
	FMLP	Cockcroft (1991)
	Fluoride	Bokoch and Gilman (1984)
HL60 cells	GTP-γ-S	Nielson et al. (1991)
(diff.)	FMLP	
FRTL-5 cells	Adrenaline	Burch et al. (1986)
	GTP-γ-S	
Fibroblasts	Bradykinin	Burch and Axelrod (1987)
	GTP-γ-S	
	Mastoparan	Gil et al. (1991)
Rod outer segments	Light	Jeselma (1987)
	β-subunits	Jeselma and Axelrod (1987)
Aplysia neurones	FMRF-amide	Volterra and Siegelbaum (1988)
	GTP-γ-S	
Platelets	H$_1$-histamine	Murayama et al. (1990)
	GTP-γ-S	Kajiyama et al. (1989)
	Fluoride	Silk et al. (1989)
Mesangial cells	LPS	Wang et al. (1988)

In all these cell types the receptor-mediated PLA$_2$ stimulation can be inhibited by pertussis toxin pretreatment indicating that the G protein involved belongs to the G$_{i/o}$ family in all cases.

FMLP stimulates a strong PLA$_2$ response in comparison to ATP (Cockcroft and Strutchfield, 1989a).

In human neutrophils, ATP-γ-S is equally potent at stimulating secretion as FMLP but is not as good at releasing AA. Clearly, the extent of activation of PLA$_2$ is not a function of the peak increases in cytosol Ca^{2+} and other controlling factors regulate the degree of PLA$_2$ activation by agonists.

The evidence that PLA$_2$ is activated by receptors via a G protein [designated G$_a$ (Burch et al., 1986)] and is not a direct consequence of the products of PLC activation is now substantial. However, Ca^{2+} is of major importance in allowing the PLA$_2$ to translocate to the membrane. This would mean that a rise in cytosol Ca^{2+} is an obligatory feature of this transmembrane signalling system and puts it downstream to PLC activation, one of the key events that regulates Ca^{2+} mobilization.

4.3   SECOND MESSENGER ROLE FOR ARACHIDONATE

What does AA do in neutrophils? Apart from it being the substrate for the lipoxygenase for the synthesis of leukotrienes, arachidonate appears to have a modulatory role in exocytosis (Cockcroft and Stutchfield, 1989a; Cockcroft, 1991) as well as activation and maintenance of the NADPH oxidase activity (Seifert et al., 1986; Henderson et al., 1989). Whilst the precise site of action of AA within neutrophils remains to be delineated,

activation of a subtype of PKC (γ-form) has been suggested (Shearman et al., 1989). However, the γ-subspecies is only expressed in central nervous tissues and is absent in neutrophils (Shearman et al., 1989).

5.   Inter-relationship Between the Three Phospholipases

FMLP can stimulate the activation of three phospholipases in intact neutrophils and studies on the regulation of the individual phospholipases reveal that all three lipases may be under the regulation of G proteins. Are the three lipases independently activated or is there a hierarchy of activation in the signalling pathway? Temporal studies do not readily permit one to discern the primary signals from secondary signals (Thompson et al., 1990). The Ca^{2+} dependence provides some indication of a hierarchy. Figure 8.7 illustrates the activation of the three phospholipases as well as exocytosis stimulated by GTP-γ-S in permeabilized HL60 cells. Of the three phospholipases, PI-PLC and PLD activation are clearly apparent at pCa 7. Activation of PLA$_2$ is only significant at Ca^{2+} levels above 300 nM. We can thus eliminate PLA$_2$ activation as a primary signal and are concerned with the inter-dependence of PLC and PLD.

MgATP has been used to distinguish the interdependence of PLD and PLC. In the absence of MgATP, PLC activation can be totally suppressed but PLD activation is still clearly stimulated by GTP-γ-S in permeabilized HL60 cells. From this, it is clear that PLD and PLC are independently regulated by G proteins. However, Ca^{2+} in the micromolar range greatly enhances the response. Obviously in intact cells, the rise in cytosol Ca^{2+} due to the activation of PLC, will amplify the PLD signal. This indicates a hierarchy of phospholipase activation. The primary event is PLC followed by PLD and PLA2.

In neutrophils/HL60 cells CB is known to enhance many of the physiological responses whilst inhibiting others (Honeycutt and Niedel, 1986). Both the secretory response and the respiratory burst are potentiated if intact cells are pretreated with CB. The basis of the action of CB is ill-understood but is most likely to do with the cytoskeletal network. The granules can get complete access to the plasma membrane when CB is present. (In permeabilized cell preparations, there is no need for CB.)

CB has been used to distinguish between events that are directly coupled to the receptor and events that occur downstream (Bennett *et al.*, 1980). For example, CB does not potentiate PLC activation, clearly establishing this event to be upstream to events that are potentiated by CB. In contrast, both PLD and PLA2 activation are substantially potentiated by CB (Honeycutt and Niedel, 1986; Billah *et al.*, 1989a). This again puts PLD and PLA2 activation downstream to PLC.

Although PLD and PLA2 activation are downstream to PLC activation, nonetheless the coupling of the individual phospholipases to the receptor appears to be an independent event. Does a single G protein mediate all three events, or are multiple G proteins involved? For FMLP to activate the three phospholipases independently via G proteins, the agonist should also be able to activate multiple G proteins. A single FMLP-occupied receptor is capable of catalysing the binding of labelled GTP-γ-S, and thus the activation of, up to 20 G proteins in native HL60 plasma membranes (Gierschik *et al.*, 1991). Thus the potential for individual G proteins to activate the three phospholipases independently is there.

Pertussis toxin is widely used to assess the involvement of the G_i family in signal transduction. Although pertussis toxin can inhibit all three lipases when stimulated in the intact cell, the inhibition of PLD and PLA2 may only reflect the fact that the G protein coupling the FMLP receptor to PLC is pertussis toxin-sensitive, but not the G-proteins coupling PLD and PLA2. An implication of this observation is that there is an obligatory requirement for PLC activation before PLD or PLA2 can be activated.

Figure 8.6 provides two alternative schemes regarding the control of the three phospholipases by an agonist. Either a single G protein regulates all three phospholipases (Scheme A) or specific G proteins regulate the individual phospholipases (Scheme B). In this case G_p regulates PLC, G_a regulates PLA2 and G_d regulates PLD. In all these cases the putative G protein needs to be identified definitively. Model B is our preferred model since it fits better with many of the observations regarding phospholipase activation in both intact and permeabilized cells.

6. Activation by FMLP of Phosphatidylinositol-3-kinase

In addition to the stimulation of the three phospholipases, FMLP also stimulates the phosphorylation of inositol-containing lipids, PI, PI-4-P and PI-4,5-P2 at the 3-hydroxyl position on the inositol ring to form PI-3-P, PI-3,4-P2 and PI-3,4,5-P3 (Traynor-Kaplan *et al.*, 1989; Stephens *et al.*, 1991). The enzyme responsible for this phosphorylation is PI-3-kinase, an enzyme that appears to utilize all three inositol lipids in an *in vitro* assay. Like PLC, its cellular target is not clear but has been suggested to be PI-4,5-P2. Purified PI-3-kinase from bovine brain is a heterodimeric complex that contains 85 kD and 110 kD proteins. The purified p85 subunit has no detectable PI-3-kinase activity, but associates tightly to PDGF receptor tyrosine kinase by virtue of possessing SH2 domains (these domains regulate protein–protein interactions by recognizing peptide sequences that encompass tyrosine phosphorylation sites (Escobedo *et al.*, 1991; Koch *et al.*, 1991; Otsu *et al.*, 1991; Skolnik *et al.*, 1991)). This suggests that p85 may be a regulatory subunit responsible for binding to tyrosine kinases, whereas p110 is probably the catalytic element.

Since receptor-mediated activation of neutrophils leads to tyrosine phosphorylation of several proteins (Gomez-Cambronero *et al.*, 1991), it is conceivable that the mode of activation of PI-3-kinase in neutrophils is similar to that described for growth factors discussed above. The most prominent proteins that are tyrosine phosphorylated are p41, p54, p66, p104 and p116. How do G-protein-coupled receptors stimulate tyrosine phosphorylation? Either activation of a tyrosine kinase or inhibition of tyrosine phosphatase will potentially lead to the accumulation of tyrosine-phosphorylated proteins. Tyrosine phosphorylation can be partially inhibited in pertussis toxin-treated neutrophils (Huang *et al.*, 1988) and since GTP-γ-S is also able to induce tyrosine phosphorylation in permeabilized neutrophils (Nasmith *et al.*, 1989; Grinstein and Furuya, 1991), it is likely that tyrosine phosphorylation is downstream to PLC activation. Moreover, it is also enhanced by CB (Huang *et al.*, 1988). It is most likely that soluble tyrosine kinases belonging to the *src* family are involved. Partial characterization of tyrosine kinase and phosphotyrosine phosphatase activity in neutrophils has been reported (Berkow *et al.*, 1989; Badwey *et al.*, 1991).

On stimulation with FMLP or A23187, translocation of CD45, a tyrosine phosphatase, has been shown to occur in neutrophils and differentiated HL60 cells (Lacal *et al.*, 1988; Caldwell *et al.*, 1991) and could be partially responsible for the accumulation of tyrosine-phosphorylated proteins.

7. Control of Functional Responses by Phospholipase-derived Second Messengers

Considering that FMLP can stimulate at least five intracellular signalling systems, the three lipases, PI-3-kinase and tyrosine phosphorylation, the question that follows is that which of these signalling pathways are important for the various functions of the neutrophil. The neutrophil responds in a complex fashion. The main functional responses that this cell can orchestrate are chemotaxis, cell–cell interactions, adherence, phago-cytosis, exocytosis and the oxidative burst. How do these multiple signalling pathways regulate any of these responses? Two of the functional responses that have been intensively studied in the recent years are exocytosis and the activation of NADPH oxidase.

Before we consider in detail any relationship between intracellular signals and functional responses, it should be understood that the relationship between the level of the second messenger and the output response does not have to be linear. In other words, the generation of the second messenger may increase as more catalytic units are recruited but the output signal may saturate when only a fraction of second messenger molecules are available. Two of the neutrophil functions where our under-standing has increased in the last few years is exocytosis and the respiratory burst. Progress in these two areas has occurred mainly because of availability of cell-free and permeabilized cell systems where the intracellular machinery can be probed without any constraint due to the plasma membrane.

7.1 NADPH OXIDASE

Phagocytic white blood cells produce a substantial amount of superoxide, and the enzyme complex respon-sible for converting O_2 into O_2^- contains several com-ponents including a low-potential b-type cytochrome which is also a flavoprotein, a 67 kD protein, a 47 kD phosphoprotein and a small GTP-binding protein, Rac1 associated with the GDP-dissociation inhibitor, Rho-GDI (Clark et al., 1990b; Abo et al., 1991; Heyworth et al., 1991) (see Chapter 3). In unstimulated cells the oxidase system is dormant and dissociated, with components residing in both cytosol and the membrane. Upon stimu-lation, there is a translocation of the soluble components to the membrane where the active oxidase is assembled (Clark et al., 1990b; Teahan et al., 1990; Heyworth et al., 1991). Phosphorylation of the 47 kD protein is closely associated with the activation process (Segal et al.,

1985; Heyworth and Segal, 1986; Heyworth et al., 1989; Lomax et al., 1989).

The 47 kD protein is phosphorylated when neutrophils are stimulated by a wide range of agents including PMA and FMLP. The kinetics of NADPH oxidase activation correspond well with the kinetics of phosphorylation of this protein. In cell-free systems it is possible to recon-stitute the NADPH oxidase by providing membranes, cytosolic protein factors, Mg^{2+} and an anionic lipid (e.g. SDS, fatty acids, phosphatidate) (Ligati et al., 1989; Aharoni and Pick, 1990). Phosphatidate is more effective at low concentrations than AA in triggering this system (Bellavite et al., 1988). In these cell-free systems, super-oxide production is potentiated by GTP or GTP-γ-S (Seifert et al., 1986; Ligati et al., 1989; Aharoni and Pick, 1990). This observation has led to the speculation that a G protein might be involved in the activation of neutrophil NADPH oxidase by AA or SDS under cell-free conditions.

The principal evidence in support of G-protein parti-cipation in the activation of the NADPH oxidase is the following: non-hydrolysable analogues of GTP and fluoride enhanced oxidase activation by arachidonate in cell-free systems which is inhibitable by GDP-β-S (Seifert et al., 1986; Gabig et al., 1987; Doussiere et al., 1988. Seifert et al., 1988; Ligati et al., 1989; Aharoni and Pick, 1990; Lu and Grinstein, 1990). The G protein proposed to participate was reported to be insensitive to both pertussis and cholera toxins (Gabig et al., 1987).

The cytochrome b_{245} of the oxidase system has been found to be associated with a membrane-bound small GTP-binding protein, p21^{rap1}, with which it co-purifies and cross-immunoprecipitates (Quinn et al., 1989). The proposed involvement of Rap1 in the oxidase was purely dependent on its association with the cytochrome b and did not include functional studies. More recently, a new cytosolic factor that is required for the stimulation of the oxidase in the cell-free system has been identified (Abo et al., 1991). This factor was identified to be a small GTP-binding protein, Rac1. Rac1 co-purified with the GDP-dissociation inhibitor, RhoGDI. Recombinant Rac1 could substitute for the purified Rac1 in the cell-free system confirming the functional requirement for this protein. Interestingly, Rac1 was only active provided that it was liganded to GTP-γ-S (Abo et al., 1991). Like Rac1, Rac2 can also regulate the NADPH oxidase in a cell-free activation system (Knaus et al., 1991). Interestingly, Rac2 mRNA is expressed only in cells of myeloid origin and has been found to increase 7–9-fold when HL60 cells are induced to differentiate with dibutyryl cAMP (Didsbury et al., 1989). Clearly, these results are con-sistent with the considerable body of evidence in support of the involvement of a GTP-binding protein in the cell-free system.

In the intact neutrophils, what drives the recruitment of the cytosolic components to the membrane to form the active complex of NADPH oxidase? From studies utilizing pharmacological tools, it is clear that curtailment of either PLA₂ or PLD activity is inhibitory to superoxide production upon stimulation by FMLP (Kusunoki *et al.*, 1992). Clearly then, one of the products, i.e. PA or AA, may be required for activation. In the cell-free system both support the activity of the NADPH oxidase. Is tyrosine- or PKC-mediated phosphorylation essential? There are many questions that still need to be answered before the intracellular machinery that *triggers* the activation of the NADPH oxidase can be fully understood.

7.2 EXOCYTOSIS

Unlike the NADPH oxidase system, no cell-free system is as yet available to study the components that make up the secretory system. However, the use of permeabilized cell systems has opened the way for the identification of intracellular effectors that regulate exocytosis (Barrowman *et al.*, 1986, 1987; Smolen and Stoehr, 1986; Smolen

et al., 1986; Stutchfield and Cockcroft, 1988; Cockcroft, 1991; Smolen *et al.*, 1991). Neutrophils contain at least two kinds of secretory granules whose release may be controlled by different mechanisms (Barrowman *et al.*, 1987; Smolen *et al.*, 1991).

Since the FMLP receptor is a G-protein-coupled receptor, it is not surprising that addition of GTP-γ-S to permeabilized neutrophils/HL60 cells induces secretion (Figure 8.7). Secretion induced by GTP-γ-S requires Ca²⁺ in the micromolar range and MgATP for optimal secretion (Stutchfield and Cockcroft, 1988; Cockcroft, 1991). Under these conditions, GTP-γ-S will stimulate PLC, PLD and PLA₂ activation maximally (Figure 8.7). PLA₂ activation by GTP-γ-S only occurs in neutrophils/differentiated HL60 cells and not in undifferentiated HL60 cells. Nonetheless, undifferentiated HL60 cells will release their secretory contents when GTP-γ-S is added to permeabilized cells (Stutchfield and Cockcroft, 1988). This eliminates products of the PLA₂ pathway from being essential for the exocytotic event. It does not,

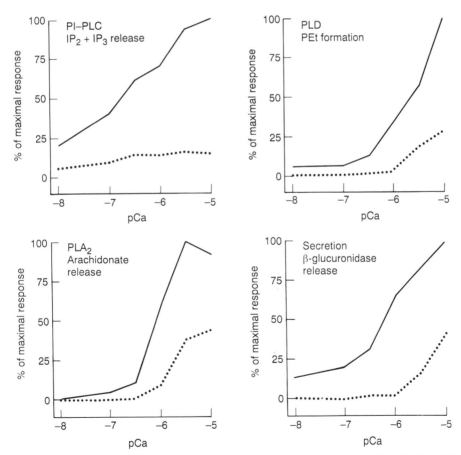

Figure 8.7 A comparison of the Ca²⁺ dependence of the GTP-γ-S-mediated stimulation of PLC, PLD, PLA₂ and secretion from permeabilized differentiated HL60 cells. HL60 cells were permeabilized with streptolysin O (0.4 iu/ml) in the presence of MgATP (1 mM) and calcium buffered with 3 mM EGTA in the range indicated in the figure in the presence or absence of GTP-γ-S (30 μM). The dotted lines denote incubations in the absence of GTP-γ-S and the solid lines denote incubations in the presence of GTP-γ-S.

however, exclude this pathway from playing a modulatory role (Cockcroft and Stutchfield, 1989a).

Secretion stimulated by GTP-γ-S is accompanied by both PLC and PLD activation in undifferentiated HL60 cells. If activation of PLC is abrogated by removing MgATP, secretion due to GTP-γ-S still occurs but at a reduced level. In the early work on neutrophils, the observation that secretion could still be induced by GTP-γ-S under conditions where G-protein-mediated activation of PLC was suppressed led to the proposal that two G proteins, G_p and G_e (e for exocytosis), were involved in exocytosis (Barrowman et al., 1986). G_p controlled PLC and G_e controlled an unidentified step. The involvement of a second G protein in exocytosis has been observed in a number of other cell types (see Gomperts, 1990, for review).

In neutrophils and differentiated HL60 cells, addition of Ca^{2+} at pCa 5 (but not pCa 6) into permeabilized cells also triggers secretion provided that MgATP is present. This response to Ca^{2+} is dependent on a G protein (G_e) since it can be blocked by GDP-β-S. Presumably the role of MgATP is to make available GTP by transphosphorylation, rather than have its effect via its receptor present on the cell-surface. This conclusion is supported by the observation that GTP can replace ATP.

The possibility that G_e controls the effector, PLD, is attractive. The observation that interference with the PLD pathway with ethanol affects secretion from intact cells further supports the view that the secretory pathway requires the activation of PLD for optimal activation. Many of the characteristics of PLD activation in permeabilized cells are similar to the characteristics for exocytosis. For example, PMA pretreatment for 5 min reduces the Ca^{2+} requirement for both exocytosis as well as for PLD activation (Stutchfield and Cockcroft, 1988).

Although much of the work on exocytosis has been done using GTP analogues, it is important to stress that the ligand, FMLP, can also stimulate secretion from permeabilized cells, and there is evidence that multiple G proteins are also involved, i.e. G_p and G_e (Cockcroft, 1991). Since under these conditions, GTP-γ-S is unable to stimulate PLC (because MgATP is absent and the cells are metabolically inhibited), GTP-γ-S must be interacting with a second G protein, presumably G_e.

The possibility that a small GTP-binding protein, analogous to that required for the activation of the NADPH oxidase, is also involved cannot be excluded. Many small GTP-binding proteins have been identified on the secretory granules. The role of many of the small GTP-binding proteins is in targeting specific vesicles to fuse with the appropriate membrane and therefore it is to be expected that one of these proteins may also be responsible for targeting secretory granules to the plasma membrane.

8. Finale

The picture that clearly emerges from studies about regulation of phospholipases is that the FMLP receptor recruits multiple phospholipases from the cytsosol via G protein(s). Figure 8.6 provides two alternative schemes. In Scheme A, a single G protein regulates all three phospholipases and in Scheme B, activation of the three phospholipases is controlled by three different G proteins. However, the primary event in both schemes is considered to be PLC activation and the associated increase in cytosol Ca^{2+} and PKC can activate PLD and PLA_2 downstream. The G protein(s) can also directly activate PLD and PLA_2 and synergistic activation of the downstream phospholipases can occur due to the simultaneous activation of a G protein, and an increase in Ca^{2+} and PKC activity. In Scheme A, it is envisaged that a single G protein, G_p is responsible for activating all three phospholipases. In Scheme B, three separate G proteins are responsible: G_p regulates PLC, G_a regulates PLA_2 and G_d regulates PLD. G_e has been previously defined as the G protein regulating exocytosis by an unidentified effector system (Barrowman et al., 1986; Cockcroft et al., 1987; Stutchfield and Cockcroft, 1988). It is suggested that the effector system that is regulated by G_e may be PLD, i.e. G_d is equivalent to G_e. This needs to be rigorously established but, from the current data available, many of the characteristics of PLD activation and exocytosis from permeabilized HL60 cells triggered by GTP-γ-S correlate very well.

Activation of phospholipases presents us with new problems that are different from the activation of adenylate cyclase by G_s where the catalytic unit is a transmembrane protein. In contrast to adenylate cyclase, all the three phospholipases have been found predominantly in the cytosol. Future studies will have to concentrate on the mechanisms of recruitment of the individual phospholipases by the activated receptor. Are there docking proteins that allow for membrane association of the phospholipases? What are the domains in the phospholipases that allow for targeting to membranes where the substrates reside? Many of these questions will need the availability of purified phospholipases and antibodies against them to study the translocation and activation by G-proteins, Ca^{2+}/PKC and tyrosine phosphorylation.

Development of different reconstitution systems, both based on native membranes and those based on purified components reconstituted in vitro will be essential to establish which phospholipases are regulated by which G proteins. New G proteins are still being discovered as are new isoforms of phospholipases. Clearly, the next few years will be an exciting period for the study of intracellular phospholipases.

9. Acknowledgement

Work in the author's laboratory has been financed by grants from the MRC, the Wellcome Trust and The Lister Institute over the last seven years.

10. References

Abo, A., Pick, E., Hall, A., Totty, N., Teahan, C.G and Segal, A.W. (1991). Activation of the NADPH oxidase involves the small GTP-binding protein p 21^{rac1}. Nature 353, 668–670.

Agwu, D.E., McPhail, L.C., Chabot, M.C., Daniel, L.W., Wykle, R.L. and McCall, C.E. (1989). Choline-linked phosphoglycerides. A source of phosphatidic acid and diglycerides in stimulated neutrophils. J. Biol. Chem. 264, 1405–1413.

Agwu, D.E., McCall, C.E. and McPhail, L.C. (1991). Regulation of phospholipase D-induced hydrolysis of choline-containing phosphoglycerides by cAMP in human neutrophils. J. Immunol. 146, 3895–3903.

Aharoni, I. and Pick, E. (1990). Activation of the superoxide-generating NADPH oxidase of macrophages by sodium dodecyl sulphate in a soluble cell-free system: evidence for involvement of a G protein. J. Leukocyte Biol. 48, 107–115.

Alonso, F., Henson, P.M. and Leslie, C.C. (1986). A cytosolic phospholipase in human neutrophils that hydrolyzes arachidonyl-containing phosphatidylcholine. Biochim. Biophys. Acta 878, 273–280.

Amatruda, T.T., Steele, D.A., Slepak, V.Z. and Simon, M.I. (1991). Gα16, a G protein α subunit specifically expressed in hematopoietic cells. Proc. Natl Acad. Sci. USA 88, 5587–5591.

Anthes, J.C., Billah, M.M., Cali, A., Egan, R.W. and Siegel, M.I. (1987). Chemotactic peptide, calcium and guanine nucleotide regulation of phospholipase C activity in membranes from DMSO-differentiated HL60 cells. Biochem. Biophys. Res. Comm. 145, 825–833.

Anthes, J.C., Wang, P., Siegel, M.I., Egan, R.W. and Billah, M.M. (1991). Granulocyte phospholipase D is activated by a guanine nucleotide dependent protein factor. Biochem. Biophys. Res. Comm. 175, 236–243.

Aridor-Piterman, O., Lavie, Y. and Liscovitch, M. (1992). Bimodal distribution of phosphatidic acid phosphohydrolase in NG108-15 cells. Modulation by the amphiphilic lipids oleic acid and sphingosine. Eur. J. Biochem. 204, 561–568.

Asano, T., Katada, T., Gilman, A.G. and Ross, E.M. (1984). Activation of the inhibitory GTP-binding protein of adenylate cyclase, G_i, by β-adrenergic receptors in reconstituted phospholipid vesicles. J. Biol. Chem. 259, 9351–9354.

Ashkenazi, A., Peralta, E.G., Winslow, J.W., Ramachandran, J. and Capon, D.J. (1989). Functionally distinct G proteins selectively couple different receptors to PI hydrolysis in the same cell. Cell 56, 487–493.

Axelrod, J. (1990). Receptor-mediated activation of phospho-lipase A_2 and arachidonic acid release in signal transduction. Biochem. Soc. Trans. 18, 503–507.

Badwey, J.A., Erickson, R.W. and Curnutte, J.T. (1991). Staurosporine inhibits the soluble and membrane-bound protein tyrosine kinases of human neutrophils. Biochem. Biophys. Res. Comm. 178, 423–429.

Bairoch, A. and Cox, J.A. (1990). EF-hand motifs in inositol phospholipid-specific phospholipase C. FEBS Lett. 269, 454–456.

Bakalyar, H.A. and Reed, R.R. (1990). Identification of a specialized adenylyl cyclase that may mediate odorant detection. Science 250, 1403–1406.

Balch, W.E. (1990). Small GTP-binding proteins in vesicular transport. Trends Biochem. Sci. 15, 473–477.

Baldassare, J.J., Knipp, M.A., Henderson, P.A. and Fisher, G.J. (1988). GTPγ-S-stimulated hydrolysis of phosphatidylinositol-4,5-bisphosphate by soluble phos-pholipase C from human platelets requires soluble GTP-binding protein. Biochem. Biophys. Res. Comm. 154, 351–357.

Balsinde, J., Diez, E. and Mollinedo, F. (1988a). Phosphatidylinositol-specific phospholipase D: a pathway for generation of a second messenger. Biochem. Biophys. Res. Comm. 154, 502–508.

Balsinde, J., Diez, E., Schuller, A. and Mollinedo, F. (1988b). Phospholipase A_2 activity in resting and activated human neutrophils. Substrate specificity, pH dependence, and subcellular localization. J. Biol. Chem. 263, 1929–1936.

Balsinde, J., Diez, E., Fernandez, B. and Mollinedo, F. (1989). Biochemical characterization of phospholipase D activity from human neutrophils. Eur. J. Biochem. 186, 717–724.

Banno, Y., Nakashima, S., Tohmatsu, T., Nozawa, Y. and Lapetina, E.G. (1986). GTP and GDP will stimulate platelet cytosolic phospholipase C independently of Ca^{2+}. Biochem. Biophys. Res. Comm. 140, 728–734.

Banno, Y., Nakashima, T., Kumada, T., Ebisawa, K., Nonomura, Y. and Nozawa, Y. (1992). Effects of gelsolin on human platelet cytosolic phosphoinositide-phospholipase C isozymes. J. Biol. Chem. 267, 6488–6494.

Banno, Y., Yada, Y. and Nozawa, Y. (1988). Purification and characterization of membrane-bound phospholipase C specific for phosphoinositides from human platelets. J. Biol. Chem. 263, 11459–11465.

Banno, Y., Yu, A., Nakashima, T., Homma, Y., Takenawa, T. and Nozawa, Y. (1990). Purification and characterization of a cytosolic phosphoinositide-phospholipase C (γ2-type) from human platelets. Biochem. Biophys. Res. Comm. 167, 396–401.

Barrowman, M.M., Cockcroft, S. and Gomperts, B.D. (1986). Two roles for guanine nucleotides in the stimulus secretion sequence of neutrophils. Nature 319, 504–507.

Barrowman, M.M., Cockcroft, S. and Gomperts, B.D. (1987). Differential control of azurophilic and specific granule exo-cytosis in Sendai virus permeabilised rabbit neutrophils. J. Physiol. (Lond.) 383, 115–124.

Becker, E.L., Kermode, J.C., Naccache, P.H., Yassin, R., Marsh, M.L., Munoz, J.J. and Sha'afi, R.J. (1985). The inhibition of neutrophil granule secretion and chemotaxis by pertussis toxin. J. Cell Biol. 100, 1641–1646.

Bellavite, P., Corso, F., Dusi, S., Grzeskowiak, Della-Bianca, M. and Rossi, F. (1988) Activation of NADPH-dependent superoxide production in plasma membrane extracts of pig neutrophils by phosphatidic acid. J. Biol. Chem. 263, 8210–8214.

Ben-Av, P. and Liscovitch, M. (1989). Phospholipase D activation by the mitogens platelet-derived growth factor and 12-O-tetradeconylphorbol 13-acetate in NIH-3T3 cells. FEBS Lett. 259, 64–66.

Benistant, C. and Rubin, R. (1990). Ethanol inhibits thrombin-induced secretion by human platelets at a site distinct from phospholipase C or protein kinase C. Biochem. J. 269, 489–497.

Bennett, C.F. and Crooke, S.T. (1987). Purification and characterisation of a phosphoinositide-specific phospholipase C from guinea pig uterus: phosphorylation by protein kinase in vivo. J. Biol. Chem. 262, 13789–13797.

Bennett, J.P., Cockcroft, S. and Gomperts, B.D. (1980). Use of cytochalasin B to distinguish between early and late events in neutrophil activation. Biochim. Biophys. Acta 601, 584–591.

Benthin, G., Anggard, E., Gustavsson, L. and Alling, C. (1985). Formation of phosphatidylethanol in frozen kidneys from ethanol-treated rats. Biochim. Biophys. Acta 835, 385–389.

Berkow, R.L., Dodson, R.W. and Kraft, A.S. (1989). Human neutrophils contain distinct cytosolic and particulate tyrosine kinase activities: possible role in neutrophil activation. Biochim. Biophys. Acta 997, 292–301.

Billah, M.M. and Anthes, J.C. (1990). The regulation and cellular functions of phosphatidylcholine hydrolysis. Biochem. J. 269, 281–291.

Billah, M.M. and Siegel, M.I. (1987). Phospholipase A_2 activation in chemotactic peptide-stimulated HL60 granulocytes: synergism between diacylglycerol and Ca^{2+} in a protein kinase C-independent mechanism. Biochem. Biophys. Res. Comm. 144, 683–691.

Billah, M.M., Eckel, S., Myers, R.F. and Siegel, M.I. (1986). Metabolism of platelet-activating factor (1-O-alkyl-2-acetyl-sn-glycero-3-phosphocholine) by human promyelocytic leukemia HL60 cells. J. Biol. Chem. 261, 5824–5831.

Billah, M.M., Eckel, S., Mullman, T.J., Egan, R.W. and Siegel, M.I. (1989a). Phosphatidylcholine hydrolysis by phospholipase D determines phosphatidate and diglyceride levels in chemotactic peptide-stimulated human neutrophils. J. Biol. Chem. 264, 17069–17077.

Billah, M.M., Pai, J.-K., Mullmann, T.J., Egan, R.W and Siegel, M.A. (1989b). Regulation of phospholipase D in HL-60 granulocytes. Activation by phorbol esters, diglyceride, and calcium ionophore via protein kinase C-independent mechanisms. J. Biol. Chem. 264, 9069–9076.

Birnbaumer, L., Abramowitz, J. and Brown, A.M. (1990). Receptor–effector coupling by G-proteins. Biochim. Biophys. Acta 1031, 163–224.

Blank, J.L., Ross, A.H. and Exton, J.H. (1991). Purification and characterization of two G-proteins that activate the β_1-isozyme of phosphoinositide-specific phospholipase C. J. Biol. Chem. 266, 18206–18216.

Bocckino, S.B., Blackmore, P.F., Wilson, P.B. and Exton, J.H. (1987). Phosphatidate accumulation in hormone-treated hepatocytes via a phospholipase D mechanism. J. Biol. Chem. 262, 15309–15315.

Bocckino, S.B., Wilson, P.B. and Exton, J.H. (1991). Phosphatidate-dependent protein phosphorylation. Proc. Natl Acad. Sci. USA 88, 6210–6213.

Bokoch, G.M. (1987). The presence of free G protein β/γ subunits in human neutrophils results in suppression of adenylate cyclase activity. J. Biol. Chem. 262, 589–594.

Bokoch, G.M. and Gilman, A.G. (1984). Inhibition of receptor-mediated release of arachidonic acid by pertussis toxin. Cell 39, 301–308.

Bokoch, G.M. and Quilliam, L.A. (1990). Guanine nucleotide binding properties of rap1 purified from human neutrophils. Biochem. J. 267, 407–411.

Bokoch, G.M., Parkos, C.A. and Mumby, S.M. (1988). Purification and characterisation of the 22,000-Dalton GTP-binding protein substrate for ADP-ribosylation by botulinum toxin, G_{22K}. J. Biol. Chem. 263, 16744–16749.

Bollag, W.B., Barrett, P.Q., Isales, C.M., Liscovitch, M. and Rasmussen, H. (1990). A potential role for phospholipase D in the angiotensin II-induced stimulation of aldosterone secretion from bovine adrenal glomerulosa cells. Endocrinology 127, 1436–1443.

Bonser, R.W., Thompson, N.T., Randall, R.W. and Garland, L.G. (1989). Phospholipase D activation is functionally linked to superoxide generation in the human neutrophil. Biochem. J. 264, 617–620.

Bonser, R.W., Thompson, N.T., Randall, R.W., Tateson, J.E., Spacey, G.D., Hodson, H.F. and Garland, L.G. (1991). Demethoxyviridin and wortmannin block phospholipase C and D activation in the human neutrophil. Br. J. Pharmacol. 103, 1237–1241.

Boulay, F., Tardif, M., Brouchon, L. and Vignais, P. (1990). The human N-formylpeptide receptor. Characterization of two cDNA isolates and evidence for a new subfamily of G-protein-coupled receptors. Biochemistry 29, 11123–11133.

Brandt, S.J., Dougherty, R.W., Lapetina, E.G. and Niedel, J.E. (1985). Pertussis toxin inhibits chemotactic peptide-stimulated generation of inositol phosphates and lysosomal enzyme secretion in human leukemic (HL-60) cells. Proc. Natl Acad. Sci. USA 82, 3277–3280.

Brunkhorst, B.A., Lazzari, K.G., Strohmeier, G., Weil, G. and Simons, E.R. (1991). Calcium changes in immune complex-stimulated human neutrophils. J. Biol. Chem. 266, 13035–13043.

Burch, R.M. and Axelrod, J. (1987). Dissociation of bradykinin-induced prostaglandin formation from phosphatidylinositol turnover in Swiss 3T3 fibroblasts: evidence for G protein regulation of phospholipase A_2. Proc. Natl Acad. Sci. USA 84, 6374–6378.

Burch, R.M., Luini, A. and Axelrod, J. (1986). Phospholipase A_2 and phospholipase C are activated by distinct GTP-binding proteins in response to α_1-adrenergic stimulation in FRTL5 thyroid cells. Proc. Natl. Acad. Sci. USA. 83, 7201–7205.

Caldwell, C.W., Patterson, W. P. and Yesus, Y.W (1991). Translocation of CD45RA in neutrophils. J. Leukocyte Biol. 49, 317–328.

Camps, M., Hou, C., Jacobs, K.H. and Gierschik, P. (1990). Guanosine 5'-[γ-thio]triphosphate-stimulated hydrolysis of phosphatidylinositol 4,5-bisphosphate in HL-60 granulocytes. Evidence that the guanine nucleotide acts by relieving phospholipase C from an inhibitory constraint. Biochem. J. 271, 743–748.

Camps, M., Hou, C., Sidiripoulos, D., Stock, J.B., Jacobs, K.H. and Gierschik, P. (1992). Stimulation of phospholipase C by G-protein βγ-subunits. Eur. J. Biochem. 206, 821–831.

Cerione, R.A., Staniszewaski, C., Benovic, J.L., Lefkowitz, R.J., Caron, M.G., Gierschik, P., Somers, R., Spiegel, A.M., Codina, J. and Birnbaumer, L. (1985). Specificity of the functional interactions of the β adrenergic receptor and rhodopsin with guanine regulatory proteins reconstituted in phospholipid vesicles. J. Biol. Chem. 260, 1439–1500.

Chalifa, V., Mohn, H. and Liscovitch, M. (1990). A neutral phospholipase D activity from rat brain synaptic plasma membranes. J. Biol. Chem. 265, 17512–17519.

Chalifour, R.J. and Kanfer, J.N. (1980). Microsomal phospholipase D of rat brain and lung tissues. Biochem. Biophys. Res. Comm. 96, 742–747.

Channon, J.Y. and Leslie, C.C. (1990). A calcium-dependent mechanism for associating a soluble arachidonyl-hydrolyzing phospholipase A2 with membrane in the macrophage cell line RAW 264.7. J. Biol. Chem. 265, 5409–5413.

Chilton, F.H. (1991). Assays for measuring arachidonic acid release from phospholipids. Methods Enzymol. 197, 166–183.

Chilton, F.H. and Murphy, R.C. (1986). Remodeling of arachidonate-containing phosphoglycerides within the human neutrophil. J. Biol. Chem. 261, 7771–7777.

Choudhury, G.G., Sylvia, V.L., Wang, L-M., Pierce, J. and Sakaguchi, A.Y. (1991). The kinase insert domain of colony stimulating factor-1 receptor is dispensable for CSF-1 induced phosphatidylcholine hydrolysis. FEBS Lett. 282, 351–354.

Churcher, Y., Allan, D. and Gomperts, B.D. (1990). Relationship between arachidonate generation and exocytosis in permeabilised mast cells. Biochem. J. 266, 157–163.

Clark, J.D., Milona, N., and Knopf, J.L. (1990a). Purification of a 110-kilodalton cytosolic phospholipase A2 from the human monocytic cell line U937. Proc. Natl Acad. Sci. USA 87, 7708–7712.

Clark, R.A., Volpp, B.D., Leidal, K.G., and Nauseef, W.M. (1990b). Two cytosolic components of the human neutrophil respiratory burst oxidase translocate to the plasma membrane during cell activation. J. Clin. Invest. 85, 714–721.

Clark, J.D., Lin, L.-L., Kriz, R.W., Ramesha, C.S., Sultzman, L.A., Lin, A.Y., Milona, N. and Knopf, J.L. (1991). A novel arachidonic acid-selective cytosolic PLA2 contains a Ca^{2+}-dependent translocation domain with homology to PKC and GAP. Cell 65, 1043–1051.

Cockcroft, S. (1984). Ca^{2+}-dependent conversion of phosphatidylinositol to phosphatidate in neutrophils stimulated with fMetLeuPhe or ionophore A23187. Biochim. Biophys. Acta 795, 37–46.

Cockcroft, S. (1986a). The dependence on Ca^{2+} of the guanine nucleotide-activated polyphosphoinositide phosphodiesterase in neutrophil plasma membranes. Biochem. J. 240, 503–507.

Cockcroft, S. (1986b). In "Phosphoinositides and Receptor Mechanisms," Receptor Biochemistry and Methodology, Vol. 7. (ed. J.W. Putney, Jr.), pp. 287–310. Allan R. Liss, Inc., New York.

Cockcroft, S. (1987). Polyphosphoinositide phosphodiesterase: regulation by a novel guanine nucleotide binding protein, G_p. Trends Biochem. Sci. 12, 75–78.

Cockcroft, S. (1991). Relationship between arachidonate release and exocytosis in permeabilised human neutrophils stimulated with formylmethionyl-leucyl-phenylalanine (fMetLeuPhe), guanosine 5′-[γ-thio]triphosphate (GTP[S]) and Ca^{2+}. Biochem. J. 275, 127–131.

Cockcroft, S. and Allan, D. (1984). The fatty acid composition of phosphatidylinositol, phosphatidate and 1,2-diacylglycerol in stimulated human neutrophils. Biochem. J. 222, 557–559.

Cockcroft, S. and Gomperts. B.D. (1985). Role of guanine nucleotide binding protein in the activation of polyphosphoinositide phosphodiesterase. Nature 314, 534–536.

Cockcroft, S. and Stutchfield, J. (1988a). Effect of pertussis toxin and neomycin on G-protein regulated polyphosphoinositide phosphodiesterase: a comparison between HL60 membranes and permeabilised HL60 cells. Biochem. J. 256, 343–350.

Cockcroft, S. and Stutchfield, J. (1988b). G-proteins, the inositol lipid signalling pathway, and secretion. Philos. Trans. R. Soc. Lond. Ser. B. 320, 247–265.

Cockcroft, S. and Stutchfield, J. (1989a). The receptors for ATP and fMetLeuPhe are independently coupled to phospholipase C and A2 via G-protein(s): relationship between phospholipase C and A2, activation and exocytosis in HL60 cells and human neutrophils. Biochem. J. 263, 715–723.

Cockcroft, S. and Stutchfield, J. (1989b). ATP stimulates secretion in human neutrophils and HL60 cells via a pertussis toxin-sensitive guanine nucleotide binding protein coupled to phospholipase C. FEBS Lett. 245, 25–29.

Cockcroft, S. and Thomas, G.M.H. (1992). Inositol lipid specific phospholipase C isozymes and their differential regulation by receptors. Biochem. J. 288, 1–14.

Cockcroft, S., Bennett, J.P. and Gomperts, B.D. (1980). Stimulus-secretion coupling in rabbit neutrophils is not mediated by phosphatidylinositol breakdown. Nature 288, 275–277.

Cockcroft, S., Baldwin, J.M. and Allan, D. (1984). The Ca^{2+}-activated polyphosphoinositide phosphodiesterase of human and rabbit neutrophil membranes. Biochem. J. 221, 477–482.

Cockcroft, S., Barrowman, M.M. and Gomperts, B.D. (1985). Breakdown and synthesis of polyphosphoinositides in fMetLeuPhe-stimulated neutrophils. FEBS Lett. 181, 259–263.

Cockcroft, S., Howell, T.W. and Gomperts, B.D. (1987). Two G-proteins act in series to control stimulus-secretion coupling in mast cells: use of neomycin to distinguish between G-proteins controlling polyphosphoinositide phosphodiesterase and exocytosis. J. Cell Biol. 105, 2745–2750.

Cockcroft, S., Nielson, C.P. and Stutchfield, J. (1991). Is phospholipase A2 activation regulated by G-proteins? Biochem. Soc. Trans. 19, 333–336.

Cotecchia, S., Exum, S., Caron, M.G. and Lekkowitz, R.J. (1990). Regions of the α_1-adrenergic receptor involved in coupling to phosphatidylinositol hydrolysis and enhanced sensitivity of biological function. Proc. Natl Acad. Sci. USA 87, 2896–2900.

Cowen, D.S., Baker, B. and Dubyak, G.R. (1990a). Pertussis toxin produces differential inhibitory effects on basal and chemotactic peptide-stimulated inositol phospholipid breakdown in HL-60 cells and HL-60 cell membranes. J. Biol. Chem. 265, 16181–16189.

Cowen, D.S., Sanders, M. and Dubyak, G. (1990b). P2-Purinergic receptors activate a guanine nucleotide-dependent phospholipase C in membranes from HL-60 cells. Biochim. Biophys. Acta 1053, 195–203.

Davidson, F.F. and Dennis, E.E. (1990). Evolutionary relationships and implications for the regulation of phospholipase A2: from snake venom to human secreted forms. J. Mol. Evol. 31, 228–238.

Deckmyn, H., Tu, S.-M., and Majerus, P.W. (1986). Guanine nucleotides stimulate soluble phosphoinositide-specific phospholipase C in the absence of membranes. J. Biol. Chem. 261, 16553–16558.

Della Bianca, V., Grzeskowiak, M., Lissandrini, D. and Rossi, F. (1991). Source and role of diacylglycerol formed during phagocytosis of opsonized yeast particles and associated respiratory burst in human neutrophils. Biochem. Biophys. Res. Comm. 177, 948–955.

De Togni, P., Cabrini, G. and Di Virgilio, F. (1984). Cyclic AMP inhibition of fMet-Leu-Phe-dependent metabolic responses in human neutrophils is not due to its effects on cytosolic Ca^{2+}. Biochem. J. 224, 629–635.

Dewald, B., Thelen, M. and Baggiolini, M. (1988). Two transduction sequences are necessary for neutrophil activation by receptor agonists. J. Biol. Chem. 263, 16179–16184.

Dexter, D., Rubins, J. B., Manning, E. C., Khachatrian, L. and Dickey, B.F. (1990). Compartmentalization of low molecular mass GTP-binding proteins among neutrophil secretory granules. J. Immunol. 145, 1845–1850.

Didsbury, J., Weber, R. F., Bokoch, G. M., Evans, T. and Snyderman, R. (1989). *rac*. a novel *ras*-related family of proteins that are botulinum toxin substrates. J. Biol. Chem. 264, 16378–16382.

Diez, E., and Mong, S. (1990). Purification of a phospholipase A_2 from human monocytic leukemic U937 cells. Calcium-dependent activation and membrane association. J. Biol. Chem. 265, 14654–14661.

Doussiere, J., Pilloud, M. C. and Vignais, P.V. (1988). Activation of bovine neutrophil oxidase in a cell-free system GTP-dependent formation of a complex between a cytosolic factor and a membrane protein. Biochem. Biophys. Res. Comm. 152, 993–1001.

Dubyak, G.R., Cowen, D.S. and Meuller, L.M. (1988). Activation of inositol phospholipid breakdown in HL60 cells by P2-purinergic receptors for extracellular ATP. Evidence for mediation by both pertussis toxin-sensitive and pertussis toxin-insensitive mechanisms. J. Biol. Chem. 263, 18108–18117.

Emori, Y., Homma, Y., Sorimachi, H., Kawasaki, H., Nakanishi, O., Suzuki, K., and Takenawa, T. (1989). A second type of rat phosphoinositide-specific phospholipase C containing a *src*-related sequence not essential for phosphoinositide-hydrolyzing activity. J. Biol. Chem. 264, 21885–21890.

English, D. and Taylor, G.S. (1991). Divergent effects of propranolol on neutrophil superoxide release: involvement of phosphatidic acid and diacylglycerol as second messengers. Biochem. Biophys. Res. Commun. 175, 423–429.

English, D., Taylor, G. and Garcia, J.G.N. (1991). Diacyl-glycerol generation in fluoride-treated neutrophils: involvement of phospholipase D. Blood 77, 2746–2756.

Escobedo, J.A., Navankasattusas, S., Kavanaugh, W.M., Milfay, D., Fried, V.A. and Williams, L.T. (1991). cDNA cloning of a novel 85 kd protein that has SH2 domains and regulates binding of PI3-kinase to the PDGF β receptor. Cell. 65, 75–82.

Exton, J.H. (1990). Signaling through phosphatidylcholine breakdown. J. Biol. Chem. 265, 1–4.

Falloon, J., Malech, H., Milligan, G., Unson, C., Kahn, R., Goldsmith, P. and Spiegel, A. (1986). Detection of the major pertussis toxin substrate of human leukocytes with antisera raised against synthetic peptides. FEBS Lett. 209, 352–356.

Fukui, T., Lutz, R.J. and Lowenstein, J.M. (1988). Purification of a phospholipase C from rat liver cytosol that acts on phosphatidylinositol 4,5-bisphosphate and phosphatidyl-inositol 4-phosphate. J. Biol. Chem. 263, 17730–17737.

Gabig, T.G., English, D., Akard, L.P. and Schell, M.J. (1987). Regulation of neutrophil NADPH oxidase activation in a cell-free system by guanine nucleotides and fluoride. Evidence for participation of a pertussis toxin and cholera toxin-insensitive G protein. J. Biol. Chem. 262, 1685–1690.

Geny, B. and Cockcroft, S. (1992). Synergistic activation of phospholipase D by a protein kinase C- and a G-protein-mediated pathway in streptolysin O-permeabilized HL60 cells. Biochem. J. 284, 531–538.

Geny, B., Stutchfield, J. and Cockcroft, S. (1988). Inhibition of G-protein-stimulated polyphosphoinositide phospho-diesterase by phorbol 12-myristate 13-acetate in perme-abilized HL60 cells. Cell. Signalling 1, 165–172.

Geny, B., Cost, H., Barreau, P., Basset, M., Le Peuch, C., Abita, J.-P. and Cockcroft, S. (1991). The differentiating agent, retinoic acid, causes an early inhibition of inositol lipid-specific phospholipase C activity in HL60 cells. Cell. Signalling 3, 11–23.

Gerard, N.P. and Gerard, C. (1991). The chemotactic receptor for human C5a anaphylatoxin. Nature 349, 614–617.

Gierschik, P. and Jacobs, K.H. (1987). Receptor-mediated ADP-ribosylation of a phospholipase C-stimulating G-protein. FEBS Lett. 224, 219–223.

Gierschik, P., Falloon, J., Milligan, G., Pines, M., Gallin, J.I. and Spiegel, A. (1986). Immunochemical evidence for a novel pertussis toxin substrate in human neutrophils. J. Biol. Chem. 261, 8058–8062.

Gierschik, P., Sidiropoulos, D., Spiegel, A. and Jakobs, K.H. (1987). Purification and immunochemical characterization of the major pertussis-toxin-sensitive guanine nucleotide binding protein of bovine-neutrophil membranes. Eur. J. Biochem. 165, 185–194.

Gierschik, P., Sidiropoulos, D. and Jakobs, K.H. (1989). Two distinct G_i-proteins mediate formyl peptide receptor signal transduction in human leukemia (HL-60) cells. J. Biol. Chem. 264, 21470–21473.

Gierschik, P., Moghtader, R., Straub, C., Dieterich, K. and Jakobs, K.H. (1991). Signal amplification in HL-60 granulocytes. Evidence that the chemotactic peptide receptor catalytically activates guanine-nucleotide-binding regulatory proteins in native plasma membranes. Eur. J. Biochem. 197, 725–732.

Gil, J., Higgins, T. and Rozengurt, E. (1991). Mastoparan, a novel mitogen for Swiss 3T3 cells, stimulates pertussis toxin-sensitive arachidonic acid release without inositol phosphate production. J. Cell Biol. 113, 943–950.

Goldman, D.W., Chang, F.H., Gifford, L.A., Goetzl, E.J. and Bourne, H.R. (1985). Pertussis toxin inhibition of chemotactic factor-induced calcium mobilization and function in human polymorphonuclear leukocytes. J. Exp. Med. 162, 145–156.

Goldsmith, P., Rossiter, K., Carter, A., Simonds, W., Unson, C. G., Vitensky, R. and Spiegel, A.M. (1988). Identification of the GTP-binding protein encoded by G_{i3} complementary DNA. J. Biol. Chem. 263, 6476–6479.

Gomez-Cambronero, J., Wang, E., Johnson, G., Huang, C.-K. and Sha'Afi, R.I. (1991). Platelet-activating factor induces tyrosine phosphorylation in human neutrophils. J. Biol. Chem. 266, 6240–6245.

Gomperts, B.D. (1990). G_E: a GTP-binding protein mediating exocytosis. Annu. Rev. Physiol. 52, 591–606.

Grand, R.J.A. and Owen, D. (1991). The biochemistry of *ras* p21. Biochem. J. 279, 609–631.

Grinstein, S. and Furuya, W. (1991). Tyrosine phosphorylation and oxygen consumption induced by G proteins in neutrophils. Am. J. Physiol. 260, C1019–C1027.

Gronich, J.H., Bonventre, J.V. and Nemenoff, R.A. (1990). Purification of a high molecular weight mass form of phospholipase A_2 from rat kidney activated at physiological calcium concentrations. J. Biol. Chem. 271, 37–43.

Gruchalla, R.S., Dinh, T.T. and Kennerly, D.A. (1990). An indirect pathway of receptor-mediated 1,2-diacylglycerol formation in mast cells. I. IgE receptor-mediated activation of phospholipase D. J. Immunol. 144, 2334–2342.

Hall, A. (1990). The cellular functions of small GTP-binding proteins. Science 249, 635–640.

Hattori, H. and Kanfer, J. N. (1984). Synaptosomal phospholipase D: potential role in providing choline for acetylcholine synthesis. Biochem. Biophys. Res. Comm. 124, 945–949.

Hattori, H. and Kanfer, J.N. (1985). Synaptosomal phospholipase D potential role in providing choline for acetylcholine synthesis. J. Neurochem. 45, 1578–1584.

Heller, M. (1978). Phospholipase D. Adv. Lipid Res. 16, 267–326.

Henderson, L.M., Chappell, J.B and Jones, O.T.G. (1989). Superoxide generation is inhibited by phospholipase A_2 inhibitors. Role of phospholipase A_2 in the activation of the NADPH oxidase. Biochem. J. 264, 249–255.

Heyworth, P.G. and Segal, A.W. (1986). Further evidence for the involvement of a phosphoprotein in the respiratory burst oxidase of human neutrophils. Biochem. J. 239, 723–731.

Heyworth, P.G., Karnovsky, M.L. and Badwey, J.A. (1989). Protein phosphorylation associated with synergistic stimulation of neutrophlils. J. Biol. Chem. 264, 14935–14939.

Heyworth, P.G., Curnutte, J.T., Nauseef, W.M., Volpp, B.D., Pearson, D. W., Rosen, H. and Clark, R.A. (1991). Neutrophil nicotinamide adenine dinucleotide phosphate oxidase assembly. Translocation of p47-phox requires interaction between p47-phox and cytochrome b558. J. Clin. Invest. 87, 352–356.

Hofmann, S.L. and Majerus, P.W. (1982). Identification and properties of two distinct phosphatidylinositol-specific phospholipase C enzymes from sheep seminal vesicular glands. J. Biol. Chem. 257, 6461–6469.

Holbrook, P.G., Pannell, L.K. and Daly, J.W. (1991). Phospholipase D-catalyzed hydrolysis of phosphatidylcholine occurs with a P-O bond cleavage. Biochim. Biophys. Acta 1084, 155–158.

Homma, Y., Imaki, J., Nakanishi, O. and Takenawa, T. (1988). Isolation and characterization of two different forms of inositol phospholipid-specific phosphoiipase C from rat brain. J. Biol. Chem. 263, 6592–6598.

Homma, Y., Emori, Y., Shibasaki, F., Suzuki, K. and Takenawa, T. (1990). Isolation and purification of a γ-type phosphoinositide-specific phospholipase C (PLC-γ2). Biochem. J. 269, 13–18.

Honda, Z.-I, Nakamura, M., Miki, I., Minami, M., Watanabe, T., Seyama, Y., Okado, H., Toh, H., Ito, K., Miyamoto, T. and Shimazu, T. (1991). Cloning by functional expression of platelet-activating factor receptor from guinea-pig lung. Nature 349, 342–346.

Honeycutt, P.J. and Niedel, J.E. (1986). Cytochalasin B enhancement of the diacylglycerol response in formyl

peptide-stimulated neutrophils. J. Biol. Chem. 261, 15900–15905.

Huang, C.-K., Laramee, G.R. and Casnellie, J.E. (1988). Chemotactic factor induced tyrosine phosphorylation of membrane associated proteins in rabbit peritoneal neutrophils. Biochem. Biophys. Res. Comm. 151, 794–801.

Hurst, K.M., Hughes, B.P. and Barritt, G.J. (1990). The roles of phospholipase D and a GTP-binding protein in guanosine 5'-[γ-thio]triphosphate-stimulated hydrolysis of phosphatidylcholine in rat liver plasma membranes. Biochem. J. 272, 749–753.

Iannone, M.A., Wolberg, G. and Zimmerman, T.P. (1989). Chemotactic peptide induces cAMP elevation in human neutrophils by amplification of the adenylate cyclase response to endogenously produced adenosine. J. Biol. Chem. 264, 20177–20180.

Jakobs, K.H. and Wieland, T. (1989). Evidence for receptor-regulated phosphotransfer reactions involved in activation of the adenylate cyclase inhibitory G protein in human platelet membranes. Eur. J. Biochem. 183, 115–121.

Jamal, Z., Martin, A., Gomez-Munoz, A. and Brindley, D.N. (1991). Plasma membrane fractions from rat liver contain a phosphatidate phosphohydrolase distinct from that in the endoplasmic reticulum and cytosol. J. Biol. Chem. 266, 2988–2996.

Jeselma, C.L. (1987). Light activation of phospholipase A_2 in rod outer segments of bovine retina and its modulation by GTP-binding proteins. J. Biol. Chem. 262, 163–168.

Jeselma, C.L. and Axelrod, A. (1987). Stimulation of phospholipase A_2 activity in bovine rod outer segments by the $\beta\gamma$ subunits of transducin and its inhibition by the α-subunit. J. Biol. Chem. 84, 3623–3627.

Kajiyama, Y., Murayama, T. and Nomura, Y. (1989). Pertussis toxin-sensitive GTP-binding proteins may regulate phospholipase A_2 in response to thrombin in rabbit platelets. Arch. Biochem. Biophys. 274, 200–208.

Kanaho, Y., Kanoh, H. and Nozawa, Y. (1991a). Activation of phospholipase D in rabbit neutrophils by fMet-Leu-Phe is mediated by a pertussis toxin-sensitive GTP-binding protein that may be distinct from a phospholipase C-regulating protein. FEBS Lett. 279, 249–252.

Kanaho, Y., Kanoh, H., Saitoh, K. and Nozawa, Y. (1991b). Phospholipase D activation by platelet-activating factor, leukotriene B4, and formyl-methionyl-leucyl-phenylalanine in rabbit neutrophils. J. Immunol. 146, 3536–3541.

Kanoh, H., Kanaho, Y. and Nozawa, Y. (1991). Activation and solubilization by triton X-100 of membrane-bound phospholipase D of rat brain. Lipids 26, 426–430.

Katan, M., Kriz, R.W., Totty, N., Meldrum, E., Aldape, R.A., Knopf, J.L. and Parker, P.J. (1988). Determination of the primary structure of PLC-154 demonstrates diversity of polyphosphoinositide-specific phospholipase C activities. Cell 54, 171–177.

Kater, L.A., Goetzl, E.J. and Austen, K.F. (1976). Isolation of human eosinophil phospholipase D. J. Clin. Invest. 57, 1173–1180.

Kikuchi, A., Kozawa, O., Kaibuchi, K., Katada, T., Ui, M. and Takai, Y. (1986). Direct evidence for involvement of a guanine nucleotide-binding protein in chemotactic peptide-stimulated formation of inositol bisphosphate and trisphosphate in differentiated human leukemic (HL-60) cells. J. Biol. Chem. 261, 11558–11562.

Kikuchi, A., Ikeda, K., Kozawa, O. and Takai, Y. (1987). Modes of inhibitory action of protein kinase C in the chemotactic peptide-induced formation of inositol phosphates in differentiated human leukemic (HL-60) cells. J. Biol. Chem. 262, 6766–6770.

Kim, D.K., Suh, P.G. and Ryu, S.H. (1991). Purification and some properties of a phospholipase A$_2$ from bovine platelets. Biochem. Biophys. Res. Comm. 174, 189–196.

Kim, H.K., Kim, J.W., Zilberstein, A., Margolis, B., Kim, J.G., Schlessinger, J. and Rhee, S.G. (1991). PDGF stimulation of inositol phospholipid hydrolysis requires PLC-γ1 phosphorylation on tyrosine residues 783 and 1254. Cell 65, 435–441.

Kim, J.W., Sim, S.S., Kim, U.H., Nishibe, S., Wahl, M.I., Carpenter, G. and Rhee, S.G. (1990). Tyrosine residues in bovine phospholipase C-γ phosphorylated by the epidermal growth factor receptor in vitro. J. Biol. Chem. 265, 3940–3943.

Kiss, Z. and Anderson, W. B. (1990). ATP stimulates the hydrolysis of phosphatidylethanolamine in NIH 3T3 cells. Potentiating effects of guanosine triphosphates and sphingosine. J. Biol. Chem. 265, 7345–7350.

Knaus, U.G., Heyworth, P.G., Evans, T., Curnutte, J.T. and Bokoch, G.M. (1991). Regulation of phagocyte oxygen radical production by the GTP-binding protein Rac2. Science. 254, 1512–1515.

Kobayashi, M. and Kanfer, J.N. (1991). Solubilisation and purification of rat tissue phospholipase D. Methods Enzymol. 197, 575–583.

Koch, C.A., Anderson, D., Moran, M.F., Ellis, C. and Pawson, T. (1991). SH2 and SH3 Domains: elements that control interactions of cytoplasmic signalling proteins. Science, 252, 668–674.

Kraft, A.S. and Berkow, R.L. (1987). Tyrosine kinase and phosphotyrosine phosphatase activity in human promyelocytic leukemic cells and human polymorphonuclear leukocytes. Blood 70, 356–362.

Kramer, R.M., Roberts, E.F., Manetta, J. and Putnam, J.E. (1991). The Ca^{2+}-sensitive cytosolic phospholipase A$_2$ is a 100-kDa protein in human monoblast U937 cells. J. Biol. Chem. 266, 5268–5272.

Krause, K.-H., Schlegel, W., Wollheim, C.B., Anderson, T., Waldvogel, F.A. and Lew, D.P. (1985). Chemotactic peptide activation of human neutrophils and HL-60 cells. Pertussis toxin reveals correlation between inositol trisphosphate generation, calcium ion transients, and cellular activation. J. Clin. Invest. 76, 1348–1354.

Kritz, R., Lin, L.-L., Sultzman, L., Ellis, C., Heldin, C.-K., Pawson, T. and Knopf, J. (1990). In "Proto-oncogenes in Cell Development." Ciba Foundation Symposium 150, pp. 112–127. Wiley, Chichester.

Kroll, S.D., Omri, G., Landau, E.M. and Iyengar, R. (1991). Activated α subunit of G$_o$ protein induces oocyte maturation. Proc. Natl Acad. Sci. USA 88, 5182–5186.

Kuhns, D.B., Wright, D.G., Nath, J., Kaplan, S.S. and Basford, R.E. (1988). ATP induces transient elevations of [Ca^{2+}]$_i$ in human neutrophils and primes these cells for enhanced O$_2$ generation. Lab. Invest. 58, 448–453.

Kumjian, D.A., Wahl, M.I., Rhee, S.G. and Daniel, T.O. (1989). Platelet-derived growth factor (PDGF) binding promotes physical association of PDGF receptor with phospholipase C. Proc. Natl Acad. Sci. USA 86, 8232–8236.

Kusunoki, T., Higashi, H., Hosoi, S., Hata, D., Sugie, K., Mayumi, M. and Mikawa, H. (1992). Tyrosine phosphorylation and its possible role in superoxide production by human neutrophils stimulated with FMLP and IgG. Biochem. Biophys. Res. Comm. 183, 789–796.

Lacal, P., Pulido, R., Sanchez-Madrid, F. and Mollinedo, F. (1988). Intracellular location of T200 and Mol glycoprotein in human neutrophils. J. Biol. Chem. 263, 9946–9951.

Lassegue, B., Alexander, R. W., Clark, M. and Griendling, K.K. (1991). Angiotensin II-induced phosphatidylcholine hydrolysis in cultured vascular smooth-muscle cells. Biochem. J. 276, 19–25.

Lechleiter, J., Hellmiss, R., Duerson, K., Ennulat, D., David, N., Clapham, D. and Peralta, E. (1990). Distinct sequence elements control the specificity of G protein activation by muscarinic acetylcholine receptor subtypes. EMBO J. 9, 4381–4390.

Leslie, C.C. (1991). Kinetic properties of a high molecular mass arachidonyl-hydrolyzing phospholipase A$_2$ that exhibits lysophospholipase activity. J. Biol. Chem. 266, 11366–11371.

Lew, P.D., Monod, A., Waldvogel, F.A. and Pozzan, T. (1987). Role of cytosolic free calcium and phospholipase C in leukotriene-B4-stimulated secretion in human neutrophils: comparison with the chemotactic peptide formylmethionyl-leucyl-phenylalanine. Eur. J. Biochem. 162, 161–168.

Liao, F., Shin, H.S. and Rhee, S.G. (1992). Tyrosine phosphorylation of phospholipase C-γ1 induced by cross-linking of the high affinity or low-affinity Fc receptor for IgG in U937 cells. Proc. Natl Acad. Sci. USA 89, 3659–3663.

Ligati, E., Tardif, M. and Vignais, P.V. (1989). Generation of O$_2^-$ generating oxidase of bovine neutrophils in a cell-free system. Interaction of a cytosol factor with the plasma membrane and control by G nucleotides. Biochemistry 28, 7116–7123.

Liggett, S.B., Caron, M.G., Lefkowitz, R.J. and Hnatowich, M. (1991). Coupling of a mutated form of the human β$_2$-adrenergic receptor to G$_i$ and G$_s$. J. Biol. Chem. 266, 4816–4821.

Lin, P., Wiggan, G.A. and Gilfillan, A.M. (1991). Activation of phospholipase D in a rat mast (RBL 2H3) cell line. A possible unifying mechanism for IgE-dependent degranulation and arachidonic acid metabolite release. J. Immunol. 146 1609–1616.

Liscovitch, M. (1991). Signal-dependent activation of phosphatidylcholine hydrolysis: role of phospholipase D. Biochem. Soc. Trans. 19, 402–407.

Liscovitch, M. and Eli, Y. (1991). Ca^{2+} inhibits guanine nucleotide-activated phospholipase D in neural-derived NG108-15 cells. Cell Reg. 2, 1011–1019.

Lomax, K.J., Leto, T.L., Nunoi, H., Gallin, J.I. and Malech, H.L. (1989). Recombinant 47-kilodalton cytosol factor restores NADPH oxidase in chronic granulomatous disease. Science 245, 409–412.

Lu, D. J. and Grinstein, S. (1990). ATP and guanine nucleotide dependence of neutrophil activation: evidence for the involvement of two distinct GTP-binding proteins. J. Biol. Chem. 265, 13721–13729.

Margolis, B.L., Holub, B.J., Troyer, D.A. and Skorecki, K.L. (1988). Epidermal growth factor stimulates phospholipase A$_2$ in vasopressin-treated rat glomerular mesangial cells. Biochem. J. 256, 469–474.

Margolis, B., Rhee, S. G., Felder, S., Mervic, M., Lyall, R., Levitzki, A., Ullrich, A., Zilberstein, A. and Schlessinger, J. (1989). EGF induces tyrosine phosphorylation of phospholipase C-II: a potential mechanism for EGF receptor signalling. Cell 57, 1101–1107.

Maridonneau-Parini, I. and de Gunzburg, J. (1992). Association of rap1 and rap2 proteins with the specific granules of human neutrophils. Translocation to the plasma membrane during cell activation. J. Biol. Chem. 267, 6396–6402.

Martin, T.W. (1988). Formation of diacylglycerol by a phospholipase D-phosphatidate phosphatase pathway specific for phosphatidylcholine in endothelial cells. Biochim. Biophys. Acta 962, 292–296.

Martin, T.W. and Michaelis, K.C. (1988). Bradykinin stimulates phosphodiesteratic cleavage of phosphatidylcholine in cultured endothelial cells. Biochem. Biophys. Res. Comm. 157, 1271–1279.

Martin, T.W. and Michaelis, K. (1989). P_2-purinergic agonists stimulate phosphodiesteratic cleavage of phosphatidylcholine in endothelial cells. Evidence for activation of phospholipase D. J. Biol. Chem. 264, 8847–8856.

Martinson, E.A., Goldstein, D. and Brown, J.H. (1989). Muscarinic receptor activation of phosphatidylcholine hydrolysis. Relationship to phosphoinositide hydrolysis and diacylglycerol metabolism. J. Biol. Chem. 264, 14748–14754.

Mayer, B.J., Hamaguchi, M. and Hideaburo, H. (1988). A novel viral oncogene with structural similarity to phospholipase C. Nature 332, 272–275.

McLeish, K.R., Gierschik, P., Schepers, T., Sidiropoulos, D. and Jakobs, K.H. (1989). Evidence that activation of a common H-protein by receptors for leukotriene B_4 and N-formylmethionyl-leucyl-phenylalanine in HL-60 cells occurs by different mechanisms. Biochem. J. 260, 427–434.

Meisenhelder, J., Suh, P.-G., Rhee, S. G. and Hunter, T. (1989). Phospholipase C-γ is a substrate for the PDGF and EGF receptor protein-tyrosine kinases in vivo and in vitro. Cell 57, 1109–1122.

Meldrum, E., Katan, M. and Parker, P. (1989). A novel inositol-phospholipid-specific phospholipase C. Rapid purification and characterization. Eur. J. Biochem. 182, 673–677.

Meldrum, E., Parker, P.J. and Carozzi, A. (1991). The PtdIns-PLC superfamily and signal transduction. Biochim. Biophys. Acta 1092, 49–71.

Merritt, J.E. and Moores, K.E. (1991). Human neutrophils have a novel purinergic P_2-type receptor linked to calcium mobilization. Cell. Signalling 3, 243–249.

Metz, S.A. and Dunlop, M. (1990). Stimulation of insulin release by phospholipase C. A potential role for endonenous phosphatidic acid in pancreatic islet function. Biochem. J. 270, 427–435.

Mitchell, F.M., Mullaney, I., Godfrey, P.P., Arkinstall, S.J., Wakelam, M.J.O. and Milligan, G. (1991). Widespread distribution of Gqα/G11α detected immunologically by an antipeptide antiserum directed against the predicted C-terminal decapeptide. FEBS Lett. 287, 171–174.

Mueller, H., Weingarten, R., Ransnas, L.A., Bokoch, G.M. and Sklar, L.A. (1991). Differential amplification of antagonistic receptor pathways in neutrophils. J. Biol. Chem. 266, 12939–12943.

Mullman, T.J., Siegel, M.I., Egan, R.W. and Billah, M.M. (1990a). Complement C5a activation of phospholipase D in human neutrophils. A major route to the production of phosphatides and diglycerides. J. Immunol. 144, 1901–1908.

Mullman, T.J., Siegel, M.I., Egan, R.W. and Billah, M.M. (1990b). Phorbol-12-myristate-13-acetate activation of phospholipase D in human neutrophils leads to the production of phosphatides and diglycerides. Biochem. Biophys. Res. Comm. 170, 1197–1202.

Murayama, T., Kajiyama, Y. and Nomura, Y. (1990). Histamine-stimulated and GTP-binding proteins-mediated phospholipase A_2 activation in rabbit platelets. J. Biol. Chem. 265, 4290–4295.

Murphy, P.M. and McDermott, D. (1991). Functional expression of the human formyl peptide receptor in Xenopus oocytes requires a complementary human factor. J. Biol. Chem. 266, 12560–12567.

Murphy, P.M. and Tiffany, H.L. (1991). Cloning of complementary DNA encoding a functional human interleukin-8 receptor. Science 253, 1280–1283.

Murphy, P.M., Eide, B., Goldsmith, P., Brann, M., Gierschik, P., Spiegel, A. and Malech, H.L. (1987). Detection of multiple forms of $G_{i\alpha}$ in HL60 cells. FEBS Lett. 221, 81–86.

Nakashima, S., Nagata, K.-I., Ueda, K. and Nozawa, Y. (1988). Stimulation of arachidonic acid release by guanine nucleotide in saponin-permeabilized neutrophils: evidence for involvement of GTP-binding protein in phospholipase A_2 activation. Arch. Biochem. Biophys. 261, 375–383.

Narasimhan, V., Holowka, D. and Baird, B. (1990). A guanine nucleotide-binding protein participates in IgE receptor-mediated activation of endogenous and reconstituted phospholipase A_2 in a permeabilized cell system. J. Biol. Chem. 264, 1459–1464.

Nasmith, P.E., Mills, G.B. and Grinstein, S. (1989). Guanine nucleotides induce tyrosine phosphorylation and activation of the respiratory burst in neutrophils. Biochem. J. 257, 893–897.

Nielson, C.P., Stutchfield, J. and Cockcroft, S. (1991). Chemotactic peptide stimulation of arachidonic acid release in HL60 cells, an interaction between G-protein and phospholipse C-mediated signal transduction. Biochim. Biophys. Acta 1095, 83–89.

Nishibe, S., Wahl, M.I., Rhee, S.G. and Carpenter, G. (1989). Tyrosine phosphorylation of phospholipase C-II in vitro by the epidermal growth factor receptor. J. Biol. Chem. 264, 10335–10338.

Nishibe, S., Wahl, M.I., Wedegaertner, P.B., Kim, J.J., Rhee, S.G. and Carpenter, G. (1990). Selectivity of phospholipase C phosphorylation by the epidermal growth factor receptor, the insulin receptor, and their cytoplasmic domains. Proc. Natl Acad. Sci. USA 87, 424–428.

Offermans, S., Schafer, R., Hoffmann, B., Bombien, E., Spicher, K., Hinsch, K.-D., Schultz, G. and Rosenthal, W. (1990). Agonist-sensitive binding of a photoreactive GTP analog to a G-protein α-subunit in membranes of HL-60 cells. FEBS Lett. 260, 14–18.

Ohtsuki, K. and Yokoyama, M. (1987). Direct activation of guanine nucleotide binding proteins through a high-energy phosphate transfer by nucleoside diphosphate-kinase. Biochem. Biophys. Res. Comm. 148, 300–307.

Okajima, F. and Ui, M. (1984). ADP-ribosylation of the specific membrane protein by islet-activating protein, Pertussis toxin, associated with inhibition of a chemotactic peptide-induced arachidonate release in neutrophils. J. Biol. Chem. 259, 13863–13871.

Okajima, F., Katada, T. and Ui, M. (1985). Coupling of the guanine nucleotide regulatory protein to chemotactic peptide receptors in neutrophil membranes and its uncoupling by islet-activating protein Pertussis toxin. J. Biol. Chem. 260, 6761–6768.

Olson, S.C., Bowman, E.P. and Lambeth, J. D. (1991). Phospholipase D activation in a cell-free system from human neutrophils by phorbol 12-myristate 13-acetate and guanosine 5′-O-(3-thiotriphosphate). J. Biol. Chem. 266, 17236–17242.

Omann, G.M., Traynor, A.E., Harris, A.L. and Sklar, L.A. (1987). LTB4-induced activation signals and responses in neutrophils are short-lived compared to formylpeptide. J. Immunol. 138, 2626–2632.

Otsu, M., Hiles, I., Gout, I., Fry, M.J., R.-L, F., Panayotou, G., Thompson, A., Dhand, R., Hsuan, J., Totty, N., Smith, A.D., Morgan, S.J., Courtneidge, S.A., Parker, P.J. and Waterfield, M.D. (1991). Characterization of two 85 kd proteins that associate with receptor tyrosine kinases, middle Tpp60^{c-src} complexes, and PI3-kinase. Cell 65, 91–104.

Padrell, E., Carty, D.J., Moriarty, T.M., Hildebrandt, J.D., Landau, E.M. and Iyengar, R. (1991). Two forms of the bovine brain G_o that stimulate the inositol trisphosphate-mediated C-currents in Xenopus oocytes. J. Biol. Chem. 266, 9771–9777.

Pai, J.-K., Siegel, M.I., Egan, R.W. and Billah, M.M. (1988a). Activation of phospholipase D by chemotactic peptide in HL-60 granulocytes. Biochem. Biophys. Res. Comm. 150, 355–364.

Pai, J.-K., Siegel, M.I., Egan, R.W. and Billah, M.M. (1988b). Phospholipase D catalyses phospholipid metabolism in chemotactic peptide-stimulated HL-60 granulocytes. J. Biol. Chem. 263, 12472–12477.

Pang, I.-H. and Sternweis, P.C. (1989). Isolation of the α subunits of GTP-binding regulatory proteins by affinity chromatography with immobilized $\beta\gamma$ subunits. Proc. Natl Acad. Sci. USA 86, 7814–7818.

Pepitoni, S., Mallon, R.G., Pai, J.-K., Borkowski, J.A., Buck, M.A. and McQuade, R.D. (1991). Phospholipase D activity and phosphatidylethanol formation in stimulated Hera cells expressing the human m1 muscarinic acetylcholine receptor gene. Biochem. Biophys. Res. Comm. 176, 453–458.

Philips, M.R., Abramson, S.B., Kolasinski, S.L., Haines, K.A., Weissmann, G. and Rosenfeld, M.G. (1991). Low molecular weight GTP-binding proteins in human neutrophil granule membranes. J. Biol. Chem. 266, 1289–1298.

Pike, M.C. and Arndt, C. (1988). Characterization of phosphatidylinositol and phosphatidylinostol-4-phosphate kinases in human neutrophils. J. Immunol. 140, 1967–1973.

Prossnitz, E.R., Quehenberger, O., Cochrane, C. G. and Ye, R. D. (1991). Transmembrane signalling by the N-formyl peptide receptor in stably transfected fibroblasts. Biochem. Biophys. Res. Comm. 179, 471–476.

Qian, Z. and Drewes, L.R. (1989). Muscarinic acetylcholine receptor regulates phosphatidylcholine phospholipase D in canine brain. J. Biol. Chem. 264, 21720–21724.

Qian, Z., Reddy, P.V. and Drewes, L.R. (1990). Guanine nucleotide-binding protein regulation of microsomal phospholipase D activity of canine cerebral cortex. J. Neurochem. 54, 1632–1638.

Quilliam, L.A., Lacal, J.C. and Bokoch, G.M. (1989). Identification of rho as a substrate for botulinum toxin C3-catalyzed ADP ribosylation. FEBS Lett. 247, 221–226.

Quilliam, L.A., Mueller, H., Bohl, B.P., Prossnitz, V., Sklar, L.A., der, C. J. and Bokoch, G. M. (1991). Rap1A is a substrate for cyclic AMP-dependent protein kinase in human neutrophils. J. Immunol. 147, 1628–1635.

Quinn, M.T., Parkos, C.A., Walker, L., Orkin, S.H., Dinauer, M.C. and Jesaitis, A.J. (1989). Association of a Ras-related protein with a cytochrome b of human neutrophils. Nature 342, 198–200.

Quinn, M.T., Mullen, M.L., Jesaitis, A.J. and Linner, J.G. (1992). Subcellular distribution of the Rap1A protein in human neutrophils: colocalization and cotranslation with cytochrome B559. Blood 79, 1563–1573.

Randall, R.W., Bonser, R.W., Thompson, N.T. and Garland, L.G. (1990). A novel and sensitive assay for phospholipase D in intact cells. FEBS Lett. 264, 87–90.

Randazzo, P.A., Northup, J.K. and Kahn, R.A. (1991). Activation of a small GTP binding protein by nucleoside diphosphate kinase. Science 254, 850–853.

Randriamampita, C. and Trautmann, A. (1990). Arachidonic acid activates Ca^{2+} extrusion in macrophages. J. Biol. Chem. 265, 18059–18062.

Ravtech, J.V. and Kinet, J-P. (1991). Fc receptors. Annu. Rev. Immunol. 9, 457–492.

Raymond, J.R., Albers, F.J., Middleton, J.P., Lefkowitz, R.J., Caron, M.G., Obeid, L.M. and Dennis, V.W. (1991). 5-HT$_{1A}$ and histamine H$_1$ receptors in HeLa cells stimulate phosphoinositide hydrolysis and phosphate uptake via distinct G-protein pools. J. Biol. Chem. 266, 372–379.

Rebecchi, M.J. and Rosen, O.M. (1987). Purification of a phosphoinositide-specific phospholipase C from bovine brain. J. Biol. Chem. 262, 12526–12532.

Reinhold, S.L., Prescott, S.M., Zimmerman, G.A. and McIntyre, T. M. (1990). Activation of human neutrophil phospholipase D by three separable mechanisms. FASEB J. 4, 208–214.

Rhee, S.G. (1991). Inositol phospholipid-specific phospholipase C: interaction of γ_1 isoform with tyrosine kinase. Trends Biochem. Sci. 16, 297–301.

Rhee, S.G. and Choi, K.D. (1992). Regulation of inositol phospholipid-specific phospholipase C isozymes, J. Biol. Chem. 267, 12393–12396.

Rhee, S. G., Suh, P-G., Rye, S.H. and Lee, S. Y. (1989). Studies of inositol phospholipid-specific phospholipase C. Science 244, 546–550.

Rhee, S. G., Kim, H., Suh, P-G. and Choi, W.C. (1991). Multiple forms of phosphoinositide-specific phospholipase C and different modes of activation. Biochem. Soc. Trans. 19, 337–341.

Rock, C.O. and Jackowski, S. (1987). Thrombin- and nucleotide-activated phosphatidylinositol 4,5-bisphosphate phospholipase C in human platelet membranes. J. Biol. Chem. 262, 5492–5498.

Rodaway, A.R.F., Teahan, C.G., Casimir, C.M., Segal, A.W. and Bentley, D.L. (1990). Characterization of the 47-kilodalton autosomal chronic granulomatous disease protein: tissue-specific expression and transcriptional control by retinoic acid. Mol. Cell. Biol. 10, 5388–5396.

Rollins, T.E., Siciliano, S., Kobayashi, S., Cianciarulo, D.N., Bonilla-Argudo, V., Collier, K. and Springer, M.S. (1991). Purification of the active C5a receptor from human polymorphonuclear leukocytes as a receptor-G_i complex. Proc. Natl Acad. Sci. USA 88, 971–975.

Rooney, T.A., Hager, R. and Thomas, A.P. (1991). β-Adrenergic receptor-mediated phospholipase C activation independent of cAMP formation in turkey erythrocyte membranes. J. Biol. Chem. 266, 15068–15074.

Sandmann, J., Peralta, E.G. and Wurtman, R.J. (1991). Coupling of transfected muscarinic acetylcholine receptor subtypes to phospholipase D. J. Biol. Chem. 266, 6031–6034.

Schepers, T.M., Brier, M.E. and McLeish, K.R. (1992). Quantitative and qualitative differences in guanine nucleotide binding protein activation by formyl peptide and leukotriene B4 receptors. J. Biol. Chem. 267, 159–165.

Segal, A.W., Heyworth, P.G., Cockcroft, S. and Barrowman, M.M. (1985). Stimulated neutrophils from patients with autosomal recessive chronic granulomatous disease fail to phosphorylate a Mr-44,000 protein. Nature 316, 547–549.

Seifert, R., Rosenthal, W. and Schultz, G. (1986). Guanine nucleotides stimulate NADPH oxidase in membranes of human neutrophils. FEBS Lett. 205, 161–165.

Seifert, R., Rosenthal, W., Schultz, G., Wieland, T., Gierschik, P. and Jakobs, K.H. (1988). The role of nucleoside-diphosphate kinase reactions in protein activation of NADPH oxidase by guanine and adenine nucleotides. Eur. J. Biochem. 175, 51–55.

Seifert, R., Burde, R. and Schultz, G. (1989a). Activation of NADPH oxidase by purine and pyrimidine nucleotides involves G proteins and is potentiated by chemotactic peptides. Biochem. J. 259, 813–819.

Seifert, R., Wenzel, K., Ecktsein, F. and Schultz, G. (1989b). Purine and pyrimidine nucleotides potentiate activation of NADPH oxidase and degranulation by chemotactic peptides and induce aggregation of human neutrophils via G proteins. Eur. J. Biochem. 181, 277–285.

Shearman, M.S., Naor, Z., Sekiguchi, K., Kishimoto, A. and Nishizuka, Y. (1989). Selective activation of the γ-subspecies of protein kinase C from bovine cerebellum by arachidonic acid and its lipoxygenase metabolites. FEBS Lett. 243, 177–182.

Shenker, A., Goldsmith, P., Unson, C.G. and Spiegel, A.M. (1991). The G protein coupled to the thromboxane A2 receptor in human platelets is a member of the novel Gq family. J. Biol. Chem. 266, 9309–9313.

Shukla, S.D. and Halenda, S.P. (1991). Phospholipase D in cell signalling and its relationship to phospholipase C. Life Sci. 48, 851–866.

Silk, S.T., Clejan, S. and Witcom, K. (1989). Evidence of GTP-binding protein regulation of phospholipase A2 activity in isolated human platelet membranes. J. Biol. Chem. 264, 21466–21469.

Simon, M.I., Strathmann, M.P. and Gautam, N. (1991). Diversity of G proteins in signal transduction. Science 252, 802–808.

Skolnik, E.Y., Margolis, B., Mohammadi, M., Lowenstein, E., Fischer, R., Dreppe, A., Ullrich, A. and Schlessinger, J. (1991). Cloning of PI3 kinase-associated p85 utilizing a novel method for expression cloning of target proteins for receptor tyrosine kinases. Cell 65, 83–90.

Smith, C.D., Lane, B.C., Kusaka, I., Verghese, M. W. and Snyderman, R. (1985). Chemoattractant receptor induced hydrolysis of phosphatidylinositol 4,5-bisphosphate in human polymorphonuclear leukocytes membranes: requirement for a guanine nucleotide regulatory protein. J. Biol. Chem. 260, 5875–5878.

Smith, C.D., Cox, C.C. and Snyderman, R. (1986). Receptor-coupled activation of phosphoinositide specific phospholipase C by an N protein. Science 232, 97–100.

Smolen, J.E. and Stoehr, S.J. (1986). Guanine nucleotides reduce the free calcium requirement for secretion of granule constituents from permeabilized human neutrophils. Biochim. Biophys. Acta 889, 171–178.

Smolen, J.E., Stoehr, S.J. and Boxer, L.A. (1986). Human neutrophils permeabilized with digitonin respond with lysosomal enzyme release when exposed to micromolar levels of free calcium. Biochim. Biophys. Acta 886, 1–17.

Smolen, J.E., Stoehr, S.J., Kuczyki, B., Koh, E.K. and Omann, G.M. (1991). Dual effects of guanosine 5'-[γ-thio]triphosphate on secretion by electroporated human neutrophils. Biochem. J. 279, 657–664.

Smrcka, A.V., Hepler, J.R., Brown, K.O. and Sternweis, P.C. (1991). Regulation of polyphosphoinositide-specific phospholipase C activity by purified Gq. Science 251, 804–807.

Sommermeyer, H., Behl, B., Oberdisse, E. and Resch, K. (1989). Effects of nucleotides on the activity of phospholipase C in rabbit thymus lymphocytes. J. Biol. Chem. 264, 906–909.

Stahl, M.L., Ferenz, C.R., Kelleher, K.L., Kriz, R.W. and Knopf, J.L. (1988). Sequence similarity of phospholipase C with the non-catalytic domain of src. Nature 332, 269–272.

Stephens, L.R., Hughes, K.T. and Irvine, R.F. (1991). Pathway of phosphatidylinositol(3,4,5)-trisphosphate synthesis in activated neutrophils. Nature, 351, 33–39.

Strathmann, M. and Simon, M.I. (1990). G protein diversity: a distinct class of α subunits is present in vertebrates and invertebrates. Proc. Natl Acad. Sci. USA 87, 9113–9117.

Strathmann, M.P. and Simon, M.I. (1991). Gα12 and Gα13 subunits define a fourth class of G protein α subunits. Proc. Natl Acad. Sci. USA 88, 5582–5586.

Strathmann, M., Wilkie, T.M. and Simon, M.I. (1989). Diversity of the G-protein family: sequence from five additional a subunits in the mouse. Proc. Natl Acad. Sci. USA 86, 7407–7409.

Strosberg, A.D. (1991). Structure/function relationship of proteins belonging to the family of receptors coupled to GTP-binding proteins. Eur. J. Biochem. 196, 1–10.

Stutchfield, J. and Cockcroft, S. (1988). Guanine nucleotides stimulate polyphosphoinositide phosphodiesterase and exocytotic secretion from HL-60 cells permeabilised with streptolysin O. Biochem. J. 250, 375–382.

Stutchfield, J. and Cockcroft, S. (1990). Undifferentiated HL60 cells respond to extracellular ATP and UTP by stimulating phospholipase C and exocytosis. FEBS Lett. 262, 256–258.

Stutchfield, J. and Cockcroft, S. (1991). Characterisation of fMetLeuPhe-stimulated phospholipase C in streptolysin O permeabilised cells. Eur. J. Biochem. 197, 119–125.

Suga, K., Kawasaki, T., Blank, M.L. and Snyder, F. (1990). An arachidonyl (poly-enoic)-specific phospholipase A2 activity regulates the synthesis of platelet activating factor in granulocytic HL-60 cells. J. Biol. Chem. 265, 12363–12371.

Suh, P.-G., Ryu, S.H., Moon, K.H., Suh, H.W. and Rhee, S.G. (1988). Inositol phospholipid-specific phospholipase C: complete cDNA and protein sequences and sequence homology to tyrosine kinase-related oncogene products. Proc. Natl Acad. Sci. USA 85, 5419–5423.

Sultzman, L., Ellis, C., Lin, L.-L., Pawson, T. and Knopf, J. (1991). Platelet-derived growth factor increases the in vivo activity of phospholipase C-γ1 and phospholipase C-γ2. Mol. Cell. Biol. 11, 2018–2025.

Takayama, K., Kudo, I., Kim, D.K., Nagata, K., Nozawa, Y. and Inoue, K. (1991). Purification and characterization of human platelet phospholipase A₂ which preferentially hydrolyzes an arachidonyl residue. FEBS Lett. 282, 326–330.

Takenawa, T. and Nagai, Y. (1981). Purification of phosphatidylinositol-specific phospholipase C from rat liver. J. Biol. Chem. 256, 6769–6775.

Taki, T. and Kanfer, J.N. (1979). Partial purification and properties of a rat brain phospholipase D. J. Biol. Chem. 254, 9761–9765.

Tao, W., Molski, T.F.P. and Sha'afi, R.I. (1989). Arachidonic acid release in rabbit neutrophils. Biochem. J. 257, 633–637.

Taylor, S.J. and Exton, J.H. (1991). Two α subunits of the Gq class of G-proteins simulate phosphoinositide phospholipase C-β1 activity. FEBS Lett. 286, 214–216.

Taylor, S.J., Chae, H.Z., Rhee, S.G. and Exton, J.H. (1991). Activation of the β1 isozyme of phospholipase C by α subunits of the Gq class of G-proteins. Nature 350, 516–518.

Teahan, C.G., Totty, N., Casimir, C.M. and Segal, A.W. (1990). Purification of the 47 kDa phosphoprotein associated with the NADPH oxidase of human neutrophils. Biochem. J. 267, 485–489.

Teng, D.H.F., Engele, C.M. and Venkatesh, T.R. (1991). A product of the *prune* locus of *Drosophila* is similar to mammalian GTPase-activating protein. Natures 353, 437–440.

Thomas, G.M.H., Geny, B. and Cockcroft, S. (1991). Identification of a cytosolic polyphosphoinositide-specific phospholipase C (PLC-86) as the major G-protein-regulated enzyme. EMBO J. 10, 2507–2512.

Thomas, K.M., Pyun, H.Y. and Navarro, J. (1990). Molecular cloning of the fMet-Leu-Phe receptor from neutrophils. J. Biol. Chem. 265, 20061–20064.

Thomas, K.M., Taylor, L. and Navarro, J. (1991). The interleukin-8 receptor is encoded by a neutrophil-specific cDNA clone, F3R. J. Biol. Chem. 266, 14839–14841.

Thompson, N.T., Tateson, J.E., Randall, R.W., Spacey, G.D., Bonser, R.W. and Garland, L.G. (1990). The temporal relationship between phospholipase activation, diradylglycerol formation and superoxide production in the human neutrophil. Biochem. J. 271, 209–213.

Totzke, F., Marme, D. and Hug, H. (1992). Inducible expression of human phospholipase C-γ2 and its activation by platelet-derived growth factor B-chain homodimer and platelet-derived growth factor A-chain homodimer in transfected NIH 3T3 fibroblasts. Eur. J. Biochem. 203, 633–639.

Traynor, J.R. and Authi, K.S. (1981). Phospholipase A₂ activity of lysosomal origin secreted by polymorphonuclear leukocytes during phagocytosis or on treatment with calcium. Biochim. Biophys. Acta 665, 571–577.

Traynor-Kaplan, A.E., Thompson, B.L., Harris, A.L., Taylor, P., Omann, G.M. and Sklar, L.A. (1989). Transient increase in phosphatidylinositol 3,4-bisphosphate and phosphatidylinositol trisphosphate during activation of human neutrophils. J. Biol. Chem. 264, 15668–15673.

Truett, A.P., Snyderman, R. and Murray, J.J. (1989). Stimulation of phosphorylcholine turnover and diacylglycerol production in human polymorphonuclear leukocytes. Novel assay for phosphorylcholine. Biochem. J. 260, 909–913;

Tyagi, S.R., Olson, S.C., Burnham, D.N. and Lambeth, J.D. (1991). Cyclic AMP-elevating agents block chemoattractant activation of diradylglycerol generation by inhibiting phospholipase D activation. J. Biol. Chem. 266, 3498–3504.

Uhing, R.J., Polakis, P.G. and Snyderman, R. (1987). Isolation of GTP-binding proteins from myeloid HL-60 cells: identification of two pertussis toxin substrates. J. Biol. Chem. 262, 15575–15579.

Uings, I.J., Thompson, N.T., Randall, R.W., Spacey, G.D., Bonser, R.W., Hudson, A.T. and Garland, L.G. (1992). Tyrosine phosphorylation is involved in receptor coupling to phospholipase D but not phospholipase C in the human neutrophil. Biochem. J. 281, 597–600.

Ullrich, A. and Schlessinger, J. (1990). Signal transduction by receptors with tyrosine kinase activity. Cell 61, 203–212.

Van Der Meulen, J. and Haslam, R.J. (1990). Phorbol ester treatment of intact rabbit platelets greatly enhances both the basal and guanosine 5′-[γ-thio]triphosphate-stimulated phospholipase D activities of isolated platelet membranes. Physiological activation of phospholipase D may be secondary to activation of phospholipase C. Biochem. J. 271, 693–700.

Verghese, M., Uhing, R.J. and Snyderman, R. (1986). A pertussis-choleratoxin-sensitive N-protein may mediate chemoattractant receptor signal transduction. Biochem. Biophys. Res. Comm. 138, 887–894.

Volpi, M., Molski, T.F.P., Naccache, P.H., Feinstein, M.B. and Sha'afi, R.I. (1985). Phorbol 12 myristate, 13 acetate potentiates the action of the calcium ionophore in stimulating arachidonic acid release and production of phosphatidic acid in rabbit neutrophils. Biochem. Biophys. Res. Comm. 128, 594–600.

Volterra, A. and Siegelbaum, S.A. (1988). Role of two different guanine nucleotide-binding proteins in the antagonistic modulation of the S-type K⁺ channel by cAMP and arachidonic acid metabolites in *Aplysia* sensory neurons. Proc. Natl Acad. Sci. USA 85, 7810–7814.

Wahl, M.I., Daniel, T.O. and Carpenter, G. (1988). Antiphosphotyrosine recovery of phospholipase C activity after EGF treatment of A-431 cells. Science 241, 968–970.

Wahl, M.I., Nishibe, S., Suh, P.-G., Rhee, S.G. and Carpenter, G. (1989). Epidermal growth factor stimulates tyrosine phosphorylation of phospholipase C-II independently of receptor internalization and extracellular calcium. Proc. Natl Acad. Sci. USA 86, 1568–1572.

Wahl, M.I., Nishibe, S., Kim, J.W., Kim, H., Rhee, S.G. and Carpenter, G. (1990). Identification of two epidermal growth factor-sensitive tyrosine phosphorylation sites of phospholipase C-γ in intact HSC-1 cells. J. Biol. Chem. 265, 3944–3948.

Wang, J., Kester, M. and Dunn, M.J. (1988). Involvement of a pertussis toxin-sensitive G-protein-coupled phospholipase A₂ in lipopolysaccharide-stimulated prostaglandin E₂ synthesis in cultured rat mesangial cells. Biochim. Biophys. Acta 963, 429–435.

Wang, P., Toyoshima, S. and Osawa, T. (1986). Partial purification and characterization of membrane-bound and cytosolic phosphatidylinositol-specific phospholipases C from murine thymocytes. J. Biochem. 100, 1015–1022.

Wang, P., Anthes, J.C., Siegel, M.I., Egan, R.W. and Billah, M.M. (1991). Existence of cytosolic phospholipase D. Identification and comparison with membrane-bound enzyme. J. Biol. Chem. 266, 14877–14880.

Ward, P.A., Cinningham, T.W., McCulloch, K.K. and Johnson, K.J. (1988). Regulatory effects of adenosine and adenine nucleotides on oxygen radical responses of neutrophils. Lab. Invest. 58, 438–447.

Wery, J.-P., Schevitz, R.W., Clawson, D.K., Bobbitt, J.L., Dow, E.R., Gamboa, G., Goodson, T., Hermann, R.B., Kramer, R.M., McClure, D.B., Mihelich, E.D., Putnam, J.E., Sharp, J.D., Stark, D.H., Teater, C., Warrick, M.W. and Jones, N.D. (1991). Structure of recombinant human rheumatoid arthritic synovial fluid phospholipase A$_2$ at 2.2 Å resolution. Nature 352, 79–82.

Wilkie, T.M., Scherle, P.A., Strathmann, M.P., Slepa, V.Z. and Simon, M.I. (1991). Characterization of the G-protein α subunits in the G$_q$ class: expression in murine tissues and in stromal and hematopoietic cell lines. J. Biol. Chem. 88, 10049–10053.

Wright, G.W., Ooi, C.E., Weiss, J. and Elsbach, P. (1990). Purification of a cellular (Granulocyte) and an extracellular (Serum) phospholipase A$_2$ that participate in the destruction of Escherichia coli in a rabbit inflammatory exudate. J. Biol. Chem. 265, 6675–6681.

Wu, D., Lee, C.H., Rhee, S.G. and Simon, M.I. (1992). Activation of phospholipase C by the α subunits of the G$_q$ and G$_{11}$ proteins in transfected Cos-7 cells. J. Biol. Chem. 267, 1811–1817.

Wynkoop, E.M., Broekman, M.J., Korchak, H.M., Marcus, A.J. and Weissman, G. (1986). Phospholipid metabolism in human neutrophils activated by N-formyl-methionyl-leucyl-phenylalanine. Degranulation is not required for arachidonic acid release: studies with neutrophils and neutrophil-derived cytoplasts. Biochem. J. 236, 829–837.

Xie, M. and Dubyak, G.R. (1991). Guanine nucleotide- and adenine-nucleotide-dependent regulation of phospholipase D in electropermeabilized HL-60 granulocytes. Biochem. J. 278, 81–89.

Xie, M., Jacobs. L.S. and Dubyak, G.R. (1991). Regulation of phospholipase D and primary granule secretion by P$_2$-purinergic- and chemotactic peptide-receptor agonists is induced during granulocytic differentiation of HL-60 cells. J. Clin. Invest. 88, 45–54.

Yang, S.F., Freer, S., and Benson, A.A. (1967). Trans-phosphatidylation by phospholipase D. J. Biol. Chem. 242, 477–484.

Yoshihara, Y. and Watanabe, Y. (1990). Translocation of phospholipase A$_2$ from cytosol to membranes in rat brain induced by calcium ions. Biochem. Biophys. Res. Comm. 170, 484–490.

Yuli, I., Tomonaga, A. and Snyderman, R. (1982). Chemoattractant receptor functions in human polymorphonuclear leukocytes are divergently altered by membrane fluidizers. Proc. Natl Acad. Sci. USA 79, 5906–5910.

9.   Priming of Neutrophils

Michael J. Pabst

Immunopharmacology of Neutrophils
ISBN 0–12–339250–0

1. The Concept of Priming

The responses of neutrophils depend upon their past experiences. If neutrophils "smell" bacteria in the environment, they become "angry". Such neutrophils are said to be "activated" or "primed". In the laboratory, neutrophils become primed when they are drawn from the blood stream and dropped into glass or plastic tubes. An LPS-encrusted fingerprint or reagents made from infested water often further aggravate laboratory neutrophils. It is now known that inadvertent exposure to LPS during cell isolation causes neutrophils to change shape, to aggregate and to secrete inflammatory mediators. Allowing neutrophils to adhere to surfaces also drastically

changes their behaviour. Because priming and adherence are often not adequately considered, many experiments with neutrophils provide unexpected results. It is the aim of this chapter to help those working with neutrophils to predict and control their behaviour more accurately.

However, priming is not merely a laboratory curiosity. The aggressiveness of neutrophils in the body is probably regulated by the same biochemical signal transduction pathways that produce priming in the laboratory. If priming in the body could be controlled, as it is in the laboratory, this could either enhance resistance to infection or control the tissue damage associated with chronic inflammation.

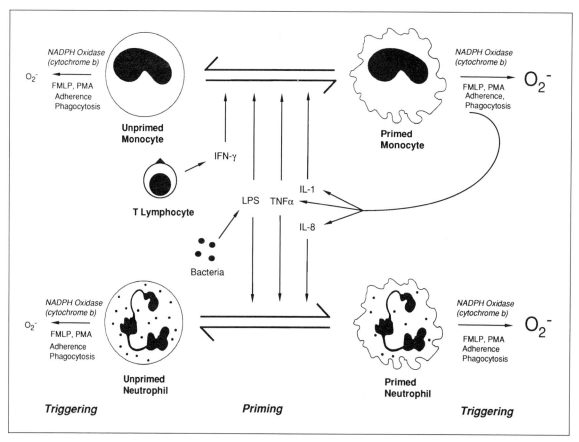

Figure 9.1 Scheme showing priming of neutrophils and monocytes by LPS and cytokines. The scheme also shows triggering by soluble stimuli (FMLP, PMA), by adherence to surfaces or by phagocytosis of microbes. Unprimed neutrophils and monocytes produce little O_2^- (small O_2^- symbols on far left) when triggered. Production of O_2^- is catalysed by the plasma membrane enzyme, NADPH oxidase, one of the components of which is cytochrome *b*. After monocytes are primed by IFNγ from T lymphocytes, by LPS from bacteria, or by TNFα and IL-1 from other primed monocytes, the monocytes produce abundant O_2^- (large O_2^- symbols on far right). Similarly, neutrophils are primed by LPS from bacteria, or by TNFα or IL-8 from primed monocytes. As indicated by the large double arrows, priming is reversible. Neutrophils and monocytes will become unprimed, if the priming agents are removed. The enhanced O_2^- release represents one of many responses that result from priming. These responses include shape change of the cells from spherical to irregular shape, aggregation, degranulation and release of hydrolytic enzymes, increased mobility and phagocytosis, and release of inflammatory mediators and cytokines.

Before proceeding with this review of priming, the terminology will be clarified, most importantly by distinguishing between the terms "activation", "priming" and "triggering".

1.1 ACTIVATION

In the context of phagocyte function, "activation" refers to enhanced antimicrobial activity of phagocytes from animals that have successfully resisted an infection (Mackaness, 1970). A key feature of the enhanced resistance to infection is that the resistance is non-specific (Mackaness, 1964). For example, animals that have survived an infection by mycobacteria show a non-specific resistance to infection by *Candida albicans*. Such activation can also be observed in animals treated with sterile bacterial products. For example, MDP (a fragment of bacterial cell walls) saves mice from an otherwise lethal infection by *Candida* (Cummings *et al.*, 1980). These experiments confirmed the work of Parant *et al.* (1978) showing that MDP protected mice against experimental *Klebsiella* infections. Peritoneal macrophages from MDP-treated mice were found to produce increased amounts of microbicidal oxygen radicals when challenged *in vitro*, which accounts in part for the non-specific resistance to infection.

1.2 PRIMING

Some aspects of "activation" can be observed in phagocytes exposed to bacterial products like LPS or MDP *in vitro* (Pabst and Johnston, 1980). Because not all aspects of activation *in vivo* are likely to be reproduced *in vitro*, the term "activation" is reserved for enhanced phagocyte functions brought about by infection in the intact animal (Karnovsky and Lazdins, 1978; North, 1978). We have promoted the term "priming" to refer to enhanced phagocyte functions brought about by exposure to bacterial products or cytokines *in vitro*. ["Priming" pairs well with "triggering" (see below). The term evokes images of muzzle-loading rifles, a metaphor appropriate to the killing functions of phagocytes. The term "specifically conditioned *in vitro*" has also been proposed (Karnovsky and Lazdins, 1978).] As an example of priming, LPS causes neutrophils to release enhanced amounts of superoxide (O_2^-), when the neutrophils are stimulated by phagocytosis or by a chemical stimulus like FMLP or PMA (Guthrie *et al.*, 1984). Priming of neutrophils and monocytes by LPS and other priming agents is illustrated in Figure 9.1. One of the points made by Figure 9.1 is that priming is a reversible process. If bacterial products are removed, then phagocytes will calm down and inflammation will subside.

Priming must eventually be explained in biochemical terms because a biochemical explanation is the only hope of managing the complexity of the experimental

observations. However, at this stage of our understanding, the concept of priming has practical value in predicting neutrophil behaviour.

Priming can be dramatic. For example, if by luck or skill, an investigator were to isolate some truly unprimed neutrophils from human blood, those neutrophils would produce almost no oxygen radicals when treated with FMLP or PMA (Figure 9.2). With respect to oxygen radical release, it is believed that if there is truly no priming, then there is also no measurable response to FMLP.

The importance of priming was also evident in work with human monocytes. If monocytes are isolated from blood under LPS-free conditions, separated from other mononuclear cells by adherence to plastic tissue culture plates and incubated for several days in LPS-free medium, almost all the monocytes become rounded and then float off the plastic into the medium. Such cells produce low amounts of superoxide when triggered with FMLP or PMA (Pabst *et al.*, 1982). These unprimed cells also release undetectable amounts of monokines like IL-1β and TNFα (Szefler *et al.*, 1989). The monocytes are not dead but they appear to have lost interest in the game in the absence of a challenge from a microbial opponent. To see a "real" macrophage, add a little LPS: 1–10 pg/ml of good LPS will do. The result will be the "typical"

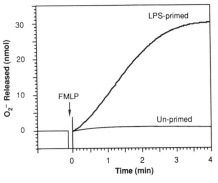

Figure 9.2 Release of O_2^- in response to FMLP requires priming by LPS. This figure shows the release of O_2^- by neutrophils (10^6 in 1 ml) in response to triggering by FMLP (0.1 μM) added at time 0. Unprimed neutrophils produced little O_2^-. In contrast, neutrophils primed with LPS (10 ng/ml) for 30 min showed a vigorous release of O_2^-. O_2^- release was measured by following reduction of the coloured protein cytochrome c (80 μM) by O_2^- in a spectrophotometer by an increase in absorbance at 550 nm. A nanomole of cytochrome c reduced corresponds to a nanomole of O_2^- released by the phagocytes. The specificity of cytochrome c reduction was confirmed by inhibiting the reduction by addition of superoxide dismutase to destroy the O_2^- before it reacted with the cytochrome c (not shown). [Adapted from Forehand (1989), with permission from the American Society for Clinical Investigation.]

cultured macrophage characterized by adherence to the plastic plate, extensive spreading, branched pseudopods and vacuoles. Such LPS-primed monocytes produce abundant O_2^- in response to FMLP and PMA, and actively secrete IL-1β and TNFα into the medium.

1.3   Triggering

"Triggering" is the application of a stimulus that produces an immediate measurable response. For example, FMLP triggers release of O_2^- by neutrophils. However, the magnitude of the response depends upon whether neutrophils had been primed before the stimulus was applied. Triggering agents can be chemicals like FMLP or PMA, surfaces like collagen or plastic, or other cells like endothelium or tumour cells.

1.4   Priming Agents

Many agents are capable of priming neutrophils: bacterial products like LPS, MDP and peptidoglycan, lipoteichoic acid and FMLP (at low concentrations); products from fungi like glucan and mannan; and cytokines like IL-8 and TNFα. Some agents, like zymosan, appear to act both as primers and as triggers. Neutrophils must respond to a variety of microbial pathogens, so their sensors and their weapons are multiple and overlapping.

1.4.1   LPS

LPS is the premier priming agent for neutrophils (Cohn and Morse, 1960) and one of the most important mediators of inflammation generally (Pabst and Johnston, 1989). The chemistry and mechanism of action of LPS has been recently reviewed (Raetz *et al.*, 1991). The structure of LPS is shown in Figure 9.3. LPS is the lipid component on the outside of the outer membrane of Gram-negative bacteria. The polysaccharide moiety of LPS extends to the world outside, while the lipid A moiety is embedded within the outer membrane, where

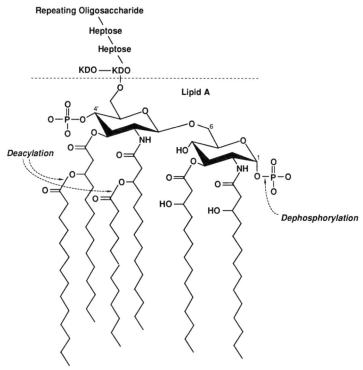

Figure 9.3 Chemical structure of LPS, showing dephosphorylation and deacylation. A complete LPS is composed of a repeating oligosaccharide, also called the O-antigen, an inner core oligosaccharide which includes unusual sugars like heptoses and ketodeoxyoctulosonic acid (KDO), and lipid A, composed of a diglucosamine backbone with N- and O-esterified β-OH myristic acid (C_{14}). Normal FAs (C_{14} and C_{12}) are attached to the β-OH groups. Phosphate groups are attached to the 4′ and 1-positions of the diglucosamine backbone. The normal FA and both phosphate groups are essential for the full immunomodulatory and toxic effects of LPS. When bacteria are phagocytosed, there are enzymes in the phagocytic vacuole that inactivate LPS. Acyloxyacyl hydrolase deacylates LPS by removing the normal FA from the β-OH groups. A phosphatase removes the phosphate group from the glycosidic linkage at the 1-position. Dephosphorylation might also occur extracellularly. This dephosphorylation, or some other chemical modification, may account for the ability of neutrophils to inactivate LPS in solution.

it contacts the normal phospholipids on the inside of the outer membrane.

A few molecules of LPS may be enough to prime neutrophils and monocytes (Pabst *et al.*, 1982). We have tried to study the effects of low concentrations of LPS on neutrophils and monocytes, but keeping an LPS-free kitchen is an essential, continuous and maddening struggle. Most researchers do not bother. They add LPS at 1, 10 or 100 μg/ml, and observe that such a million-fold excess of LPS can make cells perform, even when the system is contaminated. These experiments are useful but they must be interpreted with care. Human blood and tissues are normally LPS-free. When LPS appears in blood, the patient is near death. Experiments with neutrophils accidently exposed to LPS should be interpreted as the behaviour of neutrophils *in extremis*.

The lipid A moiety of LPS appears to contain the priming region of the LPS molecule. In recent years, the chemical structure of lipid A has been determined and biologically active lipid A has been synthesized (Galanos *et al.*, 1985, 1986). Studies with many lipid A analogues have shown that any change in lipid A chemical structure usually makes it inactive. There is a high degree of conservation of the lipid A structure among diverse species of Gram-negative bacteria (Kulshin *et al.*, 1992). Neutrophils are especially discriminating with respect to the chemical structure of lipid A, which might have important consequences for regulation of the inflammatory response, as we will see later.

1.4.2 Peptidoglycan and Muramyl Peptides

LPS is characteristic of most Gram-negative bacteria. However, neutrophils must also "smell" Gram-positive bacteria. A possible priming agent from Gram-positive bacteria is peptidoglycan and its fragments. Peptidoglycan is the "basket" that forms the cell wall of bacteria, which protects the bacterial inner membrane from osmotic shock. Almost all bacteria, except *Rickettsia* and related species, have peptidoglycan. The smallest fragment of peptidoglycan with immunomodulatory activity was found to be MDP. MDP, composed of one sugar and two amino acids, possesses the adjuvant activity of mycobacterial cells walls, the active component in Freund's complete adjuvant. MDP can prime neutrophils in whole blood (Riveau *et al.*, 1991). However, this might involve indirect priming via monocytes, because no direct priming of neutrophils by MDP (1–10 μM) was observed after 30 min incubation. In studies of rat macrophage cytotoxicity, MDP and LPS acted synergistically (Barratt *et al.*, 1991), suggesting that MDP and LPS may have separate receptors and separate intracellular signal transduction mechanisms in macrophages.

MDP shares some receptors with serotonin on various types of cells. There is an intimate integration of the nervous and immune systems, which includes priming of phagocytes by pituitary factors (Edwards *et al.*, 1991). However, priming of neutrophils by serotonin has not been observed. Nevertheless, MDP and other priming agents like LPS and TNFα are undoubtedly important as modulators of the nervous system. MDP and related peptidoglycan products are produced when macrophages digest staphylococci. When injected directly into the brain, MDP and related products induce fever and sleep (Johannsen *et al.*, 1991). However, MDP is unlikely to be the physiological inducer of sleep in healthy humans (Fox and Fox, 1991).

1.4.3 Formyl Peptides

Formyl peptides are made only by bacteria, which use formyl-methionine to initiate protein synthesis, whereas mammalian cells use ordinary methionine. FMLP is, in fact, the principal formylated peptide secreted by bacteria. Neutrophils and monocytes have receptors for FMLP and related peptides, by which they recognize the presence of bacterial metabolites in the environment. Because these receptors recycle, the phagocytes can respond to a chemical gradient of FMLP, allowing them to track down and kill bacteria. At low concentrations of 0.1–10 nM, FMLP primes neutrophils; at higher concentrations of 0.01–1 μM, FMLP triggers O_2^- release, provided that the neutrophils have been first primed by another agent like LPS.

1.4.4 Cytokines

Neutrophils respond to a number of cytokines, but it is unclear exactly which ones. In an LPS-free system, recombinant TNFα primes neutrophils for enhanced O_2^- release. The neutrophil priming activity of IL-8 has also been well-documented in several laboratories (Daniels *et al.*, 1992). LPS-primed macrophages release another cytokine, cyclophilin, so named because it binds to the anti-inflammatory drug, cyclosporin A (Sherry *et al.*, 1992). Cyclophilin is chemotactic for neutrophils, and may also be a priming cytokine.

However, contrary to some reports (Perussia *et al.*, 1987), we have not observed that recombinant IL-1β or IFNγ can prime neutrophils. There is no question that IFNγ is an important primer of monocytes. It enhances their production of oxygen radicals and increases their ability to kill microbes (Nathan *et al.*, 1983). Some cytokines might work indirectly by priming monocytes present in the neutrophil preparations to produce TNFα that can prime neutrophils. Other potential problems with cytokine experiments are that LPS may contaminate some preparations of cytokines, or LPS may be an essential cofactor for response to certain cytokines.

1.5   NEUTROPHIL RESPONSES TO PRIMING

Although the oxygen radical response has been used as the gold standard for determining whether neutrophils are primed, it is only one of many important responses.

Measuring O_2^- responses is preferred because the assay is simple and quantitative, and relates directly to the microbicidal potential of neutrophils. Some other responses to priming, including some that precede the enhanced O_2^- response in time, are discussed below.

1.5.1 Shape Change and Aggregation

One of the first responses that can be observed when neutrophils are primed is a change in shape from a sphere to a sphere with a bulge on one side. Once neutrophils change shape, they tend to aggregate and will also adhere to endothelial cells. Shape change can be observed within 30–60 min after exposure to LPS and may represent one of the most sensitive indicators of neutrophil priming (Haslett *et al.*, 1985).

1.5.2 Up-regulation of Plasma Membrane Glycoproteins

Priming up-regulates a variety of plasma membrane glycoproteins. Some glycoproteins may be stored in special granules that readily fuse with the plasma membrane when neutrophils are primed (Borregaard *et al.*, 1987). For example, the FMLP receptor is up-regulated by LPS priming (Norgauer *et al.*, 1991). The leucocyte adhesion molecules (CD11b/CD18 or Mac-1 or Mo1 or CR3) are also up-regulated by priming (Miller *et al.*, 1987). These adhesion molecules are important for enabling neutrophils to bind to endothelial cells or to bacteria (see Chapters 7 and 10).

A membrane enzyme whose activity reflects priming in neutrophils is alkaline phosphatase. Figure 9.4 shows up-regulation of alkaline phosphatase in neutrophils exposed to LPS. Up-regulation occurred in parallel with priming for enhanced O_2^-. Similar up-regulation of alkaline phosphatase has been reported in B lymphocytes responding to MDP (Souvannavong and Adam, 1990).

1.5.3 Secretion of Lipid Mediators of Inflammation

Primed neutrophils synthesize and secrete lipid mediators of inflammation, including PAF (Betz and Henson, 1980) and LTB4 (Dessein *et al.*, 1986). Priming agents might initiate these processes by binding to receptors that activate phospholipases. For example, IL-8 activates PLA$_2$ to produce PAF (Daniels *et al.*, 1992). Actual synthesis and secretion of lipid mediators may require a trigger, like the Ca^{2+} ionophore A23187, or adherence of the neutrophils to a surface. The trigger could activate PKC or some other mechanism that would turn on the machinery for secretion (McIntyre *et al.*, 1987).

LPS also primes neutrophils for enhanced production of LTB4, the principal eicosanoid product of neutrophils. Actual secretion of LTB4 *in vitro* requires a trigger like PMA or A23187 but not FMLP (Doerfler *et al.*, 1989).

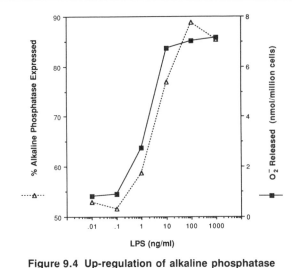

Figure 9.4 Up-regulation of alkaline phosphatase parallels priming for enhanced O_2^- release. Enhanced release of O_2^- in response to triggering by FMLP or other triggers is only one of the consequences of priming. Enhanced O_2^- release might involve migration and assembly of the components of NADPH oxidase in the plasma membrane. Many other proteins also move to the plasma membrane in response to priming. An example is alkaline phosphatase, shown here. Normally, about half of the alkaline phosphatase activity in the neutrophil is expressed on the cell surface, and half is in specialized granules. In response to LPS, almost all the alkaline phosphatase migrates to the plasma membrane. Neutrophils were primed for 30 min at 37°C with the indicated concentration of LPS in the presence of 1% autologous serum. "% alkaline phosphatase expressed" is the amount of enzyme activity found on the surface of intact cells divided by the amount measured in cells lysed with detergent. O_2^- release was triggered by FMLP (0.1 μM).

1.5.4 Protein Synthesis

At one time, neutrophils were thought to be fully functional end-stage cells that could release preformed proteins but synthesized little new protein. This misapprehension was due in part to studying neutrophils after they had been accidentally primed by LPS. We now realize that neutrophils can synthesize and secrete a variety of enzymes, cytokines and cytoplasmic proteins in response to priming agents like LPS (Djeu *et al.*, 1990; Thelen *et al.*, 1990). However, secretion may require a trigger as well.

1.5.5 Secretion of Hydrolases

Many of the enzymes that neutrophils secrete in an inflammatory site are preformed while neutrophils are developing in the bone marrow. Many granule enzymes, like elastase and cathepsin G, are in this class. For example, LPS primes neutrophils to release elastase in response to triggering by FMLP (Fittschen *et al.*, 1988).

1.5.6 Oxygen Radicals

Primed neutrophils are much more vigorous in producing oxygen radicals in response to triggers like FMLP or phagocytosis of microbes. A scheme showing oxygen radicals and related species is shown in Figure 9.5. Production of oxygen radicals is initiated by the enzyme, NADPH oxidase. This plasma membrane enzyme is normally inactive, until triggered. Then, depending upon the priming or "anger" of the neutrophil, NADPH oxidase will become active to a variable extent, using NADPH to reduce oxygen to O_2^-. This behaviour is known as the "respiratory burst" because oxygen is consumed to form O_2^- and glucose is metabolized by the hexose monophosphate shunt to provide NADPH. Two molecules of O_2^- can combine (dismutate) to form peroxide (H_2O_2) and oxygen either spontaneously or by the action of superoxide dismutase. O_2^- reacts with H_2O_2 to form $\cdot OH$ (hydroxyl radical), a powerful oxidizer that may be an important microbicidal species. This reaction is catalysed by the granule protein, lactoferrin (Ambruso and Johnston, 1981).

Neutrophils also contain an abundance of the green granule enzyme, MPO. MPO catalyses the production of hypochlorous acid (bleach) from H_2O_2 and Cl^-. MPO is mostly preformed and stored in granules, but LPS and other primers directly affect its secretion, and also affect the availability of its substrate, H_2O_2.

2. Priming by LPS

If neutrophils are carefully isolated under LPS-free conditions, and then the neutrophils are exposed to 1 ng/ml LPS, priming for enhanced FMLP-triggered O_2^- release can be detected within 15–30 min. Many other responses to LPS can also be observed within a few minutes, including shape change from spherical to oblong, aggregation, up-regulation of membrane glycoproteins and degranulation (Dahinden and Fehr, 1983). Of course, if LPS contaminates the system, then these responses might be over before experimental observation begins.

LPS and other bacterial products might be essential stimulants for proper development and function of the immune system (Bocci, 1992). A person carries around about a kilogram of bacteria so there is plenty of opportunity for exposure to LPS. What is perhaps more amazing is that blood and tissue are normally LPS-free. Although germ-free animals have normal neutrophils and monocytes, no one has produced and studied LPS-free animals, so the importance of bacterial products as

OXYGEN RADICALS

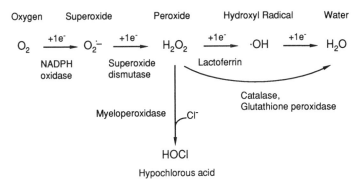

Figure 9.5 Oxygen radicals. Oxygen radicals arise from the reduction of oxygen to water. Reduction involves addition of four electrons to oxygen. In phagocytes, the first electron is added by the membrane enzyme, NADPH oxidase, which transfers an electron from NADPH to oxygen to form O_2^-, a radical with one free electron. NADPH oxidase is normally inactive in phagocytes but is triggered by soluble stimuli like FMLP or PMA, or by phagocytosis of a particle, particularly by particles opsonized with antibody that binds to Fc receptors. Once O_2^- is produced, the other oxygen radicals follow. Two molecules of O_2^- can dismutate (exchange an electron) to form H_2O_2 and oxygen. This process is catalysed by superoxide dismutase. H_2O_2 has several fates. Catalase converts two molecules of H_2O_2 to oxygen and water, neutralizing the anti-microbial activity of H_2O_2. Glutathione peroxidase reduces H_2O_2 to water, using GSH. The neutrophil granule enzyme, lactoferrin, catalyses the formation of $\cdot OH$ from H_2O_2 and O_2^-. Most organic compounds react rapidly with $\cdot OH$, which may be important in penetrating the defences of phagocytozed pathogens. MPO catalyses the formation of HOCl (bleach) from H_2O_2 and Cl^-. Normally, the oxygen radicals are delivered into the phagocytic vacuole, within which the phagocyte traps and kills offending microbes.

"vitamins" remains unclear. Certainly, in the laboratory, neutrophils and monocytes will not "perform" unless they are fed some LPS (Pabst *et al.*, 1982).

2.1   Neutrophils Respond to Minute Amounts of LPS

Neutrophils are sensitive to minute amounts of LPS (in the picogram to nanogram per millilitre range). The dose–response curve for LPS in priming neutrophils for enhanced release of superoxide in response to triggering by FMLP is shown in Figure 9.6. As discussed later, factors present in serum greatly enhance the sensitivity of neutrophils to LPS. Under optimal conditions with 1% serum present, we observed priming of neutrophils by as little as 10 pg/ml of LPS.

2.2   Dealing with LPS Contamination

LPS is everywhere! One should not believe advertisements or labels. Commercial culture media and cell-isolation reagents are often grossly contaminated with LPS and many other microbial products. Reagent

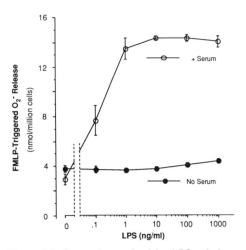

Figure 9.6 Serum is required for LPS priming. Neutrophils that had been freed of serum factors by extra washing through 50% Ficoll-Hypaque were incubated in Teflon tubes with various concentrations of LPS for 30 min in the presence or absence of 1% heat-inactivated (56°C) normal human serum. The neutrophils were then triggered by adding 0.1 μM FMLP for 10 min and the total amount of O_2^- released was determined spectrophotometrically. Teflon was used to minimize premature triggering due to attachment of the neutrophils to an artificial surface.

suppliers are slowly getting the message but their response tends to be soothing reassurances rather than extensive testing.

Neutrophils are as sensitive as the *Limulus* assay to LPS. To be sure that reagents are free of LPS, concentrated stock solutions should be tested with the Limulus assay. The water used for dilution is then the only reagent whose purity must be taken on faith. Sterile bottled water-for-irrigation should be used to make all the reagents that will come in contact with cells. It is possible to operate a closed-system glass distillation apparatus to prepare LPS-free water. The distillation apparatus should be run continuously and periodically sterilized with live steam by cutting off the flow of water to the condenser. Severe penalties should be applied to miscreants who dare to attach filthy old rubber hoses to the outlet spout. Long-term success with water purification systems involving filtration through cartridges has not been achieved in our laboratory.

When performing the *Limulus* assay, be sure always to do positive controls, in which the reagents are deliberately spiked with LPS, to confirm that the *Limulus* gels properly in the presence of the reagent to be tested. Various serum components interfere with gelation of *Limulus*. *Limulus* also will not gel if the pH is not in the neutral range.

Monocytes are sensitive to 1 pg/ml LPS, and can secrete TNFα and IL-8, which then prime neutrophils. Because most neutrophil preparations will contain at least a few percent contamination with mononuclear cells, an indirect effect of contaminating monokines on neutrophil responses should always be considered.

2.2.1   Neutrophil Exposure to LPS during Isolation

Unless special precautions are taken, neutrophils will be exposed to LPS during isolation from blood (Haslett *et al.*, 1985). This accidental exposure has profound effects on their subsequent behaviour in experiments. Cell isolation reagents like dextran and Ficoll-Hypaque are usually contaminated with LPS when they arrive from the manufacturer and addition of contaminated water from the laboratory adds to the problem. Even the act of venipuncture can release some inflammatory mediators that can prime neutrophils. Pelleting the cells by centrifugation and exposing neutrophils to unnatural plastic surfaces also makes them angry. The result is that the average neutrophil preparation is "half-primed" before the experiment starts. Half-primed cells will respond to LPS but the extent of priming will appear limited because the "control" will give the primed response to some variable extent. Even in laboratories where LPS is an obsession, occasionally a batch of neutrophils is isolated that is primed at the start of the experiment. These cells tend to adhere to plastic or to each other, sometimes even aggregating into a useless slimy mass.

Certain donors may have neutrophils that are primed in the bloodstream but this is probably not true in an overtly healthy donor. However, there may be certain stages of priming that occur in the blood of a donor, which make the neutrophils especially sensitive to LPS during isolation. Nevertheless, if the neutrophils appear to be primed in the O_2^- assay, or show a tendency to aggregate, a *Limulus* test on the reagents used to isolate the cells will almost always reveal a LPS-contaminated reagent. Usually, this reagent will come from a newly opened bottle, prominently labelled "LPS-free".

2.2.2 Techniques for Removing LPS

A number of methods can be used to remove LPS from experiments. As a rule, disposable plastic and glassware are LPS-free if delivered in sealed packages. Reusable glassware and other equipment should be baked at $180°C$ for several hours. Teflon vessels and Teflon film can also be baked. Teflon is useful in experiments where non-adherence of neutrophils is desired.

It is possible to neutralize LPS with polymyxin B. However, there are two problems with this approach. First, polymyxin B itself has powerful effects on neutrophils (Aida *et al.*, 1990). Second, if a reagent is contaminated by LPS, it is almost certainly contaminated with other material such as peptidoglycan. Removing the endotoxin will not eliminate these other bacterial agents.

In our laboratory, a method to remove LPS from protein solutions has been developed. The method, which is a modification of the procedure invented by Karplus *et al.* (1987), involves extraction of protein solutions with Triton X-114 (Aida and Pabst, 1990b). On ice, Triton X-114 in water forms a single phase. The protein solution is chilled, and Triton X-114 is added. The solution is stirred gently until it is homogeneous. The solution is then warmed to $37°C$ ($25°C$ is satisfactory for temperature-sensitive materials). The Triton X-114 forms a separate phase, taking with it the lipid-soluble materials including LPS. This method was developed to prepare LPS-free catalase and cytochrome *c* for use in assays of oxygen radical production by neutrophils under LPS-free conditions. Triton X-114, a non-ionic detergent, appears reasonably benign to enzymes like catalase. However, it is toxic to living cells so that protein solutions prepared by this method should have all traces of Triton X-114 removed by gel filtration or detergent-absorbing beads.

2.3 SERUM FACTORS ARE REQUIRED FOR PRIMING OF NEUTROPHILS BY LPS

When Dr Aida joined my laboratory, he informed me that Japanese neutrophils did not respond to LPS. He suggested that my admirable work on neutrophils might apply only in the Western hemisphere. Although I support cultural diversity, I did not support such immunological perversity. Dr Aida and I decided to go back to the beginning and reinvestigate priming of neutrophils by LPS.

The inconsistency in priming neutrophils with LPS had been noticed by other investigators (Wilson *et al.*, 1982). The primary culprit was, of course, contamination of cell isolation reagents by LPS. However, even in laboratories that invested the time to develop an LPS-free environment, priming was a variable phenomenon. A second potential complicating factor was monocyte contamination of neutrophil preparations. When it was discovered that TNFα could prime neutrophils, the potential role of TNFα produced by contaminating monocytes had to be considered. Some investigators suggested that TNFα might play an obligatory role in priming of neutrophils (Koivuranta-Vaara *et al.*, 1987).

Dr Aida and I investigated the role of monocytes and monokines in LPS priming of neutrophils. Using two-step plasma-Percoll gradients, neutrophils that contained only 0.1% monocytes were prepared. These neutrophils responded to 100 ng/ml LPS within 30 min with a five-fold increase in FMLP-triggered O_2^- release. Of course, we knew that one monocyte in 1000 B cells can make a difference in antibody responses, so we investigated further. The time course for secretion of TNFα by monocytes in response to LPS was inconsistent with requirement for TNFα as an obligatory intermediate in priming of neutrophils. Neutrophils responded to LPS within 30 min, whereas production of significant amounts of TNFα by monocytes required 60 min or longer. Furthermore, an Ab against TNFα failed to inhibit priming of neutrophils by LPS at 15, 30 and 45 min, and only produced a 15% inhibition at 60 min. By 90 minutes, the Ab made a significant difference. Our results suggested that TNFα or other factors from monocytes were not essential for priming of neutrophils by LPS (Aida and Pabst, 1990a). Of course, in an inflammatory site where monocytes are present, monokines could amplify the LPS priming effect.

If monocytes were not the unknown variable in priming of neutrophils by LPS, what was? In comparing methods for isolating neutrophils, it was suspected that Dr Aida had been washing his neutrophils too thoroughly! Thus, adding back a little serum restored the ability of neutrophils to respond to LPS. A small percentage of serum (0.1 to 1%) allowed neutrophils to respond to LPS (Figure 9.6); the amount of serum that produced half-maximal priming was 0.13%. The serum requirement was not restricted to priming for enhanced O_2^- release but also promoted up-regulation of alkaline phosphatase on the neutrophil plasma membrane in parallel fashion (Aida and Pabst, 1990a).

A role for serum in LPS priming of neutrophils had been described earlier (Wilson *et al.*, 1982). The serum factor described might also be related to a similar factor from platelets (Wright *et al.*, 1988).

Heating serum to 56°C to inactivate the complement system did not significantly affect the ability of serum to promote LPS priming. By performing every possible sequence-of-addition experiment, the serum factors were found to play two roles, which are described below.

2.3.1   Serum Protects LPS against Inactivation by Neutrophils

If a solution of LPS was exposed to neutrophils and these neutrophils were removed by centrifugation, then the LPS solution lost its power to prime fresh neutrophils. If fresh LPS was added to the solution before adding fresh neutrophils, then the fresh neutrophils responded to the fresh LPS, indicating that there was no inhibitor of priming present in the LPS solution that had been exposed to neutrophils. If LPS was exposed to neutrophils in the presence of 1% serum, then the LPS-containing supernatant was still active when tested on fresh neutrophils, suggesting that the serum protected the LPS against inactivation by the neutrophils.

Using radiolabelled LPS, the potential absorption of LPS on to the neutrophils and its removal when the neutrophils were pelleted by centrifugation was investigated. However, all the radioactivity associated with the LPS was present in solution. Furthermore, the LPS still primed monocytes, and still caused the *Limulus* lysate to gel. Thus, neutrophils were able to modify LPS so that it could no longer prime neutrophils but the LPS still retained some of its biological properties.

In contrast, monocytes did not affect the ability of LPS to prime fresh neutrophils. Thus, this apparent inactivation of LPS was neutrophil-specific in two senses. First, only neutrophils and not monocytes could cause the change in LPS. Second, only neutrophils and not monocytes could detect the change in LPS.

2.3.2   Serum "Presents" LPS to its Receptor

The second function of serum factors in LPS priming of neutrophils is to "present" the LPS to receptors on the neutrophil. One serum component capable of performing this function is LBP (Tobias, *et al.*, 1988). LBP was first identified as an "acute phase" protein, capable of binding LPS (Tobias *et al.*, 1986). An acute phase protein is a protein in serum whose concentration rises dramatically in response to infection or inflammation. LBP binds to LPS, and the complex of LBP and LPS is then recognized by the neutrophil membrane glycoprotein CD14. CD14 is a PI-anchored glycoprotein. It is not yet clear whether CD14 is itself the receptor that transduces a signal to the interior of the cell or whether CD14 forms a ternary complex with LPS and LBP which is then recognized by the true receptor whose identity is presently unknown. The idea of the ternary complex arises because there is a considerable amount of soluble CD14 present in serum. The soluble CD14 does not inhibit priming as would be expected of a receptor antagonist but rather supports priming as expected of a cofactor.

LBP does substitute for whole serum in supporting priming of neutrophils by LPS (Vosbeck *et al.*, 1990), but the magnitude of the priming does not appear to be as great as that found with whole serum, regardless of the amount of LBP used, up to 10 μg/ml (Figure 9.7). Thus, it is believed that serum contains other factors that are also critical for priming.

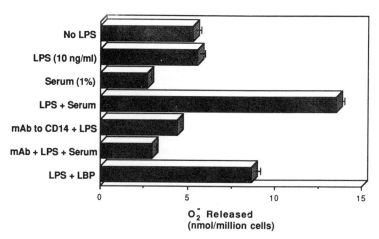

Figure 9.7 LPS priming for O$_2^-$ is blocked by mAb to CD14 and LBP partly replaces serum as an essential cofactor for LPS priming. Neutrophils were incubated for 30 min at 37°C with LPS (10 ng/ml), mAbs to CD14 (10 μg/ml), LBP (10 μg/ml) or serum (1%). Neutrophils were then triggered with FMLP in the presence of cytochrome c, and the amount of O$_2^-$ released was determined. Serum allowed LPS to prime neutrophils. Similar, but only partial, support for LPS priming was also provided by LBP. mAbs to CD14 completely blocked priming even in the presence of serum. This showed that LPS–serum or LPS–LBP complexes must interact with CD14 to prime neutrophils.

Another system in blood called "septin" may also be important. Septin is a system of proteases in blood, analogous to the complement or clotting systems, that allows neutrophils to respond more effectively to LPS (Wright *et al.*, 1992). Septin promotes binding of LPS to CD14 and also promotes priming by the LPS–CD14 complex. The septin system appears to be more important than LBP for promoting priming by LPS, particularly in the blood of healthy donors in which the concentration of LBP, an acute-phase protein, is low.

A potential antagonist of LBP is BPI (Ooi *et al.*, 1991). BPI binds to LPS but the complex does not promote priming of neutrophils (Marra *et al.*, 1990). LBP is synthesized mainly in the liver and in response to infection. BPI is synthesized and secreted by neutrophils. The two proteins share a high degree of amino-acid sequence homology. Competition for LPS between these two proteins may play an important role in moderating the response to LPS (Tobias *et al.*, 1988).

2.4 LPS PRIMES VIA THE GLYCOPROTEIN, CD14

The critical role for CD14 in the response of neutrophils to LPS can be demonstrated by the complete effectiveness of mAbs against CD14 to block priming by LPS in the presence of serum. Figure 9.7 shows that mAb against CD14 blocks priming by LPS. The role of CD14 in LPS priming is not restricted to priming for enhanced O_2^- release. LBP and CD14 are both required for up-regulation of CD11b/CD18 on neutrophils by LPS (Wright *et al.*, 1991).

2.5 NEUTROPHILS INACTIVATE LPS

As mentioned above, we observed that LPS could be inactivated by neutrophils in the absence of serum (Figure 9.8). In the absence of serum, 5 million neutrophils per ml inactivated 10 ng/ml of LPS within 5 min. Although most of the LPS-inactivating activity was associated with the cells, some inactivating activity was found in the supernatant from neutrophil suspensions.

Inactivation of LPS may involve a chemical change to the LPS, such as dephosphorylation of the lipid A moiety of LPS by a neutrophil enzyme. In Figure 9.3, which shows the chemical structure of lipid A, an arrow indicates removal of the 1-phosphate to yield monophosphoryl lipid A. Monophosphoryl lipid A does not prime neutrophils, but it does prime monocytes and has significant immunstimulatory effects on the whole animal (Chase *et al.*, 1986). However, due to the

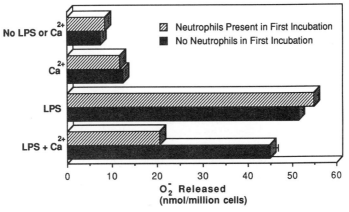

Figure 9.8 LPS inactivation requires Ca²⁺ and neutrophils. The design of this experiment was to expose LPS to neutrophils, then remove the neutrophils by centrifugation and test the LPS in the supernatant for its ability to prime fresh neutrophils. Incubation mixtures were prepared that contained neutrophils (5 × 10⁶/ml), Ca²⁺ (0.25 mM) and LPS (5 ng/ml) in various combinations in PBS with glucose (1%), but with no serum to protect LPS from inactivation. The mixtures were incubated for 30 min at 37°C to allow neutrophils to inactivate LPS. The mixtures were centrifuged to remove neutrophils, where present. The supernatants were mixed 1:1 with a suspension of fresh neutrophils to give 0.5 million fresh neutrophils in 1 ml of PBS containing 1% serum. The suspensions were incubated for 30 min to allow any active LPS present to prime the fresh neutrophils. FMLP and cytochrome c were added, and the suspensions incubated for another 5 min. The suspensions were centrifuged to remove cells, and the supernatants analysed spectrophotometrically for the amount of O₂⁻ released. In the figure, solid bars indicate samples in which there were no neutrophils present during the first incubation. Therefore, there was no opportunity for neutrophils to inactivate the LPS, if it was present, showing that inactivation required neutrophils. The striped bars indicate samples in which neutrophils were present during the first incubation. Only when Ca²⁺ was present in the medium during the first incubation were neutrophils able to inactivate LPS.

extremely low concentrations of LPS involved, dephosphorylation of LPS when it was inactivated by neutrophils has not yet been demonstrated. Therefore, other chemical or physical changes to LPS must also be considered to explain inactivation.

Another possible chemical change to lipid A involves deacylation (Hagen et al., 1991; Hall and Munford, 1983; Munford and Hunter, 1992). Deacylation is also indicated in Figure 9.3. Deacylated LPS is not active in priming neutrophils (Dal Nogare and Yarbrough, 1990).

However, in experiments using radio-labelled LPS, deacylation under conditions where LPS was inactivated was not detected (Aida and Pabst, 1990a). Nevertheless, in some infections, deacylation of LPS by macrophages may be important in limiting inflammation and LPS toxicity.

Serum lipoproteins can also inactivate LPS (Emancipator et al., 1992) but some lipoproteins might promote the effects of LPS. Low-density lipoproteins facilitate the movement of LPS through endothelium and into the tissue, where the LPS could affect tissue macrophages (Navab et al., 1988). Inactivation occurs in the absence of serum and serum lipoproteins, and serum protects LPS against inactivation.

Extracellular Ca^{2+} (>0.25 mM) is required for inactivation of LPS (Figure 9.8). It is not yet clear whether the cation acts as an enzyme cofactor, or whether it is necessary for expression of the LPS inactivating activity on the neutrophil surface. Another interesting point is that inactivated LPS does not inhibit neutrophil responses to intact LPS, although some LPS derivatives and LPS partial structures like lipid X do block priming of neutrophils by LPS and do protect animals from LPS toxicity (Danner et al., 1987).

2.6   RECEPTORS FOR LPS

There is still controversy about the true receptors for LPS in neutrophils. There are a number of candidates for membrane receptors for LPS, described in the next section. Another possibility is an intracellular receptor like those for steroid hormones or vitamin A, described in the following section.

2.6.1   Surface Membrane Receptors

The LAM, CD11b/CD18, binds to LPS but appears not capable of initiating the signal transduction events that mediate priming (Wright et al., 1990). Patients with a genetic deficiency in CD18 can respond to LPS and in normal neutrophils, mAbs against CD18 failed to inhibit priming. CD11b/CD18-deficient neutrophils treated with LPS and serum are able to produce lung injury in an animal model (Wencel et al., 1989). Thus, although CD11b/CD18 allows adherence and triggering, it is not required for LPS priming.

Another adhesion protein is L-selectin (see Chapter 7). L-Selectin is rapidly shed from the neutrophil membrane soon after the neutrophils are triggered. L-Selectin and CD11b/CD18 appear to be reciprocally regulated (Kishimoto et al., 1989). L-Selectin may be involved in adherence of unprimed neutrophils to surfaces like glass or endothelium. It is unclear whether L-selectin can recognize LPS or other bacterial surface molecules. A related molecule, P-selectin that is expressed by stimulated endothelial cells and platelets (see Chapters 7 and 10) may, in fact, inhibit neutrophil priming by LPS (May et al., 1992).

As discussed above, the membrane glycoprotein, CD14, might be the LPS receptor, or it may represent only part of a ternary complex of LPS, LBP and CD14 that binds to a true receptor on the membrane or possibly in the cytoplasm. The possibility of a membrane receptor that interacts with CD14 is supported by studies in which CD14 was transfected into a pre-B cell line. Expression of CD14 in these cells lowered the amount of LPS required to stimulate IgM expression by a factor of 10 000. However, both parental and transfected cells activated the transcription regulatory factor, NF-κB, suggesting that the CD14 interacted with, and potentiated, an existing LPS receptor and signal transduction mechanism (Lee et al., 1992).

In monocytes, blockade of CD14 with mAb almost completely blocked priming by LPS at concentrations of LPS up to 100 ng/ml (Heumann et al., 1992). Monocytes can respond to LPS in the absence of serum and thus might be able to synthesize their own serum factors. Alternatively, monocytes might have receptors that inefficiently recognize LPS in the absence of CD14. In neutrophils, there may be no access to the LPS receptor-signal transduction system in the absence of CD14.

Another neutrophil membrane protein of 73 kD has been identified as a putative LPS receptor using LPS modified with a radioactive photoaffinity label (Halling et al., 1992). Whether the labelled protein is related to the "true" receptor, or merely represents a surface protein with a proclivity for the photoaffinity label is still unclear. A number of other proteins can also be detected with the photoaffinity label. LPS binding sites have also been detected on guinea-pig peritoneal macrophages by an immunogold electron microscopy technique (Kriegsmann et al., 1991).

2.6.2   Intracellular Receptors

Like steroid hormones, LPS has the ability to induce synthesis of new mRNA for proteins. LPS is also partly lipid soluble so that it could penetrate the plasma membrane either by itself at higher concentrations or as a complex with serum factors at lower concentrations. Thus, a steroid-type intracellular receptor for LPS in neutrophils is a possibility deserving consideration. LPS has been reported to bind to a microtubule associated protein and some of the effects of LPS are mimicked by the microtubule-active agent, taxol (Ding et al., 1992).

This might be an important mechanism of LPS action because movement of proteins to the cell membrane is a prominent feature of priming by LPS.

2.7 INTRACELLULAR SIGNAL TRANSDUCTION IN LPS PRIMING

Several intracellular signal transduction events have been identified in LPS priming for enhanced superoxide release. The signal transduction mechanisms affected by LPS are complex and have been difficult to decipher, compared with, for example, the signal transduction pathways involved in triggering by FMLP. Some of the signal transduction elements that might be involved in priming by LPS are described below.

2.7.1 Phospholipases and G Proteins

PLA_2, PLC and PLD have been implicated in priming by LPS. The phospholipases are linked to membrane receptors by G proteins, as shown by the migration of G protein to the plasma membrane in response to LPS-serum complexes binding to CD14 (Yasui et al., 1992). In another example, IL-8 activates PLA_2 to produce lyso-PC, which is converted to PAF (Daniels et al., 1992). Because the evidence for involvement of the PLC, DAG and IP_3 pathway in FMLP signal transduction is strong (see Chapter 8) and because FMLP and LPS have quite different effects, it is likely that LPS works via a different pathway from that of FMLP. In rat mesangial cells, lipid A stimulates PLD via a G protein to hydrolyse phosphatidylethanolamine to phosphatidic acid which can be converted to DAG (Harris and Bursten, 1992). The DAG produced by the PLD pathway might stimulate PKC but might also prime by a mechanism bypassing PKC (Bass et al., 1987). Phosphatidic acid may itself be involved in signal transduction (Channon et al., 1987).

2.7.2 Cytosolic Ca^{2+}

The extent of FMLP-stimulated O_2^- release in neutrophils correlates with the concentration of free Ca^{2+} in the cytosol (Lew et al., 1984). FMLP causes a rapid increase in cytosolic Ca^{2+}, which, if blocked, interferes with the O_2^- response. This phenomenon may be related to priming. Priming can be produced in neutrophils by exposing them to ionomycin, a calcium ionophore (Finkel et al., 1987). Using various concentrations of ionomycin, priming was shown to be proportional to the level of cytosolic Ca^{2+}. The response to these artificially induced increases in cytosolic Ca^{2+} was reminiscent of adding a substrate to its enzyme. At low concentrations of cytosolic Ca^{2+}, the O_2^- response was directly proportional to the Ca^{2+} concentration but the priming approached a maximum corresponding to V_{max} at higher cytosolic Ca^{2+} concentrations (Figure 9.9). It should be noted that, even in primed neutrophils, the cytosolic

concentration of Ca^{2+} is still in the micromolar range, which is 1/1000th of the extracellular Ca^{2+} concentration. Another line of evidence supporting cytosolic Ca^{2+} as a mediator of priming are the experiments in which priming was inhibited by MAPTAM, an intracellular Ca^{2+} chelator (Forehand et al., 1989).

2.7.3 Protein Kinases

Both serine/threonine kinases and tyrosine kinases have been implicated in priming for enhanced release of O_2^- and other primed responses. Agents like PMA that trigger O_2^- release cause translocation of PKC from the cytoplasm to the plasma membrane. The plasma membrane is the location of NADPH oxidase, the enzyme responsible for generating oxygen radicals. PMA acts like an analogue of DAG, the endogenous lipid mediator derived from the hydrolysis of PI by PLC. PMA and DAG activate PKC, which demonstrates a role for protein phosphorylation in triggering of O_2^- release. Activation of PKC involves its movement from the cytoplasm to the plasma membrane, where it loses its regulatory subunit and becomes active in protein phosphorylation. Several components of NADPH oxidase are thought to be targets of this phosphorylation, although a role for phosphorylation in triggering NADPH oxidase has not been proven conclusively. Because activation of PKC has been so strongly connected with triggering, it seems unlikely that activation of PKC by DAG would be the mechanism of action of priming by LPS. However, because PKC also

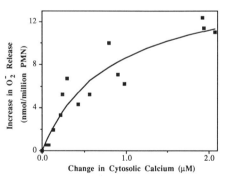

Figure 9.9 Priming is regulated by cytosolic Ca^{2+}. Neutrophils were exposed to various concentrations of the Ca^{2+} ionophore, ionomycin. Then the neutrophil samples were split in half for measurement of FMLP-triggered O_2^- release and for determination of cytosolic free Ca^{2+}, using the fluorescent indicator fura-2. The results show that priming for enhanced FMLP-triggered O_2^- release was proportional to the cytosolic free Ca^{2+} concentration, until a maximum priming response was attained. [Reproduced from Finkel (1987), with permission from the American Society for Biochemistry and Molecular Biology.].

requires Ca^{2+} for activity, protein phosphorylation by PKC could be enhanced if LPS increased the intracellular concentration of Ca^{2+}. Thus, activation of PKC by increased Ca^{2+} could be at least part of the mechanism of priming by LPS.

In human monocytes, an inhibitor of priming, sulphatide from *Mycobacterium tuberculosis*, was shown to affect protein phosphorylation (Brozna *et al.*, 1991). However, while sulphatide blocked or reversed priming for enhanced O_2^- release, it promoted synthesis of IL-1β and TNFα. In fact, this combination of effects is just what the mycobacteria want, causing suppression of oxygen radical-dependent killing, with promotion of inflammation, leading to formation of granulomata. In contrast to its inhibitory effects on priming in monocytes, sulphatide does not inhibit priming in neutrophils. Rather, sulphatide acts like a slow trigger in neutrophils (Zhang *et al.*, 1991). This complexity of response indicates that the signal transduction mechanisms controlling priming are unlikely to be agreeably simple.

In neutrophils, TNFα and LPS induce the synthesis and myristoylation of a substrate for PKC (Thelen *et al.*, 1990). Myristoylation (addition of a C_{14} FA) causes this protein substrate to move to the plasma membrane to meet PKC. PKC translocates to the membrane in response to the triggering signal, where it then phosphorylates this substrate. This substrate, called MARCKS, might function in regulation of genes whose expression is controlled by LPS.

2.7.4 Gene Expression and Protein Synthesis

Many of the priming effects of LPS, like enhanced O_2^-, do not require protein synthesis, and are unaffected by inhibitors like cycloheximide. Nevertheless, neutrophils and monocytes can produce new proteins in response to LPS. In monocytes, there are regulatory proteins like NF-$\varkappa$B and AP-1 that bind to DNA upstream from the genes for cytokines and for tissue factor of coagulation, and appear to control their transcription (Mackman *et al.*, 1991). Genes regulated by NF-$\varkappa$B respond to LPS by increasing transcription (Vincenti *et al.*, 1992). The regulatory proteins, in turn, might be controlled by signal transduction factors like Ca^{2+} and calmodulin (Ohmori and Hamilton, 1992). NF-$\varkappa$B works through a mechanism that does not appear to involve PKC (Vincenti *et al.*, 1992), but may in fact be inhibited by protein kinases (Hohmann *et al.*, 1992). One possibility is that these transcription factors are regulated through a PLA$_2$ pathway (Mohri *et al.*, 1990).

2.8 NADPH OXIDASE PROTEIN SUBUNITS

There are at least four genes, coding for four proteins, needed for the function of NADPH oxidase, the critical enzyme that initiates production of O_2^- and the other

oxygen radicals (Nunoi *et al.*, 1988; Volpp *et al.*, 1988). Defects in any of these proteins result in some form of CGD (see Chapter 3). In CGD, patients' phagocytes cannot make O_2^-, and the patients suffer frequent severe infections. Two of the components constitute cytochrome *b*, a membrane-associated flavoprotein (Rotrosen *et al.*, 1992). The amount of cytochrome *b* present in neutrophils or monocytes can be determined spectrophotometrically. In both monocytes and neutrophils, priming by LPS does not affect the concentration of cytochrome *b* inside the cells, measured spectrophotometrically. IFNγ and LPS do increase mRNA and protein levels for the heavy-chain subunit of cytochrome *b* but there is no increase in mRNA for the light chain subunit (Cassatella *et al.*, 1990). This suggests that priming for enhanced O_2^- may not be due principally to synthesis of more NADPH oxidase. Of course, some other component, perhaps one not yet recognized, might be the limiting factor in NADPH oxidase activity. LPS and other factors (1,25-dihydroxy-vitamin D_3 and lipoteichoic acid) increase expression of subunits of NADPH oxidase in monocytes, particularly the cytoplasmic p47 component (Levy and Malech, 1991). However, the evidence to date suggests that priming for enhanced O_2^- has more to do with alteration in signal transduction pathways, than with new protein synthesis. Signal transduction events alter the enzyme kinetics of NADPH oxidase, which could control O_2^- production by greatly increasing the catalytic efficiency of NADPH oxidase (Sasada *et al.*, 1983; Tsunawaki and Nathan, 1986). The activity of NADPH oxidase might be controlled by regulating the assembly of its subunits in the plasma membrane (Ambruso *et al.*, 1990). Priming may represent movement of NADPH oxidase subunits to the plasma membrane or at least may represent an alert to the transport mechanism.

3. Priming by Cytokines and Mediators

In addition to microbial products, neutrophils and monocytes express and respond to a variety of hormones or intercellular messengers. These include the protein cytokines described below and lipid mediators of inflammation described in the next section.

3.1 CYTOKINES

Cells of the immune system can prime neutrophils by secreting cytokines like TNFα and IL-8. This led to speculation that LPS might work by inducing synthesis of cytokines by neutrophils, with the neutrophils then being primed by the cytokines in an autocrine loop. However, blocking cytokine production with glucocorticoids did not interfere with priming of the O_2^- response by LPS (Szefler *et al.*, 1989). Nevertheless, a number of cytokines undoubtedly do play a role in telegraphing the message that microbes have invaded.

3.1.1 TNFα

TNFα primes neutrophils for enhanced FMLP-triggered O_2^- response (Berkow et al., 1987; Shalaby et al., 1987). Unlike priming by LPS, priming of neutrophils by TNFα does not require serum. In our work (Aida and Pabst, 1990a) and in other laboratories (Berger et al., 1988), TNFα appeared to be the most important neutrophil-priming monokine produced by human monocytes. TNFα also affects endothelial cells and fibroblasts, leading to the production of collagenase and inflammatory mediators (Dayer et al., 1985). TNFα-primed neutrophils produce abundant oxygen radicals and release proteases like elastase and CatG. When these agents are combined with secretion of collagenase by fibroblasts and a rich soup of other inflammatory mediators from both cells, it is not surprising that chronic production of TNFα can cause extensive destruction of connective tissue.

3.1.2 IL-8

IL-8 primes neutrophils for enhanced oxygen radical release. IL-8 also primes neutrophils for enhanced adhesion and phagocytosis (Detmers et al., 1991). IL-8 was identified by several laboratories as a neutrophil-priming protein produced by monocytes in response to LPS (Schröder et al., 1987; Walz et al., 1987). The protein was shown to be different from IL-1 and TNFα, and was subsequently purified, sequenced and cloned (Baggiolini et al., 1989).

In response to IL-1β, TNFα or LPS, endothelial cells also produce a variant form of IL-8. This IL-8 is then proposed to regulate migration of neutrophils through endothelium, by stimulating neutrophils to up-regulate CD11b/CD18 (Huber et al., 1991). By this IL-8 mechanism, and by chemotaxis to FMLP and LPS, neutrophils are recruited into sites of inflammation in connective tissue. In addition, the integrity of the endothelium may be compromised by primed neutrophils, leading to leakage of inflammatory factors from serum into the tissue.

3.1.3 G-CSF and GM-CSF

G-CSF (Kitagawa et al., 1987) and GM-CSF (Weisbart et al., 1985; Lopez et al., 1986) have been reported to prime neutrophils. We have not examined these factors, so the reservations expressed below concerning IFNγ and IL-1 may apply as well to the colony stimulating factors.

3.1.4 IFNγ and IL-1β

IFNγ and IL-1β were not active in priming neutrophils for enhanced O_2^- release in our experiments but others have reported that they can prime neutrophils (Perussia et al., 1987; Shalaby et al., 1987). The effect of IL-1β on neutrophils has been confirmed (Sullivan et al., 1989)

and denied (Georgilis et al., 1987). One potential caution is the possibility of contamination of neutrophils with monocytes. Another problem is the ever-present possibility of LPS contamination of the cytokines. These cytokines may synergize with low concentrations of contaminating LPS. Although IFNγ and IL-1β might or might not directly prime neutrophils, there is no dispute about their power to promote inflammation which will lead to priming of neutrophils by multiple indirect mechanisms.

3.2 LIPID MEDIATORS

In addition to the cytokines, which are protein mediators of inflammation, a number of lipid mediators of inflammation are also able to prime neutrophils. Among these are PAF, a phospholipid, and LTB$_4$, a derivative of AA. Because neutrophils both produce PAF and LTB$_4$ and also become primed in response to these lipids, PAF and LTB$_4$ may be important factors in the rapid progression of inflammation.

3.2.1 PAF

PAF enhances O_2^- release by neutrophils triggered by soluble stimuli like PMA, FMLP and C5a (Englberger et al., 1987). Indeed, PAF might be a mediator in LPS priming (Worthen et al., 1988). Much of the PAF produced in response to LPS is not secreted but remains within the neutrophil, suggesting a role for PAF in signal transduction in response to LPS (Ludwig et al., 1985). PAF is also produced rapidly, before priming for enhanced O_2^- release can be detected (Daniels et al., 1992). Thus, the time course is also consistent with a mediator role for PAF in LPS priming of neutrophils. Inhibitors of PAF synthesis can block priming by LPS, suggesting that PAF may be a mediator of LPS shock (Terishita et al., 1985). A PAF antagonist, WEB2170, attenuated neutrophil priming by factors in the sera from burn patients (Pitman et al., 1991). Neutrophils, responding to sepsis, may contribute to organ injury in burn patients.

3.2.2 Leukotrienes

Neutrophils can also be primed by LTB$_4$. Leukotrienes and other metabolites of AA arise by the action of PLA$_2$ on PC, generating AA and, through acyltransferase, PAF. Thus, if PAF is involved in priming, LTB$_4$ and other AA metabolites are probably also involved (Chilton et al., 1984).

3.3 PROTEASES

In earlier work with monocytes, it was found that brief exposure of monocytes to a variety of proteases could prime the monocytes for enhanced O_2^- release. The principal proteases secreted by neutrophils, elastase and CatG, were particularly effective in priming monocytes (Speer *et al.*, 1984). Proteases may destroy an inhibitory factor on the surface of the plasma membrane of monocytes because internalization of the protease was not essential for priming (Bryant *et al.*, 1986). Such an inhibitory factor in neutrophils might be lipocortin, a membrane protein that regulates the activity of phospholipases and a protein that is, in turn, regulated by phosphorylation (Hirata, 1981). Lipocortin is induced by glucocorticoids, which are known to suppress neutrophil functions (Webb and Roth, 1987). The possibility that there is a negative regulator of priming is reinforced by the observations of Bromberg and Pick (1985) that NADPH oxidase can be triggered in cell homogenates by the detergent SDS, which may dissociate a regulator protein from the enzyme. The idea of a negative regulator makes sense. Neutrophils and monocytes must confront unknown pathogens with little time for preparation. It would be easier if the weapons were all preassembled and ready for firing, with only the need to flick the safety switch.

Proteases secreted by neutrophils could be important inflammatory signals because neutrophils usually precede monocytes into an inflammatory site. Later, monocytes appear, primed for battle by the neutrophil proteases. Proteases from other sources like the complement and clotting systems might also be involved in priming. The recent discovery of the septin system in blood presents the possibility that proteases from neutrophils might promote priming by potentiating LPS priming, as does the septin system of endogenous plasma proteases.

4.   *Priming and Triggering by Surfaces*

Once we had made progress in controlling some of the variables involved in priming of neutrophils, like LPS contamination, monocyte contamination and the effect of serum, we attacked another conspicuous variable, the effect of adherence on neutrophil function (Aida and Pabst, 1991). Adherence is known to have a profound effect on neutrophil functions and on neutrophil responses to LPS (Dahinden *et al.*, 1983). In our philosophy, we think of adherence as a triggering event. This idea may be especially relevant with respect to adherence to artificial surfaces like tissue culture plastic. We know that adherence to plastic alone can trigger release of O_2^-. However, the amount of O_2^- released might be rather small, if the neutrophils have not been previously primed. In many experiments, LPS contamination will ensure a significant O_2^- response.

4.1   ARTIFICIAL SURFACES: PLASTIC, GLASS, TEFLON

Neutrophils readily adhere to glass or plastic surfaces. Adherence can be prevented to a large extent by

continuous stirring, or by keeping the neutrophils in Teflon. However, if neutrophils are primed, they up-regulate surface adherence molecules that allow the neutrophils to stick, even to Teflon! When neutrophils are primed by LPS, a large number of surface glycoproteins are up-regulated, including enzymes like alkaline phosphatase and glycoproteins like CD11b/CD18. As mentioned above, such up-regulation by LPS does require serum cofactors. CD11b/CD18 is one of the LAMs and also functions as CR3. This glycoprotein is one of the leucocyte integrins, a family of dimeric molecules that span the plasma membrane. CD11b/CD18 allows neutrophils to bind to endothelial cells and allows neutrophils to bind bacteria by directly interacting with LPS on the surface of the bacteria (Wright and Jong, 1986). CD11b/CD18 plays an important role in response to infection, as dramatically illustrated by patients who are genetically deficient in the LAMs. These patients suffer frequent severe infections, including rampant periodontal disease (Anderson *et al.*, 1985) (see Chapter 7).

However, as mentioned earlier, CD11b/CD18 is not the receptor that responds to priming by LPS. Neutrophils and monocytes from patients who are totally deficient in these molecules respond normally to LPS in priming for enhanced O_2^- response. A complex of LPS with serum proteins like LBP interact with CD14, a lipid-anchored glycoprotein, which probably then interacts with an unidentified transmembrane or intracellular receptor. Nevertheless, CD11b/CD18 can mediate adherence and act as a trigger for oxygen radical release (Anderson *et al.*, 1986; Shappell *et al.*, 1990).

Neutrophils are triggered to release O_2^- when they adhere to artificial surfaces (Figure 9.10). Primed cells can even adhere to surfaces like Teflon, a material to which unprimed cells do not adhere (Figure 9.11). In this situation, LPS not only primes but also enables a non-triggering surface to become a triggering surface. Priming up-regulates CD11b/CD18, allowing adherence to Teflon or serum-coated glass (Aida and Pabst, 1991). The adherence of primed cells to Teflon or serum-coated glass can be blocked by mAb directed against CD18. The mAb does not affect binding of unprimed cells to glass or plastic. Thus, the membrane glycoproteins involved in adherence to surfaces vary according to the nature of the surface and the state of priming of the neutrophil.

4.2   BIOLOGICAL SURFACES: ENDOTHELIAL CELLS, MATRIX PROTEINS

In health, neutrophils do not adhere to endothelial cells or connective tissue components. They would not do so *in vitro*, if not for a little LPS in the experiments. In response to LPS, endothelial cells up-regulate the membrane glycoprotein CD54 (intercellular adhesion

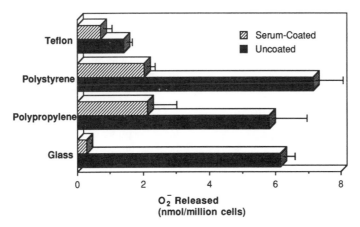

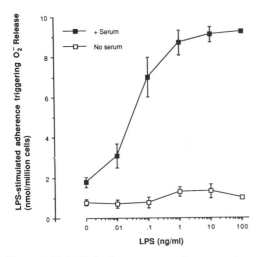

Figure 9.10 Adherence triggers neutrophils to release O_2^-. Neutrophils were incubated in various types of tubes for 30 min in the presence of LPS-free cytochrome c to measure release of O_2^- triggered by adherence of the neutrophils to the tubes. The solid bars show untreated tubes. The striped bars indicate tubes that had been filled with 1% heat-inactivated normal human serum, which was then washed out with PBS. The results showed that glass and plastic tubes triggered neutrophils to release O_2^-, but that this effect could be minimized by coating the tubes with serum beforehand. Other experiments showed that the O_2^- response was proportional to the number of cells that adhered to the tube (all tubes contained the same total number of cells during the experiment). [Reproduced from Aida and Pabst (1991), with permission.]

Figure 9.11 LPS, in the presence of serum, allows neutrophils to adhere to Teflon and to produce O_2^-. Neutrophils were incubated with various concentrations of LPS, in the presence or absence of 1% heat-inactivated autologous serum, in Teflon, at 37°C for 90 min in the presence of LPS-free cytochrome c to detect the release of O_2^-. [Reproduced from Aida and Pabst (1991), with permission.]

molecule or ICAM-1), which is recognized by CD11b/CD18 on neutrophils (see Chapter 7). Thus, LPS in infected tissue promotes adherence of neutrophils to endothelial cells by up-regulating "sticky" molecules on both cells (Nathan et al., 1989; Seifert et al., 1991).

When TNFα primes neutrophils, it up-regulates CD11b/CD18, allowing the neutrophils to attach to biological surfaces like fibrinogen or laminin (Nathan et al., 1989). When primed neutrophils attach to biological surfaces, the surface triggers a strong oxygen radical response (Nathan, 1987). For example, cardiac myocytes are damaged by primed neutrophils that recognize CD54 (ICAM-1) on the myocytes that has been up-regulated by LPS (Smith et al., 1991).

4.3 RECIPROCAL RELATIONSHIP BETWEEN PRIMING AND TRIGGERING

Some reports have described triggering of neutrophils by LPS, rather than priming, as I have described so far. In these experiments, neutrophils were given LPS (usually at high concentrations), and production of O_2^- was observed without any additional stimulus or trigger being deliberately added. However, aggregation of neutrophils or adherence to plastic might have constituted unintended triggers. In my interpretation, the actual trigger for O_2^- release is either aggregation or adherence to a surface, and LPS is the priming agent that allows a sufficient response to the trigger such that O_2^- release can be measured.

If neutrophils were triggered by a stimulus, such as adherence to plastic, then they could not be primed. Conversely, if the neutrophils were stirred to prevent them from adhering, then they were primed by LPS (Aida and Pabst, 1991). Thus, if cells are adherent, agents that are considered primers, like LPS, TNFα, G-CSF or

GM-CSF, might look like triggers (Nathan, 1989). This "priming–triggering" nomenclature is not worth arguing over, because biochemical understanding should eventually explain all.

5. *Medical Significance of Priming*

Proper control of the aggressiveness of neutrophils and monocytes is critical for health. Like soldiers, most neutrophils live their entire life without ever seeing the enemy. As important as it is for neutrophils to be able to kill bacteria efficiently, it is equally important for most neutrophils to be well disciplined and keep their weapons in check. For example, in diseases like ARDS and periodontal disease, a militant response can result in destroying the village in order to save it from the enemy.

5.1 CHRONIC INFECTIONS AND INFLAMMATIONS

ARDS may result from unrestrained priming of alveolar macrophages and infiltrating neutrophils in the lung by LPS (Harmsen, 1988). In a rat lung model, LPS-primed, FMLP-triggered neutrophils promoted lung injury through a mechanism involving PAF (Anderson *et al.*, 1991). The lung injury could be blocked by a PAF receptor antagonist.

Idiopathic pulmonary fibrosis may be due to a related mechanism in which alveolar macrophages secrete excessive IL-8 which recruits neutrophils into the lung and primes them (Carré *et al.*, 1991) (see Chapter 13). TNFα from alveolar macrophages and from blood monocytes would also promote neutrophil infiltration (Gamble *et al.*, 1985). Infiltration of primed neutrophils could damage lung endothelium. In experiments *in vitro*, endothelial cells were damaged by LPS-primed, FMLP-triggered neutrophils. The damage could be prevented by an inhibitor of neutrophil elastase (Smedly *et al.*, 1986).

The kidney is also susceptible to such injury, which is mediated by oxygen radicals and elastase (Linas *et al.*, 1991). Both priming by LPS and triggering by FMLP are needed to cause the kidney damage. Similarly, infusion of non-lethal doses of LPS primes neutrophils and Kupffer cells, leading to liver damage (Mayer and Spitzer, 1991). The brain may also be affected. Rat microglia, which are monocyte-like cells in the brain, up-regulate Fc receptors in response to TNFα, IL-1, IFNγ and LPS (Loughlin *et al.*, 1992). Other glycoproteins may be up-regulated and inflammatory mediators may be released in this situation.

5.2 PERIODONTAL DISEASE

The mouth and particularly the periodontal tissue is a battleground. In a healthy mouth, 10^5–10^6 neutrophils/min migrate from the bloodstream through the periodontal connective tissue into the gingival sulcus and into the mouth where they are swallowed. This surprisingly large number of neutrophils moving through the mouth was determined from the concentration of the neutrophil enzyme, MPO, present in saliva (Bozeman *et al.*, 1990; Thomas and Cook, 1991). During their passage, the neutrophils detect bacteria by smelling formyl peptides or LPS. The neutrophils track down the bacteria, phagocytose and kill them. This process goes on continuously, without producing a classical inflammatory reaction. Any LPS that is present will be rapidly inactivated by the neutrophils, thereby limiting the inflammatory response, and avoiding tissue damage.

If anything happens to impair the effectiveness of neutrophils in controlling periodontal bacteria, then a chronic inflammation develops. Serum components leak into the tissue. In the presence of serum, neutrophils fail to inactivate LPS. More neutrophils and monocytes are called from the bloodstream into the periodontal tissues. LPS-primed neutrophils, triggered by FMLP, adhere and damage fibroblasts isolated from the periodontal ligament (Deguchi *et al.*, 1990). Monocytes are called into the site. Once monocytes become activated, they secrete monokines like IL-1β and TNFα. Primed neutrophils can also synthesize TNFα (Djeu *et al.*, 1990). One of the important biological activities of IL-1 is "osteoclast activating factor", which causes breakdown of bone. TNFα also stimulates bone resorption by enhancing the production of a factor from osteoblasts that stimulates osteoclasts to break down bone (Thomson *et al.*, 1987). IL-1 also stimulates fibroblasts to produce collagenase (Postlethwaite *et al.*, 1983). Thus, oral pathogens cause neutrophils and monocytes to release cytokines. These cytokines cause fibroblasts and osteoclasts to break down connective tissue, so that the periodontal ligament and the alveolar bone, which hold the teeth in place, are destroyed. The situation resolves when the teeth all fall out, or the victim succumbs to the infection.

Some benign bacteria, like *Helicobacter pylori*, normally express a dephosphorylated LPS (Muotiala *et al.*, 1992). (Experimentally, care must be taken to ensure that inactive LPS is not the result of damage to the LPS during isolation.) However, pathogens like *Porphyromonas gingivalis* might also produce an LPS that could fail to prime neutrophils. The problem of dealing with such an organism would then fall to monocytes, which are capable of recognizing monophosphoryl lipid A. Unfortunately, by the time monocytes get involved in fighting an infection, tissue damage is likely to result.

5.3 ENDOTOXIC SHOCK

When LPS primes neutrophils systemically, then shock results. Normally, efficient mechanisms exist to destroy LPS in blood, but when there is an overwhelming infection in the bloodstream, priming can get out of control.

Several approaches are currently being investigated to block or reverse endotoxic shock. LPS and TNFα and neutrophils are all required to produce shock in animal models (Bauss *et al.*, 1987; Mathison *et al.*, 1988; Rothstein and Schreiber, 1988), so that neutralizing any one of these factors should prevent shock.

In some systems, mAbs directed against LPS have protected animals from death by septicaemia. One important effect of anti-LPS Abs may be to prevent synthesis of TNFα (Vacheron *et al.*, 1992). In peritoneal infections of mice with *E. coli*, antibodies to TNFα were compared with Abs against LPS. Only Abs that recognized LPS were effective. In contrast, when the bacteria were given intravenously, antibodies against TNFα were also effective in preventing death (Zanetti *et al.*, 1992). Therefore, the importance of TNFα may depend on the nature or location of the infection and indeed TNFα may have a protective effect against lethal infection (Eskandari *et al.*, 1992).

IL-1 may also be a key ingredient in shock, because an IL-1 receptor antagonist prevents *E. coli*-induced septic shock in rabbits (Wakabayashi *et al.*, 1991). IL-1 receptor antagonist also inhibited IL-8 production in LPS-treated whole blood (DeForge *et al.*, 1992).

In addition to antibodies, other factors that recognize LPS could be important as drugs for combating shock.

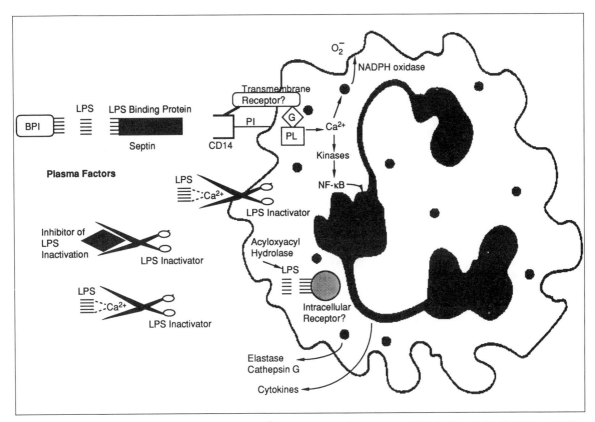

Figure 9.12 Priming of neutrophils by LPS and inactivation of LPS by neutrophils. LBP and Septin interact with LPS to form a complex that is recognized by CD14. Because CD14 is anchored to the membrane only by PI linkage, there is probably another membrane protein involved which might be a transmembrane receptor. Activation of this receptor sends a signal through a G protein (G) to a phospholipase (PL) or other membrane-associated enzyme. By generating IP_3 or some other agent, the phospholipase increases cytosolic Ca^{2+} which is known to control priming for enhanced O_2^- release. Higher Ca^{2+} activates Ca^{2+}-dependent protein kinases, leading to transport of granule proteins to the cell surface or exterior, including alkaline phosphatase and components of NADPH oxidase. Phosphorylation of transcription regulating factors like NF-κB leads to new synthesis of cytokines and enzymes. There may also be an intracellular receptor for LPS that could activate transcription. Among the secreted substances is BPI, which competes for binding of LPS with LBP and Septin, and which tends to moderate the response to LPS. Of course, if there were a great amount of LPS present, then BPI would be ineffective. LPS might also be taken up into the neutrophil, where it could be destroyed by acyloxyacyl hydrolase. An LPS inactivating enzyme, possibly a phosphatase, exists on the surface of the neutrophil and is also present in the medium (scissors symbol). The activity of this enzyme is blocked by serum factors, which might or might not be related to LBP and Septin.

An anti-LPS factor isolated from *Limulus* amoebocytes protected rabbits from shock produced by LPS from *Neisseria meningitidis* (Alpert *et al.*, 1992). The *Limulus* factor increased blood pressure and survival in the animals, warranting further evaluation as an agent for treating septic shock.

Soluble CD14 might compete with cell-bound CD14 on neutrophils and monocytes by binding and neutralizing LPS. Soluble CD14 inhibited LPS-induced oxygen radical-dependent chemiluminescence (Schütt *et al.*, 1992). Monocytes release soluble CD14 in response to LPS, which might represent a natural protective mechanism. However, the role of soluble CD14 requires further investigation. The complex of LPS with soluble CD14 might still be active in binding to a receptor on neutrophils.

The neutrophil granule protein BPI is currently being tested as an LPS-neutralizing factor. For example, LPS complexed with BPI is not pyrogenic in rabbits (Marra *et al.*, 1992).

Inactive analogues of LPS, like monophosphoryl lipid A, deacylated lipid A, or lipid A precursors like lipid X, might be used to counteract LPS in shock (Golenbock *et al.*, 1991; Lynn *et al.*, 1991). Monophosphoryl lipid A primes monocytes, which could improve non-specific resistance to infection; and this agent could make animals tolerant to the inflammatory effects of LPS (Carpati *et al.*, 1992; Gustafson and Rhodes, 1992). Monophosphoryl lipid A reportedly inhibits priming of neutrophils by LPS (Heiman *et al.*, 1990). However, in our experience, monophosphoryl lipid A at 1:1 failed to block priming of neutrophils by native lipid A. Another possibility is deacylated LPS which might be used to compete with native LPS. The LPS deacylating enzyme, acyloxyacyl hydrolase, might also be useful in inactivating LPS, while perhaps maintaining the beneficial immunostimulatory effects of LPS (Munford and Hall, 1986; Peterson and Munford, 1987). This enzyme may be an important agent to control inflammation resulting from infection (McDermott *et al.*, 1991). The enzyme has recently been cloned (Hagen *et al.*, 1991), leading to the possibility of therapeutic use.

Some types of naturally non-toxic LPS, like those isolated from *Bacteroides fragilis* (Magnuson *et al.*, 1989) or *Rhodopseudomonas sphaeroides* (Qureshi *et al.*, 1991), might be useful LPS antagonists. There are also chemically detoxified forms of LPS that might antagonize native LPS (McIntire *et al.*, 1976). LPS can stimulate its own catabolism in macrophages (Hampton and Raetz, 1991). Perhaps a non-toxic LPS could be used to stimulate the breakdown of toxic LPS.

Lastly, there may be a therapeutic application for the LPS-inactivating activity of neutrophils. This activity is presumably an enzyme present on the neutrophil surface. Part of the activity also appears to be shed into the medium. Whether or not this enzyme proves to dephosphorylate lipid A, it might prove useful for inactivating LPS in septic shock.

6. *Model of Neutrophil Priming by LPS*

A model summarizing the proposed interactions between LPS and neutrophils is shown in Figure 9.12. As the figure indicates, the response of neutrophils to LPS is greatly facilitated by factors from serum, LBP and Septin, which help the neutrophil to respond to infection. However, to limit tissue damage, the neutrophil has a variety of mechanisms for turning off its responses to LPS, including BPI, acyloxyacyl hydrolase and the LPS inactivating enzyme.

As shown in Figure 9.13, the integrity of the endothelium may be critical in determining the response of neutrophils to LPS. Loss of integrity of endothelium allows LBP and Septin into tissues, where they promote priming by LPS. Leakage of plasma factors through damaged endothelium is common at inflammatory sites. For example, the fluid found in the crevice between the tooth and inflamed gingiva (gums) in periodontal disease usually contains 70–90% of the concentration of plasma proteins found in blood. Primed neutrophils release hydrolases like elastase and CatG, oxygen radicals like O_2^-, and mediators like PAF which promote inflammation. Neutrophils also release BPI to neutralize LPS. If the bacteria are killed and the LPS neutralized, then inflammation subsides and repair begins. If the bacteria are winning, more neutrophils and monocytes are called in, and tissue damage is likely.

I notice that these figures are getting complicated. As I wrote at the beginning, the simple idea of priming is really inadequate to explain the complex behaviour of neutrophils. These cells respond to many different stimuli with a wide variety of behaviour. Many of us have been nicked by Occam's razor because we expected simple explanations from a life-form as complicated as the neutrophil. Let a thousand flowers bloom in studies of neutrophils and may each receive the appropriate monetary fertilizer!

7. *Acknowledgements*

I thank my mentors, Floyd McIntire, who introduced me to LPS, and Richard Johnston, who introduced me to phagocytes. I thank my students and colleagues, Yoshitomi Aida, Jonella Rademacher, Randy Forehand, Demin Wang, Stanley Szefler, Terri Finkel, Nancy Cummings, Holly Hedegaard, Daniel Ambruso and Sandy Bryant who kept me going and did most of the real work. Finally, I thank my wife and scientific colleague, Karen Pabst, for performing many long and difficult experiments, and for carefully reading this chapter.

The work from my laboratory reported herein was supported by grant DE05494 from the National Institute of Dental Research, National Institutes of Health, United States Public Health Service.

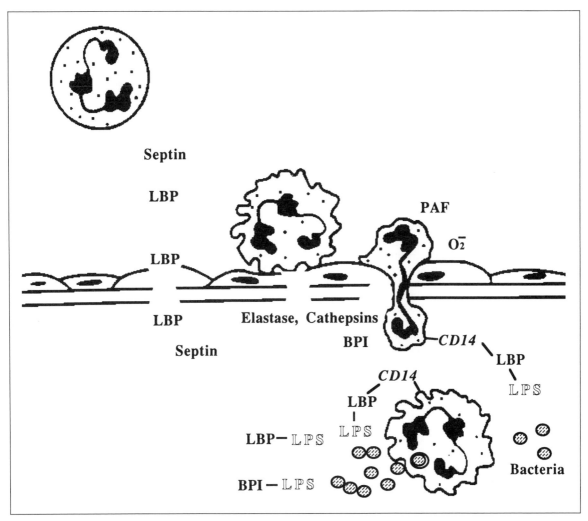

Figure 9.13 Loss of integrity of endothelium allows LBP and Septin into tissue, where they promote priming of neutrophils by LPS. Neutrophils fail to respond to LPS in the absence of the serum factors LBP and Septin. These would not normally be present in tissue, except at sites where inflammation damaged the endothelium. Primed neutrophils release hydrolases like elastase and CatG, oxygen radicals like O_2^-, and mediators like PAF which damage endothelium and promote inflammation. Neutrophils also release BPI to neutralize LPS. However, if there is too much LPS, inflammation continues, endothelium is further damaged, more serum factors leak into tissue and a vicious cycle can result leading to tissue destruction.

8. References

Aida, Y. and Pabst, M.J. (1990a). Priming of neutrophils by lipopolysaccharide for enhanced release of superoxide. Requirement for plasma but not for tumor necrosis factor-α. J. Immunol. 145, 3017–3025.

Aida, Y. and Pabst, M.J. (1990b). Removal of endotoxin from protein solutions by phase separation using Triton X-114. J. Immunol. Meth. 132, 191–195.

Aida, Y. and Pabst, M.J. (1991). Neutrophil responses to lipopolysaccharide. Effect of adherence on triggering and priming of the respiratory burst. J. Immunol. 146, 1271–1276.

Aida, Y., Pabst, M.J., Rademacher, J.M., Hatakeyama, T. and Aono, M. (1990). Effects of polymyxin B on superoxide anion release and priming in human polymorphonuclear leukocytes. J. Leuk. Biol. 47, 283–291.

Alpert, G., Baldwin, G., Thompson, C., Wainwright, N., Novitsky, T.J., Gillis, Z., Parsonnet, J., Fleisher, G.R. and Siber, G.R. (1992). Limulus antilipopolysaccharide factor protects rabbits from meningococcal endotoxin shock. J. Infect. Dis. 165, 494–500.

Ambruso, D.R. and Johnston, R.B., Jr (1981). Lactoferrin enhances hydroxyl radical production by human neutrophils, neutrophil particulate fractions, and an enzymatic generating system. J. Clin. Invest. 67, 352–360.

Ambruso, D.R., Bolscher, B.G., Stokman, P.M., Verhoeven, A.J. and Roos, D. (1990). Assembly and activation of the NADPH:O₂ oxidoreductase in human neutrophils after stimulation with phorbol myristate acetate. J. Biol. Chem. 265, 924–930.

Anderson, B.O., Poggetti, R.S., Shanley, P.F., Bensard, D.D., Pitman, J.M., Nelson, D.W., Whitman, G.J., Banerjee, A. and Harkin, A.H. (1991). Primed neutrophils injure rat lung through a platelet activating factor-dependent mechanism. J. Surg. Res. 50, 510–514.

Anderson, D.C., Schmalstieg, F.C., Finegold, M.J., Hughes, B.J., Rothlein, R., Miller, L.J., Kohl, S., Tosi, M.F., Jacobs, R.L., Waldrop, T.C., Goldman, A.S., Shearer, W.T. and Springer, T.A. (1985). The severe and moderate phenotypes of heritable Mac-1, LFA-1 deficiency: their quantitative definition and relation to leukocyte dysfunction and clinical features. J. Infect. Dis. 152, 668–689.

Anderson, D.C., Miller, L.J., Schmalstieg, F.C., Rothlein, R. and Springer, T.A. (1986). Contributions of the Mac-1 glycoprotein family to adherence-dependent granulocyte functions: structure–function assessments employing subunit-specific monoclonal antibodies. J. Immunol. 137, 15–27.

Baggiolini, M., Walz, A. and Kunkel, S.L. (1989). Neutrophil-activating peptide-1/interleukin 8, a novel cytokine that activates neutrophils. J. Clin. Invest. 84, 1045–1049.

Barratt, G.M., Raddassi, K., Petit, J.F. and Tenu, J.P. (1991). MDP and LPS act synergistically to induce arginine-dependent cytostatic activity in rat alveolar macrophages. Int. J. Immunopharmacol. 13, 159–165.

Bass, D.A., Gerard, C., Olbrantz, P., Wilson, J., McCall, C.E. and McPhail, L.C. (1987). Priming of the respiratory burst of neutrophils by diacylglycerol: independence from activation or translocation of protein kinase C. J. Biol. Chem. 262, 6643–6649.

Bauss, F., Dröge, W. and Männel, D.N. (1987). Tumor necrosis factor mediates endotoxic effects in mice. Infect. Immun. 55, 1622–1625.

Berger, M., Wetzler, E.M. and Wallis, R.S. (1988). Tumor necrosis factor is the major monocyte product that increases complement receptor expression on mature human neutrophils. Blood 71, 151–158.

Berkow, R.L., Wang, D., Larrick, J.W., Dodson, R.W. and Howard, T.H. (1987). Enhancement of neutrophil superoxide production by preincubation with recombinant human tumor necrosis factor. J. Immunol. 139, 3783–3791.

Betz, S.J. and Henson, P.M. (1980). Production and release of platelet-activating factor (PAF): dissociation from degranulation and superoxide production in the human neutrophil. J. Immunol. 125, 2756–2763.

Bocci, V. (1992). The neglected organ – bacterial flora has a crucial immunostimulatory role. Perspectives Biol. Med. 35, 251–260.

Borregaard, N., Miller, L.J. and Springer, T.A. (1987). Chemo-attractant-regulated mobilization of a novel intracellular compartment in human neutrophils. Science 237, 1204–1206.

Bozeman, P.M., Learn, D.B. and Thomas, E.L. (1990). Assay of the human leukocyte enzymes myeloperoxidase and eosinophil peroxidase. J. Immunol. Meth. 126, 125–133.

Bromberg, Y. and Pick, E. (1985). Activation of NADPH-dependent superoxide production in a cell-free system by sodium dodecyl sulfate. J. Biol. Chem. 260, 13539–13545.

Brozna, J.P., Horan, M., Rademacher, J.M., Pabst, K.M. and Pabst, M.J. (1991). Monocyte responses to sulfatide from Mycobacterium tuberculosis: inhibition of priming for enhanced release of superoxide, associated with increased secretion of interleukin-1 and tumor necrosis factor alpha, and altered protein phosphorylation. Infect. Immun. 59, 2542–2548.

Bryant, S.M., Guthrie, L.A., Pabst, M.J. and Johnston R.B., Jr (1986). Macrophage membrane proteins: possible role in the regulation of priming for enhanced respiratory burst activity. Cell. Immunol. 103, 216–223.

Carpati, C.M., Astiz, M.E., Rackow, E.C., Kim, J.W., Kim, Y.B. and Weil, M.H. (1992). Monophosphoryl lipid A attenuates the effects of shock in pigs. J. Lab. Clin. Med. 119, 346–353.

Carré, P.C., Mortenson, R.L., King, T.E., Noble, P.W., Sable, C.L. and Riches, D.W.H. (1991). Increased expression of the interleukin-8 gene by alveolar macrophages in idiopathic pulmonary fibrosis: a potential mechanism for the recruitment and activation of neutrophils in lung fibrosis. J. Clin. Invest. 88, 1802–1810.

Cassatella, M.A., Bazzoni, F., Flynn, R.M., Dusi, S., Trinchieri, G. and Rossi, F. (1990). Molecular basis of interferon-γ and lipopolysaccharide enhancement of phagocyte respiratory burst capability. Studies on the gene expression of several NADPH oxidase components. J. Biol. Chem. 265, 20241–20246.

Channon, J.Y., Leslie, C. and Johnston, R.B., Jr (1987). Zymosan-stimulated production of phosphatidic acid by macrophages: relationship to release of superoxide anion and inhibition by agents that increase intracellular cyclic AMP. J. Leuk. Biol. 41, 450–453.

Chase, J.J., Kubey, W., Dulek, M.H., Holmes, C.J., Salit, M.G., Pearson, F.C., III and Ribi, E. (1986). Effect of monophosphoryl lipid A on host resistance to bacterial infection. Infect. Immun. 53, 711–712.

Chilton, F.H., Ellis, J.M, Olson, S.C. and Wykle, R.L. (1984). 1-O-Alkyl-2-arachidonoyl-sn-glycero-3-phosphocholine: a common source of platelet-activating factor and arachidonate in human polymorphonuclear leukocytes. J. Biol. Chem. 259, 12014–12019.

Cohn, Z.A. and Morse, S.I. (1960). Functional and metabolic properties of polymorphonuclear leukocytes. II. The influence of a lipopolysaccharide endotoxin. J. Exp. Med. 111, 689–704.

Cummings, N.P., Pabst, M.J. and Johnston, R.B., Jr (1980). Activation of macrophages for enhanced release of superoxide anion and greater killing of Candida albicans by injection of muramyl dipeptide. J. Exp. Med. 152, 1659–1669.

Dahinden, C. and Fehr, J. (1983). Granulocyte activation by endotoxin. II. Role of granulocyte adherence, aggregation, and effect of cytochalasin B, and comparison with formylated chemotactic peptide-induced stimulation. J. Immunol. 130, 863–868.

Dahinden, C.A., Fehr, J. and Hugli, T.E. (1983). Role of cell surface contact in the kinetics of superoxide production by granulocytes. J. Clin. Invest. 72, 113–121.

Dal Nogare, A.R. and Yarbrough, W.C., Jr (1990). A comparison of the effects of intact and deacylated lipopolysaccharide on human polymorphonuclear leukocytes. J. Immunol. 144, 1404–1410.

Daniels, R.H., Finnen, M.J., Hill, M.E. and Lackie, J.M. (1992). Recombinant human monocyte IL-8 primes NADPH oxidase and phospholipase A_2 activation in human neutrophils. Immunology 75, 157–163.

Danner, R.L., Joiner, K.A. and Parrillo, J.E. (1987). Inhibition of endotoxin-induced priming of human neutrophils by lipid X and 3-aza-lipid X. J. Clin. Invest. 80, 605–612.

Dayer, J.-M., Beutler, B. and Cerami, A. (1985). Cachectin/tumor necrosis factor stimulates collagenase and prostaglandin E_2 production by human synovial cells and dermal fibroblasts. J. Exp. Med. 162, 2163–2168.

DeForge, L.E., Tracey, D.E., Kenney, J.S. and Remick, D.G. (1992). Interleukin-1 receptor antagonist protein inhibits interleukin-8 expression in lipopolysaccharide-stimulated human whole blood. Am. J. Pathol. 140, 1045–1054.

Deguchi, S., Hori, T., Creamer, H. and Gabler, W. (1990). Neutrophil-mediated damage to human periodontal ligament-derived fibroblasts: role of lipopolysaccharide. J. Periodont. Res. 25, 293–299.

Dessein, A.J., Lee, T.H., Elsas, P., Ravalese, J., III, Silberstein, D., David, J.R., Austen, K.F. and Lewis, R.A. (1986). Enhancement by monokines of leukotriene generation by human eosinophils and neutrophils stimulated with calcium ionophore A23187. J. Immunol. 136, 3829–3838.

Detmers, P.A., Powell, D.E., Walz, A., Clark-Lewis, I., Baggiolini, M. and Cohn, Z.A. (1991). Differential effects of neutrophil-activating peptide 1/IL-8 and its homologues on leukocyte adhesion and phagocytosis. J. Immunol. 147, 4211–4217.

Ding, A.H., Sanchez, E., Tancinco, M. and Nathan, C. (1992). Interactions of bacterial lipopolysaccharide with microtubule proteins. J. Immunol. 148, 2853–2858.

Djeu, J.Y., Serbousek, D. and Blanchard, D.K. (1990). Release of tumor necrosis factor by human polymorphonuclear leukocytes. Blood 76, 1405–1409.

Doerfler, M.E., Danner, R.L., Shelhamer, J.H. and Parrillo, J.E. (1989). Bacterial lipopolysaccharides prime human neutrophils for enhanced production of leukotriene B_4. J. Clin. Invest. 83, 970–977.

Edwards, C.K., III, Yunger, L.M., Lorence, R.M., Dantzer, R. and Kelley, K.W. (1991). The pituitary gland is required for protection against lethal effects of Salmonella typhimurium. Proc. Natl Acad. Sci. USA 88, 2274–2277.

Emancipator, K., Csako, G. and Elin, R.J. (1992). In vitro inactivation of bacterial endotoxin by human lipoproteins and apolipoproteins. Infect. Immun. 60, 596–601.

Englberger, W., Bitter-Suermann, D. and Hadding, U. (1987). Influence of lysophospholipids and PAF on the oxidative burst of PMNL. Int. J. Imrnunopharmacol. 9, 275–282.

Eskandari, M.K., Bolgos, G., Miller, C., Nguyen, D.T., DeForge, L.E. and Remick, D.G. (1992). Anti-tumor necrosis factor antibody therapy fails to prevent lethality after cecal ligation and puncture or endotoxemia. J. Immunol. 148, 2724–2730.

Finkel, T.H., Pabst, M.J., Suzuki, H., Guthrie, L.A., Forehand, J.R., Phillips, W.A. and Johnston, R.B., Jr (1987). Priming of neutrophils and macrophages for enhanced release of superoxide anion by the calcium ionophore ionomycin. Implications for regulation of the respiratory burst. J. Biol. Chem. 262, 12589–12596.

Fittschen, C., Sandhaus, R.A., Worthen, G.S. and Henson, P.M. (1988). Bacterial lipopolysaccharide enhances chemoattractant-induced elastase secretion by human neutrophils. J. Leukocyte Biol. 43, 547–556.

Forehand, J.R., Pabst, M.J., Phillips, W.A. and Johnston, R.B., Jr (1989). Lipopolysaccharide priming of human neutrophils for an enhanced respiratory burst. Role of intracellular free calcium. J. Clin. Invest. 83, 74–83.

Fox, A. and Fox, K. (1991). Rapid elimination of a synthetic adjuvant peptide from the circulation after systemic administration and absence of detectable natural muramyl peptides in normal serum at current analytical limits. Infect. Immun. 59, 1202–1205.

Galanos, C., Lüderitz, O., Rietschel, E.Th., Westphal, O., Brade, H., Brade, L., Freudenberg, M., Schade, U., Imoto, M., Yoshimura, H., Kusumoto, S. and Shiba, T. (1985). Synthetic and natural Escherichia coli free lipid A express identical endotoxic activities. Eur. J. Biochem. 148, 1–5.

Galanos, C., Lüderitz, O., Freudenberg, M., Brade, L., Schade, U., Rietschel, E.Th., Kusumoto, S. and Shiba, T. (1986). Biological activity of synthetic heptaacyl lipid A representing a component of Salmonella minnesota R595 lipid A. Eur. J. Biochem. 160, 55–59.

Gamble, J.R., Harlan, J.M., Klebanoff, S.J. and Vadas, M.A. (1985). Stimulation of the adherence of neutrophils to umbilical vein endothelium by human recombinant tumor necrosis factor. Proc. Natl Acad. Sci. USA 82, 8667–8671.

Georgilis, K., Schaefer, C., Dinarello, C.A. and Klempner, M.S. (1987). Human recombinant interleukin 1β has no effect on intracellular calcium or on functional responses of human neutrophils. J. Immunol. 138, 3403–3407.

Golenbock, D.T., Hampton, R.Y., Qureshi, N., Takayama, K. and Raetz, C.R.H. (1991). Lipid A-like molecules that antagonize the effects of endotoxins on human monocytes. J. Biol. Chem. 266, 19490–19498.

Gustafson, G.L. and Rhodes, M.J. (1992). A rationale for the prophylactic use of monophosphoryl lipid A in sepsis and septic shock. Biochem. Biophys. Res. Commun. 182, 269–275.

Guthrie, L.A., McPhail, L.C., Henson, P.M. and Johnston, R.B., Jr (1984). Priming of neutrophils for enhanced release of oxygen metabolites by bacterial lipopolysaccharide. Evidence for increased activity of the superoxide-producing enzyme. J. Exp. Med. 160, 1656–1671.

Hagen, F.S., Grant, F.J., Kuijper, J.L., Slaughter, C.A., Moomaw, C.R., Orth, K., O'Hara, P.J. and Munford, R.S. (1991). Expression and characterization of recombinant human acyloxyacyl hydrolase, a leukocyte enzyme that deacylates bacterial lipopolysaccharides. Biochemistry 30, 8415–8423.

Hall, C.L. and Munford, R.S. (1983). Enzymatic deacylation of the lipid A moiety of Salmonella typhimurium lipopolysaccharides by human neutrophils. Proc. Natl Acad. Sci. USA 80, 6671–6675.

Halling, J.L., Hamill, D.R., Lei, M.G. and Morrison, D.C. (1992). Identification and characterization of lipopolysaccharide-binding proteins on human peripheral blood cell populations. Infect. Immun. 60, 845–852.

Hampton, R.Y. and Raetz, C.R.H. (1991). Macrophage catabolism of lipid A is regulated by endotoxin stimulation. J. Biol. Chem. 266, 19499–19509.

Harmsen, A.G. (1988). Role of alveolar macrophages in lipopolysaccharide-induced neutrophil accumulation. Infect. Immun. 56, 1858–1863.

Harris, W.E. and Bursten, S.L. (1992). Lipid A stimulates phospholipase D activity in rat mesangial cells via a G protein. Biochem. J. 281, 675–682.

Haslett, C., Guthrie, L.A., Kopaniak, M.M., Johnston, R.B., Jr and Henson, P.M. (1985). Modulation of multiple neutrophil functions by preparative methods or trace concentrations of bacterial lipopolysaccharide. Am. J. Path. 119, 101–109.

Heiman, D.F., Astiz, M.E., Rackow, E.C., Rhein, D., Kim, Y.B. and Weil, M.H. (1990). Monophosphoryl lipid A inhibits neutrophil priming by lipopolysaccharide. J. Lab. Clin. Med. 116, 237–241.

Heumann, D., Gallay, P., Barras, C., Zaech, P., Ulevitch, R.J., Tobias, P.S., Glauser, M.P. and Baumgartner, J.D. (1992). Control of lipopolysaccharide (LPS) binding and LPS-induced tumor necrosis factor secretion in human peripheral blood monocytes. J. Immunol. 148, 3505–3512.

Hirata, F. (1981). The regulation of lipomodulin, a phospholipase inhibitory protein, in rabbit neutrophils by phosphorylation. J. Biol. Chem. 256, 7730–7733.

Hohmann, H.P., Remy, R., Aigner, L., Brockhaus, M. and van Loon, A.P.G.M. (1992). Protein kinases negatively affect nuclear factor-κB activation by tumor necrosis factor-α at two different stages in promyelocytic HL60 cells. J. Biol. Chem. 267, 2065–2072.

Huber, A.R., Kunkel, S.L., Todd, R.F., III and Weiss, S.J. (1991). Regulation of transendothelial neutrophil migration by endogenous interleukin-8. Science 254, 99–102.

Johannsen, L., Wecke, J., Obal, F., Jr and Krueger, J.M. (1991). Macrophages produce somnogenic and pyrogenic muramyl peptides during digestion of staphylococci. Am. J. Physiol. 260, R126–133.

Karnovsky, M.L. and Lazdins, J.K. (1978) Biochemical criteria for activated macrophages. J. Immunol. 121, 809–813.

Karplus, T.E., Ulevitch, R.J. and Wilson, C.B. (1987). A new method for reduction of endotoxin contamination from protein solutions. J. Immunol. Meth. 105, 211–220.

Kishimoto, T.K., Jutila, M.A., Berg, E.L. and Butcher, E.C. (1989). Neutrophil Mac-1 and Mel-14 adhesion proteins inversely regulated by chemotactic factors. Science 245, 1238–1241.

Kitagawa, S., Yuo, A., Souza, L.M., Saito, M., Miura, Y. and Takaku, F. (1987). Recombinant human granulocyte colony-stimulating factor enhances superoxide release in human granulocytes stimulated by the chemotactic peptide. Biochem. Biophys. Res. Comm. 144, 1143–1146.

Koivuranta-Vaara, P., Banda, D. and Goldstein, I.M. (1987). Bacterial-lipopolysaccharide-induced release of lactoferrin from human polymorphonuclear leukocytes: role of monocyte-derived tumor necrosis factor α. Infect. Immun. 55, 2956–2961.

Kriegsmann, J., Neser, F., Bräuer, R. and Waldmann, G. (1991). Demonstration of lipopolysaccharide (LPS) binding sites on the cell surface of guinea pig peritoneal macrophages by means of immunogold technique. Exp. Pathol. 43, 233–237.

Kulshin, V.A., Zähringer, U., Lindner, B., Frasch, C.E., Tsai, C.M., Dmitriev, B.A. and Rietschel, E.T. (1992). Structural characterization of the lipid A component of pathogenic Neisseria meningitidis. J. Bacteriol. 174, 1793–1800.

Lee, J.D., Kato, K., Tobias, P.S., Kirkland, T.N. and Ulevitch, R.J. (1992). Transfection of CD14 into 70Z/3 cells dramatically enhances the sensitivity to complexes of lipopolysaccharide (LPS) and LPS binding protein. J. Exp. Med. 175, 1697–1705.

Levy, R. and Malech, H.L. (1991). Effect of 1,25-dihydroxyvitamin D3, lipopolysaccharide, or lipoteichoic acid on the expression of NADPH oxidase components in cultured human monocytes. J. Immunol. 147, 3066–3071.

Lew, P.D., Wollheim, C.B., Waldvogel, F.A. and Pozzan, T. (1984). Modulation of cytosolic-free calcium transients by changes in intracellular calcium-buffering capacity: correlation with exocytosis and O_2^- production in human neutrophils. J. Cell Biol. 99, 1212–1220.

Linas, S.L., Whittenburg, D. and Repine, J.E. (1991). Role of neutrophil derived oxidants and elastase in lipopolysaccharide-mediated renal injury. Kidney Int. 39, 618–623.

Lopez, A.F., Williamson, D.J., Gamble, J.R., Begley, C.G., Harlan, J.M., Klebanoff, S.J., Waltersdorph, A., Wong, G., Clark, S.C. and Vadas, M.A. (1986). Recombinant human granulocyte–macrophage colony-stimulating factor stimulates in vitro mature human neutrophil and eosinophil function, surface receptor expression, and survival. J. Clin. Invest. 78, 1220–1228.

Loughlin, A.J., Woodroofe, M.N. and Cuzner, M.L. (1992). Regulation of Fc receptor and major histocompatibility complex antigen expression on isolated rat microglia by tumor necrosis factor, interleukin-1 and lipopolysaccharide: effects on interferon gamma induced activation. Immunology 75, 170–175.

Ludwig, J.C., Hoppens, C.L., McManus, L.M., Mott, G.E. and Pinckard, R.N. (1985). Modulation of platelet-activating factor (PAF) synthesis and release from human polymorphonuclear leukocytes (PMN): role of extracellular albumin. Arch. Biochem. Biophys. 241, 337–347.

Lynn, W.A., Raetz, C.R., Qureshi, N. and Golenbock, D.T. (1991). Lipopolysaccharide-induced stimulation of CD11b/CD18 expression on neutrophils. Evidence of specific receptor-based response and inhibition by lipid A-based antagonists. J. Immunol. 147, 3072–3079.

Mackaness, G.B. (1964). The immunological basis of acquired cellular resistance. J. Exp. Med. 120, 105–120.

Mackaness, G.B. (1970). In "Infectious Agents and Host Reactions" (ed. S. Mudd), pp. 61–75. W.B. Saunders Co., Philadelphia.

Mackman, N., Brand, K. and Edgington, T.E. (1991). Lipopolysaccharide-mediated transcriptional activation of the human tissue factor gene in THP-1 monocytic cells requires both activator protein 1 and nuclear factor-κB binding sites. J. Exp. Med. 174, 1517–1526.

Magnuson, D.K., Weintraub, A., Pohlman, T.H. and Maier, R.V. (1989). Human endothelial cell adhesiveness for neutrophils, induced by Escherichia coli lipopolysaccharide in vitro, is inhibited by Bacteroides fragilis lipopolysaccharide. J. Immunol. 143, 3025–3030.

Marra, M.N., Wilde, C.G., Griffith, J.E., Snable, J.L. and Scott, R.W. (1990). Bactericidal/permeability-increasing protein has endotoxin-neutralizing activity. J. Immunol. 144, 662–666.

Marra, M.N., Wilde, C.G., Collins, M.S., Snable, J.L., Thornton, M.B. and Scott, R.W. (1992). The role of bactericidal/permeability-increasing protein as a natural inhibitor of bacterial endotoxin. J. Immunol. 148, 532–537.

Mathison, J.C., Wolfson, E. and Ulevitch, R.J. (1988). Participation of tumor necrosis factor in the mediation of Gram negative bacterial lipopolysaccharide-induced injury in rabbits. J. Clin. Invest. 81, 1925–1937.

May, G.L., Dunlop, L.C., Sztelma, K., Berndt, M.C. and Sorrell, T.C. (1992). GMP-140 (P-selectin) inhibits human neutrophil activation by lipopolysaccharide: analysis by proton magnetic resonance spectroscopy. Biochem. Biophys. Res. Comm. 183, 1062–1069.

Mayer, A.M.S. and Spitzer, J. A. (1991). Continuous infusion of Escherichia coli endotoxin in vivo primes in vitro superoxide anion release in rat polymorphonuclear leukocytes and Kupffer cells in a time-dependent manner. Infect. Immun. 59, 4590–4598.

McDermott, C.M., Cullor, J.S. and Fenwick, B.W. (1991). Intracellular and extracellular enzymatic deacylation of bacterial endotoxin during localized inflammation induced by Escherichia coli. Infect. Immun. 59, 478–485.

McIntire, F.C., Hargie, M.P., Schenck, J.R., Finley, R.A., Sievert, H.W., Rietschel, E.Th. and Rosenstreich, D.L. (1976). Biologic properties of nontoxic derivatives of a lipopolysaccharide from Escherichia coli K235. J. Immunol. 117, 674–678.

McIntyre, T.M., Reinhold, S.L., Prescott, S.M. and Zimmerman, G.A. (1987). Protein kinase C activity appears to be required for the synthesis of platelet-activating factor and leukotriene B4 by human neutrophils. J. Biol. Chem. 262, 15370–15376.

Miller, L.J., Bainton, D.F., Borregaard, N. and Springer, T.A. (1987). Stimulated mobilization of monocyte Mac-1 and p150,95 adhesion proteins from an intracellular vesicular compartment to the cell surface. J. Clin. Invest. 80, 535–544.

Mohri, M., Spriggs, D.R. and Kufe, D. (1990). Effects of lipopolysaccharide on phospholipase A2 activity and tumor necrosis factor expression in HL-60 cells. J. Immunol. 144, 2678–2682.

Munford, R.S. and Hall, C.L. (1986). Detoxification of bacterial lipopolysaccharides (endotoxins) by a human neutrophil enzyme. Science 234, 203–205.

Munford, R.S. and Hunter, J.P. (1992). Acyloxyacyl hydrolase, a leukocyte enzyme that deacylates bacterial lipopolysaccharides, has phospholipase, lysophospholipase, diacylglycerollipase, and acyltransferase activities in vitro. J. Biol. Chem. 267, 10116–10121.

Muotiala, A., Helander, I.M., Pyhälä, L., Kosunen, T.U. and Moran, A.P. (1992). Low biological activity of Helicobacter pylori lipopolysaccharide. Infect. Immun. 60, 1714–1716.

Nathan, C.F. (1987). Neutrophil activation on biological surfaces. Massive secretion of hydrogen peroxide in response to products of macrophages and lymphocytes. J. Clin. Invest. 80, 1550–1560.

Nathan, C.F. (1989). Respiratory burst in adherent human neutrophils: triggering by colony-stimulating factors CSF-GM and CSF-G. Blood 73, 301–306.

Nathan, C.F., Murray, H.W., Wiebe, M.E. and Rubin, B.Y. (1983). Identification of interferon-γ as the lymphokine that activates human macrophage oxidative metabolism and antimicrobial activity. J. Exp. Med. 158, 670–689.

Nathan, C., Srimal, S., Farber, C., Sanchez, E., Kabbash, L., Asch, A., Gailit, J. and Wright, S.D. (1989). Cytokine-induced respiratory burst of human neutrophils: dependence on extracellular matrix proteins and CD11b/CD18 integrins. J. Cell Biol. 109, 1341–1349.

Navab, M., Hough, G.P., Van Lenten, B.J., Berliner, J.A. and Fogelman, A.M. (1988). Low density lipoproteins transfer bacterial lipopolysaccharides across endothelial monolayers in a biologically active form. J. Clin. Invest. 81, 601–605.

Norgauer, J., Eberle, M., Fay, S.P., Lemke, H.D. and Sklar, L.A. (1991). Kinetics of N-formyl peptide receptor up-regulation during stimulation in human neutrophils. J. Immunol. 146, 975–980.

North, R.J. (1978). The concept of the activated macrophage. J. Exp. Med. 121, 806–809.

Nunoi, H., Rotrosen, D., Gallin, J.I. and Malech, H.L. (1988). Two forms of autosomal chronic granulomatous disease lack distinct neutrophil cytosol factors. Science 242, 1298–1301.

Ohmori, Y. and Hamilton, T.A. (1992). Ca^{2+} and calmodulin selectively regulate lipopolysaccharide-inducible cytokine mRNA expression in murine peritoneal macrophages. J. Immunol. 148, 538–545.

Ooi, C.E., Weiss, J., Doerfler, M.E. and Elsbach, P. (1991). Endotoxin-neutralizing properties of the 25 kD N-terminal fragment and a newly isolated 30 kD C-terminal fragment of the 55–60 kD bactericidal/permeability-increasing protein of human neutrophils. J. Exp. Med. 174, 649–655.

Pabst, M.J. and Johnston, R.B., Jr (1980). Increased production of superoxide anion by macrophages exposed in vitro to muramyl dipeptide or lipopolysaccharide. J. Exp. Med. 151, 101–114.

Pabst, M.J. and Johnston, R.B., Jr (1989). In "Handbook of Inflammation", Vol. 6, "Mediators of the Inflammatory Process" (eds P.M. Henson and R.C. Murphy), pp. 361–393. Elsevier Science Publishers BV, Amsterdam.

Pabst, M.J., Hedegaard, H.B. and Johnston, R.B., Jr (1982). Cultured human monocytes require exposure to bacterial products to maintain an optimal oxygen radical response. J. Immunol. 128, 123–128.

Parant, M., Parant, F. and Chedid, L. (1978). Enhancement of the neonate's nonspecific immunity to Klebsiella infection by muramyl dipeptide, a synthetic immunoadjuvant. Proc. Natl Acad. Sci. USA 75, 3395–3399.

Perussia, B., Kobayashi, M., Rossi, M.E., Anegon, I. and Trinchieri, G. (1987). Immune interferon enhances functional properties of human granulocytes: role of Fc receptors and effect of lymphotoxin, tumor necrosis factor, and granulocyte–macrophage colony-stimulating factor. J. Immunol. 138, 765–774.

Peterson, A.A. and Munford, R.S. (1987). Dephosphorylation of the lipid A moiety of Escherichia coli lipopolysaccharide by mouse macrophages. Infect. Immun. 55, 974–978.

Pitman, J.M., III, Thurman, G.W., Anderson, B.O., Ketch, L.L., Hartford, C.E., Harken, A.H. and Ambruso, D.R. (1991). WEB2170, a specific platelet-activating factor antagonist, attenuates neutrophil priming by human serum after clinical burn injury. J. Burn Care Rehabil. 12, 411–419.

Postlethwaite, A.E., Lachman, L.B., Mainardi, C.L. and Kang, A.H. (1983). Interleukin 1 stimulation of collagenase production by cultured fibroblasts. J. Exp. Med. 157, 801–806.

Qureshi, N., Takayarna, K. and Kurtz, R. (1991). Diphosphoryl lipid A obtained from the nontoxic lipopolysaccharide of Rhodopseudomonas sphaeroides is an endotoxin antagonist in mice. Infect. Immun. 59, 441–444.

Raetz, C.R.H., Ulevitch, R.J., Wright, S.D., Sibley, C.H., Ding, A. and Nathan, C.F. (1991). Gram-negative endotoxin: an extraordinary lipid with profound effects on eukaryotic signal transduction. FASEB J. 5, 2652–2660.

Riveau, G.J., Brunel-Riveau, B.G., Audibert, F.M. and Chedid, L.A. (1991). Influence of a muramyl dipeptide on human blood leukocyte functions and their membrane antigens. Cell. Immunol. 134, 147–156.

Rothstein, J.L. and Schreiber, H. (1988). Synergy between tumor necrosis factor and bacterial products causes hemorrhagic necrosis and lethal shock in normal mice. Proc. Natl Acad. Sci. USA 85, 607–611.

Rotrosen, D., Yeung, C.L., Leto, T.L., Malech, H.L. and Kwong, C.H. (1992). Cytochrome b$_{558}$: the flavin-binding component of the phagocyte NADPH oxidase. Science 256, 1459–1462.

Sasada, M., Pabst, M.J. and Johnston, R.B., Jr (1983). Activation of mouse peritoneal macrophages by lipopolysaccharide alters the kinetic parameters of the superoxide-producing NADPH oxidase. J. Biol. Chem. 258, 9631–9635.

Schröder, J.-M., Mrowietz, U., Morita, E. and Christophers, E. (1987). Purification and partial biochemical characterization of a human monocyte-derived, neutrophil-activating peptide that lacks interleukin 1 activity. J. Irnmunol. 139, 3474–3483.

Schütt, C., Schilling, T., Grunwald, U., Schönfeld, W. and Krüger, C. (1992). Endotoxin-neutralizing capacity of soluble CD14. Res. Immunol. 143, 71–78.

Seifert, P.S., Haeffner-Cavaillon, N., Appay, M.D. and Kazatchkine, M.D. (1991). Bacterial lipopolysaccharides alter human endothelial cell morphology in vitro independent of cytokine secretion. J. Lab. Clin. Med. 118, 563–569.

Shalaby, M.R., Palladino, M.A., Hirabayashi, S.E., Eessalu, T.E., Lewis, G.D., Shepard, H.M. and Aggarwal, B.B. (1987). Receptor binding and activation of polymorphonuclear neutrophils by tumor necrosis factor-alpha. J. Leukocyte Biol. 41, 196–204.

Shappell, S.B., Toman, C., Anderson, D.C., Taylor, A.A., Entman, M.L. and Smith, C W. (1990). Mac-1 (CD11b/CD18) mediates adherence-dependent hydrogen peroxide production by human and canine neutrophils. J. Immunol. 144, 2702–2711.

Sherry, B., Yarlett, N., Strupp, A. and Cerami, A. (1992). Identification of cyclophilin as a proinflammatory secretory product of lipopolysaccharide-activated macrophages. Proc. Natl Acad. Sci. USA 89, 3511–3515.

Smedly, L.A., Tonnesen, M.G., Sandhaus, R.A., Haslett, C., Guthrie, L.A., Johnston, R.B., Jr, Henson, P.M. and Worthen, G.S. (1986). Neutrophil-mediated injury to endothelial cells: enhancement by endotoxin and essential role of neutrophil elastase. J. Clin. Invest. 77, 1233–1243.

Smith, C.W., Entman, M.L., Lane, C.L., Beaudet, A.L., Ty, T.I., Youker, K., Hawkins, H.K. and Anderson, D.C. (1991). Adherence of neutrophils to canine cardiac myocytes in vitro is dependent on intercellular adhesion molecule-1. J. Clin. Invest. 88, 1216–1223.

Souvannavong, V. and Adam, A. (1990). Increased expression of alkaline phosphatase activity in stimulated B lymphocytes by muramyl dipeptide. Immunol. Lett. 24, 247–251.

Speer, C.P., Pabst, M.J., Hedegaard, H.B., Rest, R.F. and Johnston, R.B., Jr (1984). Enhanced release of oxygen metabolites by monocyte-derived macrophages exposed to proteolytic enzymes: activity of neutrophil elastase and cathepsin G. J. Immunol. 133, 2151–2156.

Sullivan, G.W., Carper, H.T., Sullivan, J.A., Murata, T. and Mandell, G.L. (1989). Both recombinant interleukin-1 (beta) and purified human monocyte interleukin-1 prime human neutrophils for increased oxidative activity and promote neutrophil spreading. J. Leukocyte Biol. 45, 389–395.

Szefler, S.J., Norton, C.E., Ball, B., Gross, J.M., Aida, Y. and Pabst, M.J. (1989). IFN-γ and LPS overcome glucocorticoid inhibition of priming for superoxide release in human monocytes. Evidence that secretion of IL-1 and tumor necrosis factor-α is not essential for monocyte priming. J. Immunol. 142, 3985–3992.

Terishita, Z., Imura, Y., Nishikawa, K. and Sumida, S. (1985). Is platelet activating factor (PAF) a mediator of endotoxin shock? Eur. J. Pharmacol. 109, 257–261.

Thelen, M., Rosen, A., Nairn, A.C. and Aderem, A. (1990). Tumor necrosis factor α modifies agonist-dependent responses in human neutrophils by inducing the synthesis and myristoylation of a specific protein kinase C substrate. Proc. Natl Acad. Sci. USA 87, 5603–5607.

Thomas, E.L. and Cook, G.S. (1991). Leukocyte myeloperoxidase and salivary lactoperoxidase in whole human saliva. J. Dent. Res. 70, 541.

Thomson, B.M., Mundy, G.R. and Chambers, T.J. (1987). Tumor necrosis factors α and β induce osteoblastic cells to stimulate osteoclastic bone resorption. J. Immunol. 138, 775–779.

Tobias, P.S., Soldau, K. and Ulevitch, R.J. (1986). Isolation of a lipopolysaccharide-binding acute phase reactant from rabbit serum. J. Exp. Med. 164, 777–793.

Tobias, P.S., Mathison, J.C. and Ulevitch, R.J (1988). A family of lipopolysaccharide binding proteins involved in responses to Gram-negative sepsis. J. Biol. Chem. 263, 13479–13481.

Tsunawaki, S. and Nathan, C.F. (1986). Macrophage deactivation. Altered kinetic properties of superoxide-producing enzyme after exposure to tumor cell-conditioned medium. J. Exp. Med. 164, 1319–1331.

Vacheron, F., Mandine, E., Lenaour, R., Smets, P., Zalisz, R. and Guenounou, M. (1992). Inhibition of production of tumor necrosis factor by monoclonal antibodies to lipopolysaccharides. J. Infect. Dis. 165, 873–878.

Vincenti, M.P., Burrell, T.A. and Taffet, S.M. (1992). Regulation of NF-$_k$B activity in murine macrophages: effect of bacterial lipopolysaccharide and phorbol ester. J. Cell. Physiol. 150, 204–213.

Volpp, B.D., Nauseef, W.M. and Clark, R.A. (1988). Two cytosolic neutrophil oxidase components absent in autosomal chronic granulomatous disease. Science 242, 1295–1297.

Vosbeck, K., Tobias, P., Mueller, H., Allen, R.A., Arfors, K.E., Ulevitch, R.J. and Sklar, L.A. (1990). Priming of polymorphonuclear granulocytes by lipopolysaccharides and its complexes with lipopolysaccharide binding protein and high density lipoprotein. J. Leukocyte Biol. 47, 97–104.

Wakabayashi, G., Gelfand, J.A., Burke, J.F., Thompson, R.C. and Dinarello, C.A. (1991). A specific receptor antagonist for interleukin 1 prevents Escherichia coli-induced shock in rabbits. FASEB J. 5, 338–343.

Walz, A., Peveri, P. Aschauer, H. and Baggiolini, M. (1987). Purification and amino acid sequencing of NAF, a novel neutrophil-activating factor produced by monocytes. Biochem. Biophys. Res. Commun. 149, 755–761.

Webb, D.S.A. and Roth, J.A. (1987). Relationship of glucocorticoid suppression of arachidonate metabolism to alteration of neutrophil function. J. Leukocyte Biol. 41, 156–164.

Weisbart, R.H., Golde, D.W., Clark, S.C., Wong, G.G. and Gasson, J.C. (1985). Human granulocyte–macrophage colony stimulating factor is a neutrophil activator. Nature 314, 361–363.

Wencel, M.L., Morganroth, M.L., Schoeneich, S.O., Gannon, D.E., Varani, J., Todd, R.F., III, Ryan, U.S. and Boxer, L.A. (1989). Cytoplasts and Mo1-deficient neutrophils pretreated with plasma and LPS induced lung injury. Am. J. Physiol. 256, H751–759.

Wilson, M.E., Jones, D.P., Munkenbeck, P. and Morrison, D.C. (1982). Serum-dependent and -independent effects of bacterial lipopolysaccharides on human neutrophil oxidative capacity in vitro. J. Reticuloendothelial Soc. 31, 43–57.

Worthen, G.S., Seccombe, J.F., Clay, K.L., Guthrie, L.A. and Johnston, R.B., Jr (1988). The priming of neutrophils by lipopolysaccharide for production of intracellular platelet-activating factor. Potential role in mediation of enhanced superoxide secretion. J. Immunol. 140, 3553–3559.

Wright, S.D. and Jong, M.T.C. (1986). Adhesion-promoting receptors on human macrophages recognize Escherichia coli by binding to lipopolysaccharide. J. Exp. Med. 164, 1876–1888.

Wright, G.G., Read, P.W. and Mandell, G.L. (1988). Lipo-polysaccharide releases a priming substance from platelets that augments the oxidative response of polymorphonuclear neutrophils to chemotactic peptide. J. Infect. Dis. 157, 690–696.

Wright, S.D., Detmers, P.A., Aida, Y., Adamowski, R., Anderson, D.C., Chad, Z., Kabbash, L.G. and Pabst, M.J. (1990). CD18-deficient cells respond to lipopolysaccharide in vitro. J. Immunol. 144, 2566–2571.

Wright, S.D., Ramos, R.A., Hermanowski-Vosatka, A., Rockwell, P. and Detmers, P.A. (1991). Activation of the adhesive capacity of CR3 on neutrophils by endotoxin: dependence on lipopolysaccharide binding protein and CD14. J. Exp. Med. 173, 1281–1286.

Wright, S.D., Ramos, R.A., Patel, M. and Miller, D.S. (1992). Septin: a factor in plasma that opsonizes lipopolysaccharide-bearing particles for recognition by CD14 on phagocytes. J. Exp. Med. 176, 719–727.

Yasui, K., Becker, E.L. and Sha'afi, R.I. (1992). Lipopolysaccharide and serum cause the translocation of G-protein to the membrane and prime neutrophils via CD14. Biochem. Biophys. Res. Comm. 183, 1280–1286.

Zanetti, G., Heumann D., Gerain, J., Kohler, J., Abbet, P., Barras, C., Lucas, R., Glauser, M.P. and Baumgartner, J.D. (1992). Cytokine production after intravenous or peritoneal gram negative bacterial challenge in mice. Comparative protective efficacy of antibodies to tumor necrosis factor-α and to lipopolysaccharide. J. Immunol. 148, 1890–1897.

Zhang, L., English, D. and Andersen, B.R. (1991). Activation of human neutrophils by Mycobacterium tuberculosis-derived sulfolipid-1. J. Immunol. 146, 2730–2736.

10. Mechanisms of Neutrophil Accumulation in Tissues

A.G. Rossi and P.G. Hellewell

1. Introduction

Neutrophils play a vital role in host defence and are normally the predominant leucocytes found in peripheral blood. These essential cells, once recruited at the site of tissue injury or infection, phagocytose foreign particles such as invading bacteria or the host's own unwanted products, including damaged or dead cells as well as cellular debris. The phagocytosed material is destroyed and digested by a vast array of enzymes and various oxygen metabolites. Paradoxically, it is the uncontrolled and overexuberant production of these neutrophil products released into the surrounding milieu that is partly responsible for much of the tissue damage often observed with acute inflammation, and the damage associated with chronic inflammatory diseases such as rheumatoid arthritis and psoriasis. It is therefore of no great surprise that the mechanisms responsible for the accumulation of these cells in tissues has been the focus of much attention in recent years. Neutrophils, in order to fulfil their primary function of host defence, firstly have to interact with the blood vessel wall, traverse the endothelial cell layer, penetrate the basement membrane and move through the interstitial medium to reach the affected area (Figure 10.1).

2. Historical Perspective

Although the ancient Egyptians and Greeks had some understanding of the inflammatory process, it was Cornelius Celcus, a Roman writer of the first century AD

Immunopharmacology of Neutrophils
ISBN 0-12-339250-0

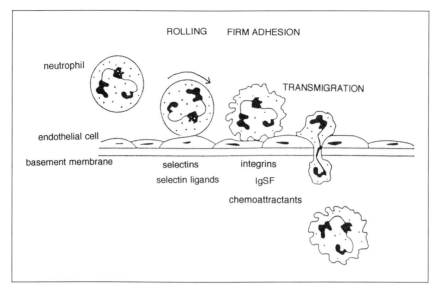

Figure 10.1 Schematic representation of the various processes involved in neutrophil accumulation in tissues showing at which stage the different families of cell adhesion molecules are involved. See text for full details.

who highlighted, with remarkable precision, the major clinical hallmarks of inflammation (redness and swelling with heat and pain). It was not until the 1800s, with the aid of the light microscope, that the involvement of white blood cells in the above process became apparent. By observing the passage of blood through the transparent tails of tadpoles, Trochet (1824) first documented the adherence of white blood cells to blood vessels and their emigration through tissues. Building on the work of Addison (1843) and Waller (1846a, 1846b), Julius Cohnheim, a pupil of the founder of modern cellular pathology, Rudolph Virchow, examined microscopically inflammatory responses in the cornea, mesentery and tongue of live frogs or rabbits (Cohnheim, 1867, 1873, 1889). He noted that white cells adhere preferentially to venular blood vessels rather than to arteriolar vessels where the blood flow was much faster (Cohnheim, 1889). Cohnheim believed that it was changes on the blood vessel wall that were responsible for the adherence and subsequent emigration of the leucocytes and not the directed movement of these cells.

This latter theory was promoted by Pfeffer who investigated the directed movement of microorganisms towards chemical stimuli (Pfeffer, 1884, 1888) and by the German ophthalmologist, Theodore Leber, who first described chemotaxis of leucocytes (Leber, 1888, 1891). Leber studied the directional movement of leucocytes in inflammatory reactions in the cornea induced by injecting, through fine capillary tubes, microorganisms or chemical substances into the anterior chamber of rabbit eyes. It was, however, the Russian biologist, Elie Metchnikoff, who made sense of Leber's observations by elegantly describing the fate and purpose of the emigrated white blood cells. Using intravital microscopy on a

number of transparent invertebrates, Metchnikoff noted that leucocytes showed a capacity to engulf foreign material such as bacteria which he referred to as "cellular eating" (Metchnikoff, 1893). Furthermore, he demonstrated that bacteria, whether dead or alive, injected into the peritoneal cavity could induce an inflammatory response manifested by the accumulation of leucocytes into the cavity. Thus, the main thesis of Metchnikoff and others was that leucocytes emigrated to sites of infection or damaged tissue because of their ability to exhibit directed movement. Chemotaxis *in vitro* was subsequently investigated by time-lapse cinematography (Comandon, 1917) and by the micropore chamber technique (Boyden, 1962). For comprehensive reviews on chemotaxis see Zigmond (1978), Valerius (1984), Wilkinson (1982) and Movat (1985).

Elegant intravital studies by the Clarks showed emigration of leucocytes from the microvasculature of frog tails towards locally applied starch grains and from new blood vessels that formed in ear chambers in rabbits using croton oil as a stimulus (Clark and Clark, 1920, 1922, 1935). Similar observations were made by Allison *et al.* (1955) who showed the rolling, sticking and emigration of leucocytes in the rabbit ear chamber induced by thermal injury. Other important contributions were made by Marchesi and Florey (1960) who presented electron microscopic evidence for the emigration of leucocytes in the rat mesentery preparations and by Atherton and Born (1972) who quantified the adhesiveness of leucocytes to blood vessels. For comprehensive reviews on adherence and emigration of leucocytes see Grant (1973) and Movat (1985).

With the observations made by the above investigators and many others, Celsus's description of inflammation could now at least partly be explained; vasodilatation could account for the redness, the increased blood flow for the heat, the exudation of tissue fluid for the swelling. These processes taken together could presumably result in the sensation of pain. In addition, the involvement of white blood cells in the inflammatory process was now certain. These studies also provided a detailed account of the interaction between the leucocyte and the micro-vasculature, highlighting the rolling phenomenon of these cells on the venular vessel wall as well as the adherence of neutrophils to each other and to venular endothelial cells. Furthermore, it is now apparent that Cohnheim's idea that changes in the endothelial cells of the microvasculature and Metchnikoff's view that directed movement of leucocytes and their ability to phagocytose all play important roles in the inflammatory response. The molecular mechanisms underlying the above processes were, however, not forthcoming until recently due to the merging disciplines of biology and medicine together with rapidly developing technology which has led to the discovery of CAMs (see Chapter 7). The essential role of these molecules in the accumulation of neutrophils into the inflammatory locus has now become apparent.

3. Mediators of Neutrophil Responsiveness

As outlined in the introduction, the neutrophil, in order to fulfil its primary function of host defence, has to reach the inflammatory stimulus in the tissue. Consequently, this cell has evolved rather complex mechanisms for detection of the diverse types of inflammatory stimuli. The neutrophil, like many other cells, can be visualized as containing numerous receptors on its plasmalemma (see Chapter 6 for an account of neutrophil chemo-attractant receptors). Ligand–receptor interactions trigger highly specialized signal transduction pathways which ultimately result in changes in neutrophil respon-siveness (see Chapter 8). A list of mediators known to affect neutrophils is given in Table 10.1.

3.1   MICROBE-DERIVED FACTORS

3.1.1   FMLP

Detection of invading bacteria by the neutrophil is of primary importance. It was known for some time that prokaryotic organisms or their products were chemo-tactic for neutrophils but the causative stimuli remained elusive. It was Schiffmann who realized that these organisms synthesized peptides using an N-terminus of formyl methionine and that it was the N-formyl peptide fragments that were chemotactic (Schiffmann et al.,

Table 10.1   Mediators of neutrophil responsiveness

Mediator	Primary effect
Microbe-derived factors	
FMLP	Stimulation
Endotoxin	Priming
Host-derived factors	
C5a	Stimulation
LTB$_4$ and related lipids	Stimulation/priming
PAF	Stimulation/priming
IL-8	Stimulation/priming
TNFα/IL-1/IFNγ/GM-CSF	Priming
PGs	Inhibition
β-Adrenergic agonists	Inhibition
Adenosine	Inhibition

1975). The discovery of the highly potent chemotactic tripeptide, FMLP, led to the demonstration and eventual characterization of FMLP receptors on neutrophils (see Chapter 6). The tripeptide not only activates neutrophils in vitro (Becker, 1987; Omann et al., 1987) but also causes neutrophil-dependent oedema formation and neutrophil accumulation in vivo (Issekutz, 1981a, 1981b; Wedmore and Williams, 1981a; Hellewell et al., 1989).

3.1.2   Endotoxin

The cell wall of most Gram-negative bacteria contains on its outer membrane LPS molecules, often referred to as endotoxin. The chemical structure of these molecules, which is thought to possess the majority of its biological activity, is the lipid A domain. Endotoxin is believed to be the main cause of shock induced by bacterial infection and in endotoxaemia in pregnancy. When injected intravenously, endotoxin causes amongst other effects a profound hypotensive state and a transient neutropaenia (Worthen et al., 1987a; Rietschel and Brade, 1992). When administered intradermally into rabbit skin, it causes a dose-dependent neutrophil accumulation (Cybulsky et al., 1988). Many of the effects of endotoxin are thought to be due to the generation of cytokines such as TNFα and IL-1. Typical endotoxin-mediated haemorrhagic and inflammatory lesions are the generalized and local Shwartzman reactions (Bronza, 1990). There is evidence to suggest that these lesions are dependent on circulating neutrophils (Becker, 1948; Stetson and Good, 1951; Thomas and Good, 1952) and that cytokines may be involved (Beck et al., 1986; Billiau et al., 1987; Movat et al., 1987; Heremans et al., 1990). In vitro, endotoxin does not appear to exhibit many direct neutrophil acti-vating properties, but it is very effective at priming them for enhanced responses when stimulated by other agonists (see Chapter 9).

3.2 Host-derived Factors

3.2.1 Complement Fragments

Mediators can be produced in the host's tissue fluid or by the host's cells. A prime example of the former type of mediator is C5a produced by the activation of the complement system. The complement system is activated by two pathways; the classical pathway and the alternative pathway (for review, see Jose, 1987). The former pathway is predominantly activated by immune complexes produced by immunoglobulin antibodies (e.g. IgG and IgM) binding with antigens on the microbe or on microbe products. The vasculitis associated with the Arthus reaction is a typical example of an inflammatory response mediated by antigen–antibody complexes resulting in the activation of the classical pathway (Cochrane and Janoff, 1974). Polysaccharides found in yeast cell walls (e.g. zymosan) activate the alternative pathway. The pivotal event in activation of the complement cascade by both pathways is the formation of C3a and C3b from the cleavage of C3. The smaller fragment, C3a, is capable of liberating histamine from mast cells (Jose, 1987). C3b and iC3b bind covalently to microbes and render them more palatable to neutrophils (opsonization). Neutrophils recognize these opsonized microbes by possessing plasmalemmal receptors for C3b and iC3b (CR1 and CR3; CR3 is also known as Mac-1 or CD11b/CD18, see Chapter 7). The fragment C3b also facilitates the formation of C5a and C5b by cleaving C5. Other complement fragments C6–C9 spontaneously combine with C5b and the resultant complexes are partly responsible for inducing cell lysis. This cellular lysis is just one of the host organism's defence mechanisms against invading bacteria.

The most important complement-derived fragment, as far as neutrophil chemoattraction is concerned, is the 74-amino-acid polypeptide C5a. The effect of C5a on neutrophil responsiveness *in vitro* has been well characterized; it causes aggregation, degranulation and superoxide release by binding to specific and saturable receptors on the plasmalemma (Hugli, 1986). The G-protein and PLC-linked C5a receptor was the first chemoattractant receptor to be sequenced and cloned (Gerard and Gerard, 1991, Chapter 6). *In vivo*, C5a, or its less active metabolite, C5a des Arg, has been detected in large quantities in certain inflammatory models (Jose *et al.*, 1983). C5a production is essential for immune-complex mediated inflammatory reactions (e.g. Arthus reaction): if animals have had their complement system depleted by intravenous cobra venom factor or if their capacity to generate C5a locally has been compromised by administration of soluble complement receptor type 1, the reaction is severely attenuated (Cochrane *et al.*, 1970; Cochrane and Janoff, 1974; Yeh *et al.*, 1991; Rossi *et al.*, 1992). Neutralizing antibodies to C5a also abrogate the reaction (Hellewell *et al.*, 1988). Similarly, inflammatory reactions induced by zymosan, which primarily activates the alternative pathway, are also inhibited by such experimental procedures. Moreover, C5a or zymosan-activated plasma (a source of preformed C5a) when intradermally injected alone or in the presence of vasodilators such as PGE_2 and CGRP will cause a marked oedema and neutrophil accumulation at the skin site (Williams, 1978; Issekutz, 1981a, 1981b; Wedmore and Williams, 1981a; Williams and Jose, 1981; Buckley *et al.*, 1991). Thus, the involvement of C5a in neutrophil attraction is well established.

3.2.2 Cellular-derived Mediators

3.2.2.1 LTB₄ and Related Lipids

One of the most potent cellular derived mediators of neutrophil accumulation *in vivo* and neutrophil activation *in vitro* is the dihydroxy lipid, LTB_4 (Ford-Hutchinson *et al.*, 1980; O'Flaherty, 1982; Samuelsson *et al.*, 1987; Nourshargh, 1992; Rossi *et al.*, 1993). Arachidonic acid, liberated from phospholipids by the action of PLA_2, is enzymatically oxygenated to a variety of bioactive products. In the neutrophil, for example, arachidonic acid is predominantly oxygenated by 5-LO resulting in the production of 5(S)-HETE and LTB_4. In other cells and to a lesser extent, in the neutrophil, arachidonic acid is oxygenated by 12-LO and/or 15-LO yielding 12- and 15-hydroxy derivatives. These products have their own biological profile (Samuelsson *et al.*, 1987). Alternatively, LTA_4, an intermediate of 5-LO activity, is converted to the sulphidopeptido-leukotrienes, LTC_4, LTD_4 and LTE_4 (Samuelsson *et al.*, 1987).

LTB_4 activates neutrophils by interacting with specific plasmalemmal receptors (Kreisle and Parker, 1983; Goldman and Goetzl, 1984; O'Flaherty *et al.*, 1986). *In vitro*, like FMLP, LTB_4 induces the repertoire of neutrophil responses and *in vivo* causes neutrophil-dependent oedema and neutrophil accumulation. There is evidence to suggest that LTB_4 may be an important mediator of various inflammatory conditions such as rheumatoid arthritis, ulcerative colitis, psoriasis and ischaemia/reperfusion injury (Nourshargh, 1992; Chapter 11).

3.2.2.2 PAF

PAF, an ether phospholipid produced by *de novo* synthesis or by the consecutive enzymatic actions of PLA_2 and acetyl transferase, is produced by many cell types including the neutrophil (Snyder, 1989). PAF stimulates neutrophils by interacting with specific receptor sites; these receptors have recently been sequenced and cloned (see Chapter 6). *In vivo*, PAF causes the accumulation of neutrophils into lungs and into skin sites when administered exogenously (Humphrey *et al.*, 1982; Issekutz and Szpejda, 1986; Chung, 1992). In rabbit skin, PAF causes a rapid neutrophil-independent oedema formation; neutropaenic animals still give an oedematous response to i.d.

PAF (Wedmore and Williams, 1981b). Although PAF does stimulate neutrophil accumulation *in vivo* and activates these cells *in vitro*, it seems that the predominant effect of this lipid, at least in rabbits, is to act directly on endothelial cells to cause an increase in vascular permeability. In the dog trachea, PAF-induced increases in microvascular permeability are partially reduced in neutropaenic animals and restored when neutrophils are infused into the isolated tracheal microcirculation (Lien *et al.*, 1992).

Using specific PAF antagonists, PAF has been shown to play an important role in immune-complex mediated reactions (Hellewell and Williams, 1986; Warren *et al.*, 1989; Hellewell, 1990; Rossi *et al.*, 1992; Pons *et al.*, 1993). PAF, like LTB4, stimulates neutrophils and is synthesized by activated neutrophils and has therefore the capacity to act as a positive feedback stimulus to cause further activation of the neutrophil. There is considerable information in the literature demonstrating interactions between the various lipids. For example, the monohydroxy acid, 5(S)-HETE, produced in large quantities by stimulated neutrophils, exerts little direct neutrophil-activating effect *per se* but can augment neutrophil responses induced by PAF (Rossi and O'Flaherty, 1991; Rossi *et al.*, 1991). Whether this particular interaction has any relevance *in vivo* remains to be established.

3.2.2.3 IL-8

IL-8, a polypeptide of approximately 8 kD, was originally shown to be a potent chemoattractant for neutrophils produced by endotoxin-stimulated monocytes (Walz *et al.*, 1987; Yoshimura *et al.*, 1987). It has now been shown to be produced by many cells, including neutrophils themselves (Baggiolini and Clark-Lewis, 1992; see Chapter 5). The IL-8 receptor has recently been cloned and sequenced (Murphy and Tiffany, 1991; Chapter 6). Neutrophil IL-8 receptor occupancy results in cellular activation via turnover of the PI cycle and elevation of cytosolic free Ca^{2+} (Baggiolini and Clark-Lewis, 1992). *In vivo*, IL-8 causes a marked neutrophil accumulation and plasma exudation when intradermally injected into skin of many species including man (Rampart *et al.*, 1989; Collins *et al.*, 1991; Leonard *et al.*, 1991; Swensson *et al.*, 1991). In addition, IL-8 has been shown to be produced in an *in vivo* experimental model of peritonitis (Beaubien *et al.*, 1990; Collins *et al.*, 1991). Zymosan particles injected i.p. induce an inflammatory exudate in the cavity. After 1–2 h the predominant inflammatory mediator present is C5a (Collins *et al.*, 1991). When the exudate is examined after longer time periods, the majority of the inflammatory activity appears to be due to IL-8 (Beaubien *et al.*, 1990) and a related cytokine, MGSA (Jose *et al.*, 1991). Furthermore, IL-8 and related cytokines have been detected in psoriatic skin and in the synovial fluid of arthritic joints (Brennan *et al.*, 1990; Nickoloff *et al.*, 1991; Seitz *et al.*, 1991). Thus, this intriguing family of cytokines may play an important role in both acute and chronic inflammatory reactions.

3.2.2.4 Other Cytokines

There are a number of other cytokines such as TNFα and IL-1 which, when injected into skin, cause a marked neutrophil accumulation (Cybulsky *et al.*, 1988; Rampart and Williams, 1988; Von Uexkull *et al.*, 1992). Whether these cytokines directly influence these cells to cause their accumulation *in vivo* is unknown. They do, however, appear to influence neutrophil responsiveness directly *in vitro*: they, for example, "prime" neutrophils for enhanced superoxide anion release and degranulation in response to other agonists such as LTB4, PAF or FMLP (O'Flaherty *et al.*, 1991; see Chapter 9). The mechanism underlying this priming phenomenon is as yet unknown and is the subject of intense investigation (Chapter 9). Despite these reported effects on neutrophils, perhaps the overwhelming effect of these cytokines is not to influence neutrophils directly *per se*, but to up-regulate cellular adhesion molecules on microvascular endothelial cells (see Chapter 7, and Section 4 of this chapter).

3.3 NEUTROPHIL MODULATORS

It is important to note that there are a number of biological substances capable of modulating or inhibiting neutrophil function. For example, it has been demonstrated that certain PGs (mainly PGE_2 and PGD_2), generated from the action of cyclo-oxygenase activity on AA, can inhibit neutrophil responses such as chemotaxis, aggregation, degranulation and superoxide anion generation. These PGs presumably interact with specific neutrophil PG receptor subtypes (Rossi and O'Flaherty, 1989) linked to AC resulting in an elevation of cAMP (Coleman and Humphrey, 1993). The precise mechanisms whereby cAMP renders the neutrophil less responsive are unknown, but there is evidence to suggest that other second-messenger systems are influenced (Della Bianca *et al.*, 1986; Takenawa *et al.*, 1986).

The situation with regard to PGs *in vivo* is, however, more confusing. Depending on the route of administration, PGs can either be pro-inflammatory or anti-inflammatory. For example, a marked oedema formation is produced in rabbit skin when PGs are coinjected with permeability-increasing substances such as bradykinin, histamine, FMLP or LTB4 (Williams and Peck, 1977; Williams, 1979; Wedmore and Williams, 1981a). This pro-inflammatory effect is thought to be due to the vasodilator properties of the PGs; arterioles become dilated thereby augmenting intralumenal hydrostatic pressure downstream in venules where the plasma leakage occurs (Majno and Palade, 1961). On the other hand, when given i.v. at a sub-vasodepressor dose, PGs can selectively inhibit oedema formation induced by i.d. injections of neutrophil-dependent agonists (e.g. FMLP or LTB$_4$) whilst responses to neutrophil-independent stimuli (e.g. histamine or bradykinin) remain unaffected (Rampart and Williams, 1986). A plausible explanation for this anti-inflammatory effect may be that i.v. PGs are directly influencing neutrophil responsiveness and thereby reducing plasma exudation. There are many animal models where PGs have been shown to be either pro-inflammatory or anti-inflammatory (Hellewell and Williams, 1988).

Neutrophils also possess AC-linked β adrenergic receptors which, when activated, suppress neutrophil function (Dulis and Wilson, 1980; Mueller et al., 1988). However, the significance of this in inflammatory situations is unclear. Certainly β agonists show anti-inflammatory properties in animal models of inflammation, but it is not known which is the target cell (Spector and Willoughby, 1960; Green, 1972; Whelan and Johnson, 1992).

It has been suggested that endogenously released adenosine, a purine nucleoside, may be an important regulator of the inflammatory response. Indeed, there is evidence showing the existence of at least two types of adenosine receptors on the neutrophil; occupancy of the adenosine A$_1$ receptors increases agonist-induced chemotaxis or adherence to endothelial cells, whereas occupancy of A$_2$ receptors results in an inhibition of agonist-induced superoxide anion release and adherence (Cronstein et al., 1992). In vivo adenosine agonists have been shown to inhibit inflammation in the carrageenin-induced pleural response in rats (Schrier et al., 1990).

The above incomplete list and brief description of neutrophil agonists and inhibitors is included merely to highlight the chemical diversity of the mediators of neutrophil function, and to stress the importance of possible interactions between mediators and their involvement in the recruitment of neutrophils to inflammatory sites.

4. Mechanisms of Leucocyte Accumulation

4.1 General Observations

Our understanding of the processes by which leucocytes accumulate at sites of inflammation has advanced greatly over the last 10 years. In the decade before, great advances were made as a result of improvements in tissue culture techniques and successful isolation and culture of vascular endothelial cells (Jaffe et al., 1973; Gimbrone et al., 1978). Thus, from the late 1970s to mid-1980s pioneering studies were conducted which established that neutrophils isolated from peripheral blood could adhere to and migrate through cultured endothelial cells (Beesley et al., 1978, 1979; Pearson et al., 1979; Tonnesen et al., 1984; Harlan, 1985). However, the

molecular basis for these interactions was not established until the last decade. The different families of endothelial and leucocyte cell adhesion molecules are discussed in Chapter 7. Tables 10.2 and 10.3 show summaries of the molecules involved in leucocyte adhesion to endothelium. Observations in the living microcirculation using intravital microscopy have shown that the process of leucocyte accumulation primarily occurs in the post-capillary venules (Clark and Clark, 1935; see Section 2). This appears to be the case for the majority of microcirculations, the exception being the pulmonary circulation where the capillary appears to be the predominant site of cell interaction and migration (discussed below).

Table 10.2 Leucocyte adhesion molecules

Family	Cell distribution
Integrins	
β_2 CD11a/CD18 (LFA-1)	All leucocytes
β_2 CD11b/CD18 (Mac-1, CR3)	All leucocytes
β_2 CD11c/CD18 (p150,95)	Neutrophils, eosinophils, monocytes
β_1 CD29/CD49d (VLA-4)	All except neutrophils
Selectins	
L-selectin	All leucocytes
Carbohydrates	
SLe^x	All, but only some lymphocytes
Immunoglobulin superfamily	
ICAM-3	All leucocytes

Table 10.3 Endothelial cell adhesion molecules

Family	Basal expression	Agonists which enhance expression	Kinetics of expression
IgSF			
ICAM-1	Yes	IL-1, TNF-α, LPS, IFNγ	Hours
ICAM-2	Yes[a]	non-inducible	Constitutive
VCAM-1	Yes[b]	IL-1, TNF, LPS, IL-4	Hours
Selectins			
P-Selectin	No	Thrombin, histamine	Minutes
E-Selectin	No	IL-1, TNF, LPS	Hours
Others			
L-Selectin ligand	No	IL-1, TNF	Hours

[a] Higher level than ICAM-1.
[b] Lower level than ICAM-1.

4.2   THE ROLE OF SELECTINS

In post-capillary venules, leucocytes have been observed to roll slowly along the wall of the vessel sticking transiently and cells flattened against the vessel wall appeared to stick with greater avidity (Atherton and Born, 1972). Hydrodynamic mechanisms appear to play an important role in allowing rolling to occur by maintaining the marginal position of leucocytes while red blood cells remain in the centre of the vessel. This process is also known as margination.

Rolling of leucocytes is thought to be absent in normal tissue and its presence in the exposed microcirculation (e.g. mesentery) is likely to be a result of the mild surgical trauma necessary to expose the tissue for intravital microscopy (Fiebig et al., 1991). Infusion of anti-CD18 mAbs is unable to prevent this rolling of leucocytes (Arfors et al., 1987; Von Andrian et al., 1991) suggesting that the mechanisms that govern the rolling response are CD18 independent. Observations by a number of groups (see below) have extended these studies by providing convincing evidence that selectins (Table 10.2) are responsible for "capturing" or "tethering" leucocytes in post-capillary venules, allowing the cells to roll along the vessel wall (this first step in the process of leucocyte accumulation is depicted in Figure 10.1). For example, infusion of anti-L-selectin antibodies virtually abolishes leucocyte rolling in both rat and rabbit mesentery (Ley et al., 1991; Von Andrian et al., 1991) and murine L cells stably transfected with human L-selectin cDNA are able to roll in rat mesenteric venules in vivo (Ley et al., 1993). In vitro studies have also revealed the importance of L-selectin in mediating the CD18-independent adhesion that occurs under shear forces in studies designed to mimic the conditions of flow in the microcirculation. However, the shear rates at which adhesion via L-selectin occurs are calculated to be only 10–20% of those in post-capillary venules (Smith et al., 1991), under shear forces similar to those calculated to exist in vivo, then the conditions appear to be too extreme to allow adhesion to occur in vitro. This apparent discrepancy remains to be resolved but might be explained if multiple selectins were induced in vivo, and all were contributing to leucocyte rolling (i.e. L-selectin on the neutrophil binding to its ligand on the endothelial cell and P- or E-selectin on the endothelial cell binding to carbohydrate determinants on the leucocyte). In vitro studies in which the relative abilities of selectins, in isolation or in combination, to mediate rolling of different leucocytes under flow have yet to be carried out.

Certainly P-selectin functions as an adhesion molecule for neutrophils in vitro and under shear conditions that render ICAM-1 completely ineffective (Lawrence and Springer, 1991). Recent preliminary studies have shown that leucocyte rolling in mesenteric venules is impaired in P-selectin "knockout" mice (Wagner, 1993). While the leucocyte ligand for P-selectin is known to be a carbohydrate (see Chapter 7; Table 10.4), the endothelial ligand that binds L-selectin is unknown. Some studies have suggested that neutrophil L-selectin is coated with SLe^x and can therefore bind E-selectin (Picker et al., 1991) while others have identified a heavily glycosylated ligand, GlyCAM-1, on HEV that binds lymphocyte L-selectin and may be involved in lymphocyte recirculation (Lasky et al., 1992). However, there is no evidence for expression of GlyCAM-1 on post-capillary venules nor for it binding to neutrophil L-selectin. There have been two reports of an L-selectin ligand expressed on cultured endothelial cells (Spertini et al., 1991a; Brady et al., 1992). This molecule is inducible by cytokines but the kinetics of expression dissociate it from E- or P-selectin. Additional studies are required to resolve the identity of this potentially important molecule, generate reagents that block its function and ascertain its role in neutrophil accumulation in inflammation.

Selectins are thought to support adhesion of leucocytes, including neutrophils, in the presence of shear stress by virtue of the interaction being governed by the kinetics rather than the affinity of binding. Thus, while selectins bind their ligands with relatively low affinity compared with, for example, the interaction of a chemoattractant with its neutrophil receptor, they are thought to do so very rapidly and form multiple interactions (Williams, 1991; Tozeren and Ley, 1992). In addition, upon neutrophil stimulation, L-selectin appears to undergo a rapid but transient up-regulation in its affinity for an artificial ligand polyphosphomonoester (PPME) (Spertini et al., 1991b). It will be interesting to examine whether a similar increase in L-selectin affinity for the novel endothelial ligand for L-selectin also occurs. Following this activation step, L-selectin is shed from the cell surface, concomitant with increased expression of β_2 integrins. This "release" mechanism may be important in allowing firm adhesion, spreading, movement and transmigration to occur (see below). The shedding of L-selectin appears to be a proteolytic process and a neutrophil protease (chymotrypsin-like) has been implicated as an endogenous regulator (Jutila et al., 1991; see Chapter 4).

Table 10.4   Cell adhesion molecule pairs involved in leucocyte binding to endothelium

Leucocyte CAM	Endothelial cell CAM	Function
L-Selectin	L-Selectin ligand, E-selectin?	Leucocyte rolling
SLe^x	E-Selectin, P-selectin	Leucocyte rolling
CD11a/CD18	ICAM-1, ICAM-2	Firm adhesion
CD11b/CD18	ICAM-1	Firm adhesion
CD11c/CD18	Unknown	Firm adhesion
CD29/CD49d (VLA-4)	VCAM-1	Firm adhesion

4.3   THE ROLE OF INTEGRINS AND IMMUNOGLOBULIN SUPERFAMILY MEMBERS

There is good evidence, therefore, that the first step in leucocyte accumulation is mediated by selectins. However, this event by itself does not necessarily lead to cells moving out of blood vessels. For example, observations in the microcirculation have shown that a rolling leucocyte can be washed off by the passing blood. In addition, histamine can induce several changes in the microcirculation that would favour neutrophil accumulation: degranulation of cultured endothelial cells such that they rapidly express P-selectin on the cell surface (Geng *et al.*, 1990) and support neutrophil adhesion; histamine-treated HUVECs also support the adhesion of neutrophils under flow conditions *in vitro* and this is abrogated by an anti-P-selectin antibody (C.W. Smith, unpublished data); infusion of histamine induces leucocyte rolling in mesenteric venules (K. Ley, unpublished data). However, despite these observations, histamine is a poor inducer of neutrophil accumulation in tissues *in vivo* at doses that cause a large increase in microvascular permeability leading to oedema formation (Figure 10.2).

Thus, once rolling has occurred, a second stimulus that activates the leucocyte integrins is required before leucocyte accumulation can occur. This activation process is thought to be the result of a conformational change from a non-adhesive form to an adhesive one. At least for the neutrophil, activation of β_2 integrins (CD11/CD18) appears to be under the regulation of a novel neutrophil-derived lipid, IMF (Hermanowski-Vosatka *et al.*, 1992). As a result of integrin activation, neutrophils are able to adhere to ICAM-1 and/or ICAM-2 (expressed constitutively or that have been up-regulated by cytokines; Table 10.3) and adhesion is "strengthened" (or becomes firmer) so that the leucocyte is less susceptible to being washed off by the passing blood. Traditionally, the neutrophil has been thought to flatten against the vessel wall as a prelude to migration between adjacent endothelial cells (Figure 10.1). However, there is little evidence to show that flattening really does occur; rather it may be that the neutrophil surface in contact with the endothelial cell becomes larger but without the leucocyte becoming discoid.

As far as the stimuli that activate β_2 integrins, there are several examples and these have already been discussed in Section 3 of this chapter. For example, the stimulus can be endothelial cell associated such as PAF or IL-8 (Kuijpers *et al.*, 1992), tissue generated such as C5a or LTB$_4$, or bacterial derived such as FMLP. Recent studies have indicated that other adhesion molecules, in particular CD44, can act as an anchor for chemotactic peptides (including chemokines such as MIP-1β) allowing the appropriate leucocyte receptor to interact with its ligand (Tanaka *et al.*, 1993). The chemokine IL-8

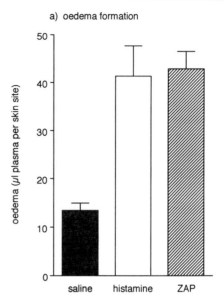

a) oedema formation

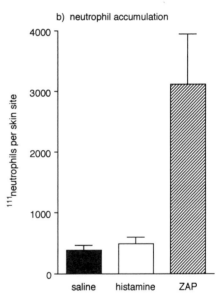

b) neutrophil accumulation

Figure 10.2 Local inflammation in guinea-pig skin induced by intradermal injection of histamine or ZAP. Oedema formation (a) and accumulation of ^{111}In-labelled neutrophils (b) were assessed simultaneously in guinea-pig skin in response to i.d. injection of histamine (2.5×10^{-8} moles/site) or ZAP (zymosan-activated plasma, as a source of C5a des Arg). Responses were measured after 2 h according to published methods (Teixeira *et al.*, 1993). Histamine and ZAP caused substantial oedema formation above the saline control (a) but only ZAP induced the significant accumulation of ^{111}In-labelled neutrophils (b). Values are means ± SEM of five experiments.

binds to endothelial cells of post-capillary venules in tissue sections and this may also involve CD44 or other proteoglycans (Rot, 1992a, 1992b). Thus, the leucocyte is envisaged as "sniffing and licking" the endothelial surface as it rolls on selectins. If it likes the smell or taste, i.e. the appropriate chemoattractant molecules are bound to proteoglycans, then the neutrophil's integrins (CD11/CD18) can up-regulate their affinity for their appropriate immunoglobulin superfamily ligands (ICAM-1, ICAM-2) expressed on the endothelial cell surface and the cell can adhere firmly to the vessel wall (Table 10.4). Leucocytes that express the β_1 integrin VLA-4 (i.e. monocytes, lymphocytes, eosinophils, basophils) can also respond to appropriate stimuli by increasing the affinity of this molecule for the endothelial ligand VCAM-1 (Table 10.4). Once firm adhesion has occurred, the process of cell emigration takes place (Figure 10.1). *In vivo* this occurs rapidly (10–15 min) and also appears to involve CAMs, in particular CD11/CD18 and ICAM-1. Exactly how these molecules interact to allow cell movement after the cells have firmly adhered remains to be resolved. One important aspect could be the "shedding" of L-selectin from the leucocyte surface (Kishimoto *et al.*, 1989) induced by the same chemoattractant that leads to activation of the integrins. Loss of L-selectin may allow the cells to crawl along the endothelium as a prelude to migrating between the cell junctions.

ICAM-1 expressed at endothelial cell junctions appears to be important for neutrophil emigration, at least *in vitro* (Smith *et al.*, 1989; Furie *et al.*, 1991, 1992). There is also evidence that E-selectin can mediate migration of neutrophils across endothelial cells (Luscinskas *et al.*, 1991), although other studies do not support these findings (Hakkert *et al.*, 1991; Kishimoto *et al.*, 1991; Furie *et al.*, 1992). Differences between the studies have been attributed to the *in vitro* techniques used. Other studies of migrating neutrophils have suggested that, in response to repeated stimulation with low doses of chemoattractant, intracellular pools of CD11b replenish surface CD11b which is transported to the uropod and filopodia of the neutrophil during migration (Francis *et al.*, 1989; Hughes *et al.*, 1992). Newly expressed CD11b is found at the leading edge of the cell and recent studies suggest that this new CD11b is used during adherence-dependent migration (Hughes *et al.*, 1992). In order for this process to function, a concentration gradient of chemoattractant is required and this may well be surface attached as discussed above.

4.4 THE MARGINATED POOL

It has been recognized for some time that a so-called marginated pool of neutrophils exists in the lung which is in dynamic equilibrium with the circulating pool (Hogg, 1987; Worthen *et al.*, 1987b; MacNee and Selby, 1993). The observations that neutrophils are released into the circulation when cardiac output is increased by infusion of adrenaline and, conversely, are retained in the lung when cardiac output is decreased

suggests that the lung plays an important role in the control of neutrophil kinetics. From direct observations of lung capillaries and manipulation of cardiac output, it has been suggested that the marginating pool is a reflection of different transit times of leucocytes as they pass through the capillary networks of the pulmonary circulation.

While there are many studies which demonstrate accumulation of leucocytes via post-capillary venules in the systemic circulation (see above), the situation in the pulmonary circulation is less clear. In part this relates to methodological difficulties in studying this site but there are several notable differences between the two microcirculations: intravascular pressure in the pulmonary circulation is approximately 10-fold lower than systemic (Von Euler and Liljestrand, 1946); flow in the pulmonary microvessels is pulsatile leading to conditions of stop-flow which favour capillary localization of passing leucocytes (Lee and DuBois, 1955; Hogg, 1987); the mean diameter of pulmonary capillaries is 5.5 μm (Guntheroth *et al.*, 1982) whereas that of the neutrophil is 7–8 μm (Schmidt-Schonbein *et al.*, 1985; Downey *et al.*, 1990). Thus, the neutrophil will have to deform to pass through a capillary, a process that is likely to slow its progress and may not involve adhesive interactions. In addition, for a neutrophil to emigrate via either arterioles or post-capillary venules to gain access to the alveolus would involve movement over long distances through the interstitium. Teleologically, this does not make sense. Observations in several animal models have suggested the capillary to be the major site of migration from the pulmonary circulation into the airspaces (Shaw, 1980; Meyrick and Brigham, 1984; Lien *et al.*, 1991; Downey *et al.*, 1993).

Exposure of neutrophils to chemoattractant molecules or LPS reduces their deformability and renders them less able to squeeze through capillaries (Downey and Worthen, 1988; Erzerum *et al.*, 1992). Studies of neutrophil retention in model capillaries have shown that CD18-dependent adhesion is not required for this process but reorganization of the neutrophil cytoskeleton with accompanying increases in cell stiffness appears to play a key role (Downey and Worthen, 1988; Worthen *et al.*, 1989; Selby *et al.*, 1991). Evidence that this mechanism is important *in vivo* comes from studies in which FMLP-induced retention of neutrophils in rabbit lungs was attenuated by pretreatment of the cells with cytochalasin D which prevents actin polymerization (Worthen *et al.*, 1989). Importantly, this has also been demonstrated in lungs of humans (Selby *et al.*, 1991). Indirect evidence that retention of neutrophils in the lungs is independent of β_2 integrins comes from the observation that LAD patients show a normal neutrophilia in response to adrenaline administration (Buchanan *et al.*, 1982; Haslett and Warren, 1990). Nevertheless, while a decrease in neutrophil deformability may allow the cell to be retained in capillaries, it is likely that the cell must become more deformable in order to penetrate the capillary wall. Thus, it may be that a decrease in neutrophil deformability allows that neutrophil to become sequestered initially, analogous to the tethering of leucocytes by selectins in post-capillary venules.

5. Modulation of Experimental Inflammation with Monoclonal Antibodies Directed Against Cell Adhesion Molecules

From the preceding overview, it is apparent that there are a number of potential sites for targeting leucocyte accumulation in inflammation. These are: generation and action of signals (i.e. inflammatory mediators); expression of CAMs; blocking of rolling or activation of integrins; interaction with extracellular matrix. *In vivo* investigations to date have been carried out using blocking mAbs to the integrin, immunoglobulin and selectin families of CAMs. All studies indicate that blocking CAM function *in vivo* has profound effects on the inflammatory process and on the outcome of experimental models of vascular and tissue injury. Rather than list all the models in which anti-CAM Abs have been shown to inhibit inflammation, the different tissues/organs in which anti-inflammatory effects of these reagents has been demonstrated are summarized in Table 10.5. For an extensive list the reader is referred to an excellent recent review (Harlan *et al.*, 1992). However, a few examples will be discussed below.

5.1 STUDIES IN THE PERIPHERAL MICROCIRCULATION

The first indication that CD18 was important for accumulation of neutrophils at sites of inflammation *in vivo* was from a study by Arfors *et al.* (1987) in which intravenous administration of the mAb 60.3 suppressed the accumulation of neutrophils into skin sites injected with chemoattractants. Direct visual observation of the microcirculation (by intravital microscopy) showed that 60.3 also prevented stimulated neutrophil adherence to endothelium (Arfors *et al.*, 1987); thus, while neutrophil adherence in the venules and migration into the tissues (in response to extravascular chemoattractant) was inhibited, rolling of neutrophils along the venular endothelium was unaffected. However, inhibitors of L-selectin do prevent leucocyte rolling *in vivo* (Ley *et al.*, 1991; Von Andrian *et al.*, 1991, 1992). Together with *in vitro* data, these observations led to the proposed mechanism of leucocyte accumulation discussed above.

The expected outcome of inhibiting L-selectin-mediated rolling *in vivo* is that neutrophil accumulation at

sites of inflammation will be abrogated. Indeed, systemic administration of the anti-murine L-selectin mAb MEL-14 has demonstrated the importance of L-selectin in regulating the extravasation of neutrophils from the bloodstream into the inflamed peritoneal cavity of the mouse (Lewisohn *et al.*, 1987; Jutila *et al.*, 1989). The inhibition was not a consequence of neutrophils being removed from the circulation as a result of antibody administration. Suppression of neutrophil accumulation into the inflamed peritoneum has also been shown in the mouse using a soluble immunoglobulin chimaera of human L-selectin (Watson *et al.*, 1991).

In view of the inhibitory activity of both anti-β_2 integrin and anti-L-selectin mAbs on neutrophil accumulation, we studied the relative contribution of these adhesion molecules to neutrophil accumulation in a model of carageenan-induced pleurisy in the mouse (Henriques *et al.*, 1990). Four hours after intrapleural administration of carageenan, an intense neutrophil influx into the cavity is observed. However, neutrophil accumulation was abrogated in mice pretreated with either the anti-CD11b mAb 5C6 or the anti-L-selectin mAb MEL-14 (Figure 10.3) (Henriques, Williams and Hellewell, unpublished data). These *in vivo* observations add support to the concept that neutrophil accumulation involves selectins and integrins but also suggest that the processes that utilize these molecules (i.e. rolling and firm adhesion/migration) are independent events, and that inhibiting either is effective at abrogating the inflammatory response.

In other studies, Hernandez *et al.* (1987) were the first to show that neutrophil adhesion via β_2 integrins was a critical event in reperfusion injury. Thus, pretreatment of cats with the anti-CD18 mAb 60.3 provided protection against ischaemia-induced microvascular injury of the gut. Subsequent studies have shown that anti-CD18 mAb-mediated inhibition of granulocyte adherence is effective at reducing injury in myocardial and whole-animal models of reperfusion injury, supporting the proposition that granulocytes play an important role in reperfusion injury (see Chapter 11; Mullane and Smith, 1990). However, in all these studies mAbs were administered before the onset of ischaemia. The clinically relevant situation would be to provide treatment after the onset of the ischaemic event but before reperfusion.

Nevertheless, Vedder *et al.* (1990) have shown that treatment with an anti-CD18 mAb either before or after ischaemia, but prior to reperfusion, did result in the same degree of significant protection against microvascular injury in the rabbit ear. In a similarly designed study, organ injury (particularly in the gut) after haemorrhagic shock in rhesus monkeys was dramatically protected by administration of 60.3 just prior to fluid-induced resuscitation. Perhaps the most noticeable observation was that, in the treated group, all animals survived for up to 72 h whereas 40% of the control animals died (Mileski *et al.*, 1990).

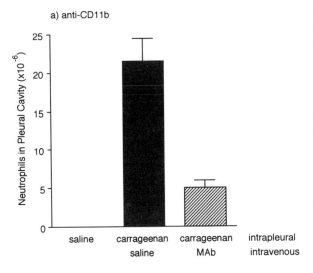

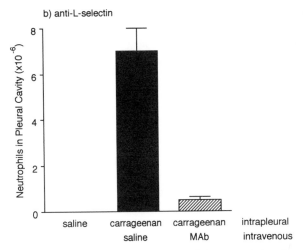

Figure 10.3 Suppression of neutrophil accumulation in experimental pleurisy in the mouse by either (a) an anti-CD11b mAb or (b) an anti-L-selectin mAb. Mice received either saline or mAb i.v. followed by an intrapleural injection of saline or carrageenan (300 μg). Neutrophil migration into the cavity was assessed after 4 h. The anti-murine CD11b mAb 5C6 was injected at 1 mg per mouse and the anti-murine L-selectin mAb MEL-14 at 100 μg per mouse. These doses had no effect on circulating neutrophil numbers. Values are means ± SEM of four experiments.

More recently, clinically relevant studies have shown that anti-CD18 mAbs prevent tissue injury in two extreme forms of microvascular damage in which ischaemia plays an important role, burns and frostbite. In thermal injury an area of irreversible injury is surrounded by a marginal zone of reduced blood flow. Anti-CD18 mAbs and an anti-ICAM-1 mAb improved microvascular perfusion in this zone of stasis which resulted in accelerated re-epithelialization (Bucky *et al.*, 1991;

Mileski *et al.*, 1992). In frostbite, administration of an anti-CD18 mAb (60.3) at the time of rewarming a frozen foot dramatically reduced swelling and tissue loss (Mileski *et al.*, 1993). Delaying the administration of 60.3 for 30 min after the start of rewarming was much less effective.

Interestingly, the non-immune, haemorrhagic and inflammatory lesion, the Shwartzman reaction, produced in rabbit skin is inhibited by systemic administration of Abs directed against ICAM-1, CD18 and CD11b but not by CD11a (Argenbright *et al.*, 1992). In addition, the immune-complex mediated vasculitis associated with a reversed passive Arthus reaction in rabbit skin is abolished by i.v. administration of an anti-CD18 mAb but only partly attenuated by i.v. injection of an anti-ICAM-1 mAb (Norman *et al.*, 1994). The elegant studies by Mulligan, Ward and co-workers on immune-complex mediated inflammation in the rat lung have shown a role for E-selectin, VLA-4, ICAM-1, CD18, CD11a and CD11b adhesion molecules (Mulligan *et al.*, 1991, 1992a, 1992b, 1993a, 1993b; Table 10.5). Despite this work, the precise role and the complex interactions of these adhesion molecules in the above inflammatory reactions remains to be fully elucidated. Furthermore, our understanding of their role will depend upon obtaining a clearer insight into which cells and cytokines are involved in these inflammatory models.

The β_1 integrin VLA-4 (or CD29/CD49d) is not found on neutrophils and therefore blocking Abs would not be expected to have any effect on neutrophil accumulation. In contrast, pretreating guinea-pig eosinophils with the anti-VLA-4 mAb HP1/2 prevents their accumulation at sites of inflammation in guinea-pig skin (Weg *et al.*, 1993). However, in a model of contact hypersensitivity in the mouse ear, systemic administration of an anti-VLA-4 mAb not only reduced ear swelling and lymphocyte accumulation but also attenuated neutrophil infiltration (Chisholm *et al.*, 1993). This suggests that neutrophil accumulation is somehow dependent on VLA-4 expressing cells or perhaps murine neutrophils express this integrin.

5.2 SEPSIS AND SAFETY

Neutrophil activation is a common feature of sepsis; thus, inhibition of neutrophil accumulation may be an effective therapeutic strategy in septic shock and ARDS (see Chapter 13). Indeed, CD11b has been shown to be up-regulated on neutrophils from pigs treated with LPS (Simms *et al.*, 1991) and Abs against this integrin reduce endotoxin-induced neutrophil-mediated tissue damage in liver and lung (Jaeschke *et al.*, 1991; Burch *et al.*, 1993; Miotla *et al.*, 1993). In addition, an anti-CD11b mAb increased survival of mice following endotoxin challenge (Burch *et al.*, 1993).

Survival of rabbits with septic shock was also significantly increased by treatment with an anti-CD18 mAb,

Table 10.5 Effects of mAbs to cell adhesion molecules on neutrophil accumulation in experimental inflammation

CAM blocked	Effects in model	Organ/tissue
CD11a	Inhibition of accumulation of neutrophils	Skin,[1] lung[2,3]
CD11b	Inhibition of accumulation of neutrophils (and monocytes)	Peritoneum,[4,5] lung,[2,3,6,7] pleural cavity,[8] foot pad,[9] heart,[10] skin,[1,5] kidney[11]
CD18	Inhibition of accumulation of neutrophils (and eosinophils and monocytes); inhibition of oedema formation	Skin,[5,12–16] intestine,[17] heart,[18–20] peritoneum,[5,21] lung,[5,22–26] eye,[27] knee joint,[28] meninges,[29,30] foot,[31] ear[32]
VLA-4	Inhibition of accumulation of neutrophils	Ear,[33] lung[2]
ICAM-1	Inhibition of accumulation of neutrophils (eosinophils and T lymphocytes)	Skin,[34] intestine,[35] lung,[2,3,24,36] kidney,[11,37] airways,[38] heart[20,39]
L-Selectin	Inhibition of accumulation of neutrophils (and monocytes)	Skin,[40] peritoneum,[41,42] pleural cavity[8]
P-Selectin	Inhibition of accumulation of neutrophils and associated tissue injury	Lung[43]
E-Selectin	Inhibition of accumulation of neutrophils and associated tissue injury	Lung,[44,45] peritoneum,[44] skin[44]

[1]Issekutz and Issekutz (1992); [2]Mulligan et al. (1993a); [3]Mulligan et al. (1993b); [4]Rosen and Gordon (1987); [5]Mulligan et al. (1992b); [6]Rosen and Gordon (1990); [7]Miotla et al. (1993); [8]Henriques, Williams and Hellewell, unpublished data; [9]Rosen et al. (1989b); [10]Simpson et al. (1988); [11]Mulligan et al. (1993c); [12]Arfors et al. (1987); [13]Price et al. (1987); [14]Rampart and Williams (1988); [15]Nourshargh et al. (1989); [16]Lindbom et al. (1990); [17]Hernandez et al. (1987); [18]Winquist et al. (1990); [19]Williams et al. (1990); [20]Byrne et al. (1992); [21]Mileski et al. (1990); [22]Doerschuk et al. (1990); [23]Horgan et al. (1990); [24]Barton et al. (1989); [25]Mulligan et al. (1992a); [26]Lo et al. (1992); [27]Till et al. (1992); [28]Jasin et al. (1992); [29]Tuomanen et al. (1989); [30]Saez-Llorens et al. (1991); [31]Mileski et al. (1993); [32]Vedder et al. (1990); [33]Chisholm et al. (1993); [34]Rampart et al. (1991); [35]Granger et al. (1991); [36]Wegner et al. (1992); [37]Cosimi et al. (1990); [38]Wegner et al. (1990); [39]Ma et al. (1992); [40]Lewinsohn et al. (1987); [41]Jutila et al. (1989); [42]Watson et al. (1991); [43]Mulligan et al. (1992c); [44]Mulligan et al. (1991); [45]Gundel et al. (1991).

although increases in lung vascular permeability in the same animals were not attenuated (Thomas et al., 1992). One of the major concerns with this type of treatment for sepsis is that it may interfere with the important function of neutrophils in recognizing and removing bacteria from the body. Thus, any protection may be countered by the risk of uncontrolled bacterial infection. For example, pretreatment of mice with an anti-CD11b mAb resulted in a substantial increase in mortality following infection with *Listeria monocytogenes* (Rosen et al., 1989a), However, in the rabbit, a short treatment period with 60.3 did not increase mortality rates in abdominal sepsis (Mileski et al., 1991), did not alter bacterial growth in a model of meningitis (Tuomanen et al., 1989; Sáez-Llorens et al., 1991) and did not increase abscess size or incidence following subcutaneous administration of clinically relevant numbers of *Staphylococcus aureus* (Sharar et al., 1991). In contrast, inoculation with high numbers of bacteria resulted in overwhelming abscess formation in skin when animals were treated with the same mAb (Sharar et al., 1991). The major worry, therefore, is that treatment of patients with these antibodies may prove problematic because of the infection risk. An alternative route for treatment in sepsis may be with blockers of selectins. For example, E-selectin is expressed in most tissues following septic shock in baboons, while hypovolaemic shock does not provide such a stimulus (Redl et al., 1991; Engelberts et al., 1992).

5.3 LUNG INFLAMMATION

In the lung there are two microvascular beds to consider; the large pulmonary circulation that is involved in gas exchange and intimately associated with leucocytes (see Section 4.3), and the smaller bronchial circulation that supplies the airways.

In asthma, which is essentially a disease of the conducting airways, it is the bronchial circulation that is considered to be the most important. The group at Boehringer Ingelheim have carried out an excellent series of studies with mAbs to cell adhesion molecules in their primate model of asthma. In the first studies, antigen-induced bronchial hyper-responsiveness and bronchial eosinophil influx were significantly attenuated by systemic administration of the anti-ICAM-1 mAb R6.5 (Wegner et al., 1990). Neutrophil numbers were not measured in these experiments. Since airway epithelial cells express ICAM-1 in this model and may be the subject of eosinophil-mediated damage, the efficacy of inhaled anti-ICAM-1 was also determined. Daily nebulization of the mAb inhibited the antigen-induced airway responsiveness (Wegner et al., 1991) suggesting that this route of administration could be exploited in asthma. In the same model, intravenous administration of CL2, an anti-E-selectin (human) mAb, which cross-reacts with primate E-selectin, had no such inhibitory effect (Gundel et al., 1991). However, when the anti-E-selectin mAb CL2 was studied in primate following a single challenge with antigen, neutrophil influx and the late-phase airway obstruction were abrogated (Gundel *et al.*, 1991). This suggests that the late-phase response may be the result of an influx of neutrophils into the airways dependent on E-selectin. Interestingly, the anti-ICAM-1 mAb had no effect on neutrophil accumulation which is surprising in view of the inhibitory effect of anti-ICAM-1 mAbs on neutrophil trans-migration *in vitro* (Smith *et al.*, 1989) and accumulation *in vivo* in other studies (Rampart *et al.*, 1991; Table 10.5).

Another example of CD18/ICAM-1-independent neutrophil accumulation was demonstrated in studies of whole-animal models of reperfusion injury. While tissue damage in gut and liver was attenuated by anti-CD18 mAbs, lung injury in the same animals did not appear to be suppressed (Vedder *et al.*, 1988). Further studies revealed that neutrophil accumulation from pulmonary capillaries in the lung can occur via CD18-dependent and CD18-independent mechanisms that appear to depend on the stimulus (Doerschuk *et al.*, 1990). Thus, intrabronchial instillation of *Streptococcus pneumoniae* or hydrochloric acid induced neutrophil accumulation in the lung that was not inhibited by the anti-CD18 mAb 60.3. In contrast, neutrophil accumulation induced by intrabronchial PMA or *E. coli* was reduced by 70–99% by 60.3. In the skin of the same animals, neutrophil accumulation induced by the same stimuli was abolished (i.e. inhibited by >98%) by 60.3 treatment.

Lung injury in the rat, as assessed by increases in vascular permeability and haemorrhage, induced by intravenous cobra venom factor or by intra-alveolar deposition of immune complexes is reported to be partially reduced by an anti-CD18 mAb (Mulligan *et al.*, 1992a, 1992b). Neutrophil accumulation as assessed by tissue myeloperoxidase was also reduced by anti-CD18 treatment (Mulligan *et al.*, 1992b). The response to cobra venom factor and immune complexes is comple-ment dependent, C5a being the major mediator. The response to C5a itself was not examined, although others have shown that C5a-induced neutrophil accumulation in rabbit lung is largely CD18 independent (Hellewell and Henson, 1991; Hellewell *et al.*, 1994). The anti-E-selectin mAb CL-3 that cross-reacts with the rat has also been shown to reduce neutrophil accumulation in the lung in response to immune complexes (Mulligan *et al.*, 1991). Lung injury was also attenuated as judged by inhibition of vascular permeability and haemorrhage (Mulligan *et al.*, 1991).

How C5a itself induces neutrophil accumulation in the lung remains to be determined. It is unlikely to be via E-selectin since *in vitro* studies have shown that C5a is unable to up-regulate endothelial CAMs; it is possible that C5a stimulates resident lung cells such as macro-phages to generate TNF and there is some *in vitro* evidence to support this idea (Okusawa *et al.*, 1988). These studies with C5a also indicate that the process of

cell migration is CD18 independent which is intriguing because *in vitro* evidence to date indicates that CD18 is essential for cell emigration to occur (Smith *et al.*, 1988, 1989). Neutrophils from LAD patients (CD18 deficient) can adhere to activated endothelium via E-selectin but they cannot migrate (Smith *et al.*, 1988). However, post-mortem examination of lungs from LAD patients shows clear evidence of neutrophil migration into the air spaces at foci of bronchopneumonia (Hawkins *et al.*, 1992). While the retention of neutrophils in the pulmonary microcirculation may be occurring via E-selectin it suggests that alternative mechanisms for retention and migration of granulocytes exist (Worthen *et al.*, 1989; MacNee and Selby, 1993). The role of neutrophil deformability was discussed above.

Evidence for a role for P-selectin in mediating neutro-phil accumulation in lung tissue has also been published (Mulligan *et al.*, 1992c). In these experiments, the anti-P-selectin mAb PNB1.6 reduced cobra venom factor-induced neutrophil infiltration into rat lung as assessed by lung total myeloperoxidase content. The effect of anti-P-selectin on neutrophil emigration into the air spaces was not assessed, although two other indices of lung injury, permeability index and haemorrhage, were attenuated by the mAb.

There is also evidence that VLA-4 plays a role in neutrophil accumulation in certain types of lung injury. Mulligan *et al.* (1993b) found that an anti-rat VLA-4 mAb was very effective at inhibiting neutrophil accumu-lation into lung tissue and into the airspaces in models of lung inflammation induced by intratracheal instillation of IgG or IgA immune complexes. Blocking VLA-4 may interfere with functions of pulmonary macrophages that are important for the development of lung injury in these models, e.g. production of cytokines or toxic products from oxygen and L-arginine.

6.   Concluding Comments

In this chapter we have reviewed current knowledge on the mechanisms by which neutrophils accumulate at sites of inflammation in tissues. It is clear that there is still much to be learned about how neutrophil migration is controlled and that more undiscovered mediators probably exist which will have effects on this process. There may even be more adhesion molecules waiting to be discovered that are involved in neutrophil accumu-lation, for example, in capillaries of the lung. When one considers that, in the setting of inflammation, there are likely to be multiple mediators and adhesion pathways, all of which can interact in complex ways, deciding which of these is important and thus the potential target for therapy is daunting. Nevertheless, the prospects look favourable for novel anti-inflammatory drugs in the future.

7. Acknowledgements

A. Rossi is supported by the Wellcome Trust and P.G. Hellewell by the National Asthma Campaign and the British Lung Foundation.

8. References

Addison, W. (1843). Experimental and practical researches on the structure and function of blood corpuscle: on inflammation; and on the origin and nature of tubercles in the lung. Prov. Med. Surg. Ass. Trans. 11, 233–306.

Allison, F., Smith, M.R. and Wood, W.B. (1955). Studies on the pathogenesis of acute inflammation. The action of cortisone on the inflammatory response to thermal injury. J. Exp. Med. 102, 669.

Arfors, K.-E., Lundberg, C., Lindbom, L., Lundberg, K., Beatty, P.G. and Harlan, J.M. (1987). A monoclonal antibody to the membrane glycoprotein complex CD18 inhibits polymorphonuclear leukocyte accumulation and plasma leakage in vivo. Blood 69, 338–340.

Argenbright, L.W. and Barton, R.W. (1992). Interactions of leukocyte integrins with intercellular adhesion molecule 1 in the production of inflammatory vascular injury in vivo. The Shwartzman reaction revisited. J. Clin. Invest. 89, 259–272.

Atherton, A. and Born, G.V.R. (1972). Quantitative investigations of the adhesiveness of circulating polymorphonuclear leucocytes to blood vessel walls. J. Physiol. 222, 447–474.

Baggiolini, M. and Clark-Lewis, I. (1992). Interleukin-8, a chemotactic and inflammatory cytokine. FEBS Lett. 307, 97–101.

Barton, R.W., Rothlein, R., Ksiazer, J. and Kennedy, C. (1989). The effect of anti-intercellular adhesion molecule-1 on phorbol-ester-induced rabbit lung inflammation. J. Immunol. 143, 1278–1282.

Beaubien, B.C., Collins, P.D., Jose, P.J., Totty, N.F., Waterfield, M.D., Hsuan, J. and Williams, T.J. (1990). A novel neutrophil chemoattractant generated during an inflammatory reaction in the rabbit peritoneal cavity in vivo: purification, partial amino acid sequence and structural relationship to interleukin 8. Biochem. J. 271, 797–801.

Beck, G., Habicht, G.S., Benach, J.L. and Miller, F. (1986). Interleukin 1: a common endogenous mediator of inflammation and the local Shwartzman reaction. J. Immunol. 136, 3025–3031.

Becker, E.L. (1987). The formal peptide receptor of the neutrophil. A search and conserve operation. Am. J. Pathol. 129, 16–24.

Becker, R.M. (1948). Suppression of local tissue reactivity (Shwartzman Phenomenon) by nitrogen mustard, benzol and x-ray irradiation. Proc. Soc. Exp. Biol. Med. 69, 247–250.

Beesley, J.E., Pearson, J.D., Carleton, J.S., Hutchings, A. and Gordon, J.L. (1978). Interaction of leukocytes with vascular cells in culture. J. Cell Sci. 33, 85–101.

Beesley, J.E., Pearson, J.D., Hutchings, A., Carleton, J.S. and Gordon, J.L. (1979). Granulocyte migration through endothelium in culture. J. Cell Sci. 38, 237–248.

Billiau, A., Heremans, H., Vandekerckhove, F. and Dillen, C. (1987). Anti-interferon-gamma antibody protects mice against the generalized Shwartzman reaction. Eur. J. Immunol. 17, 1851–1854.

Boyden, S.V. (1962). The chemotactic effect of mixtures of antibody and antigen on polymorphonuclear leukocyte adherence. J. Cell Biol. 82, 347–368.

Brady, H.R., Spertini, O., Jimenez, W., Brenner, B.M., Marsden, P.A. and Tedder, T.F. (1992). Neutrophils, monocytes, and lymphocytes bind to cytokine-activated kidney glomerular endothelial cells through L-selectin (LAM-1) in vitro. J. Immunol. 149, 2437–2444.

Brennan, F.M., Zachariae, C.O.C., Chantry, D., Larsen, C.G., Turner, M., Maini, R.N., Matsushima K. and Feldmann, M. (1990). Detection of interleukin 8 biological activity in synovial fluids from patients with rheumatoid arthritis and production of interleukin 8 mRNA by isolated synovial cells. Eur. J. Immunol. 20, 2141–2144.

Bronza, J.P. (1990). Shwartzman reaction. Sem. Thromb. Hemo. 16, 326–332.

Buchanan, M.R., Crowley, C.A., Rosin, R.E., Gimbrone, M.A. and Babior, B.M. (1982). Studies on the interaction between GP-180-deficient neutrophils and vascular endothelium. Blood 60, 160–165.

Buckley, T.L., Brain, S.D., Collins, P.D. and Williams, T.J. (1991). Inflammatory edema induced by interactions between interleukin-1 and the neuropeptide calcitonin gene-related peptide. J. Immunol. 146, 3424–3430.

Bucky, L.P., Vedder, N.B., Hong, H.-Z., May, J.W. and Ehrlich, H.P. (1991). A monoclonal antibody which blocks neutrophil adhesion prevents second degree burns from becoming third degree. Proc. Am. Burn Assoc. 23, 133.

Burch, R.M., Noronha-Blob, L., Bator, J.M., Lowe, V.C. and Sullivan, J.P. (1993). Mice treated with a leumedin or antibody to Mac-1 to inhibit leukocyte sequestration survive endotoxin challenge. J. Immunol. 150, 3397–3403.

Byrne, J.G., Smith, W.J., Murphy, M.P., Couper, G.S., Appleyard, R.F. and Cohn, L.H. (1992). Complete prevention of myocardial stunning, contracture, low-reflow, and edema after heart transplantation by blocking neutrophil adhesion molecules during reperfusion. J. Thorac. Cardiovasc. Surg. 104, 1589–1596.

Chisholm, P.L., Williams, C.A. and Lobb, R.R. (1993). Monoclonal antibodies to the integrin α-4 subunit inhibit the murine contact hypersensitivity response. Eur. J. Immunol. 23, 682–688.

Chung, K.F. (1992). Platelet-activating factor in inflammation and pulmonary disorders. Clin. Sci. 63, 127–138.

Clark, E.R. and Clark, E.L. (1920). Reactions of cells in the tail of amphibian larvae to injected croton oil (aseptic inflammation). Am. J. Anat. 27, 221.

Clark, E.R. and Clark, E.L. (1922). The reaction of living cells in the tadpole's tail toward starch, agar-agar, gelatin and gum arabic. Anat. Rec. 24, 137.

Clark, E.R. and Clark, E.L. (1935). Observations on changes in blood vascular endothelium in the living animal. Am. J. Anat. 57, 385–438.

Cochrane, G.C. and Janoff A. (1974) The Arthus reaction: a model of neutrophil and complement mediated inury. In "The Inflammatory Process" (eds B.W. Zweifach, L. Grant and R.T. McCluskey), pp. 85–162. Academic Press, New York.

Cochrane, C.G., Muller-Eberhard, H.J. and Aikin, B.S. (1970). Depletion of plasma complement in vivo by a protein of cobra venom: its effect on various immunologic reactions. J. Immunol. 105, 55–69.

Cohnheim, J. (1867). Ueber entzundung und eiterung. Virchows Arch. Path. Anat. Physiol. 40, 1–79.

Cohnheim, J. (1873). Neuere untersuchungen uber die entzundung. Hirschwald, Berlin 1–85.

Cohnheim, J. (1889). "Inflammation". Lectures in General Pathology, Vol. 1, pp. 242–382. New Syderman Society, London.

Coleman, R.A. and Humphrey, P.P.A. (1993). In "Therapeutic Applications of Prostaglandins" (eds J. Vane and J. O'Grady). Edward Arnold, London.

Collins, P.D., Jose, P.J. and Williams, T.J. (1991). The sequential generation of neutrophil chemoattractant proteins in acute inflammation in the rabbit in vivo: relationship between C5a and a protein with the characteristics of IL-8. J. Immunol. 146, 677–684.

Comandon, J. (1917). Phagocytose in vitro des hematozoaires du Calfat. Comp. rend. hibdom. seances memoires Soc. Biol. 80, 314–316.

Cosimi, A.B., Conti, D., Delmonico, F.L., Preffer, F.I., Wee, S.-L., Rothlein, R., Faanes, R. and Colvin, R.B. (1990). In vivo effects of monoclonal antibody to ICAM-1 (CD54) in nonhuman primates with renal allografts. J. Immunol. 144, 4604–4612.

Cronstein, B.N., Levin, R.J., Philips, M., Hirschhorn, R., Abramson, S.B. and Weissmann, G. (1992). Neutrophil adherence to endothelium is enhanced via adenosine A$_1$ receptors and inhibited via adenosine A$_2$ receptors. J. Immunol. 148, 2201–2206.

Cybulsky, M.I., Chan, M.K.W. and Movat, H.Z. (1988) Acute inflammation and microthrombosis induced by endotoxin, interleukin-1, and tumor necrosis factor and their implication in gram-negative infection. Lab. Invest. 58, 365–378.

Della Bianca, V.D., De Togni, P., Grzeskowiak, M., Vicentini, L.M. and Di Virgilio, F. (1986). Cyclic AMP inhibition of phosphoinositide turnover in human neutrophils. Biochim. Biophys. Acta 886, 441–447.

Doerschuk, C.M., Winn, R.K., Coxson, H.O. and Harlan, J.M. (1990). CD18-dependent and -independent mechanisms of neutrophil emigration in the pulmonary and systemic microcirculation of rabbits. J. Immunol. 144, 2327–2333.

Downey, G.P. and Worthen, G.S. (1988). Neutrophil retention in model capillaries: deformability, geometry, and hydrodynamic forces. J. Appl. Physiol. 65, 1861–1871.

Downey, G.P., Doherty, D.E., Schwab, B., Elson, E.L., Henson, P.M. and Worthen, G.S. (1990). Retention of leukocytes in capillaries: role of cell size and deformability. J. Appl. Physiol. 69, 1767–1778.

Downey, G.P., Worthen, G.S., Henson, P.M. and Hyde, D.M. (1993). Neutrophil sequestration and migration in localized pulmonary inflammation. Capillary localization and migration across the interalveolar septum. Am. Rev. Respir. Dis. 137, 168–176.

Dulis, B.H. and Wilson, I.B. (1980). The β-adrenergic receptor of live human polymorphonuclear leukocytes. J. Biol. Chem. 255, 1043–1048.

Engelberts, I., Samyo, S.K., Leeuwenberg, J.F., van der Linden, C.J. and Buurman, W.A. (1992). A role for ELAM-1 in the pathogenesis of MDF during septic shock. J. Surg. Res. 53, 136–144.

Erzurum, S.C., Downey, G.P., Doherty, D.E., Schwab, B., Elson, E.L. and Worthen, G.S. (1992). Mechanisms of lipopolysaccharide-induced neutrophil retention. Relative contributions of adhesive and cellular mechanical properties. J. Immunol. 149, 154–162.

Fiebig, E., Ley, K. and Arfors, K.-E. (1991). Rapid leukocyte accumulation by "spontaneous" rolling and adhesion in the exteriorized rabbit mesentery. Int. J. Microcirc. 10, 127–144.

Ford-Hutchinson, A.W., Bray, M.A., Doig, M.V., Shipley, M.E. and Smith, M.J.H. (1980). Leukotriene B, a potent chemokinetic and aggregating substance released from polymorphonuclear leukocytes. Nature 286, 264–265.

Francis, J.W., Todd, R.F., Boxer, L.A. and Petty, H.R. (1989). Sequential expression of cell surface C3bi receptors during neutrophil locomotion. J. Cell Physiol. 140, 519–523.

Furie, M.B., Tancinco, M.C.A. and Smith, C.W. (1991). Monoclonal antibodies to leukocyte integrins CD11a/CD18 and CD11b/CD18 or intercellular adhesion molecule-1 inhibit chemoattractant-stimulated neutrophil transendothelial migration in vitro. Blood 78, 2089–2097.

Furie, M.B., Burns, M.J., Tancinco, M.C.A., Benjamin, C.D. and Lobb, R.R. (1992). E-Selectin (endothelial-leukocyte adhesion molecule-1) is not required for the migration of neutrophils across IL-1-stimulated endothelium in vitro. J. Immunol. 148, 2395–2404.

Geng, J.-G., Bevilacqua, M.P., Moore, K.L., McIntyre, T.M., Prescott, S.M., Kim, J.M., Bliss, G.A., Zimmerman, G.A. and McEver, R.P. (1990). Rapid neutrophil adhesion to activated endothelium mediated by GMP-140. Nature 343, 757–760.

Gerard, N.P. and Gerard, C. (1991). The chemotactic receptor for human C5a anaphylatoxin. Nature 349, 614–617.

Gimbrone, M.A., Shefton, E.J. and Cruise, S.A. (1978). Isolation and priming culture of endothelial cells from human umbilical vessels. Tissue Culture Assoc. Manual 4, 813–817.

Goldman, D.W. and Goetzl, E.J. (1984). Heterogeneity of human polymorphonuclear leukocyte receptors for leukotriene B$_4$. J. Exp. Med. 159, 1027–1041.

Granger, D.N., Russell, J., Arfors, K.-E., Rothlein, R. and Anderson, D.C. (1991). Role of CD11/CD18 and ICAM-1 in ischemia–reperfusion induced leukocyte adherence and emigration in mesenteric venules. FASEB J. 5, A1753.

Grant, L. (1973). The sticking and migration of white blood cells in inflammation. In "The Inflammatory Process" (eds B.W. Zweifach, L. Grant and R.T. McCluskey), pp. 205–249. Academic Press, New York.

Green, K.L. (1972). The anti-inflammatory effect of catecholamines in the peritoneal cavity and hind paw of the mouse. Br. J. Pharmacol. 45, 322–332.

Gundel, R.H., Wegner, C.D., Torcellini, C.A., Clarke, C.C., Haynes, N., Rothlein, R., Smith, C.W. and Letts, L.G. (1991). Endothelial leukocyte adhesion molecule-1 mediates antigen-induced acute airway inflammation and late phase airway obstruction in monkeys. J. Clin. Invest. 88, 1407–1411.

Guntheroth, W.G., Luchtel, D.L. and Kawabori, I. (1982). Pulmonary microcirculation: tubules rather than sheet and post. J. Appl. Physiol. 53, 510–515.

Hakkert, B.C., Kuijpers, T.W., Leeuwenberg, J.F.M., van Mourik, J.A. and Roos, D. (1991). Neutrophil and monocyte adherence to and migration across monolayers of cytokine-activated endothelial cells: the contribution of CD18, ELAM-1 and VLA-4. Blood 78, 2721–2726.

Harlan, J.M. (1985). Leukocyte–endothelial interactions. Blood 65, 513–525.

Harlan, J.M., Winn, R.K., Vedder, N.B., Doerschuk, C.M. and Rice, C.L. (1992). In "Adhesion. Its Role in Inflammatory Disease" (eds J.M. Harlan and D.Y. Liu), p. 117. W.H. Freeman and Company, New York.

Haslett, C. and Warren, J.B. (1990). In "The Endothelium: An Introduction to Current Research" (ed. J.B. Warren), p. 187. Wiley-Liss Inc., New York.

Hawkins, H.K., Heffelfinger, S.C. and Anderson, D.C. (1992). Leukocyte adhesion deficiency: clinical and postmortem observations. Pediat. Path. 12, 119–130.

Hellewell, P.G. (1990). In "Platelet-activating Factor in Endotoxin and Immune Diseases" (eds D.A. Handley, R.N. Saunders, W.J. Houlihan and J.C. Tomesch), pp. 367–386. Marcel Dekker Inc., New York.

Hellewell, P.G. and Henson, P.M. (1991). In "Vascular Endothelium: Interactions with Circulating Cells" (ed J.L. Gordon), pp. 143–160. Elsevier Science Publishers, Amsterdam.

Hellewell, P.G. and Williams, T.J. (1986). A specific antagonist of platelet-activating factor suppresses oedema formation in an Arthus reaction but not oedema induced by leukocyte chemoattractants in rabbit skin. J. Immunol. 137, 302–307.

Hellewell, P.G. and Williams T.J. (1988). In "Eicosanoids in Inflammatory Conditions of the Lung, Skin and Joint" (eds K.K. Church and C. Robinson), pp. 43–66. MTP, Lancaster.

Hellewell, P.G., Jose, P.J. and Williams, T.J. (1988). Effect of anti-C5a antibodies on oedema formation and PMN leukocyte accumulation in allergic inflammation in the rabbit. Br. J. Pharmacol. 95, 531P.

Hellewell, P.G., Yarwood, H. and Williams, T.J. (1989). Characteristics of oedema formation induced by FMLP in rabbit skin. Br. J. Pharmacol. 97, 181–189.

Hellewell, P.G., Young, S.K., Henson, P.M. and Worthen, G.S. (1994). Disparate role of the β_2 integrin CD18 in the local accumulation of neutrophils in pulmonary and cutaneous inflammation in the rabbit. Am. J. Resp. Cell. Mol. (in press).

Henriques, M.G.M.O., Weg, V.B., Martins, M.A., Silva, P.M.R., Fernandes, P.D., Cordeiro, R.S.B. and Vargaftig, B.B. (1990). Differential inhibition by two hetrazepine PAF antagonists of acute inflammation in the mouse. Br. J. Pharmacol. 99, 164–168.

Heremans, H., Van Damme, J., Dillen, C., Dijkmans, R. and Billiau, A. (1990). Interferon gamma, a mediator of lethal lipopolysaccharide-induced Shwartzman-like shock reactions in mice. J. Exp. Med. 171, 1853–1869.

Hermanowski-Vosatka, A., Van Strijp, J.A.G., Swiggard, W.J. and Wright, S.D. (1992). Integrin modulating factor-1: a lipid that alters the function of leukocyte integrins. Cell 68, 341–352.

Hernandez, L.A., Grisham, M.B., Twohig, B., Arfors, K.E., Harlan, J.M. and Granger, D.N. (1987). Role of neutrophils in ischemia–reperfusion-induced microvascular injury. Am. J. Physiol. 253, 699–703.

Hogg, J.C. (1987). Neutrophil kinetics and lung injury. Physiol. Rev. 67, 1249–1295.

Horgan, M.J., Wright, S.D. and Malik, A.B. (1990). Antibody against leukocyte integrin (CD18) prevents reperfusion-induced lung vascular injury. Am. J. Physiol. 259, L315–L319.

Hughes, B.J., Hollers, J.C., Crockett-Torabi, E. and Smith, C.W. (1992). Recruitment of CD11b/CD18 to the neutrophil surface and adherence-dependent cell locomotion. J. Clin. Invest. 90, 1687–1696.

Hugli, T.E. (1986). Biochemistry and biology of anaphylatoxins. Complement 3, 111–127.

Humphrey, D.M., Hanahan, D.J. and Pinckard, R.N. (1982). Induction of leukocytic infiltrates in rabbit skin by acetyl glyceryl ether phosphorylcholine. Lab. Invest. 47, 227–234.

Issekutz, A.C. (1981a). Vascular responses during acute neutrophilic inflammation. Their relationship to in vitro neutrophil emigration. Lab. Invest. 45, 435–441.

Issekutz, A.C. (1981b). Effect of vasoactive agents on polymorphonuclear leukocyte emigration in vivo. Lab. Invest. 45, 234–240.

Issekutz, A.C. and Issekutz, T.B. (1992). The contribution of LFA-1 (CD11a/CD18) and MAC-1 (CD11b/CD18) to the in vivo migration of polymorphonuclear leucocytes to inflammatory reactions in the rat. Immunology 76, 655–661.

Issekutz, A.C. and Szejda, M. (1986). Evidence that platelet activating factor may mediate some acute inflammatory responses. Studies with the platelet activating factor antagonist, CV3988. Lab. Invest. 54, 275–281.

Jaeschke, H., Farhood, A. and Smith, C.W. (1991). Neutrophil-induced liver cell injury in endotoxin shock is a CD11b/CD18-dependent mechanism. Am. J. Physiol. 261, G1051–G1056.

Jaffe, E.A., Hoyer, L.W. and Nachman, R.L. (1973). Synthesis of antihemophilic factor antigen by cultured human endothelial cells. J. Clin. Invest. 52, 2757–2764.

Jasin, H.E., Lightfoot, E., Davis, L.S., Rothlein, R., Faanes, R.B. and Lipsky, P.E. (1992). Amelioration of antigen-induced arthritis in rabbits treated with monoclonal antibodies to leukocyte adhesion molecules. Arthritis Rheum. 35, 541–549.

Jose, P.J. (1987). Complement-derived peptide mediators of inflammation. Br. Med. Bull. 43, 336–349.

Jose, P.J., Forrest, M.J. and Williams, T.J. (1983). Detection of the complement fragment C5a in inflammatory exudates from the rabbit peritoneal cavity using radioimmunoassay. J. Exp. Med. 158, 2177–2182.

Jose, P.J., Collins, P.D., Perkins, J.A., Beaubien, B.C., Totty, N.F., Waterfield, M.D., Hsuan, J. and Williams, T.J. (1991). Identification of a second neutrophil chemoattractant cytokine generated during an inflammatory reaction in the rabbit peritoneal cavity in vivo: purification, partial amino acid sequence and structural relationship to melanoma growth stimulatory activity. Biochem. J. 278, 493–497.

Jutila, M.A., Rott, L., Berg, E.L. and Butcher, E.C. (1989). Function and regulation of the neutrophil MEL-14 antigen in vivo: comparison with LFA-1 and MAC-1. J. Immunol. 143, 3318–3324.

Jutila, M.A., Kishimoto, T.K. and Finken, M. (1991). Low-dose chymotrypsin treatment inhibits neutrophil migration into sites of inflammation in vivo: effects of Mac-1 and MEL-14 adhesion protein expression and function. Cell. Immunol. 132, 201–214.

Kishimoto, T.K., Jutila, M.A., Berg, E.L. and Butcher, E.C. (1989). Neutrophil Mac-1 and MEL-14 adhesion proteins inversely regulated by chemotactic factors. Science 245, 1238–1241.

Kishimoto, T.K., Warnock, R.A., Jutila, M.A., Butcher, E.C., Lane, C., Anderson, D.C. and Smith, C.W. (1991).

Antibodies against human neutrophil LECAM-1 (LAM-1/ Leu-8/DREG-56 antigen) and endothelial cell ELAM-1 inhibit a common CD18-independent adhesion pathway in vitro. Blood 78, 805–811.

Kreisle, R.A. and Parker, C.W. (1983). Specific binding of leukotriene B₄ to a receptor on human polymorphonuclear leukocytes. J. Exp. Med. 157, 628–641.

Kuijpers, T.W., Hakkert, B.C., Hart, M.H.L. and Roos, D. (1992). Neutrophil migration across monolayers of cytokine-prestimulated endothelial cells: a role for platelet-activating factor and IL-8. J. Cell Biol. 117, 565–572.

Lasky, L.A., Singer, M.S., Dowbenko, D., Imai, Y., Henzel, W.J., Grimley, C., Fennie, C., Gillett, N., Watson, S.R. and Rosen, S.D. (1992). An endothelial ligand for L-selectin is a novel mucin-like molecule. Cell 69, 927–938.

Lawrence, M.B. and Springer, T.A. (1991). Leukocytes roll on a selectin at physiologic flow rates: distinction from and prerequisite for adhesion through integrins. Cell 65, 859–873.

Leber, T. (1888) . Uber die entstehung der entizundung und die wirkung der entizudungerregenden schadlichkeiterz. Fortschr. Med. 4, 460–464.

Leber, T. (1891). "Die entstehung der entizundung. Die wirkung der entizudungerregenden schadlichkeiten nach vorzugsweise am auge angestellten undersuchungen". pp. 1–535. Engelmann, Leipzig.

Lee, G. de J. and DuBois, A.B. (1955). Pulmonary capillary blood flow in man. J. Clin. Invest. 34, 1380–1390.

Leonard, E.J., Yoshimura, T., Tanaka, S. and Raffeld, M. (1991). Neutrophil recruitment by intradermally injected neutrophil attractant/activation protein-1. J. Invest. Dermatol. 96, 690–694.

Lewinsohn, D.M., Bargatze, R.F. and Butcher, E.C. (1987). Leukocyte-endothelial cell recognition: evidence of a common molecular mechanism shared by neutrophils, lymphocytes, and other leukocytes. J. Immunol. 138, 4313–4321.

Ley, K., Gaehtgens, P., Fennie, C., Singer, M.S., Lasky, L.A. and Rosen, S.D. (1991). Lectin-like cell adhesion molecule 1 mediates leukocyte rolling in mesenteric venules in vivo. Blood 77, 2553–2555.

Ley, K., Tedder, T.F. and Kansas, G.S. (1993). L-selectin can mediate leukocyte rolling in untreated mesenteric venules in vivo independent of E- or P-selectin. Blood 82, 1632–1638.

Lien, D.C., Henson, P.M., Capen, R.L., Henson, J.E., Hanson, W.L., Wagner, W.W. and Worthen, G.S. (1991). Neutrophil kinetics in the pulmonary microcirculation during acute inflammation. Lab. Invest. 65, 145–159.

Lien, D.C., Worthen, G.S., Henson, P.M. and Bethel, R.A. (1992). Platelet-activating factor causes neutrophil accumulation and neutrophil-mediated increased vascular permeability in canine trachea. Am. Rev. Respir. Dis. 145, 693–700.

Lindbom, L., Lundberg, C., Prieto, J., Raud, J., Nortamo, P., Gahmberg, C.G. and Patarroyo, M. (1990). Rabbit leukocyte adhesion molecules CD11/CD18 and their participation in acute and delayed inflammatory responses and leukocyte distribution in vivo. Clin. Immunol. Immunopath. 57, 105–119.

Lo, S.K., Everitt, J., Gu, J. and Malik, A.B. (1992). Tumor necrosis factor mediates experimental pulmonary edema by ICAM-1 and CD18-dependent mechanisms. J. Clin. Invest. 89, 981–988.

Luscinskas, F.W., Cybulsky, M.I., Kiely, J.-M., Peckings, C.S., Davis, V.M. and Gimbrone, M.A. (1991). Cytokine-activated human endothelial monolayers support enhanced neutrophil transmigration via a mechanism involving both endothelial-leukocyte adhesion molecule-1 and intercellular adhesion molecule-1. J. Immunol. 146, 1617–1625.

Ma, X.-L., Lefer, D.J., Lefer, A.M. and Rothlein, R. (1992). Coronary endothelial and cardiac protective effects of a monoclonal antibody to intercellular adhesion molecule-1 in myocardial ischemia and reperfusion. Circulation 86, 937–946.

MacNee, W. and Selby, C. (1993). Neutrophil traffic in the lungs: role of haemodynamics, cell adhesion, and deformability. Thorax 48, 79–88.

Majno, G. and Palade, G.E. (1961). Studies on inflammation. 1. The effect of histamine and serotonin on vascular permeability: an electron microscopic study. J. Biol. Phys. Biochem. Cytol. 11, 571–605.

Marchesi, V. and Florey, H.W. (1960). Electron micrographic observations on the emigration of leucocytes. Q. J. Exp. Physiol. 45, 343–374.

Metchnikoff, E. (1893). "Lectures on the Comparative Pathology of Inflammation". Kegan, Paul, Trench, Trubner & Co., London.

Meyrick, B. and Brigham, K.L. (1984). The effect of a single infusion of zymosan-activated plasma on the pulmonary microcirculation of sheep. Am. J. Pathol. 114, 32–45.

Mileski, W., Borgstrom, D., Lightfoot E., Rothlein, R., Faanes, R., Lipsky, P. and Baxter, C. (1992). Inhibition of leukocyte-endothelial adherence following thermal injury. J. Surg. Res. 52, 334–339.

Mileski, W.J., Winn, R.K., Vedder, N.B., Pohlman, T.H., Harlan, J.M. and Rice, C.L. (1990). Inhibition of CD18-dependent neutrophil adherence reduces organ injury after hemorrhagic shock in primates. Surgery 108, 206–212.

Mileski, W.J., Winn, R.K., Harlan, J.M. and Rice, C.L. (1991). Transient inhibition of neutrophil adherence with the anti-CD18 monoclonal antibody 60.3 does not increase mortality rates in abdominal sepsis. Surgery 109, 497–501.

Mileski, W.J., Raymond, J.F., Winn, R.K., Harlan, J.M. and Rice, C.L. (1993). Inhibition of leukocyte adherence and aggregation for treatment of severe cold injury in rabbits. J. Appl. Physiol. 74, 1432–1436.

Miotla, J.M., Lorimer, S., Williams, T.J., Hellewell, P.G. and Jeffery, P.K. (1993). Neutrophil-dependent acute lung injury is suppressed by blockade of CD11b/CD18 adhesion molecule mice. Am. Rev. Respir. Dis. 147, A69.

Movat, H.Z. (1985). "The Inflammatory Reaction". Elsevier, Amsterdam.

Movat, H.Z., Burrowes, C.E., Cybulsky, M.I. and Dinarello, C.A. (1987). Acute inflammation and a Schwartzman-like reaction induced by interleukin-1 and tumor necrosis factor. Am. J. Pathol. 129, 463–476.

Mueller, H., Motulsky, H.J. and Sklar, L.A. (1988). The potency and kinetics of the β-adrenergic receptors on human neutrophils. Mol. Pharmacol. 34, 347–353.

Mullane, K.M. and Smith, C.W. (1990). In "Pathophysiology of Severe Ischemic Myocardial Injury" (ed. H.M. Piper), pp. 239–267. Kluwer Academic Publishers, Amsterdam.

Mulligan, M.S., Varani, J., Dame, M.K., Lane, C.L., Smith, C.W., Anderson, D.C. and Ward, P.A. (1991). Role of endothelial-leukocyte adhesion molecule 1 (ELAM-1) in neutrophil-mediated lung injury in rats. J. Clin. Invest. 88, 1396–1406.

Mulligan, M.S., Polley, M.J., Bayer, R.J., Nunn, M.F., Paulson, J.C. and Ward, P.A. (1992a). Neutrophil-dependent acute lung injury. Requirement for P-selectin (GMP-140). J. Clin. Invest. 90, 1600–1607.

Mulligan, M.S., Varani, J., Warren, J.S., Till, G.O., Smith, C.W., Anderson, D.C., Todd, R.F. and Ward, P.A. (1992b). Roles of β_2 integrins of rat neutrophils in complement and oxygen radical-mediated acute inflammatory injury. J. Immunol. 148, 1847–1857.

Mulligan, M.S., Warren, J.S., Smith, C.W., Anderson, D.C., Yeh, C.G., Rudolph, A.R. and Ward, P.A. (1992c). Lung injury after deposition of IgA immune complexes. Requirements for CD18 and L-Arginine. J. Immunol. 148, 3086–3092.

Mulligan, M.S., Smith, C.W., Anderson, D.C., Todd, R.F., Miyasaka, M., Tamatani, T., Issekutz, T.B. and Ward, P.A. (1993a). Role of leukocyte adhesion molecules in complement-induced lung injury. J. Immunol. 150, 2401–2406.

Mulligan, M.S., Wilson, G.P., Todd, R.F., Smith, W.C., Anderson, D.C., Varani, J., Issekutz, T.B., Myasaka, M., Tamatam, T., Rusch, J.R., Vaporciyan, A.A. and Ward, P.A. (1993b). Role of β_1, β_2 integrins and ICAM-1 in lung injury after deposition of IgG and IgA immune complexes. J. Immunol. 150, 2407–2417.

Mulligan, M.S., Johnson, K.J., Todd, R.F., Issekutz, T.B., Miyasaka, M., Tamatani, T., Smith, C.W., Anderson, D.C. and Ward, P.A. (1993c). Requirements for leukocyte adhesion molecules in nephrotoxic nephritis. J. Clin. Invest. 91, 577–587.

Murphy, P.M. and Tiffany, H.L. (1991). Cloning of complementary DNA encoding a functional human interleukin-8 receptor. Science 253, 1280–1283.

Nickoloff, B.J., Karabin, G.D., Barker, J.N.W., Griffiths, C.E.M., Sarma, V., Mitra, R.S., Elder, J.T., Kunkel, S.L. and Dixit, V.M. (1991). Cellular localization of interleukin-8 and its inducer, tumor necrosis factor-alpha in psoriasis. Am. J. Pathol. 138, 129–140.

Norman, K.E., Argenbright, L.W., Williams, T.J. and Rossi, A.G. (1993). The role of the adhesion glycoprotein CD18 and intercellular adhesion molecule-1 in complement mediated reactions of rabbit skin. Br. J. Pharmacol. (in press).

Nourshargh, S. (1992). In "Advances in Rheumatology and Inflammation", Vol. 2 (eds J. Fritsch and R. Muller-Peddinghaus), pp. 39–47. Eular Publishers, Basel.

Nourshargh, S., Rampart, M., Hellewell, P.G., Jose, P.J., Harlan, J.M., Edwards, A.J. and Williams, T.J. (1989). Accumulation of ^{111}In-neutrophils in rabbit skin in allergic and non-allergic inflammatory reactions in vivo: inhibition by neutrophil pretreatment in vitro with a monocol antibody recognising the CD18 antigen. J. Immunol. 142, 3193–3198.

O'Flaherty, J., Kosfeld, S. and Nishihira, J. (1986). Binding and metabolism of leukotriene B4 by neutrophils and their subcellular organelles. J. Cell Biol. 126, 359–370.

O'Flaherty, J.T. (1982). Biology of disease. Lipid mediators of inflammation and allergy. Lab. Invest. 47, 314–329.

O'Flaherty, J.T., Rossi, A.G., Redman, J.F. and Jacobson, D.P. (1991). Tumor necrosis factor-α regulates expression of receptors for formyl-methionyl-leucyl-phenylalanine, leukotriene B4, and platelet-activating factor. Dissociation from priming in human polymorphonuclear neutrophils. J. Immunol. 147, 3842–3847.

Okusawa, S., Yancey, K.B., van der Meer, J.W.M., Endres, S., Lonnemann, G., Hefter, K., Frank, M.M., Burke, J.F., Dinarello, C.A. and Gelfand, J.A. (1988). C5a stimulates secretion of tumor necrosis factor from human mononuclear cells in vitro. Comparison with secretion of interleukin 1β and interleukin 1α. J. Exp. Med. 168, 443–448.

Omann, G.M., Allen, R.A., Bokoch, G.M., Painter, R.G., Traynor, A.E. and Sklar, L.A. (1987). In "Physiological Reviews" (eds G.H. Giebisch and W.F. Boron), pp. 285–322, Vol. 67. Physiological Reviews, Bethesda.

Pearson, J.D., Carleton, J.S., Beesley, J.E., Hutchings, A. and Gordon, J.L. (1979). Granulocyte adhesion to endothelium in culture. J. Cell Sci. 38, 225–235.

Pfeffer, W. (1884). Locomotorishe richtungsbewegungen durch chemische. Reize. Unters. botan. Inst. Tubingen 1, 363–482.

Pfeffer, W. (1888). Uber chemotaktische bewegungen von bacterien, flagellaten und volvocineen. Unters. botan. Inst. Tubingen 2, 582–661.

Picker, L.J., Warnock, R.A., Burns, A.R., Doerschuk, C.M., Berg, E.L. and Butcher, E.C. (1991). The neutrophil selectin LECAM-1 presents carbohydrate ligands to the vascular selectins ELAM-1 and GMP-140. Cell 66, 921–933.

Pons, F., Rossi, A.G., Norman, K.E., Williams, T.J. and Nourshargh, S. (1993). Role of platelet-activating factor in platelet accumulation in rabbit skin. Effect of the novel long-acting PAF antagonist, UK-74,505. Br. J. Pharmacol. 109, 234–242.

Price, T.H., Beatty, P.G. and Corpuz, S.R. (1987). In vivo inhibition of neutrophil function in the rabbit using monoclonal antibody to CD18. J. Immunol. 139, 4174–4177.

Rampart, M. and Williams, T.J. (1986). Polymorphonuclear leukocyte-dependent plasma leakage in the rabbit skin is enhanced or inhibited by prostacyclin, depending on the route of administration. Am. J. Pathol. 124, 66–73.

Rampart, M. and Williams, T.J. (1988). Evidence that neutrophil accumulation induced by interleukin-1 requires both local protein biosynthesis and neutrophil CD18 antigen expression in vivo. Br. J. Pharmacol. 94, 1143–1148.

Rampart, M., Van Damme, J., Zonnekyn, L. and Herman, A.G. (1989). Granulocyte chemotactic protein/interleukin-8 induces plasma leakage and neutrophil accumulation in rabbit skin. Am. J. Pathol. 135, 1–5.

Rampart, M., Van Osselaer, N. and Herman, A.G. (1991). ICAM-1 (CD54)-mediated neutrophil emigration is not associated with increased vascular permeability. J. Leukocyte Biol. Suppl. 2, 46.

Redl, H., Dinges, H.P., Buurman, W.A., van der Linden, C.J., Pober, J.S., Cotran, R.S. and Schlag, G. (1991). Expression of endothelial leucocyte adhesion molecule-1 in septic but not traumatic/hypovolemic shock in the baboon. Am. J. Pathol. 139, 461–466.

Rietschel, E.T. and Brade, H. (1992). Bacterial endotoxins. Sci. Am. 267, 26–33.

Rosen, H. and Gordon, S. (1987). Monoclonal antibody to the murine type 3 complement receptor inhibits adhesion of myelomonocytic cells in vitro and inflammatory cell recruitment in vivo. J. Exp. Med. 166, 1685–1701.

Rosen, H. and Gordon, S. (1990). The role of the type 3 complement receptor in the induced recruitment of myelomonocytic cells to inflammatory sites in the mouse. Am. J. Respir. Cell Mol. Biol. 3, 3–10.

Rosen, H., Gordon, S. and North, R.J. (1989a). Exacerbation of murine listeriosis by a monoclonal antibody specific for the type 3 complement receptor of myelomonocytic cells. J. Exp. Med. 170, 27–38.

Rosen, H., Milon, G. and Gordon, S. (1989b). Antibody to the murine type 3 complement receptor inhibits T lymphocyte-dependent recruitment of myelomonocytic cells in vivo. J. Exp. Med. 169, 535–548.

Rossi, A.G. and O'Flaherty, J.T. (1989). Prostaglandin binding sites in human polymorphonuclear neutrophils. Prostaglandins 37, 641–653.

Rossi, A.G. and O'Flaherty, J.T. (1991). Bioactions of 5-hydroxyicosatetraenoate and its interaction with platelet-activating factor. Lipids 26, 1184–1188.

Rossi, A.G., Redman, J.F., Jacobson, D.P. and O'Flaherty, J.T. (1991). Mechanisms involved in the enhancement of human neutrophil responses to platelet-activating factor by 5(S)-hydroxyicosatetraenoate. J. Lipid Mediators 4, 165–174.

Rossi, A.G., Norman, K.E., Donigi-Gale, D., Shoupe, T.S., Edwards, R. and Williams, T.J. (1992). The role of complement, platelet-activating factor and leukotriene B_4 in the reversed passive Arthus reaction. Br. J. Pharmacol. 107, 44–49.

Rossi, A.G., McIntyre, D.E., Jones, C.J.P. and MacMillan, R.M. (1993). Stimulation of human polymorphonuclear leukocytes by leukotriene B_4 and platelet-activating factor: an ultrastructural and pharmacological study. J. Leukocyte Biol. 53, 117–125.

Rot, A. (1992a). Binding of neutrophil attractant/activation protein-1 (interleukin 8) to resident dermal cells. Cytokine 4, 347–352.

Rot, A. (1992b). Endothelial cell binding of NAP-1/IL-8: role in neutrophil emigration. Immunol. Today 13, 291–294.

Saez-Llorens, X., Jafari, H.S., Severien, C., Parras, F., Olsen, K.D., Hansen, E.J., Singer, I.I. and McCracken, G.H. (1991). Enhanced attenuation of meningeal inflammation and brain edema by concomitant administration of anti-CD18 monoclonal antibodies and dexamethasone in experimental haemophilus meningitis. J. Clin. Invest. 88, 2003–2011.

Samuelsson, B., Dahlen, S.-E., Lindgren, J.A., Rouzer, C.A. and Serhan, C.N. (1987). Leukotrienes and lipoxins: structures, biosynthesis, and biological effects. Science 237, 1171–1176.

Schiffmann, E., Showell, H.J., Corcoran, B.A., Ward, P.A., Smith, E. and Becker, E.L. (1975). The isolation and partial characterization of neutrophil chemotactic factors from Escherichia coli. J. Immunol. 114, 1831–1837.

Schmidt-Schonbein, G.W., Shih, Y.Y. and Chien, S. (1985). Morphometry of human leukocytes. Blood 56, 866–875.

Schrier, D.J., Lesch, M.E., Wright, C.D. and Gilbertsen, R.B. (1990). The antiinflammatory effects of adenosine receptor agonists on the carrageenan-induced pleural inflammatory response in rats. J. Immunol. 145, 1874–1879.

Seitz, M., Dewald, B., Gerber, N. and Baggiolini, M. (1991). Enhanced production of neutrophil-activating peptide-1/interleukin-8 in rheumatoid arthritis. J. Clin. Invest. 87, 463–469.

Selby, C., Drost, E., Wraith, P.K. and MacNee, W. (1991). In vivo neutrophil sequestration within lungs of humans is determined by in vitro "filterability". J. Appl. Physiol. 71(5), 1996–2003.

Sharar, S.R., Winn, R.K., Murry, C.E., Harlan, J.M. and Rice, C.L. (1991). A CD18 monoclonal antibody increases the incidence and severity of subcutaneous abscess formation after high dose S. aureus injection in rabbits. Surgery 116, 213–219.

Shaw, J.O. (1980). Leukocytes in chemotactic-fragment-induced lung inflammation. Am. J. Pathol. 101, 283–291.

Shaw, J.O., Henson, P.M., Henson, J. and Webster, R.O. (1980). Lung inflammation induced by complement-derived chemotactic fragments in the alveolus. Lab. Invest. 42, 547–558.

Simms, H.H., D'Amico, R. and Burchard, K.W. (1991). Intraabdominal sepsis: enhanced autooxidative effect on polymorphonuclear leukocyte cell surface receptor expression. Circ. Shock 34, 356–363.

Simpson, P.J., Todd, R.F., III, Fantone, J.C., Michelson, J.K., Griffin, J.D. and Lucchesi, B.R. (1988). Reduction of experimental canine myocardial reperfusion injury by a monoclonal antibody (Anti-Mol, Anti-CD11b) that inhibits leukocyte adhesion. J. Clin. Invest. 81, 624–629.

Smith, C.W., Rothlein, R., Hughes, B.J., Mariscalco, M.M., Rudloff, H.E., Schmalstieg, F.C. and Anderson, D.C. (1988). Recognition of an endothelial determinant for CD18-dependent human neutrophil adherence and transendothelial migration. J. Clin. Invest. 82, 1746–1756.

Smith, C.W., Marlin, S.D., Rothlein, R., Toman, C. and Anderson, D.C. (1989). Co-operative interactions of LFA-1 and Mac-1 with intercellular adhesion molecule-1 in facilitating adherence and transendothelial migration of human neutrophils in vitro. J. Clin. Invest. 83, 2008–2017.

Smith, C.W., Entman, M.L., Lane, C.L., Beaudet, A.L., Ty, T.I., Youker, K., Hawkins, H.K. and Anderson, D.C. (1991). Adherence of neutrophils to canine cardiac myocytes in vitro is dependent on intercellular adhesion molecule-1. J. Clin. Invest. 88, 1216–1223.

Snyder, F. (1989). Biochemistry of platelet-activating factor: a unique class of biologically active phospholipids (42839). Soc. Exp. Biol. Med. 190, 125–135.

Spector, W.G. and Willoughby, D.A. (1960). The enzymatic inactivation of an adrenaline-like substance in inflammation. J. Pathol. Bacteriol. 80, 271–279.

Spertini, O., Kansas, G.S., Munro, J.M., Griffin, J.D. and Tedder, T.F. (1991a). Regulation of leukocyte migration by activation of the leukocyte adhesion molecule-1 (LAM-1) selectin. Nature 349, 691–694.

Spertini, O., Luscinskas, F.W., Kansas, G.S., Munro, J.M., Griffin, J.D., Gimbrone, M.A. and Tedder, T.F. (1991b). Leukocyte adhesion molecule-1 (LAM-1, L-selectin) interacts with an inducible endothelial cell ligand to support leukocyte adhesion. J. Immunol. 147, 2565–2573.

Stetson, C.A. and Good, R.A. (1951). Studies on the mechanism of the Schwartzman phenomenon. Evidence for the participation of polymorphonuclear leukocytes in the phenomenon. J. Exp. Med. 93, 49–64.

Swensson, O., Schubert, C., Christophers, E. and Schroder, J.-M. (1991). Inflammatory properties of neutrophil-activating protein-1/interleukin 8 (NAP-1/IL-8) in human skin: a light- and electronmicroscopic study. J. Invest. Dermatol. 96, 682–689.

Takenawa, T., Ishitoya, J. and Nagai, Y. (1986). Inhibitory effect of prostaglandin E_2, forskolin, and dibutyryl cAMP on arachidonic acid release and inositol phospholipid metabolism in guinea pig neutrophils. J. Biol. Chem. 261, 1092–1098.

Tanaka, Y., Adams, D.H., Hubscher, S., Hirano, H., Siebenlist, U. and Shaw, S. (1993). T-cell adhesion induced by proteoglycan-immobilized cytokine MIP-1β. Nature 361, 79–82.

Teixeira, M.M., Williams, T.J. and Hellewell, P.G. (1993). E-type prostaglandins enhance local oedema formation and neutrophil accumulation but suppress eosinophil accumulation in guinea pig skin. Br. J. Pharmacol. 110, 416–422.

Thomas, J.R., Harlan, J.M., Rice, C.L. and Winn, R.K. (1992). Role of leukocyte CD11/CD18 in endotoxic and septic shock in rabbits. J. Appl. Physiol. 73, 1510–1516.

Thomas, L. and Good, R.A. (1952). Studies on the generalized Shwartzman reaction I. General observations concerning the phenomenon. J. Exp. Med. 96, 605–623.

Till, G.O., Lee, S., Mulligan, M.S., Wolter, J.R., Smith, C.W., Ward, P.A. and Marak, G.E. (1992). Adhesion molecules in experimental phacoanaphylactic endophthalmitis. Invest. Ophthalmol. Vis. Sci. 33, 3417–3423.

Tonnesen, M.G., Smedley, L.A. and Henson, P.M. (1984). Neutrophil-endothelial cell interactions. Modulation of neutrophil adhesiveness induced by complement fragments C5a and C5a des arg and formyl-methionyl-leucyl-phenylalanine in vitro. J. Clin. Invest. 74, 1581–1592.

Tozeren, A. and Ley, K. (1992). How do selectins mediate leukocyte rolling in venules? Biophys. J. 63, 700–709.

Trochet, M.H. (1824). "Recherches, anatomiques et physiologiques sur la structure intime des animaux et des vegetaux, et sur leur motilité". Balliere et Fils, Paris.

Tuomanen, E.I., Saukkonen, K., Sande, S., Cioffe, C. and Wright, S.D. (1989). Reduction of inflammation, tissue damage and mortality in bacterial meningitis in rabbits treated with monoclonal antibodies against adhesion-promoting receptors of leucocytes. J. Exp. Med. 170, 959–968.

Valerius, N.H. (1984). Chemotaxis of neutrophil granulocytes. Measurement, cell biology and clinical significance. Dan. Med. Bull. 31, 458–474.

Vedder, N.B., Winn, R.K., Rice, C.L., Chi, E.Y., Arfors, K.E. and Harber, J.M. (1988). A monoclonal antibody to the adherence-promoting leukocyte glycoprotein, CD18, reduces organ injury and improves survival from hemorrhagic shock and resuscitation in rabbits. J. Clin. Invest. 81, 939–944.

Vedder, N.B., Winn, R.K., Rice, C.L., Chi, E.Y., Arfors, K.E. and Harlan, J.M. (1990). Inhibition of leukocyte adherence by anti-CD18 monoclonal antibody attenuates reperfusion injury in the rabbit ear. Proc. Natl Acad. Sci. USA 87, 2643–2646.

Von Andrian, U.H., Chambers, J.D., McEvoy, L.M., Bargatze, R.F., Arfors, K.-E. and Butcher, E.C. (1991). Two-step model of leukocyte–endothelial cell interaction in inflammation: distinct roles for LECAM-1 and the leukocyte β_2 integrins in vivo. Proc. Natl Acad. Sci. USA 88, 7538–7542.

Von Andrian, U.H., Hansell, P., Chambers, J.D., Berger, E.M., Filho, I.T., Butcher, E.C. and Arfors, K.-E. (1992). L-Selectin function is required for β_2-integrin-mediated neutrophil adhesion at physiological shear rates in vivo. Am. J. Physiol. 263, H1034–H1044.

Von Euler, U.S. and Liljestrand, G. (1946). Observations on the pulmonary arterial blood pressure in the cat. Acta Physiol. Scand. 12, 301.

Von Uexkull, C., Nourshargh, S. and Williams, T.J. (1992). Comparative responses of human and rabbit interleukin-1 in vivo: effect of a recombinant interleukin-1 receptor antagonist. Immunology 72, 483–487.

Wagner, D.D. (1993). Molecular genetic analysis of P-selectin function. J. Cell Biol. Suppl 17A, 324.

Waller, A. (1846a) Microscopic examination of some of the principal tissues of the animal frame, as observed in the tongue of the living frog, toad etc. Phil. Mag. J. Sci. (3rd Ser.) 29, 271–287.

Waller, A. (1846b). Microscopic observations of the perforation of the capillaries by the corpuscles of the blood, and on the origin of mucous and pus-globules. Phil. Mag. J. Sci. (3rd Ser.) 29, 397–405.

Walz, A., Peveri, P., Aschauer, H. and Baggiolini, M. (1987). Purification and amino acid sequencing of NAF, a novel neutrophil-activating factor produced by monocytes. Biochem. Biophys. Res. Comm. 149, 755–761.

Warren, J.S., Mandel, D.M., Johnson, K.J. and Ward, P.A. (1989). Evidence for the role of platelet-activating factor in immune complex vasculitis in the rat. J. Clin. Invest. 83, 669–678.

Watson, S.R., Fennie, C. and Lasky, L.A. (1991). Neutrophil influx in to an inflammatory site inhibited by a soluble homing receptor-IgG chimaera. Nature 349, 164–166.

Wedmore, C.V. and Williams, T.J. (1981a). Control of vascular permeability by polymorphonuclear leukocytes in inflammation. Nature 289, 646–650.

Wedmore, C.V. and Williams, T.J. (1981b). Platelet-activating factor (PAF), a secretory product of polymorphonuclear leukocytes, increases vascular permeability in rabbit skin. Br. J. Pharmacol. 74, 916–917P.

Weg, V.B., Williams, T.J., Lobb, R.R. and Nourshargh, S. (1993). A monoclonal antibody recognizing very late activation antigen-4 inhibits eosinophil accumulation in vivo. J. Exp. Med. 177, 561–566.

Wegner, C.D., Gundel, R.H., Reilly, P., Haynes, N., Letts, L.G. and Rothlein, R. (1990). Intercellular adhesion molecule-1 (ICAM-1) in the pathogenesis of asthma. Science 247, 456–459.

Wegner, C.D., Rothlein, R. and Gundel, R.H. (1991). Adhesion molecules in the pathogenesis of asthma. Agents Actions 34, 529–544.

Wegner, C.D., Wolyniec, W.W., LaPlante, A.M., Marschman, K., Lubbe, K., Haynes, N., Rothlein, R. and Letts, L.G. (1992). Intercellular adhesion molecule-1 contributes to pulmonary oxygen toxicity in mice: role of leukocytes revised. Lung 170, 267–279.

Whelan, C.J. and Johnson, M. (1992). Inhibition by salmeterol of increased vascular permeability and granulocyte accumulation in guinea-pig lung and skin. Br. J. Pharmacol. 105, 831–838.

Wilkinson P. (1982). "Chemotaxis and Inflammation". Churchill Livingstone, Edinburgh.

Williams, A.F. (1991). Out of equilibrium. Nature 352, 473–474.

Williams, F.M., Collins, P.D., Tanniere-Zeller, M. and Williams, T.J. (1990). The relationship between neutrophils and increased microvascular permeability in a model of myocardial ischaemia and reperfusion in the rabbit. Br. J. Pharmacol. 100, 729–734.

Williams, T.J. (1978). A proposed mediator of increased microvascular permeability in acute inflammation in the rabbit. J. Physiol. 281, 44–45P.

Williams, T.J. (1979). Prostaglandin E$_2$, prostaglandin I$_2$ and the vascular changes of inflammation. Br. J. Pharmacol. 65, 517–524.

Williams, T.J. and Jose, P.J. (1981). Mediation of increased vascular permeability after complement activation: histamine-independent action of rabbit C5a. J. Exp. Med. 153, 136–153.

Williams, T.J. and Peck, M.J. (1977). Role of prostaglandin-mediated vasodilatation in inflammation. Nature 270, 530–532.

Winquist, R., Frei, P., Harrison, P., McParland, M., Letts, G., Van, G., Andrews, L., Rothlein, R. and Hintze, T. (1990). An anti-CD18 mAb limits infarct size in primates following myocardial ischemia and reperfusion. Circulation 82, suppl. III, 701.

Worthen, G.S., Haslett, C., Rees, A.J., Gumbay, R.S., Henson, J.E. and Henson, P.M. (1987a). Neutrophil-mediated pulmonary vascular injury: synergistic effect of trace amounts of lipopolysaccharide and neutrophil stimuli on vascular permeability and neutrophil sequestration in the lung. Am. Rev. Respir. Dis. 136, 19–28.

Worthen, G.S., Lien, D.C., Tonnesen, M.G. and Hensen, P.M. (1987b). In "Pulmonary Endothelium in Health and Diseases" (ed. U.S. Ryan), pp. 123–160. Marcel Dekker, New York.

Worthen, G.S., Schwab, B., Elson, E.L. and Downey, G.P. (1989). Mechanics of stimulated neutrophils: cell stiffening induces retention in capillaries. Science 245, 183–186.

Yeh, C.G., Marsh, H.C., Carson, G.R., Berman, L., Concino, M.F., Scesney, S.M., Kuestner, R.E., Skibbens, R., Donahue, K.A. and Ip, S.H. (1991). Recombinant soluble human complement receptor type 1 inhibits inflammation in the reversed passive Arthus reaction in rats. J. Immunol. 146, 250–256.

Yoshimura, T., Matsushima, K., Tanaka, S., Robinson, E.A., Appella, E., Oppenheim, J.J. and Leonard, E.J. (1987). Purification of a human monocyte-derived neutrophil chemotactic factor that has peptide sequence similarity to other host defense cytokines. Proc. Natl Acad. Sci. USA 84, 9233–9237.

Zigmond, S.H. (1978). Chemotaxis by polymorphonuclear leukocytes. J. Cell Biol. 77, 269–287.

11. Role of Neutrophils in Reperfusion Injury

F.M. Williams

1. Introduction

Interruption of the blood supply to an area of tissue results in a reduction in the supply of oxygen and nutrients, and the accumulation of toxic waste products. Initially the cells will experience a phase of reversible injury and restoration of blood flow will result eventually in complete recovery of normal function. If, however, the duration of ischaemia is extended beyond a critical period of time, irreversible cellular injury occurs and the onset of tissue necrosis ensues. The speed with which ischaemia develops depends largely on the metabolic rate of the tissue but is also influenced by other factors such as the presence and extent of any collateral blood supply.

In tissues such as the myocardium, cell necrosis can be detected after 20 min of ischaemia (Jennings and Reimer, 1983), whereas irreversible injury in resting skeletal muscle occurs only after 4–5 h of ischaemia (Miller *et al.*, 1979).

Restoration of blood flow is essential in order to halt the process of necrosis. A frequent cause of tissue ischaemia is occlusion of arteries by platelet thrombi. This often occurs at sites where the vascular lumen has already been reduced by atherosclerotic plaque formation. In the case of myocardial ischaemia, there is a correlation between the amount of tissue which becomes necrotic and the prognosis of the patient (Harnarayan *et al.*, 1970; Page *et al.*, 1971). Consequently, there is

Immunopharmacology of Neutrophils
ISBN 0-12-339250-0

considerable interest in minimizing the region of tissue necrosis. With the advent of procedures such as percutaneous transluminal angioplasty, which allows the vessel lumen to be reopened mechanically, and thrombolysis, which causes lysis of platelet thrombi, it is now possible to restore blood flow to the affected region within hours of the ischaemic insult. A number of clinical trials have now been carried out on the use of thrombolysis to reperfuse ischaemic myocardium in patients. Reductions in both myocardial infarct size and mortality as well as improvements in left ventricular function have been reported if this procedure is carried out within hours of the onset of symptoms (ISIS-2 Collaborative Group, 1988; Van de Werf and Arnold, 1988).

However, experimental studies have shown that reperfusion of ischaemic myocardium can result in a drastic acceleration of tissue necrosis (Sommers and Jennings, 1964). Similar findings have been reported in other tissues, such as intestinal mucosa (Parks and Granger, 1986). This has led to a debate as to whether reperfusion of ischaemic tissue can exacerbate tissue injury (Braunwald and Kloner, 1985; Hearse and Bolli, 1991). What is not yet clear is whether this "reperfusion injury" simply reflects an acceleration of the rate of necrosis of irreversibly injured cells or whether additional damage is occurring. Neutrophil infiltration, generation of free radicals and calcium overload are amongst the mechanisms which have been implicated in this process. In this chapter the possible involvement of the neutrophil as a mediator of reperfusion injury will be considered. The majority of studies on the role of neutrophils in reperfusion injury have been carried out in models of myocardial ischaemia, however, this phenomenon has also been examined in other tissues including skeletal muscle, intestinal mucosa and lung. The involvement of neutrophils in reperfusion injury in different tissues will be addressed.

1.1 ISCHAEMIA AND THE INFLAMMATORY RESPONSE

When examined histologically, tissue which has undergone a prolonged period of ischaemia shows characteristic features of an acute inflammatory response with increased microvascular permeability and leucocyte infiltration. Over 50 years ago the time course for the influx of inflammatory cells into infarcted myocardium was described, using tissue taken from patients at autopsy (Mallory et al., 1939). Neutrophil infiltration is observed 12–24 h following the onset of symptoms and peaks after 3–4 days. After the first week, neutrophils begin to disappear from the infarct, being replaced by mononuclear cells such as lymphocytes and monocytes (Fishbein et al., 1978). Following extravascular migration, monocytes differentiate into macrophages, which are responsible for

the removal of effete neutrophils (see Chapter 14). The appearance of macrophages within the infarct indicates that the phase of tissue repair and reorganization has commenced, the culmination of which is the formation of a collagen-rich scar of high tensile strength.

1.2 KINETICS AND DISTRIBUTION OF NEUTROPHIL INFILTRATION FOLLOWING ISCHAEMIA AND REPERFUSION

Experimental studies have revealed that there are differences in the pattern of neutrophil infiltration following reperfusion of ischaemic tissue compared with that observed following permanent occlusion. The rate of neutrophil accumulation is markedly accelerated following reperfusion (Sommers and Jennings 1964; Engler et al., 1986). Measurements of the kinetics of neutrophil accumulation, in a canine model of acute myocardial infarction, have revealed that the rate is greatest in the first hour following reperfusion (Dreyer et al., 1991). The distribution of the leucocytes also differs. Following permanent occlusion, neutrophil infiltration is confined largely to the periphery of the infarct (Mallory et al., 1939; Fishbein et al., 1978), whereas following reperfusion these cells accumulate throughout the region of myocardium which has been rendered ischaemic (Mullane et al., 1984). However, neutrophils are reported to accumulate preferentially in the subendocardium (Go et al. 1988) and, during the first hour of reperfusion, their localization correlates inversely with the blood flow during the ischaemic period (Dreyer et al., 1991). This relationship is no longer seen, however, at later reperfusion times.

1.3 INVOLVEMENT OF NEUTROPHILS IN MYOCARDIAL REPERFUSION INJURY

Although it had been known for many years that neutrophil infiltration is a characteristic feature of tissue which has been subject to an episode of ischaemia, interest in the role of this leucocyte in tissue injury has intensified dramatically over the last 10 years. This situation arose primarily as a consequence of experimental studies carried out in animal models of acute myocardial infarction. Amongst a number of interventions examined in an attempt to reduce infarct size was the systemic depletion of circulating neutrophils. In 1983, Romson et al. reported that systemic administration of polyclonal Abs to neutrophils reduced myocardial infarct size in a canine model of coronary artery occlusion and reperfusion. Subsequent experimental studies by other investigators confirmed that myocardial infarct size could be reduced in experimental models not only by anti-neutrophil serum (Jolly *et al.*, 1986) but also by other interventions which reduce the number of circulating neutrophils, including hydroxy urea (Mullane *et al.*, 1984) and leucocyte filters (Litt *et al.*, 1989).

These observations have led to the suggestion that infiltrating neutrophils contribute to the size of the infarct. It is possible that activation of the cells and the consequent release of cytotoxic agents results in the death of reversibly injured myocytes as well as those which were irreversibly damaged. This phenomenon has been termed "bystander injury". In support of this hypothesis, certain other interventions (listed below), which have also been reported to reduce infarct size, share a common characteristic of either inhibiting the extravascular migration of neutrophils in response to inflammatory stimuli or the function of these leucocytes *in vivo*. Thus, in the early 1980s, reduction in myocardial infarct size in dogs was reported using the NSAIDs, ibuprofen and BW755C (Romson *et al.*, 1982; Mullane *et al.*, 1984). This protection did not appear to be due to the cyclo-oxygenase-inhibiting action of these compounds, since other drugs with this property such as aspirin and indomethacin were ineffective in reducing myocardial infarct size (Jugdutt *et al.*, 1979; Bonow *et al.*, 1981). A reduction in myocardial infarct size associated with diminished neutrophil infiltration has also been reported following infusion of the eicosanoids, PGE$_1$, PGI$_2$ and its more stable analogue, iloprost (Simpson *et al.*, 1987a, 1987b, 1988a).

Although there is evidence derived from a large number of experimental studies in support of a role for neutrophils in causing reperfusion injury, the case is still contentious. In some studies a protective action was not observed with anti-neutrophil interventions (Reimer *et al.*, 1985; Chatelain *et al.*, 1987). The great majority of these experimental studies have been carried out using canine models of myocardial infarction. A notable feature of canine myocardium is the presence of a relatively large, but variable, degree of myocardial collateral blood flow. This is in contrast to the situation in some other species such as rats and rabbits. In some, but not all, of the studies reporting positive results with anti-neutrophil interventions, measurements of myocardial blood flow within the ischaemic zone were not made. As a result, the presence of a higher residual blood flow within the ischaemic zone, which could contribute to a reduction in myocardial infarct size, cannot be excluded as a cause of the protective action in some studies. However, in the study of Litt *et al.* (1989) in which leucocyte filters were used to deplete circulating neutrophils in dogs, myocardial infarct size was reduced compared with controls, although the measured collateral blood flow did not differ in the two groups. Interestingly, in that study a protective effect was observed even though neutrophil depletion was instituted during the reperfusion phase only.

1.4   NEUTROPHILS AND I/R INJURY IN OTHER ORGANS

A great deal of the evidence for the role of neutrophils in reperfusion injury has come from studies carried out in the heart, however, this phenomenon has also been observed in a number of other organs. A notable feature of reperfusion injury in tissues such as intestinal mucosa and skeletal muscle is the presence of increased vascular permeability to protein resulting in oedema formation (Hernandez *et al.*, 1987; Carden *et al.*, 1990). The role of neutrophils in this process is covered in Section 5.1. In a few studies the effect on tissue necrosis of inhibiting neutrophil infiltration following reperfusion has also been examined. In a model of hepatic ischaemia and reperfusion in rats, pretreatment with a mAb to neutrophils resulted in an 86% decrease in the accumulation of these leucocytes in the affected lobe. This effect was accompanied by a significant attenuation in tissue necrosis, measured after 24 h of reperfusion, from 80% in controls to 28% in the treated group (Jaeschke *et al.*, 1990). Similarly in a model of renal ischaemia and reperfusion in anaesthetized rats, administration of an anti-neutrophil serum, resulted in a reduction in both creatinine levels and tubular necrosis (Klausner *et al.*, 1989). A reduction in the mass of myocyte necrosis, following induction of neutropaenia using X-rays, has also been reported in a model of ischaemia and reperfusion in skeletal muscle (Belkin *et al.*, 1989).

2.   *Mechanisms of Neutrophil Accumulation*

Neutrophil accumulation at sites of inflammation is dependent on the local generation or release of chemotactic agents. The mediators involved in causing neutrophil infiltration following ischaemia and reperfusion have not been definitively identified. However, there is strong evidence to implicate both the complement fragment C5a and the AA metabolite, LTB$_4$. In recent years it has become clear that certain adhesive glycoproteins expressed on the surface of both neutrophils and vascular endothelial cells have an important role to play in the extravascular migration of leucocytes at sites of inflammation.

2.1   MYOCARDIAL INFARCTION AND THE COMPLEMENT SYSTEM

There is considerable evidence indicating that acute myocardial infarction is associated with activation of the complement system. This is of relevance to neutrophil infiltration since C5a, one of the products generated during activation of the complement cascade, is a powerful neutrophil chemoattractant (Snyderman *et al.*,

1970). The nine major complement components, C1–C9, together with a number of other proteins, are present in the blood and extravascular fluid. These components are activated sequentially by one of two pathways, the classical and alternative pathways, which differ in the routes by which the pivotal component C3 is activated. Thereafter activation of the complement components is the same in both pathways. Activation of C3 results in the formation of the cleavage products, C3a and C3b. The latter causes the cleavage of C5 into C5a and C5b. Subsequent binding of C5b to the proteins C6–C9 results in the formation of the membrane attack complex C5b–C9. This macromolecular complex forms pores when inserted into the lipid bilayer of the membrane, which result in cell lysis. In addition to its action as a neutrophil chemoattractant, C5a together with C3a functions as an anaphylatoxin causing release of histamine from mast cells to produce vasodilatation and increased microvascular permeability.

In patients with acute myocardial infarction, alterations in the circulating concentrations of complement components or products of complement activation have been observed. Thus, the concentration of the complement split products, C3a and C5a, and of the terminal complex C5b-9 were increased in peripheral venous blood of patients, 16 h after the onset of symptoms (Langlois and Gawryl, 1988). In addition, C3b, C4 and the cytolytic C5b-9 complex have been detected on the surface of myocytes in the infarcted region of myocardium within 4 h of reperfusion (McManus et al., 1983; Schafer et al., 1986). Links between complement activation and myocardial neutrophil accumulation have also been found. In a model of acute myocardial infarction in the dog, C1q labelled with ^{125}I was administered intravenously in order to identify sites of complement activation. Accumulation of ^{125}I-C1q, which was observed in ischaemic myocardium within 45 min of coronary artery occlusion, was found to co-localize with infiltrating neutrophils (Rossen et al., 1985).

Studies carried out in the 1970s reported that systemic administration of cobra venom factor, which depletes circulating complement components, reduced the size of experimentally induced myocardial infarcts and inhibited the infiltration of neutrophils (Maclean et al., 1978; Maroko et al., 1978). More recently, a recombinant soluble form of CR1 (sCR1) has been developed, which inhibits complement activation by binding the C3 and C5 convertases, resulting in proteolytic inactivation of C3b and C4b. Intravenous administration of sCR1 is reported to reduce myocardial infarct size measured 7 days after reperfusion in rats (Weisman et al., 1990). This protective action of sCR1 was associated with decreased neutrophil accumulation.

Neutrophil chemoattractant activity has been detected in coronary sinus blood following myocardial ischaemia in dogs. Treatment with cobra venom factor resulted in a reduction in the activity, suggesting that a product of complement activation was involved (Hartmann et al., 1977). More recently it has been reported that neutrophil chemoattractant activity detected in lymph draining infarcted canine myocardium can be inactivated by an Ab to C5a, providing more direct evidence for the involvement of this mediator (Entman et al., 1991).

2.2 THE ROLE OF LTB₄ IN REPERFUSION INJURY

LTB_4 is another neutrophil chemoattractant likely to play a role in reperfusion injury. LTB_4 is a potent neutrophil chemoattractant *in vivo* (Ford-Hutchinson et al., 1980; Dahlen et al., 1981; Higgs et al., 1981) and is released by activated neutrophils following oxygenation of AA by the enzyme 5-LO (Borgeat and Samuelsson, 1979). Increased quantities of LTB_4 in infarcted myocardium have been reported in a model of coronary artery occlusion in the rat (Sasaki et al., 1988). The investigators observed that the concentration of the leukotriene peaked prior to maximal neutrophil infiltration implying a causal relationship.

Evidence for a role of LTB_4 in causing neutrophil infiltration in I/R tissue also comes from experimental studies in which drugs were administered that inhibit the 5-LO enzyme and consequently the generation of this LT. Inhibitors of 5-LO such as REV 5901, nafazatrom and AA-861 have been reported to cause a reduction in myocardial infarct size in experimental studies (Mullane et al., 1987; Bednar et al., 1985; Sasaki et al., 1988). The protective effect in these studies was associated with a reduction in neutrophil accumulation. Many of the available 5-lipoxygenase inhibitors have other properties such as free radical scavenging activity, so these studies do not definitively implicate the LT. More recently specific antagonists of the LTB_4 receptor have become available. In a model of splanchnic ischaemia in the rat, administration of LY 255283, an antagonist of LTB_4 receptors, has been reported to increase the survival rate and to reduce neutrophil accumulation, as measured by MPO assay (Karasawa et al., 1991). However, the results reported with these agents in models of myocardial infarction have so far been mixed. One LTB_4 antagonist was reported to be effective in a rabbit model of myocardial infarction (Taylor et al., 1989), whereas LY 255283 was ineffective in a canine model (Hahn et al., 1990). These differences may, however, simply reflect species differences in the products of the 5-LO enzyme. These studies suggest therefore that this LT may have a role in mediating neutrophil infiltration into tissue following ischaemia and reperfusion. Since neutrophils are most probably the major source of LTB_4 within infarcted tissue it seems unlikely that the initial phase of neutrophil accumulation is elicited by this mediator. However, LTB_4 may well be involved in amplifying the response.

2.3 OTHER NEUTROPHIL CHEMOATTRACTANTS

Amongst other known neutrophil chemoattractants is the cytokine IL-8 (Schroder et al., 1987; Walz et al., 1987; Yoshimura et al., 1987). This is a recently identified inflammatory mediator which has been found to be comparatively potent in eliciting neutrophil infiltration in vivo (Colditz et al., 1989). It has been reported that a homologue of IL-8 is generated in vivo, subsequent to that of C5a during the course of an inflammatory response in the rabbit peritoneal cavity (Beaubien et al., 1990; Collins et al., 1991; Jose et al., 1991). As yet there is little direct evidence for the involvement of IL-8 in reperfusion injury, although ischaemia and reperfusion of isolated blood perfused rat hearts is reported to result in increased expression of mRNA for this cytokine (Kamikubo et al., 1993).

PAF has also been implicated as a mediator of neutrophil accumulation (see Chapter 10). In a model of ischaemia and reperfusion of the intestinal mucosa, increased adhesion of neutrophils to the vascular endothelium and extravascular migration of these leucocytes were observed using intravital microscopy. Administration of WEB 2086, a PAF receptor antagonist, attenuated both these responses (Kubes et al., 1990). PAF receptor antagonists have been reported to reduce myocardial infarct size in rats and rabbits (Stahl et al., 1988; Montrucchio et al., 1990). However, in a model of coronary artery occlusion and reperfusion in anaesthetized rabbits we found that administration of WEB 2086 had no effect on the accumulation of ^{111}In-labelled neutrophils in infarcted myocardium (Williams et al., 1990).

3. Role of Adhesion Molecules in Reperfusion Injury

Extravascular migration of neutrophils in response to inflammatory mediators is dependent on an initial adhesion of these leucocytes to the vascular endothelium (Harlan, 1985). In recent years it has become evident that this interaction between neutrophils and endothelial cells is dependent on certain adhesion glycoproteins which are expressed on the surface of both cells (Springer, 1990). In the case of the neutrophil, the CD11b/CD18 complex has been found to play an important role in neutrophil adhesion (Beatty et al., 1983). Neutrophils fail to accumulate in response to inflammatory stimuli, if this complex is not expressed, as is seen in patients with LAD (Crowley et al., 1980; Arnaout et al., 1984) (see Chapter 7). Monoclonal Abs have been raised against these glycoproteins and have been used to examine their role in vivo. In experimental studies it has been shown that intravenous administration of a mAb to CD18,

60.3, inhibits neutrophil accumulation in response to inflammatory stimuli and in models of allergic inflammation (Arfors et al., 1987) (see Chapter 10). Subsequently it was shown that pretreatment of neutrophils in vitro with mAb 60.3 also inhibited their accumulation in response to inflammatory mediators (Nourshargh et al., 1989). This Ab has also been used to examine whether CD18 is involved in neutrophil infiltration into ischaemic myocardium. ^{111}In-labelled neutrophils were administered intravenously to anaesthetized rabbits undergoing coronary artery occlusion and reperfusion, and their accumulation in myocardial tissue was measured. Pretreatment of the neutrophils in vitro with mAb 60.3 markedly reduced their accumulation in ischaemic/reperfused myocardium (Williams et al., 1990). Systemic administration of another mAb to CD18 has also been reported to reduce the number of neutrophils accumulating in the myocardium of dogs undergoing coronary artery occlusion and reperfusion (Dreyer et al., 1991). Furthermore, intravenous administration of anti-CD18 Abs is reported to reduce myocardial infarct size in rabbits and cats (Seewaldt-Becker et al., 1990; Ma et al., 1991). A mAb directed against the CD11b antigen has also been reported to reduce myocardial infarct size in dogs (Simpson et al., 1988b). The vascular endothelium also expresses adhesion glycoproteins, which act as ligands for those on the surface of leucocytes (see Chapters 7 and 10). Two of the most extensively studied are E-selectin and ICAM-1, although little work has been carried out on the role of these adhesion molecules in mediating neutrophil infiltration in ischaemic/reperfused tissue. However, RR1/1, a mAb raised to ICAM-1 is reported to reduce myocardial infarct size in a rabbit model of coronary artery occlusion and reperfusion (Seewaldt-Becker et al., 1990). Neutrophil infiltration was also suppressed with this treatment. There is evidence of increased expression of adhesion molecules as a consequence of ischaemia. Dreyer et al. (1989) used a canine model of coronary artery occlusion and reperfusion in which lymph draining from the ischaemic region of myocardium could be collected. They observed that the expression of CD11b/CD18 on neutrophils present in lymph samples was elevated during reperfusion compared with levels measured prior to ischaemia. Increased expression of mRNA for both ICAM-1 and P-selectin (GMP-140) in ischaemic myocardium has also been reported (Smith et al., 1991; Manning et al., 1992).

3.1 ROLE OF ADHESION MOLECULES IN THE INTERACTION BETWEEN NEUTROPHILS AND MYOCYTES

Most studies on the role of adhesion molecules have examined the interaction between neutrophils and vascular endothelial cells (see Chapter 10). Some studies have also been carried out on the role of adhesion molecules in the attachment of neutrophils to myocytes. In a study carried out with canine neutrophils activated with ZAS, as a source of C5a, adhesion to isolated canine myocytes stimulated with IL-1 was observed (Entman *et al.*, 1990). Pretreatment of neutrophils with a mAb to CD18 inhibited not only adhesion to the myocytes but also generation of H_2O_2 by the leucocytes. In a subsequent study, a mAb to ICAM-1 was shown to inhibit this adhesion of neutrophils to myocytes, indicating that ICAM-1 was the ligand for CD18 (Smith *et al.*, 1991). Samples of lymph draining from ischaemic myocardium are also reported to induce neutrophil–myocyte adhesion. This interaction was inhibited by Abs to CD18, ICAM-1 and to IL-6 (Youker *et al.*, 1992).

3.2   ROLE OF ADHESION MOLECULES IN OTHER TISSUES

The role of adhesion molecules in reperfusion injury in organs other than the heart has also received considerable attention. In a rabbit model of haemorrhagic shock, in effect a whole body model of ischaemia and reperfusion,

restoration of blood volume following a period of hypovolaemia was associated with a high mortality together with evidence of both tissue necrosis and neutrophil accumulation in lungs, liver and gastric mucosa. Administration of the anti-CD18 mAb, 60.3, improved the survival of animals and attenuated tissue injury in the gut and liver, but not in the lungs (Vedder *et al.*, 1988). The same Ab was also reported to attenuate reperfusion injury to rabbit ear (Vedder *et al.*, 1990). An interesting feature of this study is that administration of the Ab was made during rather than prior to the period of ischaemia. However, systemic administration of mAb 60.3 did not protect against increased blood urea nitrogen and plasma creatinine concentrations induced by occlusion and reperfusion of the renal artery in rabbits (Thornton *et al.*, 1989).

4.   *Mechanisms of Tissue Damage by Neutrophils*

In order for neutrophils to be implicated in reperfusion injury, it is necessary to demonstrate that they have the

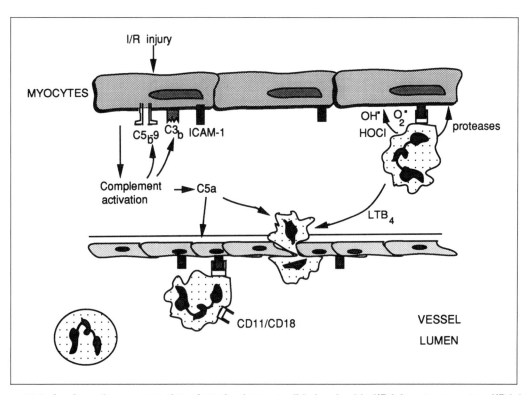

Figure 11.1 A schematic representation of mechanisms possibly involved in I/R injury to myocytes. I/R injury leads to complement activation and generation of C5a, C3b and C5b-9. C5a acts as a chemoattractant for neutrophils. These adhere to the vascular endothelium through adhesion molecules (i.e. CD11/CD18 and ICAM-1) expressed on the surface of both cell types, prior to extravascular migration. Activated neutrophils also release mediators such as LTB$_4$ which induce further leucocyte infiltration as well as proteases and ROM which may cause cellular injury.

potential to cause cell damage. Neutrophils are able to release a number of potentially injurious agents when activated and therefore fulfil this requirement. These agents fall into two main groups; reactive oxidizing chemicals (see Chapter 3) and proteolytic enzymes (see Chapter 4).

4.1   OXYGEN-DERIVED FREE RADICALS

There is a large body of research on the possible role of oxygen-derived free radicals in causing reperfusion injury but, as in the case of studies with anti-neutrophil interventions, conflicting results have been reported (Reimer et al., 1989). There are a number of metabolic pathways whereby free radicals may be generated following reperfusion but the two which have received most attention are neutrophil activation and the xanthine oxidase reaction. In the case of the neutrophil, the membrane-bound NADPH oxidase enzyme catalyses the production of superoxide anions, hydrogen peroxide and hydroxyl radicals. Although these radicals are able to react with a number of biological substrates themselves, it is thought that another product of oxidative metabolism is of greater importance in vivo. Hydrogen peroxide combines with the enzyme MPO, one of the major constituents of neutrophil granules, to form an enzyme substrate complex that oxidizes halides and in particular Cl^- to produce highly reactive toxic products such as hypochlorous acid (HOCl) (Harrison and Schultz, 1976). HOCl is now thought to be the major product of oxidative metabolism by neutrophils (Weiss, 1989). These free radicals are able to cause direct cellular injury, for instance by oxidizing nucleic acids, proteins and lipids, and thereby damaging both intracellular organelles and the cell membrane (Freeman and Crapo, 1982). In addition, these agents also affect the activity of neutrophil proteolytic enzymes as described below.

There is some experimental evidence implicating free radicals in the accumulation of neutrophils following ischaemia and reperfusion. In 1986, Grisham et al. reported that the accumulation of neutrophils into I/R intestine was reduced by administration of superoxide dismutase or allopurinol. The investigators proposed that generation of free radicals during reperfusion resulted in the generation of a neutrophil chemoattractant.

4.2   NEUTROPHIL PROTEASES

Neutrophils possess a number of enzymes stored within granules. Three of these have been of particular interest with respect to tissue damage; the serine proteinase, elastase, and the two metallo-proteases, collagenase and gelatinase. These enzymes are able to degrade key components of the extracellular matrix. Using endothelial monolayers in vitro, elastase has been shown to alter barrier properties and to cause detachment or even lysis of cells (Harlan, 1985; Harlan et al., 1985; Smedly et al., 1986). However, inhibitors of serine proteinases are present in the extracellular fluid in high concentrations in order to prevent inappropriate elastase activity. Furthermore, the metalloproteases are secreted in an inactive form (Weiss and Peppin, 1986). Despite these safeguards there is evidence to suggest that these enzymes are active at sites of inflammation (Opie, 1922) (see Chapter 4). Chlorinated oxidants are thought to inactivate α_1 proteinase inhibitor, thus destroying the anti-proteinase shield (Carp and Janoff, 1980). It has also been shown that activation of collagenase is dependent on the presence of a functional NADPH oxidase system (Weiss et al., 1985). It would appear therefore that by releasing free radicals in addition to proteolytic enzymes, the potential of neutrophils to cause tissue injury is considerably enhanced.

Elastase may also have a role in extravascular migration of neutrophils at sites of inflammation. Neutrophil accumulation in ischaemic/reperfused intestine was also significantly diminished following administration of the elastase inhibitors Eglin C and L658,758 (Zimmerman et al., 1990) suggesting that release of this enzyme is involved in the extravascular migration of these leucocytes.

5.   Neutrophils and Tissue Dysfunction following Ischaemia and Reperfusion

In addition to a possible role in causing tissue necrosis following reperfusion, neutrophils have also been implicated in other less severe changes in tissue function. These are discussed below.

5.1   THE ROLE OF NEUTROPHILS IN INCREASED VASCULAR PERMEABILITY FOLLOWING REPERFUSION

Increased microvascular permeability is a characteristic feature of an acute inflammatory reaction which is also evident following reperfusion of ischaemic tissue. A wide variety of inflammatory mediators have been shown to cause increased microvascular permeability. On the basis of studies carried out in a model of acute inflammation in the skin, it has been demonstrated that these agents can be divided into two main categories, neutrophil-dependent and neutrophil-independent mediators (Wedmore and Williams, 1981). Depletion of circulating neutrophils abolishes oedema formation in response to mediators such as C5a or LTB_4 which belong to the former category. With both types of mediator, leakage of plasma proteins occurs in the post-capillary venules

(Majno *et al.*, 1961) but, in the case of neutrophil-dependent mediators, larger venules can also be affected (Bjork *et al.*, 1982).

The possible involvement of neutrophils in causing reperfusion-induced oedema formation in tissues such as skeletal muscle and intestinal mucosa has been the subject of a number of studies. In a model of ischaemia and reperfusion in canine gracilis muscle, depletion of circulating leucocytes by filters resulted in a significant attenuation of the increase in microvascular permeability (Korthuis *et al.*, 1988). Subsequently, it was reported that in the same model administration of either a polyclonal anti-neutrophil serum or a mAb to the CD18 adhesion glycoprotein also protected against increased microvascular permeability following ischaemia and reperfusion (Carden *et al.*, 1990). Hernandez *et al.* (1987) also observed a similar protective effect in intestinal mucosa of cats using either a polyclonal anti-neutrophil serum or an anti-CD18 mAb. In the case of ischaemia and reperfusion in lung there are some conflicting results. In an *in vivo* rabbit model of 24 h pulmonary artery occlusion followed by 2 h reperfusion, administration of IB$_4$, a mAb to CD18, protected against oedema formation (Horgan *et al.*, 1990). An Ab to ICAM-1 also reduced oedema formation in this model (Horgan *et al.*, 1991). In both cases administration of the Ab was made 45 min prior to reperfusion, indicating that protection against activation of neutrophils during the occlusion phase was not required. In contrast in an *in vitro* isolated lung model of ischaemia and reperfusion, increased microvascular permeability was observed in the absence of circulating blood cells. Reperfusion with whole blood or perfusate supplemented with neutrophils did not exacerbate lung injury (Deeb *et al.*, 1990). However, this may simply reflect that neutrophil-dependent mediators of increased microvascular permeability are released in the intact lung following I/R but not in the isolated organ.

It has also been suggested that oedema formation in infarcted myocardium may be linked to the infiltration of neutrophils. Engler *et al.* (1986) reported that the increase in tissue water observed in ischaemic/reperfused myocardium was correlated with the number of accumulating neutrophils. Furthermore, depletion of circulating neutrophils inhibited oedema formation. However, the reperfusion period used in that study was very brief. In a rabbit model of coronary artery occlusion and reperfusion, systemic pretreatment with mustine hydrochloride was used to cause a 99% depletion in circulating neutrophils. This, however, had no effect on the increase in oedema formation in plasma volume, suggesting that a neutrophil-dependent mediator is not involved in this model (Williams *et al.*, 1990). It is possible therefore that this increase in vascular permeability is the result of another neutrophil-independent mediator or alternatively that it results from direct damage to the vascular endothelium.

5.2 REMOTE ISCHAEMIA-INDUCED LUNG INJURY

Under certain conditions, reperfusion of ischaemic tissue results not only in local injury but also in leucocyte sequestration in the lungs and pulmonary oedema (Anner *et al.*, 1987; Schmeling *et al.*, 1989). The development of this remote lung injury is dependent on both the mass of tissue undergoing ischaemia and the duration of the insult. It is seen with ischaemia of the legs or GI tract and has been reported in patients undergoing repair of aortic abdominal aneurysms (Paterson *et al.*, 1989). Neutrophils have been implicated in this pulmonary oedema. In a model of lower torso ischaemia and reperfusion in sheep, protection against increased pulmonary microvascular permeability was obtained by depleting circulating neutrophils using hydroxyurea (Klausner *et al.*, 1988). Administration of either an inhibitor of neutrophil elastase or of a combination of SOD and catalase is also reported to result in a reduction in lung oedema in a model of hind limb ischaemia and reperfusion in rats (Welbourn *et al.*, 1991). This suggests that endothelial injury may result from the release of these mediators from activated neutrophils. TNFα has also been implicated in remote lung injury induced by hepatic ischaemia and reperfusion. Increased plasma concentrations of this cytokine were detected following reperfusion. Administration of an Ab to TNFα resulted in a partial reduction in pulmonary neutrophil accumulation and almost complete inhibition of oedema formation (Caty *et al.*, 1990; Colletti *et al.*, 1990).

5.3 MYOCARDIAL STUNNING

Myocardial tissue that is reperfused following even a brief period of ischaemia shows evidence of impaired contractile function. This myocardial dysfunction is referred to as stunning (Heyndrickx *et al.*, 1975) and, although no sign of irreversible injury is evident either histologically or metabolically, full recovery of contractile function can take a period of hours or days depending on the duration of ischaemia (Braunwald and Kloner, 1985). The mechanisms involved in causing myocardial stunning have not yet been resolved, however, calcium overload and free radical generation have been implicated. In a few studies the role of neutrophils has also been examined. Neutrophils could contribute to myocardial dysfunction through several mechanisms, including the release of reactive oxygen species and hydrolytic enzymes or by capillary plugging. Initial evidence for a role for neutrophils in stunning came from a study carried out in a canine model of 15 min coronary artery occlusion, in which depletion of circulating neutrophils using filters was reported to alleviate the reduction in contractile function following reperfusion (Engler and Covell, 1987). This study was, however, criticised because the measurements of functional recovery in the presence and absence of neutrophils were compared in the same animal and thus entailed repeated coronary artery occlusions. A subsequent study carried out in separate control and treated dogs also reported improved recovery of contractile function following the use of leucocyte filters (Westlin and Mullane, 1989). Effective protection was observed even if leucocyte depletion was performed only on reperfusion. Furthermore, administration of the PGI$_2$ analogue, iloprost, is also reported to be protective against stunning (Farber *et al.*, 1988). Amongst the actions of iloprost that might account for its protective effect is inhibition of the neutrophil-derived superoxide burst after chemotactic stimulation. However, in other studies in which circulating neutrophils were depleted using either a polyclonal antiserum or leucocyte filters, no protection against stunning was observed (Jeremy and Becker, 1989; O'Neill *et al.*, 1989). Moreover, in a study of coronary artery occlusion and reperfusion in dog myocardium, it was observed that a short 12 min period of ischaemia was not associated with a significant accumulation of ^{111}In-labelled neutrophils (Go *et al.*, 1988). The evidence for the involvement of neutrophils in myocardial stunning is not therefore firmly established.

5.4 THE NO-REFLOW PHENOMENON

Reperfusion of tissue after a period of ischaemia is followed initially by a transient period of increased blood flow, "reactive hyperaemia", which rapidly returns to normal. Blood flow may subsequently decline over a period of hours to levels significantly lower than that prior to occlusion despite adequate perfusion pressure. This phenomenon has been termed "no-reflow" and was first described in the brain (Ames *et al.*, 1968). Subsequent studies have described the characteristic features of a slowly developing state of underperfusion following reperfusion of ischaemic tissue in a number of other organs, including heart and skeletal muscle. The mechanisms involved in this condition have not been definitively determined. Amongst the proposed mechanisms are tissue oedema causing compression of arterioles or capillaries (Flores *et al.*, 1972; Kloner *et al.*, 1974), swelling of endothelial cells causing narrowing of capillaries (Kloner *et al.*, 1974) and occlusion of microvessels by haemorrhage (Higginson *et al.*, 1982). Neutrophils have also been implicated in no-reflow. Studies carried out in a model of ischaemia and reperfusion of dog myocardium found that depletion of circulating neutrophils protected against the fall in blood flow (Schmid-Schonbein and Engler, 1986; Litt *et al.*, 1989). Neutrophils have a larger diameter than the lumen of capillaries, consequently these cells have to distort their shape in order to pass through the vessels. Furthermore, compared with red blood cells, neutrophils have a high degree of cytoskeletal stiffness, which increases when the cells are activated (Worthen *et al.*, 1989). These properties result in the transcapillary transit

time of these leucocytes being considerably greater than that of erythrocytes. It has been suggested that, under conditions of reduced perfusion pressure, neutrophils may become lodged in capillaries and thereby reduce tissue perfusion. There is some evidence in support of this hypothesis. Using carbon black, Engler *et al.* (1983) demonstrated histologically that capillaries which were not perfused with the colloid contained trapped neutrophils. In a model of haemorrhagic shock, plugging of capillaries by neutrophils was observed in skeletal muscle using intravital microscopy (Bagge *et al.*, 1980). However, there was no indication that neutrophils were firmly attached to the capillary wall in that study and, in a model of no-reflow in skeletal muscle, leucocyte plugging of capillaries was rarely observed (Menger *et al.* 1992). Furthermore, in some other studies it was reported that interventions depleting circulating neutrophils did not protect against no-reflow (de Lorgeril *et al.*, 1989) so the involvement of this leucocyte is not definitively established. As yet the clinical significance of no-reflow has not been established. A residual perfusion deficit could result in further ischaemic injury to the tissue, however, it has been shown that it only occurs in regions of tissue which have already suffered extensive damage (Ambrosio *et al.*, 1989).

6. *Conclusion*

Reperfusion injury has long been recognized in experimental models but, with the development of techniques such as thrombolysis, the clinical importance of this phenomenon has become more apparent. The large body of experimental data implicating neutrophils in the development of reperfusion injury suggests that interventions which inhibit the accumulation of these cells may provide a beneficial adjunct to thrombolytic therapy. One promising approach is the development of mAbs to adhesion molecules either on neutrophils themselves or to the ligands on the vascular endothelium. However, as yet only the acute effects of such interventions in models of ischaemia and reperfusion have been evaluated. Before such interventions could be introduced into clinical practice, it would be necessary to ensure that they had no detrimental effect on the later phases of the inflammatory response, such as monocyte infiltration, which might compromise wound repair and scar formation.

7. *References*

Ambrosio, G., Weisman, H.F., Mannisi, J.A. and Becker, L.C. (1989). Progressive impairment of regional myocardial perfusion after initial restoration of postischemic blood flow. Circ. Res. 80, 1846–1861.

Ames, A., Wright, R.L., Kowada, M., Thurston, J.M. and Majno, G. (1968). Cerebral ischemia: II. The no reflow phenomenon. Am. J. Pathol. 52, 437–453.

Anner, H., Kaufman, R.P., Kobzik, L., Valeri, C.R., Shepro, D. and Hechtman, H.B. (1987). Pulmonary leukosequestration induced by hind limb ischemia. Ann. Surg. 206, 162–167.

Arfors, K.-E., Lundberg, C., Lindbom, L., Lundberg, K., Beatty, P.G. and Harlan, J.M. (1987). A monoclonal antibody to the membrane glycoprotein complex CD18 inhibits polymorphonuclear leukocyte accumulation and plasma leakage in vivo. Blood 69, 338–340.

Arnaout, M.A., Spits, H. Terhorst, C., Pitt, J. and Todd, R.F. (1984). Deficiency of a leukocyte surface glycoprotein (LFA-1) in two patients with Mo 1 deficiency. Effects of cell activation on Mo 1/LFA-1 surface expression in normal and deficient leukocytes. J. Clin. Invest. 74, 1291–1300.

Bagge, U., Amundson, B. and Lauritzen, C. (1980). White blood cell deformability and plugging of skeletal muscle capillaries in hemorrhagic shock. Acta Physiol. Scand. 180, 159–163.

Beatty, P.G., Ledbetter, J.A., Martin, P.J., Price, T.H. and Hansen, J.A. (1983). Definition of a common leukocyte cell-surface antigen (Lp95-150) associated with diverse cell-mediated immune functions. J. Immunol. 131, 2913–2918.

Beaubien, B.C., Collins, P.D., Jose, P.J., Totty, N.F., Waterfield, M.D., Hsuan, J. and Williams, T.J. (1990). A novel neutrophil chemoattractant generated during an inflammatory reaction in the rabbit peritoneal cavity in vivo: purification, partial amino acid sequence and structural relationship to interleukin 8. Biochem. J. 271, 797–801.

Bednar, M., Smith, B., Pinto, A. and Mullane, K.M. (1985). Nafazatrom-induced salvage of ischemic myocardium in anaesthetized dogs is mediated through inhibition of neutrophil function. Circ. Res. 57, 131–141.

Belkin, M., LaMorte, W.L., Wright, J.G. and Hobson, R.W. (1989). The role of leukocytes in the pathophysiology of skeletal muscle ischemic injury. J. Vasc. Surg. 10, 14–18.

Bjork, J., Hedquist, P. and Arfors, K.-E. (1982). Increase in vascular permeability induced by leukotriene B4 and the role of polymorphonuclear leukocytes. Inflammation 6, 189–200.

Bonow, R.O., Lipson, L.C., Sheehan, F.H. Capurro, N.L. Isner, J.M., Roberts, W.C., Goldstein, R.E. and Epstein, S.E. (1981). Lack of effect of aspirin on myocardial infarct size in the dog. Am. J. Cardiol. 258–264.

Borgeat, P. and Samuelsson, B. (1979). Arachidonic acid metabolism in polymorphonuclear leukocytes: effects of ionophore A23187. Proc. Natl Acad. Sci. USA 76, 2148–2152.

Braunwald, E. and Kloner, R.A. (1985). Myocardial reperfusion: a double-edged sword? J. Clin. Invest. 76, 1713–1719.

Carden, D.L., Smith, J.K. and Korthuis, R.J. (1990) Neutrophil-mediated microvascular dysfunction in postischemic canine skeletal muscle. Role of granulocyte adherence. Circ. Res. 66, 1436–1444.

Carp, H. and Janoff, A. (1980). Potential mediator of inflammation. Phagocyte-derived oxidants suppress the elastase-inhibitory capacity of alpha1-proteinase inhibitor in vitro. J. Clin. Invest. 66, 987–995.

Caty, M.G., Guice, K.S., Oldham, K.T., Remick, D.G. and Kunkel, S.I. (1990). Evidence for tumor necrosis factor-induced pulmonary microvascular injury after intestinal ischemia–reperfusion injury. Ann. Surg. 212, 694–700.

Chatelain, P., Latour, J.-G., Tran, D., de Lorgeril, D., Dupras, G. and Bourassa, M. (1987). Neutrophil accumulation in experimental myocardial infarcts: relation with extent of injury and effect of reperfusion. Circulation 75, 1083–1090.

Colditz, I., Zwahlen, R., Dewald, B. and Baggiolini, M. (1989). In vivo inflammatory activity of neutrophil-activating factor, a novel chemotactic peptide derived from human monocytes. Am. J. Pathol. 134, 755–760.

Colletti, L.M., Remick, D.G., Burtch, G.D., Kunkel, S.L., Strieter, R.M. and Campbell, D.A. (1990). Role of tumor necrosis factor-α in the pathophysiologic alterations after hepatic ischemia/reperfusion injury in the rat. J. Clin. Invest. 85, 1936–1943.

Collins, P.D., Jose, P.J. and Williams, T.J. (1991). The sequential generation of neutrophil chemoattractant proteins in acute inflammation in the rabbit in vivo: relationship between C5a and a protein with the characteristics of IL-8. J. Immunol. 146, 677–684.

Crowley, C.A., Curnutte, J.T., Rosin, R.E., Andre-Schwartz, J., Gallin, J.I., Klempner, M., Snyderman, R., Southwick, F.S., Stossel, T.P. and Babior, B.M. (1980). An inherited abnormality of neutrophil adhesion. Its genetic transmission and its association with missing protein. N. Engl. J. Med. 302, 1163–1168.

Dahlen, S.-E., Bjork, J., Hedquist, P., Arfors, K,E. Hammarstrom, S., Lindgren, J.-A. and Samuelsson, B. (1981). Leukotrienes promote plasma leakage and leukocyte adhesion in post capillary venules. In vivo effects with relevance to the acute inflammatory response. Proc. Natl Acad. Sci. USA 78, 3887–3891.

de Lorgeril, M., Basmadjian, A., Lavallee, M., Clement, R., Millette, D., Rousseau, G. and Latour, J.-G. (1989). Influence of leukopenia on collateral flow, reperfusion flow, reflow ventricular fibrillation, and infarct size in dogs. Am. Heart J. 117, 523–532.

Deeb, G.M., Grum, C.M., Lynch, M.J., Guynn, T.P., Gallagher, K.P., Ljungman, A.G., Bolling, S.F. and Morganroth, M.L. (1990). Neutrophils are not necessary for induction of ischemia–reperfusion lung injury. J. Appl. Physiol. 68, 374–381.

Dreyer, W.J., Smith, C.W., Michael, L.H., Rossen, R.D., Hughes, B.J., Entman, M.L. and Anderson, D.C. (1989). Canine neutrophil activation by cardiac lymph obtained during reperfusion of ischemic myocardium. Circ. Res. 65, 1751–1762.

Dreyer, W.J., Michael, L.H., West, S., Smith, C.W., Rothlein, R., Rossen, R.D., Anderson, D.C. and Entman, M.L. (1991). Neutrophil accumulation in ischemic canine myocardium. Insights into time course, distribution, and mechanism of localization during early reperfusion. Circulation 84, 400–411.

Engler, R. and Covell, J.W. (1987). Granulocytes cause reperfusion ventricular dysfunction after 15-minute ischemia in the dog. Circ. Res. 61, 20–28.

Engler, R.L., Schmid-Schonbein, G.W. and Pavelec, R.S. (1983). Leukocyte capillary plugging in myocardial ischemia and reperfusion in the dog. Am. J. Pathol. 111, 98–111.

Engler, R.L., Dahlgren, M.D., Peterson, M.A., Dobbs, A. and Schmid-Schonbein, G.W. (1986). Accumulation of polymorphonuclear leukocytes during 3-h experimental myocardial ischemia. Am. J. Physiol. 251, H93–H100.

Entman, M.L., Youker, K., Shappell, S.B., Siegel, C., Rothlein, R., Dreyer, W.J., Schmalstieg, F.C. and Smith, C.W. (1990). Neutrophil adherence to isolated adult canine myocytes. Evidence for a CD18-dependent mechanism. J. Clin. Invest. 85, 1497–1506.

Entman, M.L., Michael, L., Rossen, R.D., Dreyer, W.J., Anderson, D.C., Taylor, A.A. and Smith, C.W. (1991). Inflammation in the course of early myocardial ischaemia. FASEB J. 5, 2529–2537.

Farber, N.E., Pieper, G.M., Thomas, J.P. and Gross, G.J. (1988). Beneficial effects of iloprost in the stunned canine myocardium. Circ. Res. 62, 204–215.

Fishbein, M.C., Maclean, D. and Maroko, P.R. (1978). The histopathologic evolution of myocardial infarction. Chest 73, 843–849.

Flores, J., DiBona, D.R., Beck, C.H. and Leaf, A. (1972). The role of cell swelling in ischemic renal damage and the protective effect of hypertonic solute. J. Clin. Invest. 51, 118–125.

Ford-Hutchinson, A.W., Bray, M.A., Doig, M.V., Shipley, M.E. and Smith, M.J.H. (1980). Leukotriene B, a potent chemokinetic and aggregating substance released from polymorphonuclear leukocytes. Nature 286, 264–265.

Freeman, B.A. and Crapo, J.D. (1982). Biology of disease. Free radicals and tissue injury. Lab. Invest. 47, 412–426.

Go, L.O., Murry, C.E., Richard, V.J., Weischedel, G.R., Jennings, R.B. and Reimer, K.A. (1988). Myocardial neutrophil accumulation during reperfusion after reversible or irreversible ischemic injury. Am. J. Physiol. 255, H1188–H1198.

Grisham, M.B., Hernandez, L.A. and Granger, D.N. (1986). Xanthine oxidase and neutrophil infiltration in intestinal ischemia. Am. J. Physiol. 251, G567–G574.

Hahn, R.A., MacDonald, B.R. Simpson, P.J., Potts, B.D. and Parli, C.J. (1990). Antagonism of leukotriene B$_4$ receptors does not limit canine myocardial infarct size. J. Pharmacol. Exp. Ther. 253, 58–66.

Harlan, J.M. (1985). Leukocyte-endothelial interactions. Blood 65, 513–525.

Harlan, M., Schwartz, B.R., Reidy, M.A., Schwartz, S.M., Ochs, H.D. and Harker, L.A. (1985). Activated neutrophils disrupt endothelial monolayer integrity by an oxygen radical-independent mechanism. Lab. Invest. 52, 141–150.

Harnarayan, C., Bennett, M.A., Pentecost, B.L. and Brewer, D.B. (1970). Quantitative study of infarcted myocardium in cardiogenic shock. Br. Heart J. 32, 728–732.

Harrison, J.E. and Schultz, J. (1976). Studies on the chlorinating activity of myeloperoxidase. J. Biol. Chem. 251, 1371–1374.

Hartmann, J.R., Robinson, J.A. and Gunnar, R.M. (1977). Chemotactic activity in the coronary sinus after experimental myocardial infarction: effects of pharmacologic interventions on ischemic injury. Am. J. Cardiol. 40, 550–555.

Hearse, D.J. and Bolli, R. (1991). Reperfusion-induced injury. Manifestations, mechanisms, and clinical relevance. Trends Cardiovasc. Med. 1, 233–240.

Hernandez, L.A., Grisham, M.B., Twohig, B., Arfors, K.E., Harlan, J.M. and Granger, D.N. (1987). Role of neutrophils in ischemia–reperfusion-induced microvascular injury. Am. J. Physiol. 253, 699–703.

Heyndrickx, G.R., Millard, R.W., McRitchie, R.J., Maroko, P.R. and Vatner, S.F. (1975). Regional myocardial functional and electrophysiological alterations after brief coronary artery occlusion in conscious dogs. J. Clin. Invest. 56, 978–985.

Higginson, L.A.J., White, F., Heggtveit, H.A., Sanders, T.M., Bloor, C.M. and Covell, J.W. (1982). Determinants of myocardial hemorrhage after coronary reperfusion in the anesthetized dog. Circulation 65, 62–69.

Higgs, G.A. Salmon, J.A. and Spayne, J.A. (1981). The inflammatory effects of hydroxyperoxy and hydroxy acid products of arachidonate lipoxygenase in rabbit skin. Br. J. Pharmacol. 74, 429–433.

Horgan, M.J., Wright, S.D. and Malik, A.B. (1990). Antibody against leukocyte integrin (CD18) prevents reperfusion-induced lung vascular injury. Am. J. Physiol. 259, L315–L319.

Horgan, M.J., Ge, M., Gu, J., Rothlein, R. and Malik, A.B. (1991). Role of ICAM-1 in neutrophil-mediated lung vascular injury after occlusion and reperfusion. Am. J. Physiol. 261, H1578–1584.

ISIS-2 Collaborative Group (1988). Randomised trial of intravenous streptokinase, oral aspirin, both, or neither among 17187 cases of suspected acute myocardial infarction: ISIS-2. Lancet ii, 349–360.

Jaeschke, H., Farhood, A. and Smitlh, C.W. (1990). Neutrophils contribute to ischemia/reperfusion injury in rat liver in vivo. FASEB J. 4, 3355–3359.

Jennings, R.B. and Reimer, K.A. (1983). Factors involved in salvaging ischemic myocardium: effect of reperfusion of arterial blood. Circulation 68, 25–36.

Jeremy, R.W. and Becker, L.C. (1989). Neutrophil depletion does not prevent myocardial dysfunction after brief coronary occlusion. J. Am. Coll. Cardiol. 13 1155–1163.

Jolly, S.R., Kane, W.J., Hook, B.G., Abrams, G.D., Kunkel, S.L. and Lucchesi, B.R. (1986). Reduction of myocardial infarct size by neutrophil depletion: effect of duration of occlusion. Am. Heart J. 112, 682–690.

Jose, P.J., Collins, P.D., Perkins, J.A., Beaubien, B.C., Totty, N.F, Waterfield, M.D., Hsuan, J. and Williams, T.J. (1991). Identification of a second neutrophil chemoattractant cytokine generated during an inflammatory reaction in the rabbit peritoneal cavity in vivo: purification, partial amino acid sequence and structural relationship to melanoma growth stimulatory activity. Biochem. J. 278, 493–497.

Jugdutt, B.I., Hutchins, G.M., Bulkley, B.H., Pitt, B. and Becker, L.C. (1979). Effect of indomethacin on collateral blood flow and infarct size in the conscious dog. Circulation 4, 734–743.

Kamikubo, Y. Yasuda, K. and Uede, T. (1993). Cytokines gene expression in post-ischemic reperfusion injury of cardiac tissues. J. Immunol. 150, 139A.

Karasawa, A., Guo, J.-P. Ma, X.-L. Tsao, P.S. and Lefer, A.M. (1991). Protective actions of a leukotriene B$_4$ antagonist in splanchnic ischemia and reperfusion in rats. Am. J. Physiol. 193, G191–G198.

Klausner, J.M., Anner, H., Paterson, I.S., Kobzik, L., Valeri, C.R., Shepro, D. and Hechtman, H.B. (1988). Lower torso ischemia-induced lung injury is leukocyte dependent. Ann. Surg. 208, 761–767.

Klausner, J.M., Paterson, I.S., Goldman, G., Kobzik, L., Rodzen, C., Lawrence, R., Valeri, C.R., Shepro, D. and Hechtman, H.B. (1989). Postischemic renal injury is mediated by neutrophils and leukotrienes. Am. J. Physiol. 256, F794–F802.

Kloner, R.A., Ganote, C.E. and Jennings, R.B. (1974). The "no-reflow" phenomenon after temporary coronary occlusion in the dog. J. Clin. Invest. 54, 1496–1508.

Korthuis, R.J., Grisham, M.B. and Granger, D.N. (1988). Leukocyte depletion attenuates vascular injury in post ischemic skeletal muscle. Am. J. Physiol. 254, H823–H827.

Kubes, P., Ibbotson, G., Russell, J., Wallace, J.L. and Granger, D.N. (1990). Role of platelet-activating factor in ischemia/reperfusion-induced leukocyte adherence. Am. J. Physiol. 259, G300–G305.

Langlois, P.F. and Gawryl, M.S. (1988). Detection of the terminal complement complex in patient plasma following acute myocardial infarction. Atherosclerosis 70, 95–105.

Litt, M.R., Jeremy, R.W., Weisman, H.F., Winkelstein, J.A. and Becker, L.C. (1989). Neutrophil depletion limited to reperfusion reduces myocardial infarct size after 90 minutes of ischemia. Evidence for neutrophil-mediated reperfusion injury. Circulation 80, 1816–1827.

Ma, X.-L., Tsao, P.S. and Lefer, A.M. (1991). Antibody to CD-18 exerts endothelial and cardiac protective effects in myocardial ischemia and reperfusion. J. Clin. Invest. 88, 1237–1243.

Maclean, D., Fishbein, M.C., Braunwald, E. and Maroko, P.R. (1978). Long term preservation of ischaemic myocardium after experimental coronary artery occlusion. J. Clin. Invest. 61, 541–551.

Majno, G., Schoefl, G.I. and Palade, G. (1961). Studies on inflammation. The site of action of histamine and serotonin on the vascular tree; a topographic study. J. Cell Biol. 11, 607–626.

Mallory, G.K., White, P.D. and Salcedo-Salgar, J. (1939). The speed of healing of myocardial infarction. A study of the pathologic anatomy in seventy-two cases. Am. Heart J. 18, 647–671.

Manning, A.M., Kukielka, G.L., Dore, M., Hawkins, H.K., Sanders, W.E., Michael, L.H., Entman, M.L., Smith, C.W. and Anderson, D.C. (1992). Regulation of GMP-140 mRNA in a canine model of inflammation. FASEB J. 6, 720.

Maroko, P.R., Carpenter, C.B., Chiariello, M., Fishbein, M.C., Radvany, P., Knostman, J.D. and Hale, S.L. (1978). Reduction by cobra venom factor of myocardial necrosis after coronary artery occlusion. J. Clin. Invest. 61, 661–670.

McManus, L.M., Kolb, W.P., Crawford, M.H., O'Rourke, R.A., Grover, F.L. and Pinckard, R.N. (1983). Complement localization in ischemic baboon myocardium. Lab. Invest. 48, 436–447.

Menger, M.D., Steiner, D. and Messmer, K. (1992). Microvascular ischemia–reperfusion injury in striated muscle: significance of "no reflow". Am. J. Physiol. 263, H1892–H1900.

Miller, S.H., Price, G., Buck, D., Neeley, J., Kennedy, T.J., Draham, W.P. and Davis, T.S. (1979). Effects of tourniquet ischemia and postischemic edema on muscle metabolism. J. Hand Surgery 4, 547–555.

Montrucchio, G., Alloatti, G., Mariano, F., de Paulis, R., Comino, A., Emanuelli, G. and Camussi, G. (1990). Role of platelet-activating factor in the reperfusion injury of rabbit ischemic heart. Am. J. Pathol. 137, 71–83.

Mullane, K.M. Read, N., Salmon, J.A. and Moncada, S. (1984). Role of leukocytes in acute myocardial infarction in anesthetized dogs: relationship to myocardial salvage by anti-inflammatory drugs. J. Pharmacol. Exp. Ther. 228, 510–522.

Mullane, K., Hatala, M.A., Kraemer, R., Sesa, W. and Westlin, W. (1987). Myocardial salvage induced by REV-5901: An inhibitor and antagonist of the leukotrienes. J. Cardiovasc. Pharmacol. 10, 398–406.

Nourshargh, S., Rampart, M., Hellewell, P.G., Jose, P.J., Harlan, J.M., Edwards, A.J. and Williams, T.J. (1989). Accumulation of ^{111}In-neutrophils in rabbit skin in allergic and non-allergic inflammatory reactions in vivo: inhibition by neutrophil pretreatment in vitro with a monoclonal antibody recognising the CD18 antigen. J. Immunol. 142, 3193–3198.

O'Neill, P.G., Charlat, M.L., Michael, L.H., Roberts, R. and Bolli, R. (1989). Influence of neutrophil depletion on myocardial function and flow after reversible ischemia. Am. J. Physiol. 256, H341–H351.

Opie, E.L. (1922). Intracellular digestion. The enzymes and antienzymes concerned. Physiol. Rev. 2, 552–585.

Page, D.L., Caulfield, J.B., Kastor, J.A., DeSanctis, R.W. and Sanders, C.A. (1971). Myocardial changes associated with cardiogenic shock. N. Engl J. Med. 285, 133–137.

Parks, D.A. and Granger, D.N. (1986). Contributions of ischemia and reperfusion to mucosal lesion formation. Am. J. Physiol. 250, G749–753.

Paterson, I.S., Klausner, J.M., Pugatch, R., Allen, P., Mannick, J.A., Shepro, D. and Hechtman, H.B. (1989). Noncardiogenic pulmonary edema after abdominal aortic aneurysm surgery. Ann. Surg. 209, 231–236.

Reimer, K.A., Jennings, R.B., Cobb, F.R., Murdock, R.H., Greenfield, J.C., Becker, L.C., Bulkley, B.R., Hutchins, G.M., Schwartz, R.P., Bailey, K.R. and Passamani, E.R. (1985). Animal models for protecting ischemic myocardium: results of the NHLBI cooperative study. Comparison of unconscious and conscious dog models. Circ. Res. 56, 651–665.

Reimer, K.A., Murry, C.E. and Richard, V.J. (1989). The role of neutrophils and free radicals in the ischemic-reperfused heart: why the confusion and controversy? J. Mol. Cell. Cardiol. 21, 1225–1239.

Romson, J.L., Hook, B.G., Rigot, V.H., Schork, M.A., Swanson, D.P. and Lucchesi, B.R. (1982). The effect of ibuprofen on accumulation of indium-111-labelled platelets and leukocytes in experimental myocardial infarction. Circulation 66, 1002–1011.

Romson, J.L., Hook, B.G., Kunkel, S.L., Abrams, G.D., Schork, M.A. and Lucchesi, B.R. (1983). Reduction of the extent of ischemic myocardial injury by neutrophil depletion in the dog. Circulation 67, 1016–1023.

Rossen, R.D., Swain, J.L., Michael, L.H., Weakley, S., Giannini, E. and Entman, M.L. (1985). Selective accumulation of the first component of complement and leukocytes in ischemic canine heart muscle: a possible initiator of an extramyocardial mechanism of ischemic injury. Circ. Res. 57, 119–130.

Sasaki, K., Ueno, A., Katori, M. and Kikawada, R. (1988). Detection of leukotriene B4 in cardiac tissue and its role in infarct extension through leucocyte migration. Cardiovasc. Res. 22, 142–148.

Schafer, H., Mathey, D., Hugo, F. and Bhakdi, S. (1986). Deposition of the terminal C5b-9 complement complex in infarcted areas of human myocardium. J. Immunol. 137, 1945–1949.

Schmeling, D.J., Caty, M.G., Oldham, K.T., Guice, K.S. and Hinshaw, D.B. (1989). Evidence for neutrophil-related acute lung injury after intestinal ischemia-reperfusion. Surgery 106, 195–202.

Schmid-Schonbein, G.W. and Engler, R.L. (1986). Granulocytes as active participants in acute myocardial ischemia and infarction. Am. J. Cardiovasc. Path. 1, 15–30.

Schroder, J.-M., Mrowietz, U., Morita, E. and Christophers, E. (1987). Purification and partial biochemical characterization of a human monocyte-derived, neutrophil activating peptide that lacks interleukin 1 activity. J. Immunol. 139, 3474–3483.

Seewaldt-Becker, E., Rothlein, R. and Dammgen, J.W. (1990). In "Leukocyte adhesion molecules" (eds T.A. Springer, D.C. Anderson, A.S. Rosenthal and R. Rothlein), pp. 138–148. Springer-Verlag, New York.

Simpson, P.J., Mickelson, J., Fantone, J.C., Gallagher, K.P. and Lucchesi, B.R. (1987a). Ilprost inhibits neutrophil function in vitro and in vivo and limits experimental infarct size in canine heart. Circ. Res. 60, 666–673.

Simpson, P.J., Mitsos, S.E., Ventura, A., Gallagher, K.P., Fantone, J.C., Abram, G.D., Schork, M.A. and Lucchesi, B.R. (1987b). Prostacyclin protects ischemic reperfused myocardium in the dog by inhibition of neutrophil activation. Am. Heart J. 113, 129–137.

Simpson, P.J., Mickelson, J., Fantone, J.C., Gallagher, K.P. and Lucchesi, B.R. (1988a). Reduction of experimental canine myocardial infarct size with prostaglandin E_1: inhibition of neutrophil migration and activation. J. Pharmacol. Exp. Ther. 244, 619–624.

Simpson, P.J., Todd, F.R., III, Fantone, J.C., Michelson, J.K., Griffin, J.D. and Lucchesi, B.R. (1988b). Reduction of experimental canine myocardial reperfusion injury by a monoclonal antibody (Anti-Mol, Anti-CD11b) that inhibits leukocyte adhesion. J. Clin. Invest. 81, 624–629.

Smedly, L.A., Tonnesen, M.G., Sandhaus, R.A., Haslett, C., Guthrie, L.A., Johnston, R.B., Jr., Henson, P.M. and Worthen, G.S. (1986). Neutrophil-mediated injury to endothelial cells. Enhancement by endotoxin and essential role of neutrophil elastase. J. Clin. Invest. 77, 1233–1243.

Smith, C.W., Entman, M.L., Lane, C.L., Beaudet, A.L., Ty, T.I., Youker, K., Hawkins, H.K. and Anderson, D.C. (1991). Adherence of neutrophils to canine cardiac myocytes in vitro is dependent on intercellular adhesion molecule-1. J. Clin. Invest. 88, 1216–1223.

Snyderman, R., Phillips, J. and Mergenhagen, S.E. (1970). Polymorphonuclear leukocyte chemotactic activity in rabbit serum and guinea pig serum treated with immune complexes: evidence for C5a as the major chemotactic factor. Infect. Immun. 1, 521–525.

Sommers, H.M. and Jennings, R.B. (1964). Experimental acute myocardial infarction. Histologic and histochemical studies of early myocardial infarcts induced by temporary or permanent occlusion of a coronary artery. Lab. Invest. 13, 1491–1503.

Springer, T.A. (1990). Adhesion receptors of the immune system. Nature 346, 425–434.

Stahl, G.L., Terashita, Z.-I. and Lefer, A.M. (1988). Role of platelet activating factor in propagation of cardiac damage during myocardial ischemia. J. Pharmacol. Exp. Ther. 244, 898–904.

Taylor, A.A. Gasic, A.C., Kitt, T.M., Shappell, S.B., Rui, J., Lenz, M.L., Smith, C.W. and Mitchell, J.R. (1989). A specific leukotriene B4 antagonist protects against myocardial ischemia–reflow injury. Clin. Res. 37, 528A.

Thornton, M.A., Winn, R., Alpers, C.E. and Zager, R.A. (1989). An evaluation of the neutrophil as a mediator of in vivo renal ischemic–reperfusion injury. Am. J. Pathol. 135, 509–515.

Van de Werf, F. and Arnold, A.E.R. (1988). Intravenous tissue plasminogen activator and size of infarct, left ventricular function, and survival in acute myocardial infarction. Br. Med. J. 297, 1374–1379.

Vedder, N.B., Winn, R.K., Rice, C.L., Chi, E.Y., Arfors, K.E. and Harber, J. M. (1988). A monoclonal antibody to the adherence-promoting leukocyte glycoprotein, CD18, reduces organ injury and improves survival from hemorrhagic shock and resuscitation in rabbits. J. Clin. Invest. 81, 939–944.

Vedder, N.B., Winn, R.K., Rice, C.L., Chi, E.Y., Arfors, K.E. and Harlan, J.M. (1990). Inhibition of leukocyte adherence by anti-CD18 monoclonal antibody attenuates reperfusion injury in the rabbit ear. Proc. Natl Acad. Sci. USA 87, 2643–2646.

Walz, A., Peveri, P., Aschauer, H. and Baggiolini, M. (1987). Purification and amino acid sequencing of NAF, a novel neutrophil-activating factor produced by monocytes. Biochem. Biophys. Res. Commun. 149, 755–761.

Wedmore, C.V. and Williams, T.J. (1981). Control of vascular permeability by polymorphonuclear leukocytes in inflammation. Nature 289, 646–650.

Weisman, H.F., Bartow, T., Leppo, M.K., Marsh, H.C., Carson, G.R., Concino, M.F., Boyle, M.P., Roux, K.H., Weisfeldt, M.L. and Fearon, D.T. (1990). Soluble human complement receptor type 1: in vivo inhibitor of complement suppressing post-ischemic myocardial inflammation and necrosis. Science 249, 146–151.

Weiss, S.J. (1989). Tissue destruction by neutrophils. N. Engl. J. Med. 320, 365–375.

Weiss, S.J. and Peppin, G.J. (1986). Collagenolytic metalloenzymes of the human neutrophil: characteristics, regulation and potential function in vivo. Biochem. Pharmacol. 35, 3189–3197.

Weiss, S.J., Peppin, G., Ortiz, X., Ragsdale, C. and Test, S.T. (1985). Oxidative autoactivation of latent collagenase by human neutrophils. Science 227, 747–749.

Welbourn, C.R.B., Goldman, G., Paterson, I.S., Valeri, C.R., Shepro, D. and Hechtman, H.B. (1991). Neutrophil elastase and oxygen radicals: synergism in lung injury after hindlimb ischemia. Am. J. Physiol. 260, H1852–H1856.

Westlin, W. and Mullane, K.M. (1989). Alleviation of myocardial stunning by leukocyte and platelet depletion. Circulation 80, 1828–1836.

Williams, F.M., Collins, P.D., Tanniere-Zeller, M. and Williams, T.J. (1990). The relationship between neutrophils and increased microvascular permeability in a model of myocardial ischaemia and reperfusion in the rabbit. Br. J. Pharmacol. 100, 729–734.

Worthen, G.S., Elson, E.L. and Downey, G.P. (1989). Mechanics of stimulated neutrophils: cell stiffening induces retention in capillaries. Science 245, 183–186.

Yoshimura, T., Matsushima, K., Tanaka, S., Robinson, E.A., Appella, E., Oppenheim, J.J. and Leonard, E.J. (1987). Purification of a human monocyte-derived neutrophil chemotactic factor that has peptide sequence similarity to other host defense cytokines. Proc. Natl Acad. Sci. USA 84, 9233–9237.

Youker, K., Smith, C.W., Anderson, D.C., Miller, D., Michael, L.H., Rossen, R.D. and Entman, M.L. (1992). Neutrophil adherence to isolated cardiac myocytes – induction by cardiac lymph collected during ischaemia and reperfusion. J. Clin. Invest. 89, 602–609.

Zimmerman, B.J., Grisham, M.B. and Granger, D.N. (1990). Role of oxidants in ischemia/reperfusion-induced granulocyte infiltration. Am. J. Physiol. 258, G185–G190.

12. Role of Neutrophils in Vasculitis

Caroline O.S. Savage and Andrew J. Rees

1. Introduction

Vasculitis can be defined as an inflammatory reaction affecting blood vessels. Typically it is associated with neutrophil and mononuclear leucocyte infiltration and often with necrosis of the vessel wall itself (Churg and Churg, 1989) (Figure 12.1). Vasculitis is often widespread and associated clinically with systemic disease and injury to many organs.

Vasculitis has been associated with two types of humoral (antibody) responses. Historically, serum sickness developing after repeated injections of foreign protein was characterized by widespread vasculitis both clinically and in experimental models (Dixon *et al.*, 1958). Neutrophil depletion abrogated vasculitis in such models which were believed to be caused by deposition of circulating immune complexes. There is no evidence for involvement of immune complexes in most types of systemic vasculitis including Wegener's granulomatosis, Churg–Strauss syndrome and microscopic polyarteritis, but neutrophils have recently become the focus of attention for another reason. Serum from patients with these diseases contain anti-neutrophil cytoplasm antibodies, or ANCA, that bind to components of neutrophil granules. This is in marked contrast to the situation with immune-complex-associated vasculitis. As there are no appropriate

Immunopharmacology of Neutrophils
ISBN 0–12–339250–0

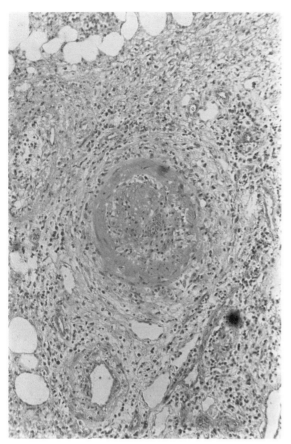

Figure 12.1 Systemic vasculitis in a patient with microscopic polyarteritis showing fibrinoid necrosis with intense neutrophil infiltration.

animal models of ANCA-associated vasculitis, almost all of the evidence for a major role of the neutrophil in these diseases has been obtained by careful clinical studies or from *in vitro* studies using human-derived material (see Note added in proof).

In this chapter, we shall focus on the role of the neutrophil in ANCA-associated primary systemic vasculitides in humans because the role of neutrophils in experimental immune-complex vasculitis has been extensively reviewed elsewhere (Cochrane and Koffler, 1973) and is of uncertain relevance to man.

2. Clinical Syndromes Associated with Vasculitis

The ANCA-associated systemic vasculitides are a group of disorders characterized by inflammation of vessel walls with neutrophil and mononuclear leucocyte infiltration and fibrinoid necrosis. Historically, the vasculitides were classified according to the presence or absence of granulomas and the size of vessel affected (Table 12.1). Interestingly, most patients classified in this way fall into

Table 12.1   Classification of systemic vasculitis

| Vessel size | Granulomas | |
	Absent	Present
Large	Takayasu's arteritis	
	Temporal arteritis	
Medium	Polyarteritis nodosa	Churg–Strauss syndrome
Small	Microscopic polyarteritis	Wegener's granulomatosis
	Kawasaki disease	
	Henoch–Schonlein purpura	

distinct clinical syndromes based on the pattern of organs involved and so the clinical classification of systemic vasculitides is reasonably consistent. However, new classifications incorporating recent data about ANCA of defined specificities is being discussed by an International Collaborative Study Group. It is worth emphasizing the aetiology of these diseases is unclear, and it is not even known whether the various clinical or pathological syndromes are caused by different agents or whether they are merely different responses to a single aetiological agent.

2.1 WEGENER'S GRANULOMATOSIS

Wegener's granulomatosis is a destructive necrotizing granulomatous vasculitis that affects the upper and lower respiratory tract as well as the kidneys (Fauci *et al.*, 1983). Other organs are often affected too as part of a multi-system disease but in some patients the disease appears to be confined to a single organ, such as the kidney ("idiopathic rapidly progressive glomerulonephritis") (Woodworth *et al.*, 1987), the lung ("limited Wegener's") (Carrington and Liebow, 1966), the eye (pseudotumour of the orbit), nasopharynx ("midline granuloma") or trachea ("subglottic stenosis") (Macfarlane *et al.*, 1983). The lungs are affected by granulomas and capillaritis affecting alveolar capillaries. Pulmonary haemorrhage is one of the more severe manifestations and the commonest cause of death in the acute stage. Renal involvement is usually manifested by focal segmental necrotizing glomerulonephritis, which frequently becomes crescentic. Clinically this results in rapidly progressive loss of renal function, associated with proteinuria, haematuria and cellular casts in the urine sediment.

In the absence of treatment, mortality from Wegener's granulomatosis is very high and more than 90% of affected individuals die within 2 years (Walton, 1958). The use of prednisolone and cyclophosphamide has dramatically changed this outlook and 5-year patient survival rates of greater than 80% are now generally achievable (Fauci *et al.*, 1983). Nevertheless, the disorder shows a strong tendency to relapse and so long-term monitoring is necessary. ANCA are valuable in the diagnosis and monitoring of Wegener's, as will be described.

2.2 MICROSCOPIC POLYARTERITIS

Microscopic polyarteritis is a multisystem necrotizing vasculitis affecting the kidney as well as other organs such as the lungs, skin, joints and eyes (Serra et al., 1984; Savage et al., 1985). The disease may be confined to the kidneys and is another cause of "idiopathic rapidly progressive glomerulonephritis". Microscopic polyarteritis differs from Wegener's granulomatosis by the absence of destructive granulomata (Rosen et al., 1991), by a lesser tendency to relapse following successful treatment of the acute episode and by the neutrophil antigenic targets that are recognized by ANCA (Gaskin et al., 1991b). Even so, treatment is with prednisolone and cyclophosphamide.

2.3 CHURG–STRAUSS SYNDROME

Churg–Strauss syndrome is the least common of the major primary systemic vasculitic syndromes associated with ANCA. This vasculitic syndrome was originally defined by the triad of fever, eosinophilia and asthma (Churg and Strauss, 1951). Although these are prominent, vasculitis may also affect the heart, gastrointestinal tract, liver, kidneys and peripheral nerves (Lanham and Churg, 1991). The affected vessels tend to be larger than in Wegener's and microscopic polyarteritis, which partly explains the different emphasis of organ involvement. Large numbers of eosinophils infiltrate vessel walls and perivascular tissues, and are associated with granulomata.

2.4 OTHER PRIMARY SYSTEMIC VASCULITIDES

Other vasculitis syndromes include classical polyarteritis nodosa, hypersensitivity vasculitis, Henoch Schonlein purpura, Kawasaki disease, temporal or giant cell arteritis and Takayasu's disease.

Classical polyarteritis nodosa has frequently been confused with microscopic polyarteritis. It is a vasculitis of predominantly medium-sized muscular arteries that causes critical ischaemia to tissues including peripheral nerves, muscles, gut and kidney. Renal cortical ischaemia and infarcts cause severe hypertension. In addition there is an association with asthma suggesting an allergic element. Polyarteritis nodosa is more prevalent in areas with a high incidence of hepatitis B and this virus has been implicated in the development of polyarteritis nodosa (Gocke et al., 1970; Trepo et al., 1974). ANCA are sometimes found in patients with classical polyarteritis nodosa when there is accompanying glomerular capillaritis and neutrophils are often present in early vasculitic lesions.

Hypersensitivity vasculitis has been used to describe many different vasculitis syndromes, including microscopic polyarteritis, but is best restricted to acute non-systemic vasculitis affecting the skin; it is often associated with sensitivity to a drug or other agent. It affects capillaries and venules whose walls are infiltrated with neutrophils and surrounded by them.

Henoch Schonlein purpura and Kawasaki disease are predominantly diseases of children. Henoch Schonlein purpura affects skin on extensor surfaces and is strongly associated with deposits of IgA within the kidney; presence of IgA ANCA has been reported (van der Wall Bake et al., 1987) but this is controversial and IgA ANCA may be artefacts due to the presence of IgA rheumatoid factor. Kawasaki disease, or mucocutaneous syndrome, is an acute illness with fever, lymphadenopathy, palmar rash, mucous membrane ulcers and coronary artery vasculitis. The coronary vasculitis may be life threatening but prompt treatment with intravenous gamma globulin has greatly improved the outlook. Antibodies to neutrophil cytoplasm determinants have been described in a proportion of patients (Savage et al., 1989).

Finally, there are two forms of vasculitis that affect large arteries, namely temporal or giant cell arteritis and Takayasu's disease. They will not be further discussed except to indicate that a number of patients with giant cell arteritis have been reported to have circulating ANCA (McHugh et al., 1990), while only occasional patients with Takayasu's arteritis have been reported to have ANCA (Cohen Tervaert et al., 1989). The significance of these antibodies associated with giant cell arteritis is less clear than for Wegener's, microscopic polyarteritis and Churg–Strauss syndrome.

3. Histological Findings

3.1 WEGENER'S GRANULOMATOSIS

The lesions of Wegener's granulomatosis include extravascular destructive granulomatous lesions and vascular lesions (Lieberman and Churg, 1991). Granulomatous lesions are particularly evident in the upper and lower respiratory tracts. Their morphology in the upper tract can be difficult to distinguish from infection which is often superimposed. Granulomata in the lung usually show central necrosis with acellular material containing fragmented neutrophils. The necrosis is bordered by inflammatory cells including neutrophils, eosinophils, macrophages, multinucleated giant cells and lymphocytes. It has been suggested that aggregates of neutrophils with necrosis constitute the earliest lesions of Wegener's granulomatosis (Mark et al., 1988).

Three types of vascular lesion can be found in patients with Wegener's granulomatosis, namely microvasculitis, granulomatous vasculitis and vasculitis with fibrinoid necrosis (Churg and Churg, 1989). Pulmonary haemorrhage is a dramatic manifestation of micro-vasculitis in the lung. Arterioles, capillaries and venules are affected with intense neutrophil infiltration. In the skin a leucocytoclastic vasculitis can occur with mono-nuclear infiltration of small vessels. Focal and segmental necrotizing glomerulonephritis with crescent formation often develops in the kidney. The earliest lesion by light microscopy is capillary thrombosis followed by segmental necrosis of the tuft. Breaks in the glomerular wall lead to spilling of blood and fibrin into Bowman's space. Fibrin deposition in Bowman's space acts as a nidus into which monocytes migrate from the glomerular tuft and is associated with proliferation of parietal epithelial cells. Immunoglobulins are scanty or absent which has given rise to the semantically inappropriate term of "pauci-immune glomerulonephritis". Granulomatous vasculitis is less common and when it occurs tends to involve muscular arteries, often adjacent to necrotizing granulo-matous foci in the lung. Less commonly vasculitis develops in larger vessels which is similar to that associated with classical polyarteritis nodosa. It is characterized by fibrinoid necrosis, which sometimes causes infarction.

Histological studies show neutrophils in large numbers in many, if not all Wegener's lesions, suggesting they play a major pathogenic role. In fact, Donald et al. (1976) in an early ultrastructural study demonstrated lysed cells within capillary lumina together with large numbers of free nuclei and cytoplasm organelles; some of these cells appeared to be monocytes and others neutrophils. Endothelial cell necrosis also occurred with deposition of fibrin on bare basement membranes and disruption of the elastic laminae. Platelet aggregates were found adjacent to the ruptured cells. This prompted the prescient obser-vation that autoantibodies against neutrophils might be responsible (Donald et al., 1976).

3.2 MICROSCOPIC POLYARTERITIS

The histological features of the microscopic form of polyarteritis are similar to those of Wegener's granulo-matosis except for the absence of granulomatous lesions. Interestingly an extensive electron microscopic analysis of the renal vasculature and glomerular lesions in microscopic polyarteritis demonstrated that endothelial injury and subendothelial fibrin formation are the first definable ultrastructural changes (D'Agati et al., 1986). These were often associated with intraluminal accumu-lation of active-looking monocytes and polymorphs, together with focal leucocyte infiltration. However, endothelial changes were also found without morpho-logical evidence of leucocyte margination or infiltration, and this observation serves as a reminder that endothelial damage may be independent of cellular cytotoxic mechanisms.

3.3 CHURG–STRAUSS SYNDROME

Churg–Strauss syndrome is characterized pathologically by tissue infiltration by eosinophils, the formation of granulomas, and necrotizing vasculitis. The granulomas begin as areas of necrosis within dense foci of eosinophils which disintegrate and release their nuclear debris. Gradually macrophages and some giant cells arrive to surround the necrotic focus. Outside of this palisade are further inflammatory cells, mainly eosinophils.

The necrotizing arteritis affects small arteries, veins and sometimes medium-sized vessels. The arteritis progresses from intimal oedema, to intimal fibrinoid deposition with infiltration by eosinophils and granuloma formation around the vessel. The fibrinoid material often contains immunoglobulins and complement. Thrombosis of the vessel and aneurysmal dilatation of the weakened wall are common. These processes can involve any organ of the body, but the severity and distribution of the lesions varies widely between individuals.

The Churg–Strauss syndrome contrasts with Wegener's granulomatosis and microscopic polyarteritis in that the predominant inflammatory cell present is the eosinophil rather than the neutrophil, yet as will be discussed, anti-bodies to neutrophil cytoplasmic components are present in both.

4. Anti-neutrophil Cytoplasm Antibodies and their Targets

ANCA were first described by Davies et al. (1982) in a group of six Australian patients with crescentic glomerulonephritis thought to be associated with arbovirus infection. Two years later, Hall et al. (1984) described ANCA in patients with glomerulonephritis and associated vasculitis but it was not until 1985 that the link with Wegener's granulomatosis was formally demon-strated (Van der Woude et al., 1985). Presence of ANCA in microscopic polyarteritis and idiopathic rapidly progressive glomerulonephritis was reported by Savage et al. (1987).

ANCA were initially detected using an indirect immunofluorescence test on ethanol-fixed smears or cytospins of normal human peripheral blood neutrophils. Two different patterns of binding were recognized and in both cases the antigen was confined to neutrophils and monocytes (Figure 12.2). "Classical" or cANCA were the first to be described. They cause granular cytoplasmic staining seen more prominently between the lobes of the nuclei. This contrasts with staining from pANCA which occurs around the nuclei. The cANCA pattern is usually caused by antibodies to PR3 and the pANCA by anti-MPO antibodies (see Table 12.2 and below).

(a)

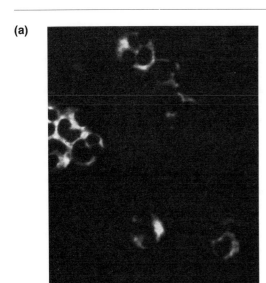

(b)

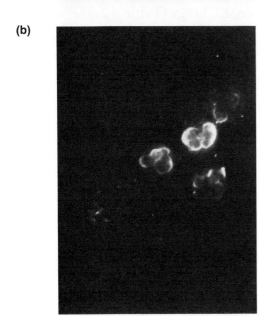

Figure 12.2 Positive tests for ANCA. (a) The typical cANCA pattern associated with specificity for PR3. (b) The pANCA pattern most frequently associated with antibodies to MPO.

Table 12.2   Major autoantigens recognized by ANCA

Immunofluorescent pattern	Antigen	Identification
pANCA perinuclear	MPO	ELISA Western blotting
cANCA cytoplasmic	PR3	Immunoprecipitation Western blotting N-terminal sequence PCR-amplification cDNA

localized in the primary (azurophilic) granules and released from cytochalasin B-treated neutrophils stimulated with chemotactic peptides such as FMLP (Goldschmeding *et al.*, 1989; Niles *et al.*, 1989; Ludemann *et al.*, 1990). Early studies showed that the 29 kD serine protease was distinct from elastase and CatG (Goldschmeding *et al.*, 1989) and subsequently, N-terminal amino-acid sequencing by Niles *et al.* (1989) and by Jenne *et al.* (1990) showed it to be the serine antibiotic protease p29b/AGP7 described by Gabay *et al.* (1989) and Wilde *et al.* (1990), and PR3 purified by Kao *et al.* (1988). PR3 had originally been described by Baggiolini *et al.* (1978) as having esterolytic activity as well as being a serine protein but this appears to have been due to contamination of his preparations with a second enzyme (Rao *et al.*, 1991). The N-terminal sequence of Kao's PR3 is identical to that of p29b described by Rao *et al.* (1991) and the only difference from the N-terminus of p29b/AGP7 is glutamic acid instead of glutamine at position 19; this is likely to be an artefact since it has not been confirmed by the p29b cDNA recently cloned from human bone marrow (Campanelli *et al.*, 1990). At the DNA level PR3 is identical to myeloblastin (Bories *et al.*, 1989) a factor involved in bone marrow cell maturation (see Section 6). The PR3 of Rao *et al.* (1991) binds cANCA (Jennette *et al.*, 1990). The antigen recognized by cANCA has also been purified to homogeneity using HPLC by Gaskin (unpublished); sequence data show that the antigen is PR3.

4.2   MYELOPEROXIDASE AS THE TARGET FOR pANCA

The autoantibodies responsible for pANCA have been shown to bind MPO by using solid phase ELISAs with purified enzyme. MPO, like PR3, is present within primary granules and so it is surprising that the fluorescence pattern was different from that associated with anti-PR3 antibodies. Falk and Jennette (1988) resolved this paradox by showing that the pattern was an *in vitro* artefact. Thus, MPO relocated to a perinuclear site within cells when neutrophils were fixed with ethanol but not when neutrophils were fixed with formalin–acetone.

4.1   PROTEINASE-3 AS THE TARGET FOR cANCA

Most cANCA bind to a 29 kD component of whole neutrophil extracts when studied by Western blotting (Goldschmeding *et al.*, 1989; Niles *et al.*, 1989). Immunochemical analysis of density-gradient fractions have shown that the 29 kD component is a DFP-binding soluble glycoprotein with serine protease activity. It is

4.3 OTHER NEUTROPHIL ANTIGENS FOR ANCA

In addition to PR3 and MPO, other neutrophil enzymes may be targets for autoantibodies developing in occasional patients with systemic vasculitis. Reactivity to elastase (Goldschmeding *et al.*, 1989), lactoferrin (Thomson and Lee, 1989; Lesavre, 1991), CAP 57 (Falk *et al.*, 1991), CatG (Flesch *et al.*, 1991), lysozyme (Hauschild, presented at the 4th International Workshop for ANCA) and eosinophil peroxidase (Dolman *et al.*, 1990) have all been described. Of these, elastase, lactoferrin and lysozyme are associated with pANCA patterns of staining, CAP 57 is associated with a cANCA pattern of staining, and CatG is associated with a homogeneous non-cANCA pattern. It is notable that lactoferrin is the only known ANCA antigen contained in specific granules.

4.4 CELLULAR SOURCES AND SUBCELLULAR LOCALIZATION OF ANCA-ASSOCIATED ANTIGENS

Double-labelling immunoelectron microscopy *in situ* has localized PR3 to the peroxidase-positive granules of neutrophils and monocytes, where it colocalizes with MPO, elastase and CatG to the azurophil granules and to the peroxidase-positive granules of monocytes (Calafat *et al.*, 1990: Csernok *et al.*, 1990). PR3 was also described in mast cells by Braun *et al.* (1991), a finding not confirmed by Goldschmeding *et al.* (1992b). PR3 is not found in eosinophils, basophils, red cells, platelets or lymphocytes. Acute myeloid leukaemia cells contain PR3 as do the promyelocytic cell line HL60, the promonocytic cell line THP1, the histiocytic promonocytic cell line U937, and the late myeloblastic cell line ML1 (Charles *et al.*, 1989; Braun *et al.*, 1991; Goldschmeding *et al.*, 1992a). Like other myeloid lysosomal enzymes, PR3 cannot be detected in tissue macrophages. Specifically, neither ANCA nor monoclonal antibodies to PR3 and MPO bind to alveolar macrophages, Kupffer cells in the liver, Langerhans cells in the skin or neuroglial cells of the central nervous system in tissue sections (Goldschmeding *et al.*, 1992b). Nor has PR3 been detected in cultured endothelial cells from umbilical cord veins (Goldschmeding *et al.*, 1992b). See Note added in proof.

5. *Specificity and Sensitivity of ANCA Tests for Vasculitis*

The classical descriptions of Wegener's granulomatosis (Wegener, 1936), polyarteritis (Kussmaul and Maier, 1866; Davson *et al.*, 1948) and of the Churg–Strauss syndrome (Churg and Strauss, 1951) were established by autopsy studies. Latterly, the diagnosis relied on clinical patterns of disease and the histology of biopsies taken from appropriate sites but there are obvious problems with this approach: clinical diagnoses are presumptive and often not confirmed by pathognomic histological findings; the diagnosis is often made late; cases of mild or atypical disease are often missed; and treatment is often delayed until significant organ damage has occurred. The association of ANCA with Wegener's granulomatosis and microscopic polyarteritis, and the development of simple assays to detect them, provided a new approach to diagnosis and to the monitoring of therapy of systemic vasculitides. The effectiveness of this approach has been demonstrated by studies of large numbers of patients with different forms of vasculitis. These have defined the sensitivity of ANCA for various types of vasculitis and clarified the relation between ANCA and disease activity.

5.1 CORRELATION OF ANCA WITH DIFFERENT FORMS OF VASCULITIS (Table 12.3)

Although there is uniformity about the histological diagnosis of the various vasculitic syndromes based on autopsies, it should be emphasized that nowadays diagnosis usually depends on clinical criteria and it is clear that these vary from one centre to another. This almost certainly explains the discrepancies with types of ANCA reported to be associated with Wegener's granulomatosis and microscopic polyarteritis by different authors.

Van der Woude *et al.* (1985) originally reported that ANCA were detected in 25 of 27 serum samples from patients with Wegener's granulomatosis who had active disease, but not in any of 500 normal blood donors or 190 disease controls. These findings were soon confirmed for Wegener's granulomatosis by Ludemann and Gross (1987), and extended to microscopic polyarteritis and idiopathic rapidly progressive glomerulonephritis in a prospective study of 100 consecutive patients by our own group (Savage *et al.*, 1987). The sensitivity and specificity of ANCA for Wegener's granulomatosis or microscopic polyarteritis was found to be 96% and 95%, respectively, in our study which used an ELISA as well as indirect immunofluorescence. Falk and Jennette (1988) distinguished between cANCA and pANCA in a study of 35 patients with idiopathic necrotizing and crescentic glomerulonephritis with and without evidence of systemic vasculitis. They also showed that pANCA was found more commonly in patients with isolated renal disease and that these antibodies bound to MPO.

Several larger studies of ANCA have followed, which confirm the early findings. Three studies were reported in 1989, all of which set out to determine the sensitivity and specificity of a classical cANCA pattern (as defined by the first ANCA Workshop in Copenhagen in 1988). Nolle *et al.* (1989) analysed 2653 serum samples from 1934 patients (277 with Wegener's granulomatosis) by indirect

Table 12.3 Clinical studies on the specificity and sensitivity of ANCA

Study	ANCA subtype	Assay system	Group studied	Study findings
Van der Woude et al. (1985)	(c)	IF	WG	First report of association between ANCA and WG
Ludemann and Gross (1987)	(c)	IF	WG	Confirmed association between ANCA and WG
Savage et al. (1987)	(c)	IF/SP	SV	ANCA have high sensitivity and specificity for SV both WG and MPA
Falk and Jennette (1988)	p	IF/SP	GN	Myeloperoxidase is a target, gives pANCA pattern
Nolle et al. (1989)	c	IF/SP	WG	cANCA have high sensitivity and specificity for WG
Cohen Tervaert et al. (1989)	c	IF	WG	cANCA have high sensitivity and specificity for WG
Specks et al. (1989)	c	IF	WG	cANCA have high sensitivity and specificity for WG
Jennette et al. (1989)	c/p	IF	SV,GN	GN with p/cANCA, WG with cANCA

(c) denotes studies involving cANCA which predated the c/p terminology; IF, indirect immunofluorescence; SP, solid phase assay; WG, Wegener's granulomatosis; GN, idiopathic necrotizing and crescentic glomerulonephritis; SV, systemic vasculitides; MPA, microscopic polyarteritis.

immunofluorescence and an ELISA which used affinity-purified antigen prepared using Wegener patients' autoantibodies. The specificity of ANCA for systemic Wegener's granulomatosis measured by indirect immunofluorescence and ELISA was 99% and 98%, respectively. Sensitivity for active localized Wegener's was 67% by immunofluorescence and 60% by ELISA, and for active generalized disease, 96% by immuno-fluorescence and 93% by ELISA. ANCA were detected in ten patients without a clinical diagnosis of Wegener's granulomatosis, eight had vasculitis (including four with microscopic polyarteritis, two with classical polyarteritis nodosa), one had rapidly progressive glomerulonephritis without evidence of systemic disease and one had rapidly progressive glomerulonephritis with pulmonary haemorrhage. Cohen Tervaert et al. (1989) also found that the specificity and sensitivity of cANCA for Wegener's granulomatosis was about 95% in a study of 103 patients (45 with active Wegener's). Two patients without a diagnosis of Wegener's had ANCA, one with Takayasu's vasculitis and one with lymphomatoid granulomatosis. Finally, Specks et al. (1989) studied 186 patients (65 with Wegener's) from the Mayo Clinic and reported a sensitivity of 84% for active generalized Wegener's granulomatosis, and 69% for active localized disease. Specificity was 98% – two of the 131 disease controls were ANCA-positive (cANCA pattern) and both had microscopic polyarteritis.

Other studies have investigated the value of ANCA more generally. Jennette et al. (1989) focused on patients with glomerulonephritis and demonstrated both cANCA and pANCA in patients with crescentic, necrotizing glomerulonephritis (without anti-glomerular basement membrane antibodies). Positive patients had a variety of clinical presentations ranging from isolated renal disease to widespread systemic vasculitis. pANCA was most frequent with renal-limited disease and cANCA when the lungs and sinuses were involved. These findings have been reinforced by a study of 70 ANCA-positive

patients by the North American Glomerular Disease Collaborative Networks (Falk et al., 1990). Cohen Tervaert et al. (1990b) has considered ANCA pattern with autoantibody specificity in a study of 35 consecutive patients with idiopathic crescentic necrotizing glomerulo-nephritis (Wegener's granulomatosis – nine biopsy-proven, 15 suspected; idiopathic rapidly progressive glomerulo-nephritis – 8; infection-related – 3). Antibodies to the 29 kD (later shown to be PR3) antigen and with a cANCA pattern by indirect immunofluorescence were present in 21 of the patients (nine biopsy-proven Wegener's, ten suspected Wegener's, two idiopathic), while antibodies to myeloperoxidase and with a pANCA pattern were present in eleven (five suspected Wegener's, six idiopathic). One patient had crescentic glomerulo-nephritis of infectious origin and a pANCA pattern without MPO specificity by ELISA.

A further paper from Cohen Tervaert et al. (1990a) examined the clinical associations of anti-myeloperoxidase antibodies in 53 sera. The patients fell into four groups: 21% had Wegener's granulomatosis, 26% idiopathic rapidly progressive glomerulonephritis, 28% systemic necrotizing vasculitis of the polyarteritis group (including classical polyarteritis nodosa and Churg–Strauss syndrome) and 25% were not classified (five were suspected of having Wegener's, three had unclassified systemic vasculitis, and three had glomerulonephritis without extrarenal manifestations). This study suggested that anti-MPO antibodies are associated with a wide range of vasculitides (at least as diagnosed clinically): these include, Wegener's granulomatosis, microscopic polyarteritis, classical polyarteritis nodosa, Churg–Strauss syndrome, and idiopathic rapidly progressive glomerulo-nephritis. It also confirmed earlier reports of ANCA in Churg–Strauss syndrome (Wathen and Harrison, 1987) and classical polyarterits nodosa (although ANCA probably only appear when there is concomitant microvascular disease). Comparison of these results to our own data illustrates the fallibility of the present clinical approaches to the diagnosis of the vasculitic syndromes. Our patients with microscopic polyarteritis have either pANCA or cANCA whereas patients with Wegener's have cANCA (Gaskin *et al.*, 1991a). The apparent inconsistencies in the results for these two studies is almost certainly caused by differences in the clinical criteria used for diagnosis. The uniformity of the association of ANCA with active vasculitis is much more important than these differences of detail. Three other observations emerge from these studies: first that not all pANCA react with myeloperoxidase; second, that some sera with an atypical cytoplasmic stain have MPO activity; and finally, exceptional ANCA do not bind to MPO or PR3 which suggests other neutrophil components may occasionally be involved.

The increasing availability of appropriate assays has led to the recognition of ANCA in other groups of patients. It is now apparent that occasional patients with anti-glomerular-basement-membrane antibody-mediated nephritis also have ANCA (Jayne *et al.*, 1990b; Pusey *et al.*, 1991; Saxena *et al.*, 1991). ANCA (both typical and atypical patterns) are found in some children with Kawasaki disease (Savage *et al.*, 1989). Atypical patterns of ANCA are found in patients with UC, Crohn's disease, sclerosing cholangitis (Snook *et al.*, 1989; Duerr *et al.*, 1991), HIV disease (Koderisch *et al.*, 1990), RA (Savige *et al.*, 1991), SLE (Gallicchio and Savige, 1991) and other connective tissue diseases.

5.2   RELATIONSHIP OF ANCA TO DISEASE ACTIVITY AND RELAPSE

Van der Woude's original report (1985) suggested that ANCA were more likely to be found in patients with active disease than in those in remission, thus ANCA were demonstrated in 25/27 patients with active Wegener's granulomatosis and only 4/32 of those in remission. Subsequently, Ludemann and Gross (1987), Nolle *et al.* (1989), and Specks *et al.* (1989) have all confirmed these observations. Van der Woude also suggested that ANCA titres correlated with disease activity and Figure 12.3 documents an example of this relationship. The phenomenon has been confirmed in a prospective study (Cohen Tervaert *et al.*, 1989) in which all 17 relapses (in 35 patients) were preceded by a rise in ANCA titre. Cohen Tervaert *et al.* (1990c) went on to ascertain whether treatment of rising ANCA titres prevented relapses. Fifty-eight with biopsy-proven Wegener's granulomatosis were studied for 24 months. ANCA titres rose in 20 patients, nine were randomly assigned to receive increased immunosuppression and 11 were not. There were clinical relapses in the group who did not receive increased treatment (six within 3 months and three later). However, there are now a lot of data which show that ANCA are not always associated with active disease (Egner & Chappell, 1990; Gaskin *et al.*,

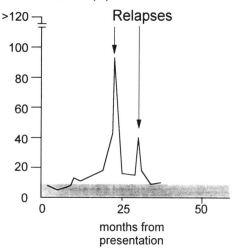

Figure 12.3 Sequential measurements of anti-MPO antibodies in a patient with Churg–Strauss syndrome. Both relapses during follow up were preceded by increasing anti-MPO antibody concentrations, assessed by ELISA. (Anti-MPO antibody concentrations are related to a standard positive serum designated 100%.)

1991a); for example, Gaskin *et al.* (1991a) reported that, although clinical relapses were confined to patients with detectable ANCA, roughly a half of treated patients with persistently positive ANCA did not relapse over a 2-year period. Nevertheless, relapses are accompanied or closely preceded by reappearance of cANCA. Based on this, our policy is to follow patients closely when ANCA titres are rising but to treat only those with clinical evidence of disease activity.

6.   *Potential Pathogenicity of ANCA*

It is clear from the clinical studies that ANCA are closely associated with the development of systemic vasculitis and that their titres frequently increase prior to relapse. This suggests that ANCA synthesis may be directly involved in the development of vasculitis, either in response to vascular injury, or as a common response to the aetiological agent responsible for injury, or because ANCA are directly responsible for injury in vasculitis. The fact that ANCA titres rise before a relapse argues in favour of their involvement in pathogenesis but this must be considered alongside the apparent paradox that ANCA can persist in some patients without clinical evidence of disease activity. Thus, if ANCA are involved in pathogenesis, other factors must also be involved. There is an increasing body of evidence to suggest that ANCA do have effects on neutrophils *in vitro* which is summarized in Table 12.4.

Table 12.4 *In vitro* effects of ANCA

Binding to neutrophil granule antigens on cell membrane surface
Neutrophil activation
   O_2^- release
   Granule release
   Chemotaxis
Promote neutrophil adherence to endothelium
Stimulate neutrophil cytotoxicity to cellular (endothelial cell) targets
Promote translocation of PKC to neutrophil cell membrane
Binding to MPO and PR3 on non-neutrophil cell surfaces (endothelial cells)
Possible effects on leucocyte maturation in bone marrow

6.1 IN VITRO STUDIES OF POTENTIAL DISEASE MECHANISMS: EFFECTS OF ANCA ON NEUTROPHIL ACTIVATION

The ability of ANCA to activate neutrophils has been studied using several of the markers described fully in Chapter 4. Falk *et al.* (1990b) measured generation of reactive oxygen species by chemiluminescence and superoxide dismutase-inhibitable reduction of ferricytochrome *c*. Thirteen ANCA-positive sera, 11 ANCA-IgG (five cANCA, six pANCA reactive with MPO), heterologous rabbit polyclonal anti-MPO, mouse monoclonal anti-MPO and MPO-ANCA-positive F(ab')$_2$ fragments were all able to stimulate greater release of reactive oxygen species compared with negative control sera, IgG and heterologous antibodies. It was also shown that O_2^- production and the chemiluminescence response to ANCA-positive F(ab')$_2$ fragments were enhanced by priming the neutrophils with TNF. Priming is the term given to a phenomenon by which an agent that itself does not activate the neutrophil, enhances subsequent neutrophil responses to substimulatory concentrations of a second agent (see Chapter 9). Keogan *et al.* (1991) also reported that ANCA-positive F(ab')$_2$ fragments can induce chemiluminescence with "unprimed" neutrophils. "Unprimed" is in parentheses since it is difficult to determine whether neutrophils that have been isolated from peripheral blood for *in vitro* studies are truly resting, especially as bacterial lipopolysaccharide, one of the most ubiquitous contaminants, can prime neutrophils at extremely low concentrations (Aida and Pabst, 1990; discussed in detail in Chapter 9). Use of Ficoll-hypaque to isolate neutrophils, the technique used by Keogan *et al.*, has also been reported to prime a proportion of the neutrophils (Haslett *et al.*, 1985).

Falk *et al.* (1990b) have examined release of granular enzymes from neutrophils and demonstrated that ANCA promote release of β-glucuronidase and N-acetyl-β-glucosaminidase from azurophilic granules. Anti-MPO antibodies (both human autoantibodies, rabbit polyclonal antibodies and mouse monoclonal antibody) have the same effect. Interestingly, the human autoantibodies were absolutely dependent on the presence of priming concentrations of TNF, whereas the effects of the heterologous polyclonal and monoclonal anti-MPO antibodies were only partly dependent on TNF.

Keogan *et al.* (1991) have also shown that ANCA promote chemotaxis without influencing random mobility or phagocytosis. The chemotactic response to FMLP was increased by five out of six ANCA F(ab')$_2$ whereas they had no effect on ZAS-induced chemotaxis.

The ability of ANCA to release reactive oxygen species and granule enzymes from neutrophils, or to increase neutrophil chemotaxis, suggests a possible role for ANCA in pathogenesis, but these observations must be linked to the major focus of inflammation and tissue injury, the vascular wall. Falk *et al.* (presented at the 4th International ANCA Workshop), as well as Keogan *et al.* (presented at the 4th International ANCA Workshop), reported that ANCA IgG and F(ab')$_2$ fragments increase neutrophil adhesion to endothelial monolayers. Adhesion was enhanced by activating the endothelium with TNF and substantially inhibited by anti-CD18 monoclonal antibodies, suggesting that integrin molecules are involved. Kiser *et al.* presented evidence at the 4th International ANCA Workshop that anti-MPO antibodies could induce permeability changes in the dermal vasculature of spontaneously hypertensive rats.

Preliminary studies on the effects of ANCA on neutrophil intracellular signalling have been reported by Fujimoto and Lockwood (1991) who demonstrated that ANCA-F(ab')$_2$ induced a shift in PKC from the cytosol to the plasma membrane, an early step in the activation of PKC, which can then lead to O_2^- production and, in the presence of a rise in intracellular calcium, degranulation (see Chapter 8).

6.2 IN VITRO STUDIES OF POTENTIAL DISEASE MECHANISMS: EFFECTS OF ANCA ON NEUTROPHIL-MEDIATED KILLING

Neutrophils can be activated to damage endothelial cell monolayers *in vitro* by mouse monoclonal antibodies to myeloperoxidase and PR3 and by human anti-MPO or anti-PR3 F(ab')$_2$ fragments (Figure 12.4) (Savage *et al.*, 1992). The effect is dependent on neutrophil priming with low doses of PMA (Savage *et al.*, 1992) or TNF (Ewert *et al.*, 1992); interestingly, endothelial cell activation with TNF also enhances the effect (Savage *et al.*, 1992).

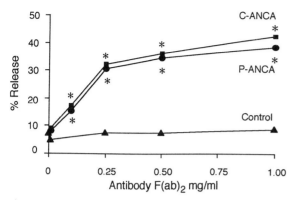

Figure 12.4 The percentage release of ^{111}In from human endothelial cells that were co-incubated with neutrophils and varying concentrations of human IgG F(ab)$_2$ containing pANCA (closed circle) or cANCA (closed square) activity. Neutrophils were primed with PMA 1 ng/ml and ionomycin 0.1 mM. The control antibody shown here was pooled normal IgG F(ab)$_2$ (triangle). The asterisks show values that were significantly different ($P < 0.05$) from the corresponding controls (control antibody with primed neutrophils or test antibody alone).

A possible model for endothelial cell injury, and conceivably injury to other types of cell, is as follows. First ANCA interact with MPO or PR3 which have transferred to the cell membrane surface of neutrophils primed by cytokines released during an intercurrent infection. The bound ANCA then leads to further neutrophil activation, enhanced neutrophil adhesion and endothelial cell damage in a process that quickly undergoes self-amplification. The necessity for neutrophil priming could explain why ANCA, both *in vitro* and *in vivo*, cannot cause tissue damage on their own.

6.3   CELL MATURATION

PR3 is identical to myeloblastin (Jenne *et al.*, 1990) which is involved in the terminal differentiation of HL60 cells into cells with a granulocyte phenotype or a monocyte–macrophage phenotype. Myeloblastin mRNA is down-regulated during this terminal differentiation of HL60 cells and inhibition of myeloblastin expression by an antisense oligodeoxynucleotide inhibited proliferation and induced differentiation (Bories *et al.*, 1989). Jenne *et al.* (1990) suggested that autoantibodies against myeloblastin/PR3 might induce such differentiation *in vivo* to cause the neutrophil leucocytosis seen in Wegener's granulomatosis. Similar mechanisms could also lead to enhanced monocyte differentiation, increased numbers of mature macrophages and to the development of multinucleate giant cells, and thus promote the granuloma formation.

6.4   CHARACTERISTICS OF THE TARGET ANTIGENS RECOGNIZED BY ANCA

As discussed earlier, PR3 accounts for more than 95% of cANCA, and cANCA have a high sensitivity and specificity for Wegener's granulomatosis but are also be found in microscopic polyarteritis. MPO is a major target for pANCA and accounts for the specificity in over 90% of pANCA in patients with microscopic polyarteritis, Churg–Strauss syndrome and idiopathic rapidly progressive glomerulonephritis. Thus ANCA of different specificities are associated with different clinical syndromes. In particular, patients with anti-PR3 have a very much greater tendency to extravascular granuloma formation, which raises the question whether the disease patterns reflect different physicochemical and functional properties of MPO and PR3.

MPO and PR3 are cationic proteases found in neutrophil azurophil granules and are released when neutrophils are activated. PR3 has a pI of 9.2 and it is a serine proteinase with anti-elastase activity; it also has anti-microbial activity which is independent of the proteolytic activity. MPO has a molecular weight of 140 kD, a pI of > 11, and is a chloride peroxidase that generates hypochlorous acid from H_2O_2 and Cl^-. It is responsible for killing of ingested bacteria, activation of latent metalloproteins, inactivation of α_1-proteinase inhibitor and for oxidative tissue injury (Weiss, 1989). α_1-Proteinase inhibitor is the main circulating inhibitor for PR3 but MPO is inactivated by products of its own peroxidase reaction.

PR3 and MPO both cause tissue injury in animal models. For example, PR3 causes emphysema when instilled into the tracheas of hamsters (Kao *et al.*, 1988). MPO, infused into isolated rat kidneys via the renal artery, binds to anionic GBM but causes little injury by itself. However, subsequent infusion of low concentrations of H_2O_2 and halides results in acute glomerular injury with proteinuria and mild proliferative changes (Johnson *et al.*, 1987). Human leucocyte elastase and CatG also localize to the GBM and cause proteinuria (Johnson *et al.*, 1987); it is likely that PR3 could do the same.

We have shown that MPO and PR3 bound to cultured endothelial cells can still be recognized by ANCA, and that MPO bound to endothelium retains enzymatic activity because in the presence of H_2O_2 and chloride ions, it causes endothelial injury and detachment; equivalent studies with PR3 have yet to be done.

Cationic proteins are also taken up more efficiently by antigen presenting accessory cells and are presented more effectively to T cells. Potentially at least, microvascular endothelial cells might present such antigens (or more accurately peptides derived from them), since there is substantial evidence that they can function as accessory cells in T-cell responses (Hughes *et al.*, 1990).

Presentation of antigens by glomerular endothelium could explain the development of a crescentic necrotizing glomerulonephritis in the absence of immunoglobulin deposition, especially as there are experimental precedents for nephritis to be induced in this way. For example, Rennke *et al.* (1990) induced a T-cell restricted immune response in rats to the cationic hapten azobenzene-arsonate, and then induced granulomatous and crescentic glomerulonephritis by perfusing one kidney with the hapten; nephritis did not develop in the contralateral kidney.

ANCA could be pathogenic in other ways. They could interact with antigens in solution to form immune complexes but there is little evidence for this in man. ANCA binding could affect MPO and PR3 activity, either by interfering with their enzymic/antimicrobial function or by interfering with their natural inhibitors. Van de Wiel *et al.* (presented at the 4th International Workshop for ANCA) have shown that cANCA IgG can inhibit the proteolytic cleavage of elastin, although cleavage of smaller synthetic substrates was inhibited to a lesser degree. cANCA IgG also inhibited formation of PR3–α_1-proteinase inhibitor complexes. These studies suggest that cANCA binding to PR3 prevents inactivation of PR3 by α_1-proteinase inhibitor and also decreases proteolytic activity of PR3 towards elastin. However, the net balance of these effects *in vivo* remains to be determined.

7. *Nature and Control of the Autoimmune Response*

The presence of ANCA puts the systemic vasculitides into the realm of autoimmune disorders. This poses the interesting question of why tolerance should be lost to myeloid lysosomal enzymes, particularly as they are not normally sequestered or hidden from the immune system.

It is likely that the antibody responses to MPO and PR3 are T-cell dependent, indeed the reported IgG1 and IgG4 subclass dominance of the ANCA response (Brouwer *et al.*, 1991; Segelman, presented at the 4th International Workshop for ANCA) supports the notion of a T-cell-driven response with repeated antigenic stimulation (Bird *et al.*, 1990). The interaction between MHC class II molecules, antigen-derived peptides and T-cell receptors is the central event in the development of an immune response and this is thought to explain the influence of HLA molecules on susceptibility to autoimmunity. Thus, it was natural to study HLA genes in patients with ANCA-associated vasculitis. Early studies suggested a slight predominance of HLA-B8 (Katz *et al.*, 1979) and HLA-DR2 (Elkon *et al.*, 1983) in patients with Wegener's granulomatosis. More recently, Spencer *et al.* (1992) described a strong association between HLA-DQw7 specificity and ANCA-associated vasculitis. The findings were similar in patients diagnosed as having

Wegener's granulomatosis and microscopic polyarteritis, and were not influenced by the type of ANCA present.

Despite the MHC associations and occasional reports of Wegener's granulomatosis occurring in siblings (Hay *et al.*, 1991), it is unusual to find more than one member of a family suffering from systemic vasculitis and identical twins have been reported to be discordant for the disease (Weiner *et al.*, 1986; Rees and Pusey, unpublished data). This suggests that an appropriate genetic background may predispose or even be necessary for development of disease, but that additional factors, some of which must be environmental, also contribute to the pathogenesis.

7.1 THE ROLE OF INFECTION

Infection is known to induce relapse in patients with systemic vasculitis (Pinching *et al.*, 1980), flu-like symptoms are often present in the prodromal period prior to acute disease (Savage *et al.*, 1985), and ANCA was first reported in a group of Australian patients with glomerulonephritis and arthralgia associated with Ross River arbovirus infection (Davies *et al.*, 1982). Interestingly, there is no clear-cut relationship between infection and ANCA titre. Despite the fact that relapse may be preceded by an intercurrent infection or by a rise in ANCA titre, ANCA titres can remain remarkably stable during intercurrent infections (personal observations). The simplest explanation for this phenomenon is that infection enhances the inflammation non-specifically as has been described in other types of nephritis, both clinically (Rees *et al.*, 1977) and experimentally (Tomosugi *et al.*, 1989).

The possibility that infection may contribute in some way to tissue injury is supported by the beneficial effect of trimethoprim-sulphamethoxazole in patients with active Wegener's granulomatosis that has been reported by DeRemee *et al.* (1985), although it is possible that the effectiveness of this antibiotic is due to an immunosuppressive rather than an antimicrobial action.

Stegeman *et al.* (abstract presented at the 4th International Workshop on ANCA) have also reported a relationship between chronic nasal carriage of *Staphylcoccus aureus* and an increased tendency to relapse in patients with Wegener's granulomatosis, but the effects of eradication have yet to be tested. In addition to the local nasal infection, carriage of staphylococci could have more widespread systemic effects on the immune system, for example, via the production of staphylococcal enterotoxins, which may act as superantigens (Fraser, 1989).

7.2 EFFECTS OF THERAPY ON THE COURSE OF DISEASE AND IMPLICATIONS FOR UNDERSTANDING PATHOGENESIS

In the absence of therapy, more than 90% of patients

with Wegener's granulomatosis are dead by 2 years (Walton, 1958). The introduction of cyclophosphamide, used in conjunction with prednisolone, dramatically improved patient and renal survival rates, and better than 80% 5-year survival rates are now achievable (Fauci *et al.*, 1983). The use of prednisolone and cyclophosphamide had a similar beneficial effect on the course of patients with microscopic polyarteritis (Savage *et al.*, 1985). The effective use of immunosuppressive drugs supported an immunological pathogenesis for systemic vasculitis even before ANCA had been described. The particular use of cyclophosphamide with its anti-B and anti-T cell effects suggested that abnormal specific immune responses were involved.

More recently, intravenous immunoglobulin has been used for treatment of patients with ANCA-positive vasculitis, leading to clinical improvement and a general reduction in ANCA titres (Jayne *et al.*, 1990a). The rationale for its use stems from its effectiveness in treatment of children with Kawasaki disease (Furusho *et al.*, 1984; Newburger *et al.*, 1986). The use of immunoglobulin further supports the notion that immune mechanisms are involved in pathogenesis. Further, it has been suggested that immune "control mechanisms" are at fault and, in particular, that there is an imbalance in the V-region idiotype network which allows autoimmunity to develop while intravenous immunoglobulin restores the network balance (Rossi *et al.*, 1989).

Finally, monoclonal anti-T cell antibodies have been used for treatment of a few patients with vasculitis. For example, Mathieson *et al.* (1990) treated a patient with ANCA-negative dermal lymphocytic vasculitis with CAMPATH-1H (directed against CDw52), and later with CAMPATH-1H and mouse monoclonal anti-CD4 antibody, inducing remission that lasted for over 1 year. This suggests that T cells may be involved in the development of some types of vasculitis lesions, although the clinical features and course of this particular patient were very different from those of most patients with ANCA-positive vasculitides.

8. Antibodies to Endothelial Cells

ANCA are not the only autoantibodies found in patients with systemic vasculitis. AECA have been reported frequently (Abbott *et al.*, 1989; Brasile *et al.*, 1989; Ferraro *et al.*, 1990; Frampton *et al.*, 1990; Savage *et al.*, 1991). However, they are found much less consistently than ANCA and do not cross-react with them. There is no consensus as to whether AECA bind complement or are cytotoxic to endothelial cells, and both cytotoxic (Brasile *et al.*, 1989) and non-cytotoxic antibodies have been reported (Savage *et al.*, 1991). Recently a few antibodies with the capacity to promote antibody-dependent cellular cytotoxicity with mononuclear cells has been reported but only in exceptional patients (Savage *et al.*, 1991).

9. Summary

Neutrophils appear to be one of the principal effector cells in patients with systemic vasculitis, and they are also the target of autoantibodies that are almost always found in serum from patients with these diseases. However, despite major developments in understanding these disorders, questions remain. These include the nature of the factor(s) responsible for the development of vasculitis and synthesis of ANCA, whether ANCA are directly pathogenic, and how disease activity may be inhibited using more specific therapy.

10. References

Abbott, F., Jones, S., Lockwood, C.M. and Rees, A.J. (1989). Autoantibodies to glomerular antigens in patients with Wegener's granulomatosis. Nephrol. Dial. Transpl. 4, 1–8.

Aida, T. and Pabst, M.J. (1990). Priming of neutrophils with lipopolysaccharide for enhanced release of superoxide. Requirement for plasma but not for tumor necrosis factor-alpha. J. Immunol. 145, 3017–3025.

Baggiolini, M., Bretz, U., Dewald, B. and Feigenson, M.E. (1978). The polymorphonuclear leucocyte. Agents Actions 8, 3–11.

Bird, P., Colvert, J.E. and Amlot, P.L. (1990). Distinctive development of IgG4 subclass antibodies in the primary and secondary responses to keyhole limpet haemocyanin in man. Immunology 69, 355–360.

Bories, D., Raynal, M.C., Solomon, D.H., Darzynkiewicz, Z. and Yvon, E.C. (1989). Down-regulation of a serine proteinase, myeloblastin, causes growth arrest and differentiation of promyelocytic leukemia cells. Cell 59, 959–968.

Brasile, L., Kremer, J.M., Clarke, J.L. and Cerilli, J. (1989). Identification of an autoantibody to vascular endothelial cell-specific antigens in patients with systemic vasculitis. Am. J. Med. 87, 74–80.

Braun, M.G., Czernok, E., Gross, W.L. and Muller-Hermelink, H.-K. (1991). Proteinase 3, the target antigen of anticytoplasmic antibodies circulating in Wegener's granulomatosis. Am. J. Pathol. 139, 831–838.

Brouwer, E., Cohen Tervaert, J.W., Horst, G., Huitema, M.G., Van der Giessen, M., Limburg, P.C. and Kallenberg, C.G.M. (1991). Predominance of IgG1 and IgG4 subclasses of anti-neutrophil cytoplasmic antibodies (ANCA) in patients with Wegener's granulomatosis and clinically related disorders. Clin. Exp. Immunol. 83, 379–386.

Calafat, J., Goldschmeding, R., Ringeling, P.L., Janssen, H. and van der Schoot, C.E. (1990). In situ localization by double-labeling immunoelectron microscopy of anti-neutrophil cytoplasmic autoantibodies in neutrophils and monocytes. Blood 75, 242–250.

Campanelli, D., Melchoir, M., Fu, Y., Nakata, M., Shuman, H., Nathan, C. and Gabay, J.E. (1990). Cloning of cDNA for proteinase 3: a serine protease, antibiotic, and autoantigen from human neutrophils. J. Exp. Med. 172, 1709–1715.

Carrington, C.B. and Liebow, A. (1966). Limited forms of angiitis and granulomatosis of Wegener's type. Am. J. Med. 41, 497–527.

Charles, L.A., Falk, R.J. and Jennette, J.C. (1989). Reactivity of anti-neutrophil cytoplasmic autoantibodies with HL-60 cells. Clin. Immunol. Immunopathol. 53, 243–253.

Churg, J. and Churg, A. (1989). Idiopathic and secondary vasculitis: a review. Modern Pathol. 2, 144–160

Churg, J. and Strauss, L. (1951). Allergic granulomatosis, allergic angiitis, and periarteritis nodosa. Am. J. Pathol. 27, 277–301.

Cochrane, C.G. and Koffler, D. (1973). Immune complex disease in experimental animals and man. Adv. Immunol. 16, 185–264.

Cohen Tervaert, J.W., van der Woude, F.J., Fauci, A.S., Ambrus, J.L., Velosa, J., Keane, W.F., Meijer, S., van der Giessen, M., The, T.H., van der Hem, G.K. and Kallenberg, C.G.M. (1989). Association between active Wegener's granulomatosis and anticytoplasmic antibodies. Arch. Intern. Med. 149, 2461–2465.

Cohen Tervaert, J.W., Goldschmeding, R., Elema, J.D., Limburg, P.C., van der Giessen, M., Huitema, M.G., Koolen, M. I., Hene, R.J., The, T.H., van der Hem, G.K., von dem Borne, A.E.G.K. and Kallenberg, C.G.M. (1990a). Association of autoantobodies to myeloperoxidase with different forms of vasculitis. Arthritis Rheum. 33, 1264–1272.

Cohen Tervaert, J.W., Goldschmeding, R., Elema, J.D., van der Giessen, M., Huitema, M.G., van der Hem, G.K., The, T.H., von dem Borne, A.E.G.K. and Kallenberg, C.G.M. (1990b). Autoantibodies against myeloid lysosomal enzymes in crescentic glomerulonephritis. Kidney Int. 37, 799–806

Cohen Tervaert, J.W., Huitema, M.G., Hene, R.J., Sluiter, W.J., The, T.H., van der Hem, G.K. and Kallenberg, C.G.M. (1990c). Prevention of relapses in Wegener's granulomatosis by treatment based on antineutrophil cytoplasmic antibody titre. Lancet 336, 709–711.

Csernok, E., Ludemann, J., Gross, W.L. and Bainton, D.F. (1990). Ultrastructural localization of proteinase 3, the target antigen of anti-cytoplasmic antibodies circulating in Wegener's granulomatosis. Am. J. Pathol. 137, 1113–1120.

D'Agati, V., Chandler, P., Nash, M.E. and Mancilla-Jimenez, R.M. (1986). Idiopathic microscopic polyarteritis nodosa ultrastructural observations on the renal vasculature and glomerular lesions. Am. J. Kid. Dis. 7, 95–110.

Davies, D.J., Moran, J.E., Niall, J.F. and Ryan, G.B. (1982). Segmental necrotizing glomerulonephritis with antineutrophil antibody: possible arbovirus aetiology? Br. Med. J. 285, 606.

Davson, J., Ball, J. and Platt, R. (1948). The kidney in periarteritis nodosa. Q. J. Med. 17, 175–205.

DeRemee, R.A., McDonald, T.J. and Weiland, L.H. (1985). Wegener's granulomatosis: observations on treatment with antimicrobial agents. Mayo Clin. Proc. 60, 27–32.

Dixon, F.J., Vazquez, J.J., Weigle, W.O. and Cochrane, C.G. (1958). Pathogenesis of serum sickness. AMA Arch. Pathol. 65, 18–28.

Dolman, K.M., Goldschmeding, R., Sonnenberg, A. and Von dem Borne, A.E.G. (1990). ANCA related antigens. Acta Pathol. Microbiol. Immunol. Scand. 98 (Suppl. 19), 28.

Donald, K.J., Edwards, R.L. and McEvoy, J.D.S. (1976). An ultrastructural study of the pathogenesis of tissue injury in limited Wegener's granulomatosis. Pathology. 8, 161–169.

Duerr, R.H., Targan, S.R., Landers, C.J., Larusso, N.F., Lindsay, K.L., Wiesner, R.H. and Shanahan, F. (1991). Neutrophil cytoplasmic antibodies: a link between primary sclerosing cholangitis and ulcerative colitis. Gastroenterology 100, 1385–1391.

Egner, W. and Chapel, H.M. (1990). Titration of antibodies against neutrophil cytoplasmic antigens is useful in monitoring disease activity in systemic vasculitis. Clin. Exp. Immunol. 82, 244–249.

Elkon, K.B., Sutherland, D.C., Rees, A.J., Hughes, G.R.V. and Batchelor, J.R. (1983). HLA frequencies in systemic vasculitis. Increase in HLA-DR2 in Wegener's granulomatosis. Arthritis Rheum. 26, 102–105.

Ewert, B.H., Jennette, J.C. and Falk, R.J. (1992). Anti-myeloperoxidase antibodies stimulate neutrophils to damage human endothelial cells. Kidney Int. 41, 375–383.

Falk, R.J. and Jennette, J.C. (1988). Anti-neutrophil cytoplasmic autoantibodies with specificity for myeloperoxidase in patients with systemic vasculitis and idiopathic necrotising and crescentic glomerulonephritis. N. Engl. J. Med. 318, 1651–1657.

Falk, R.J., Becker, M., Terrell, R. and Jennette, J.C. (1991). Antigen specificity of p-ANCA and of c-ANCA. Am. J. Kid. Dis. 18, 197 (abstract).

Falk, R.J., Hogan, S., Carey, T.S. and Jennette, J.C. (1990a). Clinical course of anti-neutrophil cytoplasmic autoantibody-associated glomerulonephritis and systemic vasculitis. Ann. Intern. Med; 113, 656–663.

Falk, R.J., Terrell, R.S., Charles, L.A. and Jennette, J.C. (1990b). Anti-neutrophil cytoplasmic autoantibodies induce neutrophils to degranulate and produce oxygen radicals in vitro. Proc. Natl. Acad. Sci. USA 87, 4115–4119.

Fauci, A.S., Haynes, B.F., Katz, P. and Wolff, S.M. (1983). Wegener's granulomatosis: prospective clinical and therapeutic experience with 85 patients for 21 years. Ann. Intern. Med. 98, 76–85.

Ferraro, G., Meroni, P.L., Tincani, A., Sinico, A., Barcellini, W., Radice, A.G.G., Froldi, M., Borghi, M.O. and Balestrieri, G. (1990). Anti-endothelial cell antibodies in patients with Wegener's granulomotosis and micropolyarteritis. Clin. Exp. Immunol. 79, 47–53.

Flesch, B.K., Lampe, M., Rautman, A. and Gross, W.L. (1991). Anti-elastase, cathepsin G, and lactoferrin antibodies in sera with c-ANCA or with atypical fluorescence staining pattern. Am. J. Kid. Dis. 18, 201 (abstract).

Frampton, G., Jayne, D.R.W., Perry, G.J., Lockwood C.M. and Cameron, J.S. (1990). Autoantibodies to endothelial cells and neutrophil cytoplasmic antigens in systemic vasculitis. Clin. Exp. Immunol. 82, 227–232.

Fraser, J.D. (1989). High-affinity binding of staphylococcal enterotoxins A and B to HLA-DR. Nature 339, 221–223.

Fujimoto, T. and Lockwood, C.M. (1991). Antineutrophil cytoplasm antibodies (ANCA) activate protein kinase C in human neutrophils and HL-60 cells. Am. J. Kid, Dis. 18, 204 (abstract).

Furusho, K., Kamiya, T., Nakano, H., Kiyosawa, N., Shinomiya, K. and Hayashidera, T. (1984). High-dose intravenous gammaglobulin for Kawasaki disease. Lancet ii, 1055–1058.

Gabay, J.E., Scott, R.W., Campanelli, D., Griffith, J., Wilde, C., Marra, M.N., Seeger, M. and Nathan, C.F. (1989). Antibiotic proteins of human polymorphonuclear leukocytes. Proc. Natl Acad. Sci. USA 86, 5610–5614.

Gallicchio, M.C. and Savige, J.A. (1991). Detection of anti-myeloperoxidase and anti-elastase antibodies in vasculitides and infection. Clin. Exp. Immunol. 84, 232–237.

Gaskin, G., Ryan, J.J., Rees, A.J. and Pusey, C.D. (1991a). ANCA specificity in microscopic polyarteritis, Churg–Strauss syndrome, and polyarteritis nodosa. Am. J. Kid. Dis. 18, 207–208.

Gaskin, G., Savage, C.O.S., Ryan, J.J., Jones, S., Rees, A.J., Lockwood, C.M. and Pusey, C.D. (1991b). Anti-neutrophil cytoplasmic antibodies and disease activity during follow-up of 70 patients with systemic vasculitis. Nephrol. Dial. Transpl. 6, 689–694.

Gocke, D.J., Hsu, K., Morgan, C., Bombardieri, S., Lockshin, M. and Christian, C.L. (1970). Association between polyarteritis and Australia antigen. Lancet ii, 1149–1153.

Goldschmeding, R., van der Schoot, C.E., ten Bokkel Huinink, D., Hack, C.E., van den Ende, M.E., Kallenberg, C.G.M. and von dem Borne, A.E.G.K. (1989). Wegener's granulomatosis autoantibodies identify a novel diisopropylfluorphosphate-binding protein in the lysosomes of normal human neutrophils. J. Clin. Invest. 84, 1577–1587.

Goldschmeding, R., van der Schoot, C.E., Calafat, J., Wyermans, P.W. and von dem Borne, A.E.G.K. (1992a). "Target Antigens of Antineutrophil Cytoplasmic Antibodies", thesis, Amsterdam. pp. 162.

Goldschmeding, R., Vroom, T.M., Tesselaar, N.A. and von dem Borne, A.E.G.K. (1992b). In "Target Antigens of Antineutrophil Cytoplasmic Antigens," thesis, Amsterdam. pp. 64.

Hall, J.B., Wadham, B.M., Wood, C.J., Ashton, V. and Adam, W.R. (1984). Vasculitis and glomerulonephritis: a subgroup with antineutrophil cytoplasmic antibody. Austin, N.Z. J. Med. 14, 277–278.

Haslett, C., Guthrie, L.A., Kopaniak, M.M., Johnston, R.B. and Henson, P.M. (1985). Modulation of multiple neutrophil functions by preparative methods or trace concentrations of bacterial lipopolysaccharide. Am. J. Pathol. 119, 101–110.

Hay, E.M., Beaman, M., Ralston, A.J., Ackrill, P., Bernstein, R.M. and Holt, P.J.L. (1991). Wegener's granulomatosis occurring in siblings. Br. J. Rheumatol. 30, 144–145.

Hughes, C.C.W., Savage, C.O.S. and Pober, J.S. (1990). The endothelial cell as a regulator of T-cell function. Immunol. Rev. 117, 85–102.

Jayne, D.R.W., Davies, M.J., Fox, C.J.V., Black, C.M. and Lockwood, C.M. (1990a). Treatment of systemic vasculitis with pooled intravenous immunoglobulin. Lancet. 337, 1137–1139.

Jayne, D.R.W., Marshall, P.D., Jones, S. and Lockwood, C.M. (1990b). Autoantibodies to GBM and neutrophil cytoplasm in rapidly progressive glomerulonephritis. Kid. Int. 37, 965–970.

Jenne, D.E., Tschopp, J., Ludemann, J., Utecht, B. and Gross, W.L. (1990). Wegener's autoantigen decoded. Nature. 346, 520.

Jennette, J.C., Wilkman, A.S. and Falk, R.J. (1989). Anti-neutrophil cytoplasmic autoantibody-associated glomerulonephritis and vasculitis. Am. J. Pathol. 135, 921–930.

Jennette, J.C., Hoidal, J.H. and Falk, R.J. (1990). Specificity of anti-neutrophil cytoplasmic autoantibodies for proteinase 3. Blood. 78, 2263–2264.

Johnson, R.J., Couser, W.G., Chi, E.Y., Adler, S. and Klebanoff, S.J. (1987). New mechanism for glomerular injury. Myeloperoxidase–hydrogen peroxide–halide system. J. Clin. Invest. 79, 1379–1387.

Kao, R.C., Wehner, N.G., Skubitz, K.M., Gray, B.H. and Hoidal, J.R. (1988). Proteinase 3. A distinct human polymorphonuclear leukocyte proteinase that produces emphysema in hamsters. J. Clin. Invest. 82, 1963–1973.

Katz, P., Alling, D.W., Haynes, B.F. and Fauci, A.S. (1979). Association of Wegener's granulomatosis with HLA-B8. Clin. Immunol. Immunopathol. 14, 268–270.

Keogan, M.T., Esnault, V.L., Green, A.J., Lockwood, C.M. and Brown, D.L. (1991). Anti-neutrophil cytoplasm antibody (ANCA) stimulates unprimed neutrophils. Am. J. Kid. Dis. 18, 203 (abstract).

Koderisch, J., Andrassy, K., Rasmussen, N., Hartmann, M. and Tilgen, W. (1990). "False-positive" anti-neutrophil cytoplasmic antibodies in HIV infection. Lancet ii, 1227–1228.

Kussmaul, A. and Maier, R. (1866). Ueber eine bisher beschriebene eigenthumliche arterienerkrankung (periarteritis nodosa), die mit morbus brightii und rapid fortschreitender allgemeiner muskellahmung einhergeht. Deutsches Arch. Kin. Med. 1, 484–517.

Lanham, J.G. and Churg, J. (1991) In "Systemic Vasculitides." (eds A. Churg and J. Churg) pp. 101–120. Igaku-Shoin Medical Publishers, Inc., New York.

Lesavre, P. (1991). Antineutrophil cytoplasmic autoantibodies antigen specificity. Am. J. Kid. Dis. 18, 159–163.

Lieberman, K. and Churg, A. (1991). "Systemic Vasculitides" (eds A. Churg and J. Churg) pp. 79–99. Igaku-Shoin Medical Publishers, Inc., New York.

Ludemann, G. and Gross, W.L. (1987). Autoantibodies against cytoplasmic structures of neutrophil granulocytes in Wegener's granulomatosis. Clin. Exp. Immunol. 69, 350–357.

Ludemann, J., Utecht, B. and Gross, W.L. (1990). Antineutrophil cytoplasm antibodies in Wegener's granulomatosis recognize an elastinolytic enzyme. J. Exp. Med. 171, 357–362.

Macfarlane, D.G., Bourne, J.T., Dieppe, P.A. and Easty, D.L. (1983). Indolent Wegener's granulomatosis. Ann. Rheum. Dis. 42, 398–407.

Mark, E.J., Matsubara, O., Tan-liu, N.S. and Fienberg, R. (1988). The pulmonary biopsy in the early diagnosis of Wegener's (pathergic) granulomatosis. Hum. Pathol. 19, 1065–1071.

Mathieson, P.W., Cobbold, S.P., Hale, G., Clark, M.R., Oliveira, D.B.G., Lockwood, C.M. and Waldmann, H. (1990). Monoclonal-antibody therapy in systemic vasculitis. N. Engl. J. Med. 323, 250–254.

McHugh, N.J., James, I.E. and Plant, G.T. (1990). Anticardiolipin and antineutrophil antibodies in giant cell arteritis. J. Rheumatol. 17, 916–922.

Newburger, J.W., Takahashi, M., Burns, J.C., Beiser, A.S., Chung, K.J., Duffy, C.E., Glode, M.P., Mason, W.H., Reddy, V., Sanders, S.P., Shulman, S.T., Wiggins, J.W., Hicks, R.V., Fulton, D.R., Lewis, A.B., Leung, D.Y.M., Colton, T., Rosen, F.S. and Melish, M.E. (1986). The treatment of Kawasaki syndrome with intravenous gamma globulin. N. Engl. J. Med. 315, 341–347.

Niles, J.L., McCluskey, R.T., Ahmad, M.F. and Arnaout, M.A. (1989). Wegener's granulomatosis autoantigen is a novel neutrophil serine proteinase. Blood 74, 1888–1893.

Nolle, B., Specks, U., Ludemann, J., Rohrbach, M.S., DeRemee, R.A. and Gross, W.L. (1989). Anticytoplasmic autoantibodies: their immunodiagnostic value in Wegener's granulomatosis. Ann. Intern. Med. 111, 28–40.

Pinching, A.J., Rees, A.J., Pussell, B.A., Lockwood, C.M., Mitchison, R.S. and Peters, D.K. (1980). Relapses in Wegener's granulomatosis: the role of infection. Br. Med. J. 281, 836–838.

Pusey, C.D., Turner, A.N., Gaskin, G., Katbamna, I., Ryan, J.J. and Rees, A.J. (1991). Specificity of anti-GBM antibodies found in patients with ANCA. Am. J. Kid. Dis. 18, 210–211.

Rao, N.V., Wehner, N.G., Marshall, B.C., Gray, W.R., Gray, B.H. and Hoidal, J.R. (1991). Characterization of proteinase-3 (PR-3), a neutrophil serine proteinase. J. Biol. Chem. 266, 9540–9548.

Rees, A.J., Lockwood, C.M. and Peters, D.K. (1977). Enhanced allergic tissue damage in Goodpasture's syndrome by intercurrent bacterial infection. Br. Med. J. 2, 723–726.

Rennke, H.G., Klein, P.S. and Mendrick, D.L. (1990). Cell mediated immunity (CMI) in hapten-induced interstitial nephritis and glomerular crescent formation in the rat. Kid. Int. 37, 428 (abstract).

Rosen, S., Falk, R.J. and Jenett, J.C. (1991). Polyarteritis nodosa, including microscopic form and renal vasculitis. In "Systemic Vasculitides" (eds J. Churg and A. Churg) pp. 57–77. Igaku-Shoin Medical Publishers Inc., New York.

Rossi, F., Dietrich, G. and Kazatchkine, M.D. (1989). Anti-idiotypes against autoantibodies in normal immunoglobulins: evidence for network regulation of human autoimmune responses. Immunol. Rev. 110, 135–150.

Savage, C.O.S., Winearls, C.G., Evans, D.J., Rees, A.J. and Lockwood, C.M. (1985). Microscopic polyarteritis: presentation, pathology and prognosis. Q. J. Med. 56, 467–483.

Savage, C.O.S., Winearls, C.G., Jones, S., Marshall, P.D. and Lockwood, C.M. (1987). Prospective study of radioimmunoassay for antibodies against neutrophil cytoplasm in diagnosis of systemic vasculitis. Lancet i, 1389–1393.

Savage, C.O.S., Tizard, J., Jayne, D., Lockwood, C.M. and Dillon, M.J. (1989). Antineutrophil cytoplasm antibodies in Kawasaki disease. Arch Dis. Child. 64, 360–363

Savage, C.O.S., Pottinger, B., Gaskin, G., Lockwood, C.M., Pusey, C.D. and Pearson, J. (1991). Vascular damage in Wegener's granulomatosis and microscopic polyarteritis: presence of anti-endothelial cell antibodies and their relation to anti-neutrophil cytoplasm antibodies. Clin. Exp. Immunol. 85, 14–19.

Savage, C.O.S., Pottinger, B.E., Gaskin, G., Pusey, C.D. and Pearson, J.D. (1992). Autoantibodies developing to myeloperoxidase and proteinase 3 in systemic vasculitis stimulate neutrophil cytotoxicity towards cultured endothelial cells. Am. J. Pathol. 141, 335–342.

Savige, J.A., Gallicchio, M.C., Stockman, A., Cunningham, T.J. and Rowley, M.J. (1991). Anti-neutrophil cytoplasm antibodies in rheumatoid arthritis. Clin. Exp. Immunol. 86, 92–98.

Saxena, R., Bygren, P., Rasmussen, N. and Wieslander, J. (1991). Circulating autoantibodies in patients with extracapillary glomerulonephritis. Nephrol Dial Transplant. 6, 389–397.

Serra, A., Cameron, J.S., Turner, D.R., Hartley, B., Ogg, C.S., Neild, G.H., Williams, D.G., Taube, D., Brown, C.B. and Hicks, J.A. (1984). Vasculitis affecting the kidney: presentation, histopathology and long-term outcome. Q.J. Med. 210, 181–207.

Snook, J.A., Chapman, R.W., Fleming, K. and Jewell, D.P. (1989). Anti-neutrophil nuclear antibody in ulcerative colitis, Crohn's disease and primary sclerosing cholangitis. Clin. Exp, Immunol. 76, 30–33.

Specks, U., Wheatley, C.L., McDonald, T.J., Rohrbach, M.S. and DeRemee, R.A. (1989). Anticytoplasmic autoantibodies in the diagnosis and follow-up of Wegener's granulomatosis. Mayo Clin. Proc. 64, 28–36.

Spencer, S.J.W., Burns, A., Gaskin, G., Pusey, C.D. and Rees, A.J. (1992). HLA class II specificities and the development and duration of small vessel. Kidney Int. 41, 1059–1063.

Thomson, R.A. and Lee, S.S. (1989). Antineutrophil cytoplasm antibodies. Lancet i, 670–671.

Tomosugi, N., Cashman, S.J., Hay, H., Pusey, C.D., Evans, D.J., Shaw, A. and Rees, A.J. (1989). Modulation of antibody-mediated glomerular injury in vivo by bacterial lipopolysaccharide, tumour necrosis factor, and interleukin-1. J. Immunol. 142, 3083–3090.

Trepo, C.G., Zuckerman, A.J., Bird, R.C. and Prince, A.M. (1974). The role of circulating hepatitis B antigen/antibody immune complexes in the pathogenesis of vascular and hepatic manifestations in polyarteritis nodosa. J. Clin. Pathol. 27, 863–868.

van der Wall Bake, A.W.L., Lobatto, S., Jonges, L., Daha, M.R. and van Es, L.A. (1987). IgA antibodies directed against cytoplasmic antigens of polymorphonuclear leukocytes in patients with Henoch–Schoenlein purpura. Adv. Exp. Med. Biol. 216b, 1593–1598.

van der Woude, F.J., Rasmussen, N., Lobatto, S., Wiik, A., Permin, H., van Es, L.A., van der Giessen, M., van der Hem, G.K. and The, T.H. (1985). Autoantibodies against neutrophils and monocytes: tool for diagnosis and marker of disease activity in Wegener's granulomatosis. Lancet i, 425–429.

Walton, E.W. (1958). Giant-cell granuloma of the respiratory tract (Wegener's granulomatosis). Br. Med. J. 2, 265–270.

Wathen, C.W. and Harrison, D.J. (1987). Circulating anti-neutrophil antibodies in systemic vasculitis. Lancet i, 1037.

Wegener, F. (1936). Ueber generalisierte, septische Gefaserkrankungen. Verhandl. Deutsch. Pathol. Gasellsch. 29, 202–210.

Weiner, S.R., Kwan, L.W., Paulus, H.E., Caro, X J. and Weisbart, R.H. (1986) Twins discordant for Wegener's granulomatosis. Clin. Exp. Rheumatol. 4, 389–390 (letter).

Weiss, S.J. (1989). Tissue destruction by neutrophils. N. Engl J. Med. 320, 365–376.

Wilde, C.G., Snable, J.L., Griffith, J.E. and Scott, R.W. (1990). Characterization of two azurophil granule proteases with active-site homology to neutrophil elastase. J. Biol. Chem. 265, 2038–2041.

Woodworth, T.G., Abuelo, J.G., Austin, H.A. and Esparza, A. (1987). Severe glomerulonephritis with late emergence of classic Wegener's Granulomatosis. Report of 4 cases and review of the literature. Medicine 66, 181–191.

Note added in proof

1. An animal model of anti-MPO-associated glomerulonephritis has been described by Brouwer et al. (1993). J. Exp. Med. 177, 905–914.
2. Presence of PR3 in endothelial cells has been described by Mayet et al. (1993) Blood 82, 1221–1229.

13. Role of Neutrophils in Adult Respiratory Distress Syndrome and Cryptogenic Fibrosing Alveolitis

Stanley Braude, Timothy W. Evans and R.M. du Bois

Immunopharmacology of Neutrophils
ISBN 0–12–339250–0

1. Adult Respiratory Distress Syndrome

1.1 INTRODUCTION

The term adult respiratory distress syndrome (ARDS) defines the condition of severe acute lung injury leading to increased pulmonary vascular permeability, alveolar oedema and refractory hypoxaemia. Since it was first described some 25 years ago (Ashbaugh *et al.*, 1967), there has been little progress in improving the 50–70% mortality associated with the syndrome, but major advances have been made in understanding its pathophysiology and clinical spectrum. In 1972 it was estimated that there were 150 000 cases of ARDS per year in the USA alone, but a recent retrospective study in a single region of the UK suggested an annual incidence for the country as a whole of between 1000–1500 established cases.

1.1.1 Pathophysiology

The initial concept that ARDS was exclusively pulmonary based has changed in recent years due to several factors. Firstly, experimental studies that examined the relationship between pulmonary and systemic capillary injury showed that granulocyte activation produced polymorphonuclear cell accumulation in many organs other than the lung, including the liver (Mizer *et al.*, 1989). Similarly, the administration of exogenous endotoxin produced significant neutrophil accumulation and increased extravascular protein, not only in the lung, but also in kidney and heart (Welsh *et al.*, 1988). Secondly, in clinical studies a positive correlation was found between extravascular lung water and urinary B_2 macroglobulin in patients with established ARDS (Kreuzfelder *et al.*, 1988). These studies suggested that the syndrome might represent only the pulmonary manifestation of a panendothelial injury. Additionally, definition of the natural history of ARDS showed clearly that most patients died not from irreversible hypoxaemia, but from sepsis and the development of multisystem organ failure (Montgomery *et al.*, 1985). These early concerns that the ARDS appellation and its strict definition (by fulfillment of specific clinical criteria) were unhelpful in advancing understanding (Murray, 1975) have been borne out subsequently. It is now accepted that ARDS is not a threshold disorder, but rather the severe end of a continuum of pathophysiological responses (Murray *et al.*, 1988). Studies revealing abnormal pulmonary microvascular permeability in patients at risk for ARDS, but failing to fulfil diagnostic criteria, have subsequently underlined the validity of this concept (Rocker *et al.*, 1989).

1.1.2 Histopathology

ARDS can arise in association with a wide variety of serious medical and surgical disorders, only some of which involve the lung directly (Table 13.1). Nevertheless,

Table 13.1 Conditions associated with ARDS

Pulmonary	Non-pulmonary
Gastric aspiration	Sepsis
Drowning	Fat embolism
Smoke inhalation	Hypovolaemia
Direct lung trauma	Head injury
Pneumonia	Disseminated intravascular coagulopathy
Drug/oxygen toxicity	Pancreatitis
	Eclampsia
	Amniotic fluid embolus

the resulting pulmonary histopathology appears to be uniform (Tomashefski, 1990). The changes arise from severe injury to the alveolar-capillary unit with inflammation, intra-alveolar oedema and haemorrhage prominent in the early exudative phase (Figures 13.1 and 13.2).

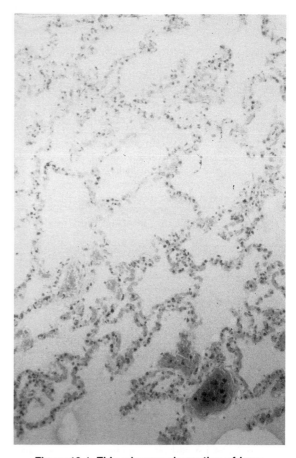

Figure 13.1 This microscopic section of lung parenchyma in ARDS shows pale staining pink proteinaceous fluid with alveoli indicating leakage of capillaries with oedema. Note the presence of dilated, congested capillaries within the interstitium between alveoli.

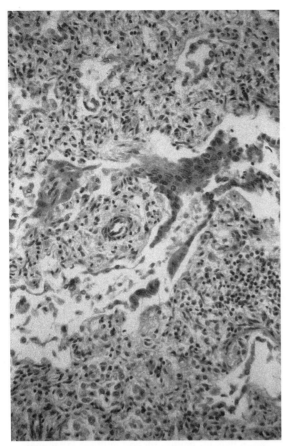

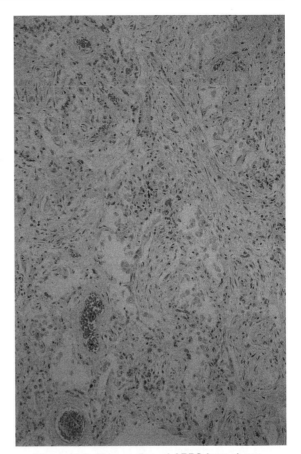

Figure 13.2 This section shows a bronchiole and accompanying artery in ARDS. There is damage to the bronchial epithelium with hyaline membrane formation and regenerating squamous type hyperplastic Type II pneumocytes lining the narrowed alveoli indicating prevous epithelial damage. The interstitium is damaged with infiltration by lymphocyte and plasma cells.

Figure 13.3 This section of ARDS lung shows obliteration of the normal architecture by dense bands of fibrous tissue within the interstitium and total destruction of gas exchanging alveoli.

Subsequently, an organization and repair phase is seen with Type II pneumocyte and fibroblast proliferation, and a relative paucity of inflammatory changes (Figure 13.3). In ventilator-dependent patients who survive beyond 3–4 weeks there is extensive interstitial fibrosis. Pulmonary vascular lesions may be thrombotic, fibroproliferative or obliterative and, similarly to the parenchymal changes, correlate with the temporal phase of lung injury. These stereotypic pathological features raise the possibility of a final common pathway of lung injury, regardless of the nature of the initial insult. In view of the complexity of the pathophysiology, it seems likely that diverse pathways of injury exist that elicit a uniform response in the lung (Repine, 1992).

To date, no drug has been shown to be useful in ARDS and treatment remains essentially supportive (Macnaughton and Evans, 1992). In recent years, research efforts have moved our understanding regarding pathogenesis away from a critical single mediator or cytokine to a complex interplay between different cells, mediators and cytokines (Figure 13.4). Meaningful therapeutic advances in future will arise only from a clearer understanding of these mechanisms. This section of the chapter addresses the important issue of the role of the neutrophil and its potentially cytotoxic products in the genesis of lung injury.

1.2 The Neutrophil as a Key Effector Cell in Lung Injury

1.2.1 Early Clinical and Experimental Studies

Interest in the neutrophil as a potential mediator of lung injury arose initially from a series of studies carried out in patients with haemodialysis-associated leukopenia in the late 1970s (Craddock et al., 1975; Craddock et al., 1977a; Craddock et al., 1977b). Dialysis was invariably associated with marked neutropenia, apparently resulting from pulmonary sequestration. Moderate hypoxaemia

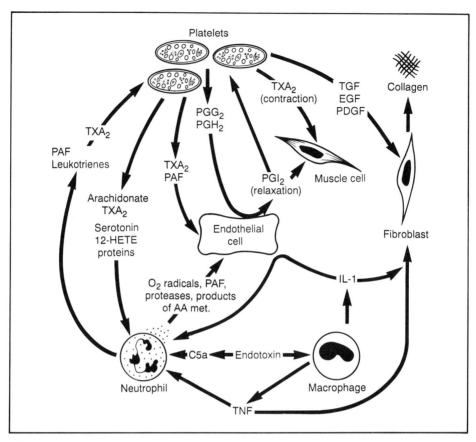

Figure 13.4 Representation of possible interplay between the endothelium, neutrophil and multiple inflammatory cascades and pathways in ARDS.

and decreased pulmonary diffusing capacity were also noted. The syndrome could be reproduced in animals by incubating autologous plasma with the cellophane dialyser membrane, or prevented by complement inactivation (Craddock *et al.*, 1977a). *In vitro* (Craddock *et al.*, 1977c) and subsequently *in vivo* studies (Hammerschmidt *et al.*, 1981) revealed the activated complement fraction to be C5a. In 1980, Hammerschmidt and colleagues published exciting data suggesting that intravascular complement activation played a similar role in ARDS, by demonstrating in humans a correlation between C5a levels and the development of lung injury. These findings were extended when, for the first time, a marked predominance of neutrophils was noted in differential cell counts of BAL fluid obtained from patients with ARDS (Lee *et al.*, 1981), a finding reproduced more recently (Fowler *et al.*, 1987). These studies suggested that complement-mediated neutrophil sequestration in pulmonary capillaries with subsequent pulmonary microvascular damage could be a unifying feature in patients with lung injury. However, complement activation was subsequently shown to occur to a similar extent both in patients at risk for ARDS and in those with the established syndrome (Duchateau *et al.*, 1984;

Weinberg *et al.*, 1984). This implied that, although still conceivably important, complement activation could not be solely responsible for the development of ARDS.

Early experimental studies also implicated the neutrophil in animal models of acute lung injury, including those mediated via endotoxin (Brigham *et al.*, 1979), hyperoxia (Shasby *et al.*, 1982) and microembolization (Johnson and Malik, 1980). Prior neutrophil depletion appeared to partially protect against lung injury in these models. An analogous clinical study examining trends in gas exchange in leukaemic patients with coincident drug-induced leukopenia and acute lung injury found that the alveolar–arterial oxygen gradient and the radiographic appearances deteriorated as the neutrophil count rose (Rinaldo and Borowetz, 1985). Nevertheless, other studies have confirmed that classical ARDS may develop in grossly neutropenic patients (Braude *et al.*, 1985; Laufe *et al.*, 1986; Maunder *et al.*, 1986; Ognibene *et al.*, 1986), suggesting that other cell types may also be involved.

1.2.2 The Role of Endotoxin

The realization that complement activation alone could not fully account for the pathogenesis of ARDS focused attention on the possible contributory role of bacterial endotoxin. Experimentally, it was shown in 1979 that endotoxin increased lung vascular permeability (Brigham et al., 1979), although at the time the mechanism was unclear. Subsequently, a significant body of experimental evidence developed to support the concept of neutrophil sequestration in the pulmonary microvasculature as an important early feature of endotoxaemia-associated lung injury (Haslett et al., 1987). Small concentrations of the LPS component of endotoxin were shown to markedly enhance C5a-stimulated release of superoxide and elastase from neutrophils (Guthrie et al., 1984; Fittschen et al., 1988). Trace amounts of LPS and other neutrophil stimuli (including complement fragments) were also found to act synergistically in promoting neutrophil sequestration and accumulation in pulmonary capillaries and airspaces, and to stimulate neutrophil-dependent increases in microvascular permeability (Worthen et al., 1987). Extrapolating the results of these studies implied that ARDS patients might not only display evidence of complement activation but also have detectable levels of circulating endotoxin. Unfortunately, in an investigation designed to test this hypothesis, complement activation was found in virtually all critically ill patients studied, irrespective of the development of ARDS (Parsons et al., 1989). However, in the same study, levels of endotoxin were significantly higher in patients with the established syndrome than those only at risk. Furthermore, those in the latter group who eventually developed ARDS had significantly higher levels of complement activation and endotoxin than those who did not. These findings suggest that complement and endotoxin levels might be helpful in predicting the development of ARDS, and might also explain certain aspects of the pathophysiology of acute lung injury. Thus, clinical and experimental synergy could result from the action of endotoxin as a neutrophil "priming" agent, which on subsequent triggering would cause enhanced release of histotoxic substances. Endotoxin can promote neutrophil sequestration in the lung (Haslett et al., 1987) and injure lung endothelial cells directly (Brigham et al., 1987), effects accentuating those mediated by complement activation.

1.2.3 Cytokines and Inflammatory Mediators

The concept that important putative mediators of lung injury might have different effects on inflammatory cells, particularly the neutrophil, is now assuming increasing importance. PAF, cytokines such as TNF and the ILs, and LPS are ineffective at low concentrations in stimulating neutrophil secretion but their "priming" effect enhances the subsequent release of injurious substances by triggering agents (Donnelly and Haslett, 1992; see Chapter 9). Typical triggering agents include C5a, LTB$_4$ and IL-8. Amplification mechanisms resulting from the combination of priming and triggering agents could be important in the understanding of the pathogenesis of lung injury.

The alveolar macrophage has a destructive capability similar to that of the neutrophil, being capable of generating and releasing reactive oxygen species, proteases and arachidonic acid derivatives (Repine, 1992). Macrophages are also an important source of cytokines (Table 13.2). Cytokines are released in response to endotoxin and other stimuli, including other cytokines and eicosanoids. TNF has now been cloned by recombinant technology and studied extensively. Experimentally, the physiological response to TNF closely parallels that to infused endotoxin, causing pulmonary sequestration of neutrophils, alveolar oedema and haemorrhage (Rinaldo and Christman, 1990). In normal individuals a small bolus of endotoxin results in a short-lived burst of TNF release (Michie et al., 1988). In patients with ARDS, TNF levels in BAL are significantly higher than those detectable in normal individuals (Hyers et al., 1991). In vitro, TNF stimulates the production of adhesive glycoproteins thereby enhancing the adherence of neutrophils to the endothelium (Rinaldo and Christman, 1990; see Chapter 10). It seems increasingly likely that TNF mediates many of the clinical features of endotoxaemia. Notwithstanding this, it is now appreciated that the interplay between inflammatory cells, cytokines and other mediators and the endothelium amplifies and regulates tissue injury, rather than individual mediators (Figure 13.4).

1.2.4 Role of Other Chemoattractants

Other neutrophil chemoattractants may have a role in causing the migration of neutrophils into the interstitium and airspaces. FMLP is released by bacteria and is a neutrophil chemoattractant; it may have a role in the accentuation of lung injury, particularly in those patients with ARDS who develop nosocomial pneumonia (Niederman and Fein, 1990). LTB$_4$ is released both from alveolar macrophages and neutrophils, and is chemotactic for neutrophils (Martin et al., 1989). It is found in the BAL fluid of ARDS patients (Stephenson et al., 1988),

Table 13.2 Cellular responses mediated by cytokines

Biological property	IL-1	TNF
Endogenous pyrogen fever	+	+
Hepatic acute phase proteins	+	+
Decreased albumin synthesis	+	+
Activation of endothelium	+	+
Hypotension	+	+
Fibroblast proliferation	+	+
Collagen production	+	+
Cytotoxicity	+	+
Neutrophil superoxide	−	+
Basophil degranulation	+	−
T/B lymphocyte activation	+	+/−

although in concentrations that are probably too low to act chemotactically.

1.3   HOW DO NEUTROPHILS CONTRIBUTE TO LUNG INJURY?

The neutrophil contains an extensive armamentarium of potentially toxic agents which can injure and destroy host tissue (Table 13.3) (Ganz, 1988; see Chapters 3 and 4). Because of this, neutrophils are assuming increasing importance as mediators of tissue injury in diverse chronic inflammatory diseases, both pulmonary (e.g. ARDS; IPF) and non-pulmonary (e.g. rheumatoid arthritis, myocardial reperfusion injury and ulcerative colitis) (Malech and Gallin, 1987; Henson and Johnson, 1987; see Chapter 11). The histotoxic agents of the neutrophil can be divided broadly into two groups, both of which may have important and interrelated roles in the pathogenesis of acute lung injury: (1) intracellular granules containing microbicidal peptides, proteins and enzymes (see Chapter 4); and (2) the NADPH oxidase enzyme, which is localized to the plasma membrane of the triggered neutrophil and is central to its ability to produce oxidizing agents (see Chapter 3).

1.3.1   Neutrophil Intracellular Granules

Lysozyme, a cationic enzyme, is present in the azurophilic and specific granules of the neutrophil (Spitznagel et al., 1974). It has a hydrolytic effect on constituents of the bacterial cell. Other antimicrobial substances released from granules include CatG, a serine protease, and lactoferrin, an iron-binding glycoprotein. Little information exists regarding their possible role in acute lung injury, although one study in patients at risk for ARDS who subsequently developed the established syndrome had higher levels of lactoferrin in BAL than those that did not (Hallgren et al., 1984). The major proteolytic enzymes of the neutrophil with the greatest potential for tissue injury are the serine protease, elastase and the metallo proteinases, collagenase and gelatinase. Significant elastolytic activity of neutrophil origin has been identified in BAL from patients with ARDS and was surprisingly associated with normal concentrations of α1-PI (Lee et al., 1981). The authors argued that these

findings pointed to inactivation of the protease inhibitor, possibly by oxidants. Subsequent studies have both confirmed (Cochrane et al., 1983) and refuted (Idell et al., 1985; Weiland et al., 1986) these findings. In a study comparing BAL neutrophil elastase concentrations in patients with lung injury and various fibrosing lung diseases, significantly higher concentrations were found in those with ARDS and IPF when compared to levels measured in BAL from normal controls and patients with sarcoidosis (Idell et al., 1985). In neither the ARDS nor IPF groups was elastolytic activity found, but there was a significant correlation between the degree of hypoxaemia and neutrophil elastase concentration in the patients with ARDS. This finding is difficult to interpret, as the investigators were unable to detect evidence of elastolytic activity. In a similar study, neutrophil elastase was present antigenically, but elastolytic activity was again uniformly absent (Weiland et al., 1986). This apparent inconsistency may be attributable to complexing of elastase with α1-PI. It is difficult to reconcile the above studies, which give conflicting results about the protease–antiprotease balance in clinical acute lung injury, but reactive oxygen species generated by high inspired oxygen concentrations may inactivate α1-PI, thus critically shifting the protease–anti-protease balance.

In contrast to elastase, neutrophil collagenase has been detected in BAL from patients with ARDS (Weiland et al., 1986). Lavage neutrophil concentrations also correlate with the severity of enhanced pulmonary microvascular permeability and the deficit in gas exchange. The finding of neutrophil collagenase activity in lavage fluid underlines the additional potential of neutrophil proteases to attack the lung extracellular connective tissue. Similar lavage collagenase activity has been found in IPF (Gadek et al., 1979).

1.3.2   The NADPH Oxidase System and Oxygen Metabolites

This membrane-associated enzyme system participates in the generation of three oxygen metabolites: superoxide anion, the hydroxyl radical and hydrogen peroxide. In stimulated neutrophils the enzyme system is rapidly activated, causing a marked increase in cellular oxygen uptake (the respiratory burst). Electrons are shuttled from cytosolic NADPH to oxygen dissolved in the extracellular fluid resulting in the generation of superoxide anion:

$$2O_2 + NADPH \ldots\ldots NADPH\ oxidase \ldots\ldots 2O_2^- + NADPH^+ + H^+$$

Two molecules of superoxide anion may in turn interact to form hydrogen peroxide (H_2O_2). However, both these oxidants are relatively innocuous, with little evidence to suggest that either are in themselves significantly cytotoxic (Weiss, 1989). Nevertheless, these metabolites have the potential to generate a third more powerful oxidant, the hydroxyl radical. This requires a

Table 13.3   Toxic products of neutrophils

Oxidants and reactive oxygen species	Proteolytic enzymes
Superoxide anion	Elastase
Hydrogen peroxide	Gelatinase
Hydroxyl radical	Hypochlorous acid
Chloramines	Lysozyme
Nitric acid	Neuraminidase
	Heparanase

suitable metal catalyst, usually iron. The best characterized biological damage caused by the hydroxyl radical is its potential to oxidize the polyunsaturated lipid of cell membrane, lipid peroxidation. MPO is an abundant component of neutrophil azurophilic granules, constituting 5% of the dry weight of the cell. In combination with hydrogen peroxide and the halide Cl^-, MPO generates the hypochlorite anion (OCl^-). This is an extremely reactive and microbicidal radical with marked *in vitro* cytotoxicity (Test and Weiss, 1986). For a detailed account of the neutrophil NADPH oxidase see Chapter 3.

1.3.3 Oxidant Involvement in Pathogenesis of Acute Lung Injury

Evidence of a role for ROS in acute lung injury is largely inferential. Because of their reactive nature, the concentration of ROS in blood cannot be measured directly. Instead, studies have examined either the effects of free radical scavengers in experimental acute lung injury, or other antioxidant cellular defence mechanisms. Various scavenging agents (mannitol, dimethylurea and dimethyl sulphoxide) have been shown to inhibit neutrophil-mediated pulmonary oedema in isolated perfused lungs (Tabe and Repine, 1983; Ward *et al.*, 1985; Brigham, 1986). Superoxide dismutase and catalase are intracellular enzymes which are theoretically protective against toxic oxygen metabolites. However, experimental administration of these agents has not conferred protection against free-radical mediated injury, probably because the molecules are too large to enter cells (Brigham, 1990). An important potential cellular defence mechanism is the glutathione system. The detoxification of newly formed hydrogen peroxide by NADPH is a glutathione-dependent process (Reed, 1969). *N*-Acetyl cysteine is a small molecule that can enter cells, increase intracellular glutathione stores and also act as a free radical scavenger. In sheep, exogenous glutathione moderates the pulmonary response to endotoxaemia (Bernard *et al.*, 1984). In patients with ARDS, red cell glutathione is depleted and *N*-acetyl cysteine has been shown to replete glutathione stores (Bernard, 1991) which improved oxygen delivery and consumption, although this was not statistically significant.

Hydrogen peroxide, although very reactive, can enter the gas phase at physiological temperatures. Baldwin and colleagues (1986) measured the hydrogen peroxide concentration of breath condensates in patients with and without ARDS, detecting significantly higher concentrations in ARDS patients compared to those patients only at risk of developing the syndrome. Although hydrogen peroxide *per se* is unlikely to be cytotoxic, it may have a potential role as part of the H_2O_2–MPO–Cl^--system.

A second approach to the assessment of lung oxidant-mediated injury involves the measurement of products of lipid peroxidation in blood. Canine cardiopulmonary bypass produces intrapulmonary neutrophil sequestration and mild lung injury. In this model, a trans-pulmonary gradient for lipid peroxidation products has been noted, implying ROS-mediated pulmonary injury was present (Quinlan *et al.*, 1992). A correlation was noted between the degree of pulmonary neutrophil sequestration, the transpulmonary gradient for lipid peroxidation products and increased pulmonary vascular permeability.

Lastly, recent work has detected evidence of ROS-mediated plasma protein damage as shown by increased protein carbonyl formation and decreased protein thiol groups in patients with established ARDS. More significantly, survivors had significantly lower total plasma protein values and higher protein thiol values than non-survivors (Braude *et al.*, 1986). Thus, notwithstanding the indirect nature of the evidence, several experimental and theoretical lines of evidence have implicated oxidant mechanisms in the pathogenesis of acute lung injury.

1.4 Neutrophil Function in ARDS

As outlined earlier, the predominance of neutrophils in BAL from patients with ARDS has been well described. Neutrophil numbers in lavage fluid correlate moderately well with the severity of the gas exchange abnormality and the lavage total protein concentration (Weiland *et al.*, 1986). Until recently, the functional activity of these "alveolar" neutrophils was poorly defined. Previous studies, which examined the functional status of circulating neutrophils in ARDS, gave conflicting results (Zimmerman *et al.*, 1983). Zimmerman and colleagues showed that pulmonary artery neutrophils produced enhanced chemiluminescence when stimulated with opsonized zymosan and also demonstrated enhanced chemotactic neutrophil responses toward a bacteria-derived chemotactic factor. These findings suggested profound activation of circulating neutrophils in ARDS patients. By contrast, other investigators have shown a significant reduction in neutrophil chemotaxis to FMLP during ARDS (Fowler *et al.*, 1984). In an effort to further define neutrophil functional activity in ARDS, Martin and co-workers (1991) examined both circulating and "air-space" neutrophils using three important antibacterial functions: the release of reactive oxygen species, microbicidal activity for *Staphylococcus aureus* and chemotaxis. The data demonstrated that alveolar neutrophils from ARDS patients had significantly impaired release of superoxide anion and hydrogen peroxide. Migration of alveolar neutrophils to a variety of stimuli was also markedly reduced, whilst microbicidal activity of the lavaged neutrophils for *Staphylococcus aureus* was also impaired. Pulmonary artery neutrophils from the same patients had normal chemotactic responses and microbicidal activity, but demonstrated some reduction in the generation of ROS. The authors argued that the apparent differences in the three studies (Zimmerman *et al.*, 1983; Fowler *et al.*, 1984, Martin *et al.*, 1991) with regard to neutrophil functional status could be ascribed in part to differences in methodology and timing. Nonetheless, the study of Martin and colleagues has been the first to provide data regarding the functional characteristics of alveolar (as opposed to circulating) neutrophils. Its potential relevance is considerable, as it suggests air-space neutrophils in ARDS are compromised in their ability to respond to microorganisms, thus placing the patient at increased risk of pulmonary nosocomial infection. The novel perspective of this study on the role of the neutrophil in ARDS is that impairment of an important physiological host-defence capability may be a complicating factor in ARDS. These findings significantly extend the previous more simplistic concept of the neutrophil as an exclusively injury-mediating cell. It also complicates the application and assessment of putative pharmacological interventions designed to limit neutrophil adherence, the respiratory burst or the inactivation or scavenging of neutrophil products (Mandel, 1988; Riva *et al.*, 1990).

1.5 MODULATION OF NEUTROPHIL FUNCTIONAL ACTIVITY – AN OVERVIEW OF NOVEL THERAPEUTIC STRATEGIES

Despite intensive research, no effective pharmacotherapy for ARDS is available and treatment remains supportive. In view of the pivotal role of the neutrophil in the pathogenesis of lung injury, agents which potentially counter its deleterious effects on the pulmonary microvascular endothelium are continually being evaluated (Bone, 1992). These include the following.

(a) *Inhibitors of neutrophil adherence to endothelium.* Pentoxifylline has pronounced anti-inflammatory effects (Seear *et al.*, 1990) to reduce the adhesiveness of activated neutrophils to endothelium and may reduce release of oxygen free radicals and lysosomal enzymes (Bessleer *et al.*, 1986). It reduces intrapulmonary neutrophil sequestration and is partially protective in diverse experimental models of acute lung injury (Ishizaka *et al.*, 1988; Welsh *et al.*, 1988; Tighe *et al.*, 1990; Liu *et al.*, 1992). As yet there are few data on its potential use clinically, although experimental evidence suggests that such a study is warranted. A further potential therapeutic approach is monoclonal antibodies to adhesive molecules relevant to neutrophil-endothelial interactions (Anderson *et al.*, 1990; discussed in detail in Chapter 10). Although these novel concepts remain to be assessed clinically, they have potentially deleterious effects in that they may reduce the neutrophil's host defence capability.

(b) *Oxygen free-radical scavengers.* Superoxide dismutase and catalase are of theoretical interest as they respectively scavenge the superoxide radical and convert hydrogen peroxide to water. However, they have not yet been demonstrated convincingly to confer protection against ROS-mediated injury. More recently, a recombinant form of superoxide dismutase has been introduced. Initial investigations in experimental sepsis suggest that the agent is without side-effect and may be beneficial (Koyama *et al.*, 1992). *N*-Acetyl cysteine has been shown to have no significant effect on gas exchange or survival in established ARDS (Jepson *et al.*, 1992). Other potential free-radical scavengers (mannitol, dimethylurea and dimethyl sulphoxide) mentioned above, have not been assessed clinically.

(c) *Protease inhibitors.* Novel antiproteases have appeared promising in initial animal studies (Okuda and Ogata, 1989; Sieback *et al.*, 1989), but no clinical trials of protease inhibitors and ARDS have been reported to date.

(d) *Steroids.* The effects of steroids on mortality in established ARDS have been disappointing (Bernard *et al.*, 1987; Bone *et al.*, 1987), but there is some suggestion that a beneficial response may be obtained in patients in the organizing (non-active) phase of the disease, even to the extent of reducing neutrophil numbers in BAL (Braude *et al.*, 1992).

1.6 CONCLUSION

More complete understanding of the role of the neutrophil in the pathogenesis of lung injury has served partly to underline its complexity. From the therapeutic viewpoint it appears increasingly unlikely that a single agent, focusing on one component of a complex inflammatory response, will be beneficial. Recent studies emphasize both the destructive and host-defence elements of the inflammatory response. The challenge for the future is to tailor drug therapy to the temporal evolution of the disease so that the most appropriate aspect of the inflammatory response can be modulated.

2. *Cryptogenic Fibrosing Alveolitis*

2.1 CFA AND NEUTROPHILS

Interstitial pulmonary fibrosis or cryptogenic fibrosing alveolitis (CFA) is a condition which is characterized by the presence of inflammation and fibrosis of the pulmonary interstitium and peripheral airspaces on histological evaluation of lung biopsy samples, and by an increase of inflammatory cells, particularly neutrophils, in samples of epithelial lining fluid obtained from the lower respiratory tract by bronchoalveolar lavage (Scadding, 1964; Crystal *et al.*, 1984; Haslam *et al.*, 1980; Weinberger *et al.*, 1978). There has accumulated a body of evidence which would support the concept that the neutrophil plays a pivotal role in the pathogenesis of the disease process, by causing endothelial, epithelial and connective tissue damage. Unlike the acute lung injury which occurs in ARDS, the time-frame of lung damage in CFA is much longer with disease occurring in a patchy fashion and evolving non-contemporaneously in different regions of the lung.

2.1.1 Clinical Features

Fibrosing alveolitis presents with progressive breathlessness on exertion and can result in respiratory failure and death. It is estimated that approximately 5/100 000 of the population suffer from fibrosing alveolitis in the United Kingdom and approximately 1400 patients die each year from the condition (Johnston et al., 1990). Disease incidence is increasing and response to treatment is poor with only 20% of patients responding objectively to corticosteroid therapy. Median survival is 5 years (Turner-Warwick et al., 1980; Watters et al., 1986; Johnson et al., 1989). Factors which indicate a poor prognosis include an excess of granulocytes, particularly neutrophils, obtained by bronchoalveolar lavage of the lower respiratory tract (Haslam et al., 1980; Turner-Warwick et al., 1980; Watters et al., 1987).

Recently developed investigations, including bronchoalveolar lavage, high-resolution CT and ^{99m}Tc DTPA scanning have provided an important window through which to assess the disease. These techniques have made it possible to detect early disease and to predict disease progression (Harrison et al., 1989; Hansell and Kerr, 1991).

The pattern and extent of abnormality on high-resolution CT correlate with the lavage cell profile: more extensive fibrotic disease is associated with an excess of neutrophils within the lower respiratory tract, whereas eosinophils are obtained when disease first becomes evident on CT images (Wells et al., 1991).

2.2 AETIOLOGY AND PATHOGENESIS

2.2.1 Aetiology

The aetiology is unknown. A pathological process similar to CFA may develop in response to inhaled organic antigens such as avian and fungal antigen and also in response to inorganic dusts such as hard metal and asbestos. A high incidence of EBV antibodies has been found in one series but other attempts to implicate virus in the aetiology have been disappointing (Vergnon et al., 1984).

In a small subset of patients, the disease process appears to be familial and, in one study of normal individuals from families in whom there has been more than one case of fibrosing alveolitis, excess neutrophils and neutrophil products were observed in the lower respiratory tract in the absence of any other clinical index of disease suggesting that the neutrophil may play a role in the early stages of pathogenesis (Bitterman et al., 1986).

In the autosomal recessive disorder, Hermansky–Pudlak syndrome, fibrosing alveolitis occurs as part of the syndrome suggesting some predisposition to lung fibrosis (Hoste et al., 1979). Studies of HLA status have been disappointing but α1AT and immunoglobulin linkage disequilibrium studies have suggested that a gene on chromosome 14 may be involved in disease pathogenesis in some individuals (Fulmer et al., 1978; Musk et al., 1986).

One problem with HLA studies in fibrosing alveolitis is that it is such a heterogeneous disease process. In a more homogeneous population of patients with systemic sclerosis, lung fibrosis was associated with a particular DR3-related haplotype (DR3, DRw52a) and also the presence of the Scl70 anti-DNA topoisomerase antibody (Briggs et al., 1991). The implications of this observation are not yet clear but could include linkage of this haplotype to genes responsible for pulmonary fibrosis, lung injury or to the involvement of a particular MHC class II haplotype in antigen presentation at the inductive phase of disease.

2.2.2 Pathology

Histological examination of lung biopsy samples shows that inflammatory cells, particularly lymphocytes and mononuclear phagocytes are present in large numbers within the interstitium (Haslam et al., 1980; Liebow et al., 1975). Eosinophils and neutrophils are relatively sparse. In the airspaces, mononuclear cells may be present and it is also within the airspaces that neutrophils are most commonly observed (Haslam et al., 1980). Variable degrees of lung damage and interstitial fibrosis are present. Type II epithelial cell proliferation is a prominent feature. Electron microscopy of lung which is normal to light microscopy reveals endothelial and epithelial cell damage with interstitial oedema suggesting that damage to these cells may be one of the critical early disease processes (Harrison et al., 1991). Loss of basement membrane may also be crucial to the further development of interstitial disease by preventing normal epithelial repair after injury (Vrako, 1972).

2.2.3 Pathogenesis

The present paradigm of cryptogenic fibrosing alveolitis involves concepts of immune response, inflammatory cell recruitment to disease sites, lung damage and fibrosis.

2.2.3.1 Triggering Events

The initial trigger is unknown. This almost certainly involves damage as shown by the ultrastructural observations. It is possible that this damage could be provoked by both external agents such as viruses or internal factors including inflammatory cells. Whatever the mechanism, tissue injury appears to be the initial event following which clinical disease evolves.

2.2.3.2   Immune Response

It is beyond the aim of this chapter to detail the evidence for the involvement of immunological mechanisms in the disease process but in summary:

(1) Multiple lymphoid follicles are present within the lung interstitium. These contain germinal centres and the immunohistological appearances of these follicles confirms that they are true secondary follicles capable of antibody production (Campbell *et al.*, 1985).

(2) The lung interstitium contains large numbers of T lymphocytes predominantly CD4+ cells bearing the CD45RO phenotype of "primed" cells. These cells are activated as shown by the presence of activation markers such as HLA-DR and IL-2R (Haslam, 1990; Wells *et al.*, 1992).

(3) Immune complexes are present in serum and bronchoalveolar lavage fluid from these patients. They are rarely observed in tissue (Dreisin *et al.*, 1978; Dall'Aglio *et al.*, 1988).

(4) HLA class II molecule expression is observed on the majority of macrophages and epithelial cells and some lymphocytes suggesting activation (Campbell *et al.*, 1985).

(5) Sera from patients with cryptogenic fibrosing alveolitis contain non-organ specific antibodies including antinuclear antibody, rheumatoid factor and antibodies to DNA topoisomerase II, an enzyme which plays an important role in gene transcription. Polyclonal increases in one or more IgG classes G, M and A are also found (Meliconi *et al.*, 1989; Turner-Warwick and Haslam, 1971; Hobbs and Turner-Warwick, 1967).

(6) Lavage cells from patients with CFA spontaneously secrete more B-cell growth factor than control lavage cell populations and lung lavage fluid contains more immunoglobulin than controls (Reynolds *et al.*, 1977; Emura *et al.*, 1990).

Immune mechanisms are, therefore, undoubtedly involved in disease pathogenesis and likely play a crucial role in macrophage activation.

2.2.3.3   The Role of Alveolar Macrophages

Alveolar macrophages are present in increased numbers in lung lavage fluid from patients with fibrosing alveolitis compared with normal individuals (Weinbeger *et al.*, 1978; Haslam *et al.*, 1980; Watters *et al.*, 1987). Using a panel of mAbs it has been shown that the macrophage population in the lower respiratory tract is heterogeneous: increased numbers of cells bear ligands identified by RFD-1, a monoclonal antibody which recognizes interdigitating cells. Other cells bear ligands associated with mature macrophages (RFD-7) and with epithelioid cells (more usually found in sarcoid granulomata) (RFD-9) (Campbell *et al.*, 1986; Noble *et al.*, 1989). The functional significance of these different phenotypes in CFA is unknown.

The functional repertoire of alveolar macrophages is extensive. Macrophage products which have been shown to be involved in the pathogenesis of cryptogenic fibrosing alveolitis are:

(1) The synthesis and secretion of pro-inflammatory cytokines which may regulate inflammatory cell traffic into the lungs, e.g. TNF-α, IL-1 (Gosset *et al.*, 1991; Nagai *et al.*, 1991).

(2) Neutrophil chemotactic factors, notably IL-8 (Merrill *et al.*, 1980; Carre *et al.*, 1991; Southcott *et al.*, 1992).

(3) Competence and progression growth factors including fibronectin, PDGF and IGF-1 (Martinet *et al.*, 1987; Yamauchi *et al.*, 1987; Rom *et al.*, 1988).

Alveolar macrophages also secrete lysosomal enzymes, proteases and release oxygen radicals which are capable of producing tissue injury (du Bois *et al.*, 1980; Cross *et al.*, 1987).

2.2.3.4   The Role of Granulocytes

In considering the role of granulocytes in CFA, three major questions emerge: (1) are they present?; (2) do they damage lung?; and (3) at what stage of disease pathogenesis are they involved? Both neutrophils and eosinophils are present in increased numbers in the lower respiratory tract of patients with cryptogenic fibrosing alveolitis. Secretory products of both cells are also present in high concentrations in lung lavage fluid removed from these patients and there is also evidence for enhanced oxygen radical generation (Gadek *et al.*, 1979; Davies *et al.*, 1984; Hallgren *et al.*, 1989).

Although the answers to the first two questions are clearly positive there are no unequivocal data to answer the third question particularly with regard to the neutrophil. Animal models and human studies provide evidence which is not entirely concordant, and the remainder of this chapter will focus on concepts of neutrophil involvement in CFA with particular emphasis on this issue.

2.3   Neutrophils and Lung Disease – General Concepts

2.3.1   Neutrophil Origin and Fate

Neutrophils are derived from bone marrow progenitor cells, 60% of which are of neutrophil lineage (Abramson *et al.*, 1991; see Chapter 2). Pro-inflammatory cytokines including the CSFs, G-CSF and GM-CSF, IL-1, TNF-α and glucocorticoids are potent stimulators of neutrophil production and release from bone marrow (Dale *et al.*, 1975; Dinarello, 1984; Beutler and Cerami, 1987). Neutrophils remain in the circulation for approximately 10 h before migrating into tissue (Golde, 1983) . Large numbers of neutrophils, estimated to be approximately

55%, are marginated, particularly in the lung which removes 20% of the 4×10^8 neutrophils passing through the lung each second (Muir *et al.*, 1984). It is clear, therefore, that a considerable potential neutrophil burden is available for traffic into the lungs following appropriate signalling.

2.4 EVIDENCE FOR THE INVOLVEMENT OF NEUTROPHILS IN FIBROSING ALVEOLITIS

2.4.1 Animal Models

A number of animal models have been developed to study the sequence of events leading to lung injury and fibrosis. Best studied examples of these models are those induced by bleomycin or asbestos. Although agents are used in these animal models which are known to produce human lung disease, the nature of the process is such that a more acute pathological process ensues which is more like ARDS than fibrosing alveolitis in terms of time scale and extent of lung involved – in CFA lung is involved in a patchy fashion and different stages of disease process are present in different parts of the lung. Despite these limitations, bleomycin-induced fibrosis has been helpful in emphasizing the mechanisms which are important in initial injury.

As with the ultrastructural studies of human lung, first evidence of injury involves epithelial and endothelial cell damage, followed by fluid leakage and activation of coagulation and complement cascades (Adamson and Bowden, 1974; Thet *et al.*, 1986). In the initial stages of disease, neutrophils are present in large numbers. Numbers then become reduced but neutrophils may still be observed a number of weeks later. Neutrophil labelling with indium-111 can be used to monitor neutrophil migration into the lungs after bleomycin instillation. Haslett *et al.* (1989) have demonstrated that intratracheal injection of 10 units/kg bleomycin induces neutrophil migration into the lung which continued for a 3-week period. Furthermore, external scintigraphy confirmed that indium-labelled neutrophil traffic correlated with quantification of neutrophils in histological sections and also with the percentage of neutrophils present in airspaces. Consistent with the concept of neutrophil products being capable of inducing lung fibrosis, studies by Nakashima have shown that repeated oxidant injury to hamster lung using mixtures of glucose, glucose oxidase and lactoperoxidase at weekly intervals produced neutrophil influx, and ultimately lung fibrosis (Nakashima *et al.*, 1991). The study would suggest that epithelial injury is capable of attracting inflammatory cells to disease sites. Further support for the concept of neutrophil-induced damage comes from studies involving the administration of α1-PI to animals treated with bleomycin (Nagai *et al.*, 1992). This reduced pulmonary fibrosis at both 7 and 30 days after bleomycin therapy, although there was no difference in the amount of elastase present within the lavage fluids of the α1-PI and control groups.

Although these studies clearly demonstrate the presence of neutrophils and their products within the lungs of animals which are in the process of developing lung fibrosis, Harris *et al.* (1991) have demonstrated that neutrophil influx alone is not sufficient to produce fibrosis. In this study repeated installation of human recombinant C5a was used to attract neutrophils to the lung but this did not result in sufficient injury to produce pulmonary fibrosis. The implication of this study is that neutrophils were not being triggered to release either oxidants or damaging proteolytic enzymes within the local milieu.

2.4.2 Human Studies

Up to 15-fold increases in neutrophil numbers are observed in lung lavage samples of the lining fluid of the lower respiratory tracts of patients with CFA (particularly cigarette smokers) (The BAL Cooperative Group Steering Committee, 1990). Neutrophils may also be observed histologically, although in lower numbers than might be expected, from the lavage findings.

Other diseases such as asbestosis and rheumatological diseases in which fibrosing alveolitis is a part are also characterized by the presence of excess numbers of neutrophils in the lower respiratory tract (Gellert *et al.*, 1985; Breit *et al.*, 1989). Of particular interest is that a subclinical neutrophil alveolitis, i.e. alveolitis which occurs in the absence of any clinical or radiographic evidence of disease, may occur in diseases such as systemic sclerosis and rheumatoid arthritis supporting the concept that neutrophils emerge into the lung at an early stage of disease (Rossi *et al.*, 1985; Garcia *et al.*, 1986; Harrison *et al.*, 1989). By contrast, neutrophils are only present in the lungs of patients with sarcoidosis, a granulomatous disease normally associated with excess numbers of lymphocytes within the lower respiratory tract, at a time when lung fibrosis has developed (Lin *et al.*, 1985).

Neutrophil secretory products are present in CFA lung lavage fluid. Gadek *et al.* (1979) found high levels of collagenase and neutral proteinase in epithelial lining fluid from patients with CFA, and a more recent observation by Hallgren *et al.*, (1989) of increased MPO in the lower respiratory tract would support the concept that neutrophil-mediated damage occurs in CFA. This conclusion is strengthened by results from two studies which have demonstrated that increased oxidized methionine residues are present in bronchoalveolar lavage-derived proteins and enhanced oxygen radical production is found in cells obtained from patients with fibrosing alveolitis by comparison with lung cells from normal individuals (Behr *et al.*, 1991; Maier *et al.*, 1991).

2.5 MECHANISMS OF RECRUITMENT AND ACTIVATION OF NEUTROPHILS TO DISEASE SITES

Alveolar macrophages from patients with fibrosing alveolitis spontaneously synthesize and secrete a lipid chemotactic factor for neutrophils which has not been fully characterized, but is probably LTB4 (Merrill et al., 1980). More recent studies have demonstrated that alveolar macrophages contain mRNA for IL-8 in increased amounts by comparison with normal macrophages, and higher concentrations of IL-8 are present in lavage fluid from the same patients by comparison with samples from control patients [IL-8 is likely to be the alveolar macrophage-derived neutrophil chemotactic factor first described by Hunninghake et al., 1980)]. Furthermore, both IL-8 and TNF-α can activate neutrophils to release oxygen radicals (Leonard and Yoshimura, 1992).

Increasing interest has been shown in adhesion molecules for inflammatory cells (discussed in detail in Chapters 7 and 10). E-selectin (ELAM-1) is now recognized as an adhesion molecule for neutrophils (Bevilacqua et al., 1989). Endothelial cell expression of E-selectin requires pro-inflammatory signals from cytokines such as TNF-α and IL-1 (Bevilacqua et al., 1989). Alveolar macrophages in CFA are known to produce TNF-α and IL-1 (Gosset et al., 1991; Nagai et al., 1991) and recent preliminary studies have identified the presence of soluble E-selectin in lavage fluid from patients with fibrosing alveolitis (du Bois et al., 1992).

The alveolar macrophage therefore is likely to play a central role in attracting neutrophils to disease sites by both increasing expression of endothelial E-selectin and providing a chemoattractant gradient whereby neutrophils are released from their vascular attachment, proceed by diapedesis between the endothelial cells, pass through the basement membrane and into the lung interstitium where they are activated in situ. The presence of high levels of IL-8 in lung lavage fluid and increased amounts of IL-8 mRNA in lavage cells might imply that there is a gradient of IL-8 chemoattraction through the interstitium and into the airspace where the majority of neutrophils are observed.

The mechanisms which activate macrophages to release IL-1, TNF-α and IL-8 have not been fully evaluated in cryptogenic fibrosing alveolitis, although a candidate could be immune complexes. Normal macrophages incubated in the presence of immune complexes are capable of releasing neutrophil chemotactic factor (Hunninghake et al., 1989) and immune complexes are present within the lungs of patients with fibrosing alveolitis (Dall'Aglio et al., 1988). It is therefore possible to speculate that antibody generated in lung lymphoid follicles reacts with local antigen resulting in the production of immune complexes which then activate macrophages to produce neutrophil chemotactic and other regulatory factors.

2.6 NEUTROPHIL INVOLVEMENT IN THE PATHOGENESIS OF FIBROSING ALVEOLITIS – EARLY OR LATE?

There is little doubt that neutrophils are involved in the pathogenesis of cryptogenic fibrosing alveolitis. They are present in increased numbers, free secretory products are present in lung epithelial lining fluid and there is evidence of oxidant generation which is neutrophil derived. Mechanisms of recruitment of neutrophils to the lungs have now been well defined and neutrophils are seen to be present within the lungs of patients with fibrosing alveolitis associated with rheumatological diseases even before chest radiography has become abnormal, suggesting a role in early disease pathogenesis. In support of this, neutrophils are the first cells to be found in excess in the lungs of patients suspected of having extrinsic allergic alveolitis following inhalation challenge with the appropriate antigen. Taken together with animal model experiments it is possible to speculate, therefore, that neutrophils are one of the key cells in the early inductive phases of disease. Despite this weight of evidence, however, no satisfactory explanation has been provided for the observations that relatively few neutrophils are seen within the lung interstitium in early disease.

Alternatively, support for the concept that neutrophils are latecomers to disease sites is provided by a recent study comparing extent of disease and relative degrees of cellularity and fibrosis assessed by high-resolution CT in a single lobe of lung with lung lavage findings from the same lobe. This study has shown that lymphocytes are present in excess even before CT abnormalities have become apparent. If up to 50% of the lavage lobe is involved in the disease process, excess numbers of eosinophils are present but it is only when more than 50% of the lung is involved that neutrophils emerge in large numbers (Wells et al., 1992). Furthermore, neutrophil numbers correlate with the extent of fibrotic change observed on CT. These observations would suggest that neutrophils are a later feature in disease pathogenesis and that they are observed only when initial damage and fibrosis has occurred.

Why are many more neutrophils present both on histological examination and in lavage in the later stages of disease, and why are larger numbers of neutrophils lavaged from the lower respiratory tract than appear to be present within lung tissue in more advanced CFA? Possible explanations for the tissue/lavage discordance include "dilution" by the abundant mononuclear cells present in the interstitium preventing accurate identification.

The presence of large numbers of neutrophils within airspaces is often interpreted as reflecting end-stage infection rather than extensive disease but this has never been confirmed bacteriologically, and may indeed be consistent with the hypothesis that advanced disease is associated with increasing neutrophil traffic to the lungs.

It is, however, intriguing to speculate that the predilection of neutrophils for the airspaces reflects a gradient of chemotaxis and that the expression of potent neutrophil chemoattractants such as IL-8 is preferentially up-regulated in airway cells. Using CT-guided lavage together with immunohistochemistry and *in situ* hybridization of lung biopsy samples to identify the spatial localization of IL-8 within the lung, it should be possible to answer these important questions.

Despite these conflicting data it is safe to conclude that neutrophils and their products play a role in CFA, and indeed their presence in excess numbers in lavage is associated with a poorer prognosis for the patient compared with those whose granulocyte numbers are normal. It is logical to conclude a priori that early acute injury, which is thought to trigger disease, is associated with a neutrophil influx, although there is no direct evidence for this in man. There is unequivocal evidence that large numbers of neutrophils are present in advanced disease. Perhaps, therefore, neutrophil-induced injury is biphasic or even multiphasic with new "waves" of cells being attracted to the lung at different time points during the evolution of disease, and as more lung becomes involved, a greater neutrophil presence is observed.

2.7 FATE OF NEUTROPHILS – EVIDENCE OF APOPTOSIS?

It has become clear in recent years that the reason neutrophils, which move to the lungs in great numbers in, for example, lobar pneumonia, do not produce extensive injury is that they undergo preprogrammed cell death, a process known as apoptosis, and are ultimately being removed from the local microenvironment by macrophages (Savill *et al.*, 1989; see Chapter 14). The precise mechanisms whereby the neutrophils undergo the preprogrammed changes are unclear but the macrophage vitronectin receptor, CD36 and thrombospondin are implicated (Savill *et al.*, 1991). Nothing is known about apoptotic regulation in chronic diseases such as fibrosing alveolitis which are characterized by persistent neutrophil presence. It is not possible to say whether neutrophil life is extended in the local milieu or if persistent neutrophilia is due to continual recruitment of neutrophils. In this regard, there have been no studies of neutrophil survival in lung lavage neutrophil samples but the persistence of neutrophil chemoattractants and adhesion molecules would certainly suggest that continuing recruitment is at least a part of the explanation.

2.8 ANALOGIES WITH RHEUMATOID ARTHRITIS

There are a number of lines of evidence which indicate that CFA is an expression of a local autoimmune disease bearing many similarities to rheumatoid arthritis, and fibrosing alveolitis may occur as part of rheumatoid disease. In CFA occurring alone, immunological mechanisms are activated. Furthermore, immunohistochemical analysis of open lung biopsy material and the concept of local generation of immune complexes activating macrophages, resulting in neutrophil chemotaxis, are also important features of the paradigm of disease pathogenesis of rheumatoid arthritis.

Rheumatoid arthritis is characterized by the presence of activated immune effector cells, notably macrophages and lymphocytes, at disease sites. Neutrophils are present in acutely inflamed joint fluid but not in quiescent joints nor within the synovial tissue itself. Locally generated immune complexes may be responsible for neutrophil chemotaxis: synovial fluid mononuclear cells spontaneously release IL-8 and this release can be enhanced by stimulation with immune complexes LPS and IL-1 (Seitz *et al.*, 1991). Rheumatoid factors containing immune complexes are also potent activators of IL-8 production and synovial fluids contain high levels of IL-8 (Brennan *et al.*, 1990; Endo *et al.*, 1991; Piechl *et al.*, 1991; Seitz *et al.*, 1991).

These common cellular and molecular biological processes emphasize that similar immunological and damaging inflammatory cell mechanisms can produce tissue damage in different disease entities. These common features also emphasize that studies of one disease can provide important novel insights into the mechanisms which produce another.

2.9 FUTURE APPROACHES

Once fibrosing alveolitis has advanced to the stage of extensive damage and fibrosis, little can be done. Future goals should be the identification of early disease, the development of prognostic indicators, and the production of specifically designed treatment which blocks disease at the inductive phase before damage and fibrosis have ensued. These future therapies will include modulation of immune mechanisms and of granulocyte-induced injury.

Treatment strategies could employ therapy which inhibits neutrophil chemotaxis or factors which trigger neutrophils *in situ* to release their damaging products. Treatment of lung disease has the added advantage of local access of drug directly to the disease site, through the inhaled route for drugs which might have an unacceptable side-effect profile if given systemically. In addition, the ease of access to lung inflammatory cell populations by fibreoptic bronchoscopy and lavage, procedures which are extremely well tolerated and safe, will allow assessments to be made of the efficacy of newer more targeted treatment of inflammation within the lung. The obvious dangers of blocking neutrophil function lie in the risk of infection but this risk already exists with the more globally acting corticosteroid and immunosuppressive therapies which are currently used to treat the disease. Further studies of the molecular and cell biology of neutrophils and their role in producing chronically injured lung will undoubtedly yield further information of importance in the management of this relentless condition.

3.   References

Abramson, L., Malech, H.L. and Gallin, J.I. (1991). In "The Lung: Scientific Foundations" (eds R.G. Crystal and J.B. West) pp. 553–563. Raven Press, New York.

Adamson, I.Y. and Bowden, D.H. (1974). The pathogenesis of bleomycin induced pulmonary fibrosis in mice. Am. J. Pathol. 77, 185–197.

Anderson, D.C., Rothlein, R., Marlin, S.D., Kraters, S.S. and Smith, C.W. (1990). Impaired transendothelial migration by neonatal neutrophils: abnormalities of MAC-1 (CD11b/CD18)-dependent adherence reactions. Blood 76, 2613–2621.

Ashbaugh, D.G., Bigelow, D.D., Petty, T.L. and Levine, B.E. (1967). Acute respiratory distress in adults. Lancet 2, 219–323.

BAL Cooperative Group Steering Committee (1990). Bronchoalveolar lavage constituents in healthy individuals, idiopathic pulmonary fibrosis and selected comparison groups. Am. Rev. Respir. Dis. 141 (Suppl. 5), S188–S192.

Baldwin, S.R., Grum, C.M., Boxer, L.A., Simon, R.H., Ketai, L.H. and Devall, L.J. (1986). Oxidant activity in expired breath of patients with adult respiratory distress syndrome. Lancet 1, 11–14.

Behr, J., Maier, K., Krombach, F. and Adelmann-Grill, B.C. (1991). Pathogenetic significance of reactive oxygen species in diffuse fibrosing alveolitis. Am. Rev. Respir. Dis. 144, 146–150.

Bernard, G.R. (1991). N-Acetylcysteine in experimental and clinical acute lung injury. Am. J. Med. 91, 545–595.

Bernard, G.R., Lucht, W.D., Niedermeyer, M.E., Snapper, J.E., Ogeltree, M.L. and Brigham, K.L. (1984). Effects of N-acetyl cysteine on the pulmonary response to endotoxin in the awake sheep and upon in vitro granulocyte function. J. Clin. Invest. 73, 1772–1784.

Bernard, G.R., Luce, J.M., Sprung, C.L., Rinaldo, J.E., Tate, R.B., Sibbald, W.J., Kariman, K., Higgins, S., Bradley, R. and Metz, C.A. (1987). High-dose corticosteroids in patients with the adult respiratory distress syndrome. N. Engl. J. Med. 317, 1565–1570.

Bessleer, H., Gilgal, R., Djaldetti, M. and Zahari, I. (1986). Effect of pentoxifylline on the phagocytic activity c-AMP levels and superanion production by monocytes and polymorphonuclear cells. J. Leukocyte Biol. 40, 747–754.

Beutler, B. and Cerami, A. (1987). Cachectin: more than a tumour necrosis factor. N. Engl. J. Med. 316, 379–385.

Bevilacqua, M.P., Staengelin, S., Gimbrone, M.A. and Seed, B. (1989). Endothelial leukocyte adhesion molecule 1: an inducible receptor for neutrophils related to complement regulatory proteins and lectins. Science 243, 1160–1165.

Bitterman, P.B., Rennard, S.I., Keogh, B.A., Wewers, M.D., Adelberg, S. and Crystal, R.G. (1986). Familial idiopathic pulmonary fibrosis. Evidence of lung inflammation in unaffected family members. N. Engl. J. Med. 314, 1343–1347.

Bone, R.C. (1992). Inhibitors of complement and neutrophils: a critical evaluation of their role in the treatment of sepsis. Crit. Care Med. 20, 891–898.

Bone, R.C., Fisher, C.J., Clemmer, T.P., Slotman, G.T. and Metz, L.A. (1987). A controlled clinical trial of high dose methylprednisolone in the treatment of severe sepsis and septic shock. N. Engl. J. Med. 317, 653–658.

Braude, S., Krausz, T., Apperley, J. and Goldman, J.M. (1985). Adult respiratory distress syndrome after allogeneic bone marrow transplantation: evidence for a neutrophil independent mechanism. Lancet i, 1239–1243.

Braude, S., Nolop, K., Taylor, K., Krausz, T. and Royston, D. (1986). Increased pulmonary transvascular protein flux after canine cardiopulmonary bypass: association with neutrophil sequestration and tissue peroxidation. Am. Rev. Respir. Dis. 134, 867–872.

Braude, S., Haslan, P., Hughes, D., MacNaughton, P.D. and Evans, T.W. (1992) Chronic adult respiratory distress syndrome – a role for corticosteroid? Crit. Care Med. 20, 1187–1190.

Breit, N., Cairns, D., Szentirmay, A., Calagan, T. et al. (1989). The presence of Sjogren's syndrome as a major determinant of the pattern of interstitial lung disease in scleroderma and other connective tissue diseases. J. Rheumatol. 16, 1043–1049.

Brennan, F.M., Zacharia, C.O., Chantry, D., Larsen, C.G., Turner, M., Maini, R.M., Matsushima, K. and Feldmann, M. (1990). Detection of IL-8 biological activity in synovial fluids from patients with rheumatoid arthritis and production of IL-8 mRNA by isolated synovial cells. Eur. J. Immunol. 20, 2141–2144.

Briggs, D., Vaughan, R., Welsh, K., Myers, A., du Bois, R.M. and Black, C. (1991). Immunogenetic prediction of pulmonary fibrosis in systemic sclerosis. Lancet 338, 661–662.

Brigham, K.L. (1986). Role of free radicals in lung injury. Chest 89, 859–863.

Brigham, K.L. (1990). Oxidant stress and adult respiratory stress syndrome. Eur. Resp. J. 3(Suppl 11), 482S–484S.

Brigham, K.L., Bowers, R. and Haynes, J. (1979). Increased sheep lung vascular permeability caused by E. coli endotoxin. Circ. Res. 45, 292–297.

Brigham, K.L., Meyrick, D., Berry, L.C. and Repine, J.E. (1987). Antioxidants protect cultured bovine lung enothelial cells from injury by endotoxin. J. Appl. Physiol. 63, 848–850.

Campbell, D.A., Poulter, L.W., Janossy, G. and du Bois, R.M. (1985). Immunohistological analysis of lung tissue from patients with cryptogenic fibrosing alveolitis suggesting local expression of immune hypersensitivity. Thorax 40, 405–411.

Campbell, D.A., Poulter, L.W. and du Bois, R.M. (1986). Phenotypic analysis of alveolar macrophages in normal subjects and in patients with interstitial lung disease. Thorax 41, 429–434.

Carre, P.C., Mortenson, R.L., King, T.E., Noble, P.W., Sable, C.L. and Riches, D.W.H. (1991). Overexpression of the interleukin 8 gene by alveolar macrophages from patients with idiopathic pulmonary fibrosis. Am. Rev. Respir. Dis. 143, A396.

Cochrane, C.G., Spragg, R. and Revak, S.D. (1983). Pathogenesis of the adult respiratory distress syndrome: evidence of oxidant activity in bronchoalveolar lavage fluid. J. Clin. Invest. 71, 754–761.

Craddock, P.R., Fehr, J., Brigham, K.L. and Jacob, H. (1975). Pulmonary capillary leucostasis: a complement mediated complication of haemodialysis. Clin. Res. 23, 402A.

Craddock, P.R., Fehr, J., Brigham, K.L., Kroneberg, R.S. and Jacob, H.S. (1977a). Complement and leucocyte mediated pulmonary dysfunction in human dialysis. N. Engl. J. Med. 296, 769–774.

Craddock, P.R., Fehr, J., Dalmasso, A.P., Brigham, K.L. and Jacob, H.S. (1977b). Human dialysis leucopenia: pulmonary vascular leucostasis resulting from complement activation by dialyser cellophane membranes. J. Clin. Invest. 59, 879–888.

Craddock, P.R., Hammerschmidt, D.E., Dalmasso, A., White, J.G. and Jacob, H.S. (1977c). Complement (C5a) induced granulocyte aggregation in vitro: a possible mechanism of complement mediated leucostasis and leucopenia. J. Clin. Invest. 260–264.

Cross, C.E., Halliwell, B., Borish, E.T., Pryor, W.A., Ames, B.N., Saul, R.L., McCord, J.M. and Harman, D. (1987). Oxygen radicals and human disease. Ann. Intern. Med. 107, 526–545.

Crystal, R.G., Bitterman, P.B., Rennard, S.T., Hance, A.J. and Keogh, B.A. (1984). Interstitial lung diseases of unknown cause: disorders characterized by chronic inflammation of the lower respiratory tract. N. Engl. J. Med. 310, 154–165, 235–244.

Dale, D.C., Fauci, A.S., Guerry, D.-P. and Wolff, S.M. (1957). Comparison of agents producing a neutrophilic leukocytosis in man. J. Clin. Invest. 56, 808–813.

Dall'Aglio, P.P., Pesci, A., Bertorelli, G., Brianti, E. and Scarpa, S. (1988). Study of immune complexes in broncho-alveolar lavage fluids. Respiration 54(Suppl. 1), 36–41.

Davies, W.B., Fells, G.A., Sun, X.H., Gadek, J.E., Venet, A. and Crystal, R.G. (1984). Eosinophil mediated injury to parenchymal cells and interstitial matrix. A possible role for eosinophils in chronic inflammatory disorders of the lower respiratory tract. J. Clin. Invest. 74, 269–278.

Dinarello, C.A. (1984). Interleukin-1 and the pathogenesis of the acute phase response. N. Engl. J. Med. 311, 1413–1418.

Donnelly, F.C. and Haslett, C. (1992). Cellular mechanisms of acute lung injury: implications for treatment in the adult respiratory distress syndrome. Thorax 47, 250–263.

Dreisin, R.B., Schwarz, M.I., Theofilopoulos, A.N. and Stanford, R.E. (1978). Circulating immune complexes in the idiopathic interstitial pneumonias. N. Engl. J. Med. 298, 353–357.

du Bois, R.M., Townsend, P.J. and Cole, P.J. (1980). Alveolar macrophage lysozomal enzyme in C3b receptors in crypto-genic fibrosing alveolitis. Clin. Exp. Immunol. 40, 60–65.

du Bois, R.M., Hellewell, P.G., Hemingway, I. and Gearing, A.J. (1992). Soluble cell adhesion molecules ICAM-1, ELAM-1 and VCAM-1 are present in epithelial lining fluid in patients with interstitial lung disease. Am. Rev. Respir. Dis. 145A.

Duchateau, J., Haas, M., Schreyen, H. et al. (1984). Comple-ment activation in patients at risk of developing the adult respiratory distress syndrome. Am. Rev. Respir. Dis. 130, 1958–1964.

Emura, M., Nagai, S., Takeuchi, M., Kitaichi, M. and Izumi, T. (1990). In vitro production of B-cell growth factor and B-cell differentiation factor by peripheral blood mononuclear cells and bronchoalveolar lavage T lymphocytes from patients with idiopathic pulmonary fibrosis. Clin. Exp. Immunol. 82, 133–139.

Endo, H., Akahoshi, T., Takagishi, K., Kashiwazaki, S. and Matsushima, K. (1991). Elevation of interleukin-8 (IL-8) levels in joint fluids of patients with rheumatoid arthritis and the induction by IL-8 of leukocyte infiltration in synovitis in rabbit joints. Lymphokine Cytokine Res. 10, 245–252.

Fittschen, C.F., Sandhaus, R.A., Worthen, G.S. and Henson, P.M. (1988). Bacterial lipopolysaccharide enhances chemo-attractant induced elastase secretion by human neutrophils. J. Leucocyte Biol. 43, 547–556.

Fowler, A.A., Fisher, B.J., Centor, R.M. and Carchman, R.A. (1984). Development of the adult respiratory distress syndrome: progressive alteration of neutrophil and chemo-taxis secretory processes. Am. J. Pathol. 116, 427–435.

Fowler, A.A., Hyers, T.M., Fisher, V.J. et al. (1987). The adult respiratory distress syndrome: cell populations and soluble mediators in the air spaces of patients with high risk. Am. Rev. Respir. Dis. 136, 1225–1231.

Fulmer, J.D., Sposovska, M.S., Von Gal, E.R. and Mittal, K.K. (1978). Distribution of HLA antigens in idiopathic pulmonary fibrosis. Am. Rev. Respir. Dis. 118, 141–147.

Gadek, J.E., Kelman, J.A., Fells, G., Weinberger, S.E., Horwitz, A.K., Reynolds, H.Y., Fulmer, J.D. and Crystal, R.G. (1979). Collagenase in the lower respiratory tract of patients with idiopathic pulmonary fibrosis. N. Engl. J. Med. 301, 737–742.

Garcia, J.G.N., Parhami, N., Garcia, P.L. and Keogh, P.A. (1986). Bronchoalveolar lavage fluid evaluation in rheumatoid arthritis. Am. Rev. Respir. Dis. 133, 450–454.

Gellert, A.R., Langford, J.A., Winter, R.J.D., Utchayakumar, S., Sinha, G. and Rudd, R.M. (1985). Asbestosis: assessment by bronchoalveolar lavage and measurement of pulmonary epithelial permeability. Thorax 40, 508–514.

Golde, D.W. (1983). In "Haematology" (eds W.J. Williams and E. Beutler) pp. 759–765. McGraw-Hill, New York.

Gossett, P., Perez, T., Lassalle, P., Duquesnoy, B., Farre, J.M., Tonnel, A.B. and Capron, A. (1991). Increased TNFα secretion by alveolar macrophages from patients with rheumatoid arthritis. Am. Rev. Respir. Dis. 143, 593–597.

Guthrie, L.A., McPhail, L.C., Henson, P.M. and Johnson, R.B. (1984). Priming of neutrophils for enhanced release of oxygen metabolites by bacterial lipopolysaccharide. J. Exp. Med. 160, 1656–1671.

Hallgren, R., Borg, T., Venge, P. and Modig, J. (1984). Signs of neutrophil and eosinophil activation in adult respiratory distress syndrome. Crit. Care Med. 12, 14–18.

Hallgren, R., Bjermer, L., Lundgren, R. and Venge, P. (1989). The eosinophil component of the alveolitis in idiopathic pulmonary fibrosis. Signs of eosinophil activation in the lung are related to impaired lung function. Am. Rev. Respir. Dis. 139, 373–377.

Hammerschmidt, D.E., Weaver, L.J., Hudson, L.D., Craddock, P.R. and Jacob, H.S. (1980). Association of complement activation and elevated plasma C5a, with adult respiratory distress syndrome. Lancet 1, 947–949.

Hammerschmidt, D.E., Harris, T.D., Wayland, J.H., Craddock, P.R. and Jacob, H.S. (1981). Complement induced granulo-cyte aggregation in vivo. Am. J. Pathol. 102, 14.

Hansell, D.M. and Kerr, I.H. (1991). The role of high resolution computed tomography in the diagnosis of inter-stitial lung disease. Thorax 46, 77–84.

Harris, J.A., Hyde, D.M., Wang, G.J., Stovall, M.Y. and Giri, S.N. (1991). Repeated episodes of C5a-induced neutrophil influx do not result in pulmonary fibrosis. Inflammation 15, 233–250.

Harrison, N.K., Glanville, A.R., Strickland, B., Haslam, P.L., Corrin, B., Addis, B.J., Lawrence, R., Millar, A.B. and Turner-Warwick, M. (1989). Pulmonary involvement in systemic sclerosis: the detection of early changes by thin section CT scan, bronchoalveolar lavage and ^{99m}Tc DTPA clearance. Respir. Med. 83, 403–414.

Harrison, N.K., Myers, A.R., Soosay, G., Dewar, A., Black, C.M., du Bois, R.M., Turner-Warwick, M. and Corrin, B. (1991). Structural features of interstitial lung disease in systemic sclerosis. Am. Rev. Respir. Dis. 144, 706–713.

Haslam, P.L. (1990). Evaluation of alveolitis by studies of lung biopsies. Lung (Suppl.) 984–992.

Haslam, P., Turton, C.W.G., Heard, B., Lukoszek, A., Collins, J.V., Salsbury, A.J. and Turner-Warwick, M. (1980). Bronchoalveolar lavage in pulmonary fibrosis: comparison of cells obtained with lung biopsy and clinical features. Thorax 35, 9–18.

Haslam, P.L., Turton, C.W.G., Lukoszek, A., Salisbury, A.J., Dewar, A., Collins, J.V. and Turner-Warwick, M. (1980). Bronchoalveolar lavage fluid cell counts in cryptogenic fibrosing alveolitis and their relation to therapy. Thorax 35, 328–339.

Haslett, C., Worthen, G.S., Giclas, P.C., Morrison, D.C., Henson, J.E. and Henson, P.M. (1987). Pulmonary vascular sequestration of neutrophils in endotoxaemia is initiated by an effect of endotoxin on the neutrophil in the rabbit. Am. Rev. Respir. Dis. 136, 9–18.

Haslett, C., Shen, A.S., Feldsien, D.C., Allen, D., Henson, P.M. and Cherniak, R.M. (1989). 111-Indium labelled neutrophil migration into the lungs of bleomycin treated rabbits assessed non-invasively by external scintigraphy. Am. Rev. Respir. Dis. 140, 756–763.

Henson, P.M. and Jonson, R.B., Jr. (1987). Tissue injury in inflammation: oxidants, proteinases and cationic proteins. J. Clin. Invest. 79, 669–674.

Hobbs, J.R. and Turner-Warwick, M. (1967). Assay of circulating immunoglobulins in patients with fibrosing alveolitis. Clin. Exp. Immunol. 2, 645–652.

Hoste, P., Williams, J., Devriendt, J., Lamont, H. and Van der Straeten, M. (1979). Familial diffuse interstitial pulmonary fibrosis associated with oculocutaneous albinism. Report of two cases with a family study. Scand. J. Respir. Dis. 60, 128–134.

Hunninghake, G.W., Gadek, J.E., Fates, H.M. and Crystal, R.G. (1980). Human alveolar macrophage-derived chemotactic factor for neutrophils. J. Clin. Invest. 60, 473–483.

Hyers, T.M., Tricomi, S.M., Dettenmeier, P.A. and Fowler, A.A. (1991). Tumour necrosis factors in serum and bronchoalveolar lavage fluid of patients with the adult respiratory distress syndrome. Am. Rev. Respir. Dis. 144, 268–271.

Idell, S., Kucich, U., Fine, A. et al. (1985). Neutrophil elastase releasing factors in bronchoalveolar lavage from patients with adult respiratory distress syndrome. Am. Rev. Respir. Dis. 132, 1098–1105.

Ishizaka, A., Wu, Z., Stephens, K.E., Harada, H., Hogue, R.S., O'Hanley, P.S. and Rajjin, T.A. (1988). Attenuation of acute lung injury in septic guinea pigs by pentoxifylline. Am. Rev. Respir. Dis. 138, 376–382.

Jepson, S., Herlevson, P., Knudson, P., Bud, M.I. and Klausen, N.-O. (1992). Antioxidant treatment with N-acetylcysteine during adult respiratory distress syndrome: a prospective, randomized, placebo-controlled study. Crit. Care Med. 20, 918–923.

Johnson. A. and Malik, A.B. (1980). The effect of granulocytopenia on extravascular lung water content after micro-embolisation. Am. Rev. Respir. Dis. 122, 561–566.

Johnson, M.A., Kwan, S., Snell, N.J.C., Nunn, A.J., Darbyshire, J.H. and Turner-Warwick, M. (1989). Randomised controlled trial comparing Prednisolone alone with Cyclophosphamide and low dose Prednisolone in combination in cryptogenic fibrosing alveolitis. Thorax 44, 280–288.

Johnston, I., Britton, J., Kinnear, W. and Logan, R. (1990). Rising mortality from cryptogenic fibrosing alveolitis. Br. Med. J. 301, 1017–1020.

Koyama, S., Kobayashi, T., Kubo, K., Sekiguchi, M. and Ueda, G. (1992). Recombinant-human superoxide dismutase attenuates cardotoxin-induced lung injury in awake sheep. Am. Rev. Respir. Dis. 145, 1404–1409.

Kreuzfelder, E., Joka, T., Keinecke, H.O., Obertacke, U., Schmit-Neuerberg, K.P., Nakhosteen, J.A., Paar, D. and Scheierman, N.L. (1988). Adult respiratory distress syndrome as a specific manifestation of a general permeability defect in trauma patients. Am. Rev. Respir. Dis. 137, 95–99.

Laufe, M.D., Simon, R.H., Flint, A. and Keller, J.B. (1986). Adult respiratory distress syndrome in neutropenic patients. Am. J. Med. 80, 1022–1026.

Lee, C.T., Fein, A.M., Lippman, M., Holtzman, H., Kimbel, T. and Weinbaum, G. (1981). Elastolytic activity in pulmonary lavage fluid from patients with adult respiratory distress syndrome. N. Engl. J. Med. 304, 192–196.

Leonard, E.J. and Yoshimura, T. (1992). Neutrophil attractant/activation protein-1 (NAP-1) (interleukin-8). Am. J. Respir. Cell. Mol. Biol. 479–486.

Liebow, A.A. (1975). In "Progress in Respiration Research" (eds F. Basset and R. Georges) pp. 1–33. Karger, New York.

Lin, Y.H., Haslam, P.L. and Turner-Warwick, M. (1985). Chronic pulmonary sarcoidosis: relationship between lung lavage cell counts, chest radiograph and results of standard lung function tests. Thorax 40, 501–507.

Lui, S.F., Dewar, A., Crawley, D.E., Barnes, P.J. and Evans, T.W. (1992). Effects of tumour necrosis factor on hypoxic pulmonary vasoconstriction and endothelium-dependent relaxation in the blood-perfused rat lung. J. Appl. Physiol. 72, 1044–1048.

Macnaughton, P.D. and Evans, T.W. (1992). Management of adult respiratory distress syndrome. Lancet 339, 466–469.

Maier, K., Leuschel, L. and Costabel, U. (1991). Increased levels of oxidized methionine residues in bronchoalveolar lavage fluid proteins from patients with idiopathic pulmonary fibrosis. Am. Rev. Respir. Dis. 143, 271–274.

Malech, L. and Gallin, J.I. (1987). Neutrophils in human diseases. N. Engl. J. Med. 317, 687–694.

Mandel, G.L. (1988). ARDS, neutrophils and pentoxifylline. Am. Rev. Respir. Dis. 138, 1103–1105.

Martinet, Y., Rom, W.N., Grotendorst, G.R., Martin, G.R. and Crystal, R.G. (1987). Exaggerated spontaneous release of platelet-derived growth factor by alveolar macrophages from patients with idiopathic pulmonary fibrosis. N. Engl. J. Med. 317, 202–209.

Martin, T.R., Pistorese, B.P., Chi, E.Y., Goodman, R.B. and Matthay, M.A. (1989). Effects of leukotriene B4 in the human lung: recruitment of neutrophils in the alveolar spaces without a change in protein permeability. J. Clin. Invest. 84, 1609–1619.

Martin, T.R., Pistorese B.P., Hudson, L.D. and Maunder, R.J. (1991). The function of lung and blood neutrophils in patients with the adult respiratory distress syndrome: implications for the pathogenesis of lung infections. Am. Rev. Respir. Dis. 144, 254–262.

Maunder, R.J., Hackman, R.F.C., Riff, E., Albert, R.K. and Springmeyer, S.C. (1986). Occurrence of the adult respiratory distress syndrome in neutropenic patients. Am. Rev. Respir. Dis. 133, 313–316.

Meliconi, R., Bestagno, M., Sturani, C., Negri, C., Galavotti, V., Sala, C., Facchini, A., Ciarrocchi, G., Gasbarrini, G. and Astaldi Ricotti, G.C.B. (1989). Autoantibodies to DNA topoisomerase II in cryptogenic fibrosing alveolitis and connective tissue disease. Clin. Exp. Immunol. 76, 184–189.

Merrill, W.W., Naegel, G.P., Matthay, R.A. and Reynolds, H.Y. (1980). Alveolar macrophage derived chemotactic factor. Kinetics of in vitro production and partial characterization. J. Clin. Invest. 65, 268–276.

Michie, H.R., Manngue, K.R., Spriggs, D.R. et al. (1988). Detection of circulating tumour necrosis factor after endotoxin administration. N. Engl. J. Med. 318, 1481–1486.

Mizer, L.A., Weisbrode, S.E. and Dorinsky, P.M. (1989). Neutrophil accumulation and structural changes in non-pulmonary organs after acute lung injury induced by phorbol myristate acetate. Am. Rev. Respir. Dis. 139, 1017–1026.

Montgomery, A.D., Stager, M.A., Carrico, C.J. and Hudson, L.D. (1985). Causes of mortality in patients with the adult respiratory distress syndrome. Am. Rev. Respir. Dis. 132, 485–489.

Muir, A.L., Cruz, M., Martin, B.A., Thommasen, H.V., Belzberg, A. and Hogg, J.C. (1984). Leukocyte kinetics in the human lung: role of exercise and catecholamines. J. Appl. Physiol. 57, 711–719.

Murray, J.F. (1975). Editorial. The adult respiratory distress syndrome. (May it rest in peace). Am. Rev. Respir. Dis. 111, 716–718.

Murray, J.F., Matthay, M.A., Luce, J.M. and Flick, M.R. (1988). An expanded definition of the adult respiratory distress syndrome. Am. Rev. Respir. Dis. 138, 720–723.

Musk, A.W., Zilko, P.J., Manners, P., Kay, P.H. and Kamboh, M.I. (1986). Genetic studies in familial fibrosing alveolitis: possible linkage with immunoglobulin allotypes (Gm). Chest 89, 206–210.

Nagai, S., Aung, H., Takeuchi, M., Kusume, K. and Izumi, T. (1991). IL-1 and IL-1 inhibitory activity in the culture supernatants of alveolar macrophages from patients with interstitial lung diseases. Chest 99, 674–680.

Nagai, A., Aoshiba, K., Ishihara, Y., Inano, H., Sakamoto, K., Yamagauchi, E., Kagawa, J. and Takizawa, T. (1992). Administration of alpha-1-proteinase inhibitor ameliorates bleomycin induced pulmonary fibrosis in hamsters. Am. Rev. Respir. Dis. 145, 651–656.

Nakashima, J.M., Levin, J.R., Hyde, D.M. and Giri, S.N. (1991). Repeated exposures to enzyme generated oxidants cause alveolitis, epithelial hyperplasia and fibrosis in hamsters. Am. J. Pathol. 139, 1485–1499.

Niederman, M.S. and Fein, A.M. (1990). Sepsis syndrome, the adult respiratory distress syndrome, and nosocomial pneumonia. Clinics Chest Med. 11, 633–656.

Noble, B., du Bois, R.M. and Poulter, L.W. (1989). The distribution of phenotypically distinct macrophage subsets in the lungs of patients with cryptogenic fibrosing alveolitis. Clin. Exp. Immunol. 76, 41–46.

Ognibene, F.P., Martin, S.E., Parker, M.M., Schlesinger, T., Roach, P., Birch, C., Shaelhamer, J.H. and Parrillo, J.E. (1986). Adult respiratory distress syndrome in patients with severe neutropenia. N. Engl. J. Med. 315, 547–551.

Okuda, Y. and Ogata, H. (1989). The effects of the protease inhibitor FUT-175 on phospholipase A_2, complement, prostaglandins and prekallikrein during endotoxin shock. Masui 38, 334–342.

Parsons, P.E., Worthen, G.S., Moir, E.E., Tate, R.M. and Henson, P.M. (1989). The association of circulating endotoxin with the development of the adult respiratory distress syndrome. Am. Rev. Respir. Dis. 140, 294–301.

Peichl, P., Ceska, M., Effenberger, F., Harberhauer, G., Broell, H. and Lindley, I.J. (1991). Presence of NAP-1/IL-8 in synovial fluids indicates a possible pathogenic role in rheumatoid arthritis. Scand. J. Immunol. 34, 333–339.

Quinlan, G.J., Evans, T.W. and Gutteridge, J.M.C. (1992). Plasma protein damage in ARDS. Crit. Care Med. (submitted).

Reed, P.W. (1969). Glutathione and hexose monophosphate shunt in phagocytosing and hydrogen peroxide treated rat leucocytes. J. Biol. Chem. 224, 2459–2464.

Repine, J.E. (1992). Scientific perspectives on adult respiratory distress syndrome. Lancet 339, 469–472.

Reynolds, H.Y., Fulmer, J.D., Kazmierowski, J.A., Roberts, W.C., Frank, M.M. and Crystal, R.G. (1977). Analysis of bronchoalveolar lavage fluid from patients with idiopathic pulmonary fibrosis and chronic hypersensitivity pneumonitis. J. Clin. Invest. 59, 165–175.

Rinaldo, J.E. and Borowetz, H. (1985). Deterioration of oxygenation and abnormal lung microvascular permeability during resolution of leukopenia in patients with diffuse lung injury. Am. Rev. Respir. Dis. 131, 579–583.

Rinaldo, J.E. and Christman, J.W. (1990). Mechanisms and mediators of the adult respiratory distress syndrome. Clinics Chest Med. 11, 621–632.

Riva, C.M., Morganroth, M.L., Ljungman, A.G., Schoeneich, S.O., Marks, R.M., Todd, R.F., Ward, P.A. and Boxer, L.A. (1990). Iloprost inhibits neutrophil induced lung injury and neutrophil to endothelial adherence monolayers. Am. J. Respir. Cell Mol. Biol. 3, 301–309.

Rocker, G.M., Pearson, D., Wiseman, M.S. and Shale, D.J. (1989). Diagnostic criteria for adult respiratory distress syndrome: time for reappraisal. Lancet i, 120–123.

Rom, W.N., Basset, P., Fells, G.A., Nukiwa, T., Trapnell, B.C. and Crystal, R.G. (1988). Alveolar macrophages release an insulin-like growth factor 1-type molecule. J. Clin. Invest. 82, 1685–1693.

Rossi, G.A., Bitterman, P.B., Rennard, S.I. and Crystal, R.G. (1985). Evidence for chronic inflammation as a component of the interstitial lung disease associated with progressive systemic sclerosis. Am. Rev. Respir. Dis. 131, 612–617.

Savill, J.S., Wyllie, A.H., Henson, J.E., Walport, M.J., Henson, P.M. and Haslet, C. (1989). Macrophage phagocytosis of aging neutrophils in inflammation. Programmed cell death in the neutrophil leads to its recognition by macrophages. J. Clin. Invest. 83, 865–875.

Savill, J., Hogg, N. and Haslett, C. (1991). Macrophage vitronectin receptor, CD36, and thrombospondin co-operate in recognition of neutrophils undergoing programmed cell death. Chest 99, 6S.

Scadding, J.G. (1964). Fibrosing alveolitis. Br. Med. J. 2, 686.

Seear, N.D., Hannam, V.L., Kaapa, P., Raj, U. and O'Brodovich, H.M. (1990). Effect of pentoxifylline on haemodynamic, alveolar fluid reabsorption, and pulmonary oedema in a model of acute lung injury. Am. Rev. Respir. Dis. 142, 1083–1087.

Seitz, M., Dewald, B., Gerber, N. and Bagiolini, M. (1991). Enhanced production of neutrophil activating peptide-1/interleukin-8 in rheumatoid arthritis. J. Clin. Invest. 87, 463–469.

Shasby, D.M., Fox, R.B., Harada, R.N. and Repine, J.E. (1982). Reduction of the oedema of acute hyperoxic lung injury by granulocyte depletion. J. Appl. Physiol. 42, 1237–1244.

Sieback, M., Hoffman, H., Weipert, J. and Spannagl, M. (1989). Therapeutic effects of the combination of two protease inhibitors in endotoxin shock in the pig. Prog. Clin. Biol. Res. 308, 937–943.

Southcott, A.M., Pantelidis, P., Black, C.M. and du Bois, R.M. (1992). Is interleukin-8 mRNA expression compartmentalized in fibrosing alveolitis and systemic sclerosis? Am. Rev. Respir. Dis. 145, A465.

Spitznagel, J.K., Dalldorf, F.J. and Leffel, M.S. (1974). Characterization of azurophil and specific granules purified from human polymorphonuclear leucocytes. Lab. Invest. 30, 774–785.

Stephenson, A.H., Lonigro, A.J., Hyers, T.M., Webster, R.O. and Fowler, A.A. (1988). Increased concentrations of leukotrienes in bronchoalveolar lavage fluid of patients with ARDS or at risk for ARDS. Am. Rev. Respir. Dis. 138, 714–717.

Tabe, R.M. and Repine, J.E. (1983). Neutrophils in adult respiratory distress syndrome. Am. Rev. Respir. Dis. 128, 552–559.

Test, S.T. and Weiss, S.J. (1986). The generation and utilisation of chlorinated oxidants by human neutrophils. Adv. Free Radical Biol. Med. 2, 91–116.

Thet, L.A., Parra, S.C. and Shelbourne, J.D. (1986). Sequential changes in lung morphology during the repair of acute oxygen induced lung injury in adult rats. Exp. Lung Res. 11, 209–228.

Tighe, D., Moss, R., Hynd, J., Boyhossian, S., Al-Saady, N., Heath, M.F. and Bennett, E.D. (1990). Pre-treatment with pentoxifylline improves the haemodynamic and histologic changes and decreases neutrophil adhesiveness in a pig faecal peritonitis model. Crit. Care Med. 18, 184–189.

Tomashefski, J.F., Jr. (1990). Pulmonary pathology of the adult respiratory distress syndrome. Clin. Chest Med. 11, 593–620.

Turner-Warwick, M. and Haslam, P. (1971). Antibodies in some chronic fibrosing lung diseases. I. Non organ specific antibodies. Clin. Allergy 1, 83–95.

Turner-Warwick, M., Burrows, B. and Johnson, A. (1980a). Cryptogenic fibrosing alveolitis: clinical features and their influence on survival. Thorax 35, 171–180.

Turner-Warwick, M., Burrows, B. and Johnson, A. (1980b). Cryptogenic fibrosing alveolitis: response to corticosteroid treatment and its effect on survival. Thorax 35, 593–599

Vergnon, J.M., De The, G., Weynants, P., Vincent, M., Mornex, J.F. and Brune, J. (1984). Fibrosing alveolitis and Epstein–Barr virus: an association? Lancet i, 768–771.

Vrako, R. (1972). Signficance of basal lamina for regeneration of injured lung. Virchows Arch. Pathol. (Pathol. Anat.) 355, 264–274.

Ward, T.A., Till, G.O., Harherrill, J.R., Annersley, T.M. and Kunel, R.G. (1985). Systemic complement activation, lung injury, and products of lipid peroxidation. J. Clin. Invest. 76, 517–527.

Watters, L.C., King, T.E., Schwartz, M.I., Waldron, J.A., Stanford, R.E. and Cherniak, R.M. (1986). A clinical, radiographic, and physiologic scoring system for the longitudinal assessment of patients with idiopathic pulmonary fibrosis. Am. Rev. Respir. Dis. 133, 97–103.

Watters, L.C., Schwarz, M.I., Cherniack, R.M., Waldron, J.A., Dunn, T.L., Stanford, R.E. and King, T.E. (1987). Idiopathic pulmonary fibrosis. Pretreatment bronchoalveolar lavage cellular constituents and their relationships with lung histopathology and clinical response to therapy. Am. Rev. Respir. Dis. 135, 696–704.

Weiland, J.D., David, W.B., Holter, J.F. et al. (1986). Lung neutrophils in the adult respiratory distress syndrome: clinical and pathophysiological significance. Am. Rev. Respir. Dis. 133, 218–225.

Weinberg, P.F., Matthay, M.A., Webster, R.O. et al. (1984). Biologically active products of complement and acute lung injury in patients with a set syndrome. Am. Rev. Respir. Dis. 130, 791–796.

Weinberger, S.E., Kelman, J.A., Elson, N.A., Young, R.C., Jr, Reynolds, H.Y., Fulmer, J.D. and Crystal, R.G. (1978). Bronchoalveolar lavage in interstitial lung disease. Ann. Intern. Med. 89, 459–466.

Weiss, S.J. (1989). Tissue destruction by neutrophils. N. Engl. J. Med. 320, 365–376.

Wells, A.U., Hansell, D.M., Cullinan, P., Haslam, P.L., Black, C.M. and du Bois, R.M. (1992). High resolution computed tomography appearances correlate with bronchoalveolar lavage cell profiles in fibrosing alveolitis. Thorax 47, 218P.

Wells, A.U., Hansell, D.M., Haslam, P.L., Cullinan, P., Black, C.N. and du Bois, R.M. (1991). Bronchoalveolar lavage cell profiles and high resolution computed tomography in systemic sclerosis; a correlation. Eur. Respir. J. 4, 254S.

Wells, A.U., Lorimer, S., Jeffery, P.K., Majundar, S., Harrison, N.J., Sheppard, M.N., Corrin, B., Black, C.M. and du Bois, R.M. (1992). Fibrosing alveolitis associated with systemic sclerosis is characterized by the presence of antigen-prime T-cells in the lung interstitium. Am. Rev. Respir. Dis. 145, A466.

Welsh, C.H., Lien, D., Worthen, G.S. and Weil, J.V. (1988). Pentoxifylline decreases endotoxin induced pulmonary neutrophil sequestration and extravascular protein accumulation in the dog. Am. Rev. Respir. Dis. 138, 1106–1114.

Worthen, G.S., Haslett, C., Rees, A.J., Gumbays, R.S.,

Henson, J.E. and Henson, P.M. (1987). Neutrophil mediated pulmonary vascular injury: synergistic effect of trace amounts of lipopolysaccharide and neutrophil stimuli in vascular permeability and neutrophil sequestration in the lung. Am. Rev. Respir. Dis. 136, 19–28.

Yamauchi, K., Martinet, Y. and Crystal, R.G. (1987).

Modulation of fibronectin gene expression in human mononuclear phagocytes. J. Clin. Invest. 80, 1720–1727.

Zimmerman, G.A., Renzetti, A.D. and Hill, H.R. (1983). Functional and metabolic activity of granulocytes from patients with adult respiratory distress syndrome. Am. Rev. Respir. Dis. 127, 290–300.

14.   Fate of Neutrophils

John Savill and Christopher Haslett

1.   Introduction

The neutrophil polymorphonuclear granulocyte is the archetypal inflammatory leucocyte. A terminally differentiated cell arising from the bone marrow, its usual fate is to remain within the blood for a few hours before reaching physiological "graveyards" in macrophages of the liver and spleen. However, should infection or injury of a tissue result in the local generation of inflammatory mediators, the neutrophil is usually the first type of leucocyte to be summoned from the blood to defend the host. Neutrophils possess an impressive array of weapons with which to fight invading microorganisms. These include membrane systems which generate reactive oxygen intermediates (Chapter 3) and cytoplasmic granules containing powerful degradative enzymes (Chapter 4) and toxic cationic proteins ("defensins"), which can be discharged upon stimulation of the cell with appropriate concentrations of inflammatory mediators. However, these weapons can inflict "friendly fire" injury upon the host, and there is growing evidence that neutrophils and their toxic contents play an important role in the pathogenesis of a number of inflammatory diseases affecting the kidney, lung, joint and other vital organs (see Tables 14.1 and 14.2). Nevertheless, during resolution of inflammation, neutrophils can be removed from inflamed sites without inciting further tissue injury, demonstrating that powerful clearance mechanisms must exist which help to keep the destructive power of these cells in check. The purpose of this chapter is to describe recent advances in understanding of the fate of the neutrophil, concentrating on neutrophil clearance from inflamed sites, since this is likely be a crucial control point in the inflammatory response.

However, before going further, the size and potential significance of the problem of neutrophil fate must be emphasized. A vast army of neutrophils is available to the host – approximately 50 billion arise from the marrow each day in health (Chapter 2). In disease, much larger

Table 14.1   Neutrophil products which may injure tissue

Oxidants and radicals	Superoxide anion
	Hydrogen peroxide
	Singlet oxygen
	Hydroxyl radical
	Hypohalous acids
	N chloramines
Enzymes	Degradative
	Elastase
	CatG
	Collagenases
	Neuraminidase
	Heparanase
	MPO (generates oxidants)
Cationic proteins	Defensins
	Cationic antimicrobial proteins
Pro-inflammatory mediators	PAF
	LTB$_4$
	Cytokines (e.g. IL-1)

Adapted from Henson and Johnston (1987).

Table 14.2   Diseases in which there is evidence that neutrophils may injure tissues

Systemic	Vasculitis
Lung	ARDS
	Emphysema
	Asthma
	Brochiectasis
Kidney	Glomerulonephritis
	Interstitial nephritis
Joint	Rheumatoid arthritis
	Gout and other arthritides
Cardiac	Myocardial reperfusion injury
	Ischaemic heart disease
Gut	Inflammatory bowel disease
Others	Injury by extremes of heat and cold
	Dermatitis

Adapted from Malech and Gallin (1988).

numbers of neutrophils can be released from the marrow and these cells can be mobilized to a localized battle front in staggering numbers. For example, rough calculations suggest that a lobe of lung infected with pneumococci, in which the airspaces may be virtually filled with neutrophils, might contain over 100 billion leucocytes. Remarkably, this massive load of neutrophils and their potentially toxic contents can be removed from the lung during resolution of the inflammatory response. Furthermore, this can be achieved in a manner which may restore the normal structure and function of the affected portion of lung (Figure 14.1a and b). Indeed, given the destructive potential of the neutrophil, effective removal of leucocytes can be seen to be a prerequisite of resolution.

The ultimate fate of any cell is to die and, until recently, it has been widely assumed that the usual fate of the inflammatory neutrophil is to die *in situ* by disintegration, a process which would inevitably result in uncontrolled release of cell contents. Among these are

Figure 14.1 Neutrophil fate. (a) and (b) Histological appearance of experimental pneumococcal pneumonia showing neutrophil clearance during resolution. A fibreoptic bronchoscope was used to instill 10^8 Streptococcus pneumoniae organisms into the apical segment of the right upper lobe of the lung of rabbits. (a) At 48 h there is a profound acute inflammatory response, the alveolar spaces being packed with neutrophils and monocyte-macrophages ($\times$400). (b) By 7 days the corresponding area of lung has returned to a virtually normal appearance ($\times$100). Reproduced with permission from Haslett (1992). (c) and (d) External scintigraphy of emigration of intravenously administered ^{111}In-labelled neutrophils to experimental pneumococcal pneumonia in rabbits. (c) When a "pulse" of ^{111}In-labelled neutrophils was administered 6 h after instillation of bacteria into the right apical segment, the posterior γ-camera image taken 24 h thereafter shows accumulation of neutrophils in that region of the lung. Note also that a large proportion of administered neutrophils have met a "physiological" fate, localizing to the liver (right) and spleen (left). (d) However, if neutrophils were administered 24 h after instillation of bacteria, emigration is not detected, even though large numbers of neutrophils are known to be present in the lung [see (a)]. Reproduced with permission from Haslett (1992). (e) and (f) Neutrophil apoptosis and phagocytosis by macrophages at an inflamed site. (e) Macrophages (arrowed) in the wall of a colonic abscess containing large numbers of neutrophils ($\times$800; from original material supplied courtesy of Dr M. Alison, Royal Postgraduate Medical School). (f) Human neutrophils isolated from an inflamed human joint demonstrate typical light microscopical features of apoptosis (arrowed cells; $\times$1600). Note nuclear chromatin condensation and compare with appearances of ingested neutrophils in (e).

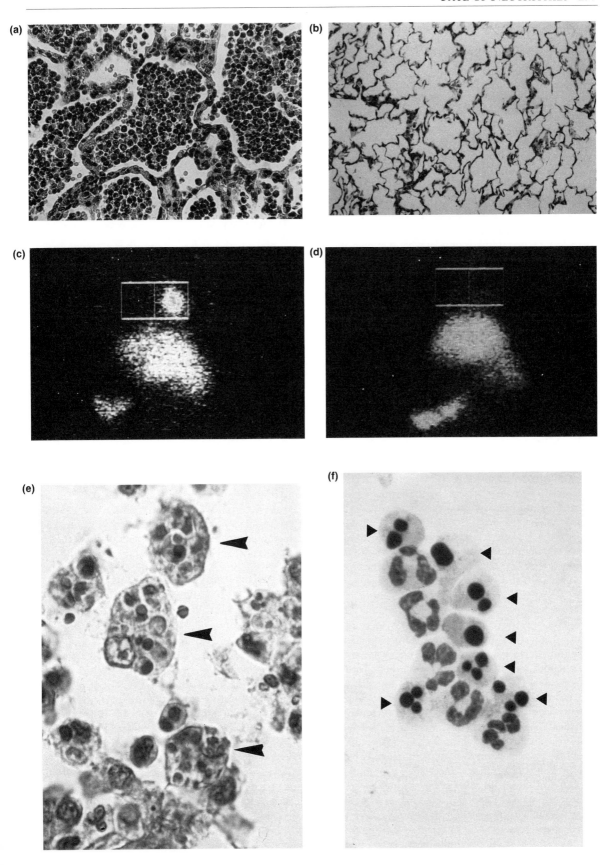

not only molecules which may directly exacerbate local tissue injury, such as the powerful proteinase elastase, but also species which may summon more leucocytes to the inflamed site. For example, neutrophils contain the chemotactic protein, CAP37, and their proteinases may degrade matrix proteins such as fibronectin to yield chemotactic fragments with potential to amplify leucocyte infiltration (Chapter 4). Therefore it can be seen that neutrophil death by necrosis or disintegration is likely to be undesirable. Recently, increasing evidence has pointed to an important role in neutrophil clearance for a much "cleaner" and more controlled form of death, apoptosis, which leads to recognition and removal by macrophages of the intact senescent granulocyte without release of potentially injurious cell contents. Before describing these data it is necessary to consider what is known about death of cells other than the neutrophil.

2.   Cell Death: Necrosis versus Apoptosis

In recent years it has become apparent that death of nucleated cells can be classified into two distinct types, "accidental" death or necrosis and "programmed" death or apoptosis (Kerr *et al.*, 1972; Wyllie *et al.*, 1980; Duvall and Wyllie, 1986). The distinguishing features of these modes of cell death are summarized below.

2.1   NECROSIS

This type of cell death is induced by gross insults to the cell such as extremes of temperature, hypoxia, high concentrations of toxins, "attack" by the terminal components of the complement cascade and lytic viruses. These stimuli inhibit membrane cation pumps or directly damage the plasma membrane, leading to abnormal permeability of the cell to ions and water, which may be usefully detected *in vitro* by failure to exclude the vital dye Trypan blue. The result of these defects is that the cell undergoes swelling and blebbing which, although initially reversible in some cases (such as osmotic shock), rapidly becomes irreversible and leads to disintegration of the cell. Every component of the cell is adversely affected. Thus the structure and function of organelles such as mitochondria are disrupted, protein synthetic pathways fail, cellular ATP levels fall and there is flocculation of nuclear chromatin which may remain in an approximately normal pattern. However, it is important to note that small loose aggregates of chromatin may marginate against the nuclear membrane, giving rise to a compacted basophilic appearance known by light microscopists as *pyknosis* while, if the nuclear membrane ruptures, these aggregates of chromatin may be dispersed within the cell ghost resulting in the appearance known as *karyorrhexis*.

The stimuli inducing necrosis usually affect large tracts of cells and so tend to result in appreciable tissue damage to the host — frostbite leading to necrosis and ultimate loss of extremities is a good example. This also emphasizes that an important result of necrosis is to incite an inflammatory response, which may exacerbate local tissue injury further. Thus, in experimental animals, cold injury may be attenuated by preventing recruitment of neutrophils into the reperfused area of damage by inhibiting leucocyte adhesion to blood vessel walls using a monoclonal antibody to CD18, the common β_2 chain of the leucocyte integrin adhesion molecules (Vedder *et al.*, 1990) (see Chapters 7 and 10). Thus, because of the capacity to trigger inflammation, cell death by necrosis can be seen to be doubly undesirable.

2.2   APOPTOSIS

By contrast with necrosis, apoptosis is a "physiological" form of cell death which results in cell removal without inciting inflammation. Rather than being an "accidental" event, apoptosis is "programmed" in two senses. Firstly, cell removal by apoptosis frequently occurs according to an organized program. A striking example is the involvement of apoptosis in developmental cell death where, during embryological remodelling or metamorphosis, "unwanted" cells are removed in an exquisitely precise manner by apoptosis (Ferguson, 1988; Cagan and Ready, 1989; Ballard and Holt, 1968). Endocrine-dependent atrophy of tissues such as those of the lactating breast represents another program of cell removal (Ferguson and Anderson, 1981), as does the elimination of potentially autoreactive T lymphocytes in the thymus (Smith *et al.*, 1989; MacDonald and Lees, 1990; Cohen, 1991). This aspect of apoptosis is evident in the meaning of the word in ancient Greek – the "falling off" as of leaves from a tree in autumn, a carefully regulated event. Apoptosis is also programmed in that cells undergoing this process display a remarkably reproducible series of structural and biochemical changes. These are now described.

2.2.1   Morphology of Apoptosis

This mode of cell death was first defined by Kerr *et al.* (1972) on the basis of a characteristic series of morphological changes (see also Wyllie *et al.*, 1980; Duvall and Wyllie, 1986). Rather than swelling, cells undergoing apoptosis shrink (indeed apoptosis was once known as "shrinkage necrosis"), because of cytoplasmic condensation and, in some cell types, detachment of cytoplasmic "blebs". There are dramatic cell surface changes, such as loss of microvilli and the development of invaginations (Morris *et al.*, 1984), but organelles such as mitochondria and cytoplasmic granules remain intact, although the endoplasmic reticulum may dilate. However, the most characteristic changes are in the nucleus. There is rapid condensation of chromatin into dense crescent-shaped aggregates at the periphery of the nucleus, which if multilobed may coalesce into a single spherical body. Alternatively, the condensed nucleus may segment and pieces of condensed chromatin may bud off from the cell in membrane-bound "apoptotic bodies". Nucleolar prominence may also be a feature. At the light microscopical level, nuclear condensation and fragmentation due to apoptosis can be confused by the unwary with the pyknosis and karyorrhexis of necrosis – electron microscopy is usually needed to verify that observed changes are indeed those of apoptosis.

In vivo, apoptotic cells and bodies are very swiftly ingested and degraded by phagocytes, so that in tissue sections apoptotic cells are usually seen to be within other cells (Alison and Sarraf, 1992). Although macrophages are the "professional" phagocytes ingesting apoptotic cells, other "semi-professional" phagocytes can participate, for example, in epithelia, apoptotic cells may be taken up by their neighbours. It is important to emphasize that the speed and efficiency of clearance of cells undergoing apoptosis renders this mode of cell death histologically inconspicuous, particularly as the process may occur apparently at random within a population of cells (rather than in sheets of contiguous cells, as is the case with necrosis) and, crucially, without inciting an inflammatory response.

2.2.2 Biochemical Features of Apoptosis

There are major differences in the metabolism of cells undergoing apoptosis when compared with those dying by necrosis (reviewed in Wyllie *et al.*, 1980; Duvall and Wyllie, 1986). Membrane ion pumps remain active and ATP levels are maintained, but perhaps the most impressive difference is that protein synthesis may be *required* for apoptosis in some situations as demonstrated by the inhibitory effect of protein synthesis inhibitors *in vitro* (Wyllie *et al.*, 1986). A number of proteins have been shown to be actively synthesized in cells undergoing apoptosis, a well-known example being clusterin (also known as SGP-2, SP40,40 or TRPM-2) which is expressed in prostatic and thymic cells undergoing apoptosis (Buttyan *et al.*, 1989: Tusurata *et al.*, 1990).

However, the most characteristic biochemical feature of apoptosis is internucleosomal cleavage of chromatin, which was first described by Wyllie (1980). Activation of an endogenous endonuclease, which selectively acts on linker DNA between nucleosomes, yields low molecular weight fragments of chromatin which are integer multiples of the 180–200 bp of DNA associated with a nucleosome (Arends *et al.*, 1990). When DNA is extracted from nuclei of apoptotic cells and subjected to agarose gel electrophoresis, a "ladder" of oligonucleosomal fragments is seen. In necrosis, probably because proteinases degrade histones and other components of the nucleosome, exposing the whole length of DNA to attack by endonucleases, DNA is cleaved into fragments with a continuous spectrum of sizes so that extracted DNA merely runs as a "smear" upon electrophoresis. It is fair to say that identification of the endonuclease responsible for the chromatin cleavage of apoptosis has been a "holy grail" for those interested in

this mode of cell death since preliminary studies indicated that this type of endonuclease activity is dependent upon Ca^{2+} and Mg^{2+}, but inhibited by Zn^{2+} (Cohen and Duke, 1984; Wyllie *et al.*, 1986; Arends *et al.*, 1990). As a number of laboratories close in on this target, it is becoming apparent that not only DNA cleaving enzymes, e.g. DNase 1 has been proposed as a candidate by Pietsch *et al.* (1993), but also proteinases may be implicated in endonuclease activity (Shi *et al.*, 1992). Exciting new developments appear likely in the near future.

2.2.3 Regulation of Apoptosis

The highly organized removal of "unwanted" cells by apoptosis strongly suggests that apoptosis is subject to careful regulation. There has been intense interest in the mechanisms responsible, regulatory molecules being defined *in vitro*, by administration to experimental animals and by the study of transgenic animals over-expressing certain genes. A detailed description of these data is beyond the scope of this chapter but some examples are shown in Table 14.3. The important principle is that cell death by apoptosis is subject to control by as yet poorly understood interplay between lineage-specific exogenous factors and the genes of the cell itself. Raff (1992) has recently made the interesting suggestion that in all cells the death program is kept in check by exogenous "survival factors"; where the supply of such factors is critical, only those cells best equipped (for example, by a relatively larger number of receptors) will survive. Much is still to be learnt about control of apoptosis, but an important stimulus to future research will be the prospect that apoptosis might be manipulated for therapeutic effect; for example, it might be possible to encourage tumour cells to kill themselves by apoptosis (Trauth *et al.*, 1989).

3. *Neutrophil Life Span*

Before any mammalian cell dies, it is born (by division of a precursor cell) and it lives for periods ranging from a few hours to many years. Thus, at any particular site, the size of a population of cells is determined by a number of dynamic variables: the rate of generation of the cell type by division; the life span of individual cells; and the rate of cell death, which must be finely tuned to the rate of division if the cell population is to remain the same size.

Neutrophils are released from the bone marrow as terminally differentiated cells apparently incapable of further division. The origin and development of neutrophils is discussed in detail in Chapter 2. Their normally short life span has been demonstrated by a number of approaches. As it has been possible for many years to prepare more or less pure populations of neutrophils from blood, the short-lived nature of the cell has been apparent in various attempts to maintain neutrophils in culture, which were

Table 14.3   Examples of regulation of apoptosis

Mechanism	Factor	Cell	Reference
Induction of apoptosis			
1. Withdrawal of growth/survival factor	Erythropoietin	Erythroid progenitors	Koury and Bondurant (1990)
	Sex hormones	Prostate and breast cells	Kyprianou et al. (1990), Walker et al. (1989)
	Neurotrophic factors	Neurons	Sendtner et al. (1990), Schubert et al. (1990)
	bFGF	Endothelial cells	Araki et al. (1990)
	IL-2	T-cell lines/lymphoblasts	Duke and Cohen (1986)
	IL-3, GM-CSF and G-CSF	Haemopoietic cells	Williams et al. (1990)
	PDGF/IGF-1	Oligodendrocytes	Barres et al. (1992)
2. Binding of cell surface structures	T-cell receptor	Thymocytes	Smith et al. (1989), MacDonald and Lees (1990)
	Surface Ig	Immature B cells	Benhamou et al. (1990), Nemazee and Buerki (1989)
	Surface Ig	Differentiating B cells	Liu et al. (1989)
	Fas	Many cell types	Itoh et al. (1991)
	APO-1	Leukaemia cells	Trauth et al. (1989)
	TGF-β_1 receptors	Hepatocytes	Oberhammer et al. (1992)
3. Oncogene expression	c-myc (+ growth factor deprivation)	Fibroblasts	Evan et al. (1992)
		Lymphoid cells	Y. Shi et al. (1992)
Prevention of apoptosis			
1. Supply of growth/survival factor	See above	Many cell types	
2. Binding of cell surface structures	LPS FMLP receptors GM-CSF	Neutrophils	Lee et al. (1989)
3. Oncogene expression	bcl-2	Many cell types	Vaux et al. (1988), Hockenberry et al. (1990), Nunez et al. (1990), Jacobson et al. (1993), Fanidi et al. (1992), Bissonnette et al. (1992)

Abbreviations: bFGF, basic fibroblast growth factor; IL-2, interleukin-2; G-CSF, granulocyte colony stimulating factor; GM-CSF, granulocyte-monocyte colony-stimulating factor; PDGF, platelet-derived growth factor; IGF-1, insulin-like growth factor-1; Ig, immunoglobulin; TGF-β, transforming growth factor-β; LPS, lipopolysaccharide.

often stimulated by a desire to perfect a technique for storage of granulocytes for later administration to neutropaenic patients (McCullough et al., 1978). The limited life span of neutrophils suggested by such in vitro studies was also apparent in studies of the kinetics in vivo of neutrophils "tagged" with radioisotopes. These are discussed later in the chapter, but a number of methods suggest that the half-time of circulating neutrophil survival is in the region of only 7 h (Athens et al., 1961b; Dancey et al., 1976; Saverymuttu et al., 1983).

However, the life span of neutrophils at inflamed sites has been obscure. Although histological study of tissue sections taken at frequent intervals during the evolution and resolution of inflammation can be used to draw inferences on neutrophil life span (i.e., this is unlikely to be much longer than the total time for which neutrophils can be seen in the tissues after application of an inflammatory stimulus), accurate kinetic data are very difficult to obtain from such "snapshots" of a dynamic process. Nevertheless, this problem can now be addressed using radiolabelled granulocytes. Ideally, labelling should not alter the normal behaviour of the cell, and this can be achieved by pulse radiolabelling the bone marrow with tritiated thymidine in order to avoid a need for manipulation of the cells ex vivo. However, this technique does not selectively label neutrophils and, because of the nature of the radioactive emitter, it is now considered unsuitable for human studies. Techniques have been developed whereby neutrophils can be purified and radiolabelled with γ-emitters without activation so that upon reinfusion they circulate with kinetics indistinguishable from those suggested by bone marrow labelling. Infusions of such neutrophils can be "tracked" by harvesting the site into which they migrate or by external scintigraphy (Figure 14.1c), which although less invasive is also less sensitive (Haslett et al., 1989a).

Clearly, at an inflamed site destined to resolve, there must come a point at which neutrophils are no longer recruited from the blood and, if this could be determined, then the "time of residence" of neutrophils at an inflamed site could then be inferred. Infusions of radio-labelled neutrophils administered at various times after an inflammatory stimulus can be used in experimental animals to determine the time course of cessation of neutrophil influx (Haslett, 1992). Remarkably, in self-limited inflammation of the rabbit knee joint, skin or lung induced by local administration of C5a and other stimuli, cessation of neutrophil influx is rapid, neutrophil migration into the site being undetectable as early as 1–4 h after inducing the response (Haslett et al., 1989b; Colditz and Movat, 1984; Clark et al., 1989). However, at 24 h after stimulation, large numbers of neutrophils are still present at the inflamed site (Figures 14.1a, c and d), indicating a life span considerably longer than that which might be inferred from data on circulating neutrophils.

Nevertheless, to develop a complete picture of the life span of extravasated neutrophils at inflamed sites, it is necessary to understand the mechanisms and rate of removal of these cells. Recent progress will now be described.

4. Neutrophil Fate at Inflamed Sites
4.1 DEATH IN SITU – THE USUAL FATE?

Disappearance of neutrophils from an inflamed site does not necessarily indicate that the cells have died. The classical work of Gowans, Ford and others on trafficking of lymphocytes illustrates that leucocytes may leave one tissue whilst still alive and migrate to another site in the body (e.g. Harris and Ford, 1964). However, in biopsy and autopsy studies, only occasional neutrophils may be seen in lymphatic vessels and nodes draining inflamed tissues which, despite the dynamic limitations of histology, strongly suggests that the lymphatics are not major routes of neutrophil disposal (Haslett and Henson, 1988). This conclusion is supported by radiolabelled neutrophil studies of patients and animals with localized inflammation where neutrophil migration consistent with "escape" of large numbers of cells via the lymphatics is not widely recognized.

There are routes other than the lymphatics by which viable neutrophils might leave an inflamed site. Although possible, there is no histological evidence to suggest that neutrophils leave an inflamed site by migrating back into the blood. Indeed, recent insights from in vitro and in vivo studies into the mechanisms by which leucocytes migrate across the vessel wall suggest that adhesion molecule expression and the influence of cytokines is very carefully co-ordinated to make the pathway of leucocyte extravasation a "one way street", so that return to the blood would seem very unlikely (see Chapters 7 and 10).

At certain anatomical sites, large numbers of intact neutrophils are removed in excreted fluids. For example, a mainstay of the clinical management of urinary tract infection and inflammation is the maintenance of a high urine flow to wash away bacteria and inflammatory cells. Direct disposal of neutrophils may also occur from the alimentary and respiratory tracts (a familiar example being the copious purulent sputum of bronchiectasis), or if an abscess discharges on to the "surface" of the host. The numerical importance of direct disposal to the outside world is unclear even in those sites where it is possible. Furthermore, there are a number of completely enclosed sites such as the joint or central nervous system from which such "escape" is impossible.

The consensus from histological study and tracking radiolabelled cells is that the majority of inflammatory neutrophils never leave the perturbed site, most cells meeting their fate and dying in situ (Hurley, 1983; Haslett and Henson, 1988). There is evidence that this fate may be either necrosis or apoptosis; our contention is that programmed death is the preferred injury limiting mechanism for removal of neutrophils from inflamed sites.

4.2 NEUTROPHIL NECROSIS IN INFLAMMATION
4.2.1 Evidence of Neutrophil Necrosis

A number of distinguished pathologists have suggested that neutrophil necrosis is the usual mechanism for clearance from inflamed sites. For example, in his 1983 treatise Hurley stated:

"Some polymorphs may leave the damaged area via lymphatics or tissue spaces and finally die at some distance from the site of inflammation. However, most die locally and liberate their granules and cytoplasmic enzymes into adjacent tissue spaces. The remnants of the dead cells are then engulfed by macrophages."

In support, there is evidence that neutrophil necrosis can occur at inflamed sites. A compelling example is offered by systemic vasculitis, where light microscopical evidence of leucocyte disintegration in tissues close to inflamed vessels is recognized as "leucocytoclastic" vasculitis, and neutrophil disintegration in this disorder was also reported in ultrastructural studies of affected renal glomeruli (Donald et al., 1976; Gammon, 1982). However, since vasculitis is a serious, often life-threatening disorder, it would be unwise to extrapolate these findings to "beneficial" inflammation in which resolution is more or less complete. This point is emphasized by the large numbers of necrotic neutrophils which can be found in the pus in the centre of an abscess, a form of termination of inflammation which is less successful than resolution (Hurley, 1983). Thus, it is possible that many of the available examples of neutrophil necrosis at inflamed sites represent situations in which the response has already become "uncontrolled" and liable to damage tissue. Indeed, in our own studies of *self-limited* inflammation in human and animal joints and lung (Savill *et al.*, 1989a; Grigg *et al.*, 1991), it is notable that neutrophils obtained from inflammatory exudates have exhibited very high viability (>98% assessed by trypan blue exclusion).

4.2.2 Neutrophil Necrosis in the Inflammatory Microenvironment

The consequences of neutrophil disintegration at inflamed sites should this occur are, at present, the subject of conjecture. A glance at Table 14.1 will remind the reader of the enormous histotoxic potential of the cell contents which would be inevitably released during neutrophil necrosis. However, it is important to note that the capacity of these molecules to injure tissue may be kept in check by a series of inhibitory mechanisms (see Chapter 4).

For example, azurophil granules contain the 35 kD molecule leucocyte elastase which is reputed to account for nearly all neutrophil-derived proteolytic activity *in vitro* (reviewed by Janoff, 1985). This potent enzyme not only has the capacity to cleave elastin (an essentially irreplaceable protein important to the function of, for example, the lung and major vessels), but also can degrade virtually all components of the extracellular matrix including fibronectin, collagen types III and IV, and proteoglycans. Furthermore, the enzyme can also cleave complement components such as C3 and C5 to yield phlogistic fragments capable of amplifying the inflammatory response. Fortunately, plasma and interstitial fluids contain a "shield" of antiproteinases in all but individuals with varying degrees of congenital deficiency (Henson *et al.*, 1988). The most potent inhibitor of elastase is α_1-PI (also known as α_1-antitrypsin), a 52 kD glycoprotein which irreversibly combines with the enzyme, achieving inactivation in milliseconds. Other inhibitors include the large (~800 kD) broad-spectrum anti-proteinase α_2-M, the small (14 kD) secretory leucoproteinase inhibitor, and at least two TIMPs. Therefore, although cell contents would be released during neutrophil necrosis, this would not inevitably be deleterious.

However, the "anti-proteinase shield" can be breached and there is abundant *in vitro* and *in vivo* evidence that neutrophils can degrade protein substrates and injure tissues in the presence of proteinase inhibitors (reviewed by Weiss, 1989). Weiss and colleagues (1986) have classified the mechanisms responsible as "oxidative" and "non-oxidative". Oxidative inhibition involves inactivation of anti-proteinases by reactive oxygen species; for example, oxidation of a critical methionine residue in α_1-PI reduces its affinity for elastase 2000-fold. However, the very reactivity of oxidants with biomolecules limits their activity to sites extremely close to that at which they are generated. Non-oxidative inhibition of anti-proteinases may be similarly circumscribed. Thus,

neutrophils can physically exclude the penetration of anti-proteinases to areas of substrate "sealed off" by surrounding points of cell contact (Campbell and Campbell, 1988) and, close to a site of neutrophil degranulation, available anti-proteinases may be overwhelmed by a vast molar excess of enzyme. Thus in the microenvironment of an inflamed site in which reactive oxygen species are being generated and cells are crowded together, the highly localized discharge of large amounts of granule enzymes from neutrophils undergoing necrosis is likely to weigh the proteinase–anti-proteinase balance in favour of tissue injury.

Furthermore, other neutrophil contents have more direct and less obviously regulated potential to injure tissue. For example, the non-enzymatic cationic antimicrobial proteins (which include the 4 kD defensins, and species of 57 kD and 37 kD) can directly injure cell membranes (Janoff and Zweifach, 1964; Ranadive and Cochrane, 1970; Spitznagel, 1990), while the abundant enzyme MPO can, in conjunction with hydrogen peroxide, oxidize chloride and other halides to produce potent hypohalous acids (Johnson *et al.*, 1987; Klebanoff, 1988). Finally, release of neutrophil contents can result in recruitment of more leucocytes to an inflamed site, potentially amplifying and prolonging the response: neutrophil enzymes can generate chemotactic fragments from complement and from matrix components, such as fibronectin (Vartio *et al.*, 1981; Doherty *et al.*, 1990), while the cationic anti-microbial protein of 37 kD (CAP37), more colourfully known as azurocidin, also has monocyte-specific chemoattractant properties (Spitznagel, 1990).

To conclude, although neutrophil necrosis can be seen at inflamed sites, there is sufficient evidence to suggest that this may be a deleterious and uncontrolled mode of clearance which is likely to favour persistence of inflammatory tissue injury rather than resolution.

4.3 NEUTROPHIL APOPTOSIS IN INFLAMMATION

4.3.1 Macrophage Phagocytosis of Senescent Neutrophils

Although there is a body of pathological opinion favouring neutrophil necrosis as the usual clearance mechanism operating in inflammation, this was not the fate of extravasated neutrophils described by Elie Metchnikoff, one of the fathers of modern histopathology. Over 100 years ago he employed vital microscopy to observe the evolution and resolution of self-limited inflammation experimentally induced in animals by injury with rosethorns or fine glass probes. During the resolution phase he observed that intact neutrophils were "englobed" by macrophages (Metchnikoff, 1893). Over the ensuing century there have been many reports in both health and disease of macrophage phagocytosis of neutrophils (Brewer, 1964; Nichols and Bainton, 1975; Kadri *et al.*, 1975; Parmely *et al.*, 1981), and of particular relevance to the resolution of inflammation is the clinical phenomenon of "Reiter's cells", neutrophil-containing macrophages found in fluid aspirated from inflamed joints of patients with Reiter's disease and other forms of arthritis (Pekin *et al.*, 1967; Spriggs *et al.*, 1978). Indeed, in situations where it is possible to sample the inflammatory exudate at frequent intervals, such as experimentally induced self-limited peritonitis, massive waves of macrophage ingestion of apparently intact neutrophils can be seen to be the dominant mode of neutrophil removal from the inflamed site during resolution (Sanui *et al.*, 1982; Chapes and Haskill, 1983). An idea of the capacity of this clearance mechanism is given by Figure 14.1e, demonstrating macrophages which have apparently "gorged" themselves with neutrophils.

However, these observations raise a fundamental biological problem – how does a macrophage determine that an intact "self" neutrophil is "unwanted"? Obviously, it would not be advantageous for macrophages to ingest neutrophils still needed to fight invading organisms, suggesting that there must be some way of marking neutrophils as "surplus" to requirements. This problem has only been addressed in the last decade, the seminal study being that of Newman *et al.* (1982). Reasoning that macrophages might recognize "old" neutrophils, an *in vitro* model of neutrophil senescence was established. Neutrophils isolated from blood and "aged" overnight were recognized and ingested, apparently whilst still intact, by macrophages obtained from human monocytes matured in the presence of autologous serum *in vitro*, or from inflamed rabbit lungs. Freshly isolated neutrophils were not ingested, needing to undergo a time-related ageing process before they could be recognized. This demonstrated that aging neutrophils must undergo changes leading to their recognition as "senescent-self", but the nature of such changes was not determined.

4.3.2 Apoptosis Determines Macrophage Recognition of Senescent Neutrophils

Employing improved methods of neutrophil isolation from blood (Haslett *et al.*, 1985), it proved possible to develop a system for neutrophil culture in which there was minimal cell loss over 24 h (Savill *et al.*, 1989a). Furthermore, these methods could be adapted to isolate human neutrophils from inflammatory joint fluid obtained from patients with sterile acute arthritis. When "aged" in culture for up to 24 h neutrophils from either blood or inflamed joints remained intact (>98% of cells excluded Trypan blue dye) and retained potentially phlogistic granule contents such as myeloperoxidase. With increasing duration of culture there was a progressive increase in the proportion of cells exhibiting condensation of nuclear chromatin and cytoplasm

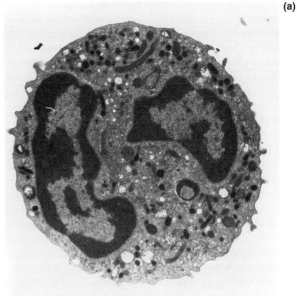

(a)

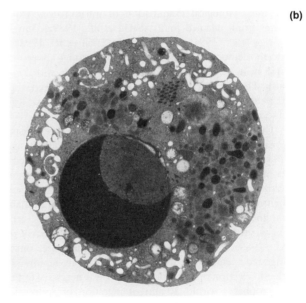

(b)

Figure 14.2 Ultrastructural appearances of (a) normal human neutrophil and (b) apoptotic human neutrophil. In (a) note the irregular outline of the cell, the loose granular appearance of the nuclear chromatin, the irregular lobed nucleus and the large numbers of cytoplasmic granules. In the apoptotic cell (b) the granules are retained and the plasma membrane is intact but apparently smooth and invaginated. The nucleus has coalesced into a single sphere, and demonstrates the typical dense crescent of heterochromatin. Transmission electron micrographs (×11 000) taken by Dr Jan Henson, National Jewish Centre for Immunology and Respiratory Medicine, Denver, Colorado, USA. Reproduced with permission from Haslett (1992).

(Figure 14.1f), and other light microscopical features typical of apoptosis, which were confirmed by electron microscopy (Figure 14.2). This increase occurred in parallel with time-related increases in the proportion of human monocyte-derived macrophages taking up cultured neutrophils in a microscopically quantified 30-min phagocytic assay, implying that apoptosis was the change in the ageing neutrophil determining recognition by macrophages. This was confirmed by using centrifugal elutriation to separate given aged neutrophil populations into fractions with varying proportions (>90% to <5%) of apoptotic cells; macrophage recognition of a given fraction was closely correlated to apoptosis. Furthermore, in apoptotic fractions, internucleosomal chromatin cleavage was demonstrated in extracted low molecular weight DNA by the typical "ladder" pattern of oligonucleosomal DNA fragments on agarose gel electrophoresis. Additionally, preferential recognition of apoptotic aged neutrophils by inflammatory macrophages freshly isolated from joint exudate was observed, confirming that this mechanism is likely to be available *in vivo*. Lastly, there is now a body of histological evidence that this mode of neutrophil clearance operates at inflamed sites *in vivo*. Cytological examination of inflammatory exudates from inflamed joints (Savill *et al.*, 1989a), lungs (Grigg *et al.*, 1991) and glomeruli (Savill *et al.*, 1992b) clearly demonstrated neutrophils undergoing apoptosis and being ingested by macrophages, which was confirmed by electron microscopy (Figure 14.3). Indeed, the ingested neutrophils seen in Figure 14.1e show typical nuclear chromatin condensation of apoptosis.

The speed and capacity of this process as a mechanism for destroying unwanted neutrophils warrants emphasis. *In vitro*, macrophage phagocytosis of apoptotic cells occurs within a few minutes of contact and, although a variable proportion of macrophages can take up aged neutrophils (on average about 45% in the case of human monocyte-derived macrophages), individual cells can ingest several neutrophils (Newman *et al.*, 1982; Savill *et al.*, 1989a 1989b; Haslett, 1992). Furthermore, once ingested, neutrophils are degraded extremely rapidly so that in electron microscopic studies it was necessary to fix macrophages within 20 min of ingestion of apoptotic cells in order to demonstrate intact neutrophils within the phagocyte. After this time ingested cells were rapidly degraded so that nuclear morphology could not be determined. However, although these studies demonstrate the efficiency of macrophage ingestion of apoptotic neutrophils as a clearance mechanism, the potential significance of the process needs further consideration.

4.3.3 "Injury-limiting" Neutrophil Clearance by Apoptosis

As discussed above, one of the hallmarks of apoptosis is that dying cells can be removed from tissues without

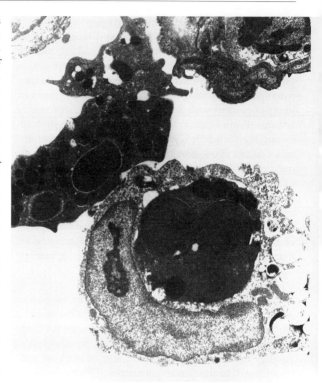

Figure 14.3 Ultrastructural demonstration of macrophage phagocytosis of apoptotic neutrophil *in vivo*. Experimental pneumococcal pneumonia in the rabbit, sampled during the phase of leucocyte clearance (72 h after instillation of bacteria into the lung). Transmission electron micrograph, × 8000. Reproduced with permission from Haslett (1992).

inciting inflammation. Given the pro-inflammatory potential of neutrophils, it is attractive to extrapolate from this observation and propose that neutrophil removal by apoptosis may be an "injury-limiting" clearance mechanism (Haslett and Henson, 1988; Haslett, 1992). Recent evidence suggests that apoptosis may constrain the tissue-damaging potential of the neutrophil in a number of ways.

Firstly, *in vitro* studies indicate that apoptosis may render the senescent neutrophil "less dangerous" by leading to loss of phlogistic functions such as superoxide production, degranulation and chemotaxis/morphological (Whyte *et al.*, 1993a). These defects appear to involve a number of changes in the cell consequent upon apoptosis, one of which is loss of the ability to bind and therefore respond to the chemoattractant FMLP. In the case of superoxide production, however, PMA (which activates neutrophils without being dependent upon cell surface receptors) was still able to elicit a "respiratory burst" comparable to that seen with freshly isolated neutrophils. These data indicate that an important consequence of apoptosis may be that the neutrophil and its pro-inflammatory mechanisms become "functionally isolated" from stimuli which would otherwise trigger responses likely to damage tissue.

However, it is apparent that if competent phagocytes are available then neutrophils undergoing apoptosis will be rapidly taken up by macrophages. This constitutes the second and more obvious facet of the injury-limiting potential of this mode of cell removal. Thus, apoptotic neutrophils retain their phlogistic contents and are ingested whilst still intact, preventing leakage of granule enzymes, etc. which would occur should the cell disintegrate before being taken up by macrophages (Savill et al., 1989a). This is emphasized by preliminary in vitro data obtained in a simple model of the inflamed site in which macrophages and neutrophils are co-cultured (Kar et al., 1993). If macrophage uptake of apoptotic neutrophils is blocked (with colchicine, for example), then rather than being ingested, the apoptotic cells disintegrate and release toxic contents such as MPO and elastase before cell fragments are taken up by macrophages.

Finally, however, macrophage phagocytosis of apoptotic neutrophils limits injury in one further, subtle manner. The usual response of macrophages to ingestion of particles in vitro is to release pro-inflammatory mediators such as eicosanoids (e.g. thromboxane), granule enzymes and cytokines. However, we found that even maximal uptake of apoptotic neutrophils failed to stimulate such release of mediators (Meagher et al., 1992). This did not reflect some toxic effect of the neutrophil upon the macrophage, since phagocytes which had ingested apoptotic cells retained their full potential to release mediators when stimulated by opsonized zymosan (yeast cell wall) particles. Furthermore, when apoptotic neutrophils were deliberately opsonized, macrophages did produce a pro-inflammatory response. These experiments prompted two important conclusions. Firstly, the "silent", histologically inconspicuous and non-inflammatory manner in which phagocytes remove apoptotic cells in vivo may reflect a selective failure to respond to such particles. Secondly, this lack of response is not a function of the particle ingested, but relates to the mechanism by which the apoptotic cell is normally ingested. This fuelled our interest in the molecular mechanisms by which macrophages normally recognize and ingest apoptotic cells.

4.3.4 Macrophage Recognition of Apoptotic Neutrophils

Although our studies showed that apoptosis is the change marking intact senescent neutrophils for removal by phagocytes, the molecular mechanisms by which the intact apoptotic cell is recognized as ripe for removal were obscure. These were important to define for reasons in addition to the inherent interest of determining how "senescent-self" is detected. Firstly, as already inferred, definition of the cell surface receptors involved in phagocytosis would be an essential step toward unravelling the signalling pathways which enable macrophages to

"uncouple" phagocytosis of an apoptotic cell from generation of pro-inflammatory mediators. However, the second reason was to understand how the clearance of apoptotic cells might be regulated. For example, molecules inhibiting this process could be sought at inflamed sites where progression to persistent inflammation and scarring occurs, or could be administered to in vivo models of self-limited inflammation to seek a pro-inflammatory effect of selectively inhibiting clearance of apoptotic cells. Alternatively, molecules stimulating uptake of senescent neutrophils might be the basis for novel anti-inflammatory therapies.

4.3.4.1 Cell Surface Molecules

The first step was to define the cell surface molecules involved in recognition and uptake, both those on the phagocyte and those on the apoptotic neutrophil. Despite considerable progress, this ambitious objective has yet to be achieved, partly because it appears that apoptotic cells may employ a number of different molecular changes to signal their "edible" status to phagocytes, while the macrophage may deploy a number of receptor mechanisms. A large body of work, primarily based upon inhibition of macrophage uptake of apoptotic cells in vitro by sugars, peptides/proteins, phospholipids and monoclonal antibodies is summarized in Figure 14.4. Although reviewed in detail elsewhere (Savill, 1992; Savill et al., 1993), no evidence has been obtained in studies of macrophage uptake of apoptotic neutrophils to support the involvement of phagocyte surface lectin recognition of apoptotic cell surface sugar residues exposed by loss of sialic acid, although this mechanism is implicated in clearance of other types of apoptotic cell (Duvall et al., 1985; Dini et al., 1992).

However, our studies demonstrated that recognition of apoptotic neutrophils occurred by a "charge-sensitive" mechanism, inhibitable by cationic molecules such as aminosugars and directly modulated by pH in a manner suggesting involvement of negatively charged residues on the neutrophil surface (Savill et al., 1989b). This implied that low pH and a particular mix of charged molecules might adversely influence clearance of apoptotic neutrophils in vivo, which was of interest as (where it has been measured) interstitial pH is indeed low in inflammation which terminates in scarring or abscess rather than resolution (Menken, 1956; Hunt et al., 1985). The inhibitory effect of aminosugars also sparked two lines of enquiry leading to definition of cell surface molecules involved in clearance of neutrophils.

Firstly, amino sugars were known to inhibit functions of certain adhesive molecules (Gartner et al., 1978; Jaffe et al., 1982; Nachman and Leung, 1982), namely members of the heterodimeric integrin superfamily of cell surface receptors (Hynes, 1987, 1992) and thrombospondin, a homotrimeric, multifunctional adhesive glycoprotein (Lawler et al., 1978; Lawler, 1986; Silverstein et al., 1986; Frazier, 1987). Involvement of

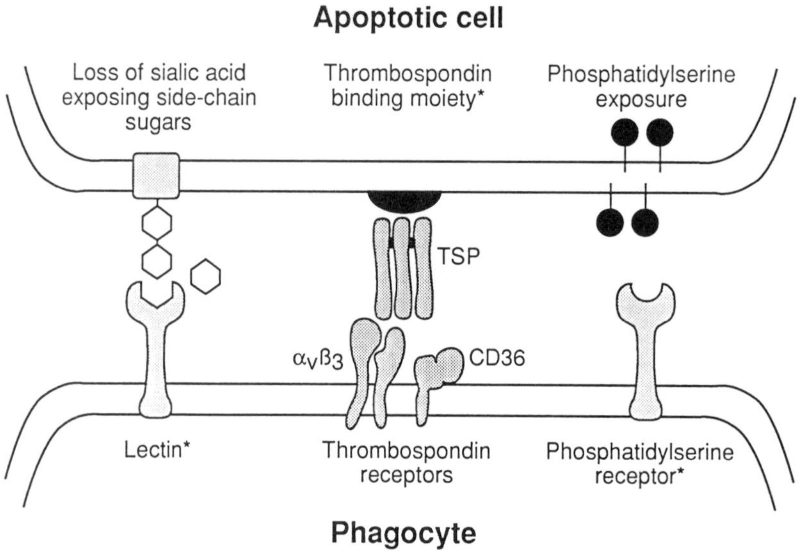

Apoptotic cell

Phagocyte

Figure 14.4 Mechanisms by which phagocytes may recognize apoptotic cells. Asterisks denote moieties that have yet to be characterized. See text for references. Left: sugar-lectin recognition. Although supporting evidence has been obtained for this mechanism in recognition of thymocytes and hepatocytes undergoing apoptosis, none has indicated a role in clearance of apoptotic neutrophils. Centre: integrin-thrombospondin. Evidence supports this mechanism in recognition of apoptotic neutrophils by human monocyte-derived macrophages, glomerular mesangial cells and fibroblasts, and by rodent bone-marrow derived macrophages. Right: recognition of exposed phosphatidylserine. Evidence supports this mechanism in clearance of apoptotic neutrophils by rodent-elicited macrophages and by cells by the human THP-1 monocyte/macrophage line. TSP, thrombospondin. Reproduced from Savill et al. (1993) with permission.

integrins and thrombospondin was sought by a number of strategies (reviewed by Savill, 1992). To date our studies (Savill et al., 1990; Savill et al., 1992b) indicate that macrophage-secreted thrombospondin acts as a "molecular glue" during the recognition process, binding unknown neutrophil surface residues to two receptors on the phagocyte surface, the $\alpha_v\beta_3$ "vitronectin receptor" integrin (which recognizes the tripeptide Arg-Gly-Asp in its ligands; Pytela et al., 1985) and an 88 kD monomer known as CD36 (which is also implicated in binding malarially parasitized erythrocytes; Asch et al., 1987; Oquendo et al., 1989). A working model of this recognition mechanism is presented in Figure 14.4. The data allow one to speculate that this system may be inhibited in vivo by fragments of fibronectin, vitronectin and thrombospondin released by uncontrolled proteolysis of the extracellular matrix at the inflamed site (Savill et al., 1992b).

Secondly, in Dr Henson's laboratory in Denver, our colleagues investigated the putative anionic sites suggested to be on the apoptotic cell surface by the inhibitory effect of cations. Their work, initially in a system of rodent macrophage recognition of rodent thymocytes induced to undergo apoptosis with glucocorticoids, elegantly demonstrated that as yet unknown receptors on phagocytes can recognize exposure of phosphatidylserine residues on the surface of apoptotic cells (Fadok et al., 1992a). These are normally asymmetrically

distributed so that they are largely limited to the inner leaflet of the lipid bilayer, but this asymmetry is lost in apoptosis (but also in other processes such as "sickling" of erythrocytes; Schwartz et al., 1985). In Fadok's system Arg-Gly-Asp peptides did not inhibit, by contrast with our studies of human monocyte-derived macrophage recognition of apoptotic neutrophils (Savill et al., 1990). Subsequently evidence indicated that this difference in use of recognition mechanisms was not a reflection of differences in the species or the lineage of the apoptotic cells, but was determined by the population of macrophages employed (Fadok et al., 1992b). Thus apoptotic neutrophils from both rodents and humans were recognized in a phosphatidylserine-dependent manner by rodent macrophages prepared by thioglycollate stimulation of the peritoneum, and phorbol ester-stimulated human phagocytes of the THP-1 line. However, rodent macrophages obtained by culture of bone marrow in vitro employed an Arg-Gly-Asp/vitronectin receptor-dependent mechanism. Clearly, therefore, neutrophils undergoing apoptosis may be recognized in different ways by different populations of macrophages (Fadok et al., 1992b; Savill et al., 1993). The significance of these differences is, at present, obscure.

4.3.4.2 Regulation of Phagocytosis of Apoptotic Cells

Definition of some of the cell surface molecules involved

in macrophage uptake of apoptotic neutrophils suggested mechanisms by which this capacity of macrophages might be regulated. In monocytic cells and other cell types, $\alpha_v\beta_3$ expression has been reported by Krissansen *et al.* (1990) and Ignotz *et al.* (1989) to be enhanced by exposure to the cytokines GM-CSF and TGFβ_1. When human monocyte-derived macrophages were preincubated for 6 h with either of these cytokines, potentiation of apoptotic neutrophil recognition was seen; in the case of GM-CSF there was a 2.4-fold increase in the proportion of macrophages ingesting senescent polymorphs (Ren and Savill, 1993). Intriguingly, increased macrophage uptake of neutrophils was stimulated by other "pro-inflammatory" cytokines known to be found at inflammatory sites, including IL-1β, TNF-α and IFNγ [see Dinarello (1989) and Arai *et al.* (1990) for review]. Since these cytokines may *amplify* inflammation by recruiting leucocytes to the inflamed site (by stimulating endothelial cell adhesion molecule expression and promoting transendothelial migration of neutrophils; see Chapters 7 and 10), it is possible that their capacity to promote *resolution* (by enhancing the ability of macrophages to remove leucocytes which have served their function and have undergone apoptosis) may represent a form of "negative feedback" control of inflammation. Furthermore, in addition to TGFβ [which attracts fibroblasts and promotes the laying down of extracellular matrix; reviewed by Sporn *et al.* (1987) and Massague (1990)], neutrophil uptake was also stimulated by a further cytokine with "reparative" properties, PDGF [which by promoting cell division promotes repair of injured sites by replacing damaged cells; see Ross (1989) for a review].

When the mechanism of the potentiating effect of GM-CSF and other cytokines upon neutrophil uptake was investigated, we were surprised to find that macrophage expression of $\alpha_v\beta_3$ (or, indeed, CD36) was not increased (Ren and Savill, 1993). Instead, these cytokines stimulated secretion of thrombospondin, which by supernatant transfer and depletion experiments was shown to account for the enhancing effect upon neutrophil recognition. It is likely that there will be further mechanisms by which macrophage clearance of apoptotic neutrophils may be regulated, but the crucial point demonstrated by these studies is that this capacity *is* subject to regulation. Thus it may prove possible to define cytokine networks which might down-regulate neutrophil clearance by macrophages, increasing the risk of neutrophil disintegration and persistent inflammation, while other networks may promote neutrophil clearance and resolution of inflammation.

4.3.5 "Semi-professional" Clearance of Apoptotic Neutrophils

As described above, apoptotic cells are not only taken up *in vivo* by the "professionals", macrophages, but are also cleared by "semi-professional" phagocytes. Apoptotic neutrophils appear to be no exception: we have recently obtained both *in vivo* and *in vitro* evidence that glomerular mesangial cells (resident smooth muscle-like cells not derived from bone marrow) can also take up large numbers of apoptotic neutrophils (Savill *et al.*, 1992a). Furthermore, fibroblasts also exhibit this property *in vitro* (Hall *et al.*, 1990).

The significance of clearance by mesangial cells and fibroblasts has yet to be studied. These interactions are of great interest, however, since they represent a direct link between the archetypal inflammatory leucocyte, the neutrophil, and two cell types implicated in tissue scarring by reason of their capacity to proliferate and lay down extracellular matrix. It will be interesting to determine if the response these cells make to uptake of apoptotic neutrophils is as benign as that exhibited by macrophages. That the response of these phagocytes might differ is suggested by preliminary data indicating that the recognition mechanisms these cells employ show differences from the macrophage; for example, fibroblasts appear to be able to use a sugar-lectin recognition mechanism in addition to an integrin (Hall *et al.*, 1990).

Furthermore, it will also be necessary to attempt to determine the relative importance of infiltrating inflammatory macrophages and resident semi-professional phagocytes in clearance of neutrophils from various inflamed sites at different stages of the response. It is possible that semi-professional phagocytes only come in to play when the capacity of inflammatory macrophages to clear apoptotic cells is overwhelmed, perhaps by repeated influx of neutrophils. Alternatively, semi-professional phagocytes may represent a tissue's first line of defence against uncontrolled release of contents of apoptotic neutrophils because monocytes must mature into macrophages before they can acquire the capacity to take up apoptotic neutrophils, a process which takes at least 3 days *in vitro* (Newman *et al.*, 1982; Savill *et al.*, 1990) but which is likely to be faster *in vivo*. Therefore, it is possible that neutrophils undergoing apoptosis before sufficient phagocytically competent monocyte-derived macrophages have matured are removed by mesangial cells, fibroblasts and other cells. Studies of inflammation *in vivo* will be needed to resolve these issues.

4.3.6 Regulation of Neutrophil Apoptosis

Another mechanism by which monocytes could be allowed time to mature before neutrophils undergo apoptosis would be if pro-inflammatory mediators were to slow neutrophil apoptosis. This is indeed the case *in vitro*, as bacterial LPS, C5a and FMLP can all slow the rate of neutrophil apoptosis (Lee *et al.*, 1989). Indeed, GM-CSF is potent at slowing apoptosis, raising the possibility that this cytokine might have a central role in coordinating the clearance mechanism, concomitantly enhancing the readiness of macrophages to remove neutrophils when they eventually undergo apoptosis.

Study of the intracellular mechanisms regulating neutrophil apoptosis is at an early stage. However, an important difference from other cell types is already apparent. In cells of the lymphocyte line elevation of intracellular Ca_i^{2+} (Ca_i^{2+}) concentration by stimuli such as calcium ionophore induces apoptosis, and apoptosis induced by other stimuli is associated with rises in Ca_i^{2+} (McConkey et al., 1989). However, in neutrophils spontaneously undergoing apoptosis during "ageing" in culture no such rises in Ca_i^{2+} were observed, and ionophore induced a dramatic slowing of apoptosis without inducing necrosis (Whyte et al., 1993b). This suggests that in different cell types rises in Ca_i^{2+} may stimulate different pathways of regulation of apoptosis. Because ionopore has only a transient effect on neutrophil Ca_i^{2+}, which rises and falls to baseline in around 1 h, and yet a much more prolonged effect on apoptosis (at 24 h only ~20% of cells are apoptotic, by contrast with ~80% in control unstimulated cultures), it is likely that in the neutrophil "downstream" intracellular pathways retarding apoptosis involve signalling dependent upon slower processes, such as synthesis of mRNA and protein. Indeed, in the neutrophil "constitutive" apoptosis is accelerated by inhibitors of RNA and protein synthesis. Effort is now being directed toward identifying the "apoptosis-retarding" genes of the neutrophil. Ultimately it might prove possible to regulate neutrophil apoptosis for therapeutic benefit.

4.3.7   Other Leucocytes may be Cleared by Apoptosis

Clearance of "unwanted" lymphocytic cells in lymphoid tissue such as lymph nodes and thymus is well recognized, as is apoptosis of unwanted cells in bone marrow (Wyllie et al., 1980; Alison and Sarraf, 1992). We have shown in vitro that eosinophils (which contain particularly toxic proteins such as eosinophil cationic protein) do undergo apoptosis in culture, although at a much slower rate than neutrophils, which can be retarded further by IL-5; eventual macrophage recognition of eosinophils appears to employ mechanisms similar to those used in neutrophil recognition (Stern et al., 1992). Others have reported that monocytes deprived of stimulation by growth factors and other cytokines undergo apoptosis (Mangan et al., 1991), but as yet the fate of inflammatory macrophages is obscure. Consequently, it appears that apoptosis may be a general mechanism for removing unwanted leucocytes from inflamed sites.

4.4   CONCLUSIONS ON NEUTROPHIL FATE IN INFLAMMATION

Neutrophil necrosis can occur at inflamed sites. Although mechanisms exist to limit tissue damage consequent upon release of neutrophil contents, it is clear that this mode of neutrophil removal is uncontrolled and carries the risk of promoting persistence rather than resolution of inflammation.

Neutrophil apoptosis leading to clearance of intact cells by macrophages and other phagocytes also occurs at inflamed sites. In vitro data emphasize that this is a controlled mode of neutrophil clearance, involving specific molecular mechanisms which are subject to fine regulation. Furthermore, apoptosis leads to "functional isolation" of neutrophils from inflammatory mediators by loss of receptors, disruption of intracellular responses involved in phlogistic responses, "packaging" of neutrophil contents for safe removal and uptake by macrophages without eliciting a pro-inflammatory response from macrophages. Thus it is clear that neutrophil apoptosis is likely to be an "injury-limiting" neutrophil disposal mechanism. We intend to test this hypothesis by a number of approaches but at the moment we feel that the available data indicate that, in common with other cells, apoptosis constitutes the preferred "physiological" mechanism of neutrophil elimination.

5.   Fate of Circulating Neutrophils

5.1   NEUTROPHIL KINETICS

To the uninitiated the study of neutrophil kinetics is a confusing and often controversial area, many of the difficulties relating to differences between the methods used to label and track neutrophils. A detailed discussion is beyond the scope of this chapter, and the interested reader is referred to reviews elsewhere (Hogg, 1987; MacNee and Selby, 1990).

However, the basics of neutrophil kinetics were apparent in the earliest studies of the problem performed by Wintrobe's group over 30 years ago (Athens et al., 1959, 1960, 1961a, 1961b). They used intravenous injections of [^{32}P]DFP to label cells of the granulocyte series in vivo and also used the same agent to label granulocytes prepared ex vivo before reinfusion. These studies showed that the total blood pool of neutrophils is normally equilibrated between a "circulating pool" and a "marginated pool" from which neutrophils can be released by exercise, adrenaline and other stimuli. The later use of infusions of autologous neutrophils prepared by "physiological" methods ex vivo and labelled with indium-111 or other γ-emitters (to facilitate external scintigraphy) confirmed these results, and supported earlier conclusions that a large proportion of "marginated" neutrophils were sequestered in the lung and, to a lesser extent, the spleen (Saverymuttu et al., 1983; Peters et al., 1985). Current concepts (Downey and Worthen, 1988) suggest that this "hold up" reflects the slow passage (relative to erythrocytes) of neutrophils through the smallest vessels of these organs; for example, the mean diameter of alveolar capillaries is about 5 μm, indicating that neutrophils (average diameter about

7 μm) must deform in order to "squeeze" through these vessels. It is easy to see why neutrophil activation, for example, by LPS (Haslett *et al.*, 1987), leads to increased sequestration, because such stimuli lead to actin polymerization and "stiffening" of the neutrophil. Indeed the reduced deformability of stimulated neutrophils by comparison with unstimulated cells has now been demonstrated by a number of techniques, most elegantly by prodding neutrophils with a "micropoker" (Worthen *et al.*, 1989).

There is also general agreement from a number of techniques that, provided cells have not been activated or damaged *ex vivo* (when they tend not to recirculate after venous injection, rapidly lodging in the liver and spleen after abnormally prolonged retention in the pulmonary circulation), neutrophils are lost from the total blood pool in an exponential fashion with a half-time of around 7 h. Although a gross oversimplification, it appears that the majority of neutrophils entering the total blood meet their fate in the liver and spleen; a smaller proportion are removed in the bone marrow (where studies with [^{32}P]DFP and tritiated thymidine also suggest that many immature cells of the granulocyte series are removed without ever having the chance to circulate). However, these studies have provided no information on the changes in blood pool neutrophils which result in their eventual retention in the reticuloendothelial system of the liver and spleen.

5.2 NEUTROPHIL CLEARANCE DIFFERS FROM CIRCULATING RED CELL REMOVAL

Although there has been little study of the mechanisms mediating clearance of circulating neutrophils, there has been more extensive study of reticuloendothelial uptake of senescent erythrocytes. The life span of these cells is measured in weeks rather than hours and, during their long sojourn in the blood, there is ample time for surface proteins of red cells to undergo a very slow non-enzymatic "Amadori" reaction with sugars to form AGEs, which *in vitro* takes several days. There is now compelling evidence that macrophages have receptors which recognize and ingest cells displaying AGE, and that this is one pathway for removal of senescent erythrocytes by the macrophages of the liver and spleen (Vlassara *et al.*, 1986, 1987). Not only is the life span of circulating neutrophils so short that there would appear to be insufficient time for AGE to form but also we failed to find evidence to support a role for AGE in human monocyte-derived macrophage recognition of human neutrophils "aged" in culture (Savill *et al.*, 1989b).

A second body of evidence suggests that senescent erythrocytes (and possibly other cell types) may be cleared because there are time-related changes in surface proteins enabling binding of autoantibodies and com-plement, which opsonize the senescent cell for macrophages (Kay, 1975). However, in our *in vitro* model of neutrophil senescence, blockade of macrophage receptors for complement and immunoglobulin with monoclonal antibodies failed to inhibit the uptake of aged neutrophils (Savill *et al.*, 1989b), casting some doubt on whether this mechanism is involved in the removal of neutrophils from the blood pool *in vivo*.

5.3 A ROLE FOR APOPTOSIS?

We have already emphasized the importance of apoptosis as a "physiological" means of elimination of extravasated neutrophils from inflamed sites. There would seem to be a *prima facie* case that apoptosis also determines elimination of circulating neutrophils, and although there has been very little study of this issue, there is support for such a role from a number of quarters.

We have observed very occasional neutrophils with typical light microscopical features of apoptosis in peripheral blood smears made immediately after venepuncture (unpublished data). Furthermore, haematologists are familiar with pyknotic neutrophils in blood samples left *ex vivo* for a period before fixation and staining (Undritz, 1973). Although colloquially known as "EDTA change" (EDTA is the anti-coagulant routinely employed) it appears likely that many cells of this appearance have in fact undergone apoptosis (which *in vitro* can proceed at room temperature, albeit at a much slower rate than at 37°C; Savill and Haslett, unpublished data). However, formal confirmation of apoptosis by electron microscopy, etc. has yet to be attempted. Although circumstantial, these observations suggest that circulating neutrophils can indeed undergo apoptosis. The infrequency of apparently apoptotic cells would be entirely consistent with the known speed and efficiency of phagocyte removal of such cells, which suggests that splenic and hepatic macrophages are likely to be able to remove such cells at first pass. Nevertheless, it is tempting to speculate that, just prior to apoptosis, changes in the neutrophil occur which favour its retention close to its presumptive reticuloendothelial graveyards.

However, there is more direct evidence that circulating neutrophils can undergo apoptosis from studies performed in 1964. Fliedner and colleagues labelled human bone marrow with tritiated thymidine *in vivo*. After the expected delay consequent upon the need for precursors to mature sufficiently to leave the marrow, autoradiography of blood smears showed appearance of label in neutrophils. A few hours later, label was seen to appear in a subset of neutrophils with pyknoytic nuclei, which accounted for less than 1% of the total neutrophils. Just as the proportion of labelled neutrophils rose with arrival of the bulk of labelled cells from the marrow, a parallel increase in the proportion of pyknotic cells bearing label was also observed several hours later. It was concluded that the pyknotic form represented a senescence phase of the circulating neutrophil (Fliedner *et al.*, 1964) and in this regard it is intriguing that the pyknotic neutrophils illustrated can now be appreciated to have light microscopic features indistinguishable from apoptosis.

Finally, we have preliminary evidence that Kupffer cells (hepatic macrophages) recognize and ingest senescent neutrophils (Staub, Savill and Haslett, unpublished data). These cells were magnetically purified from enzymatically dissociated livers of rats preinjected with colloidal iron particles. After overnight culture, rat Kupffer cells failed to ingest freshly isolated human neutrophils but succeeded in taking up 24 h-aged human neutrophils. Although as yet incomplete, elutriation experiments suggested preferential recognition of apoptotic cells by a mechanism inhibitable with aminosugars. Clearly more rigorous study of both hepatic and splenic macrophages is required, but these data point to the Kupffer cell being able specifically to recognize and ingest apoptotic neutrophils.

6. Conclusions

Much remains to be learnt of the fate of neutrophils leaving the blood pool in health or migrating to inflamed sites in disease. In view of a reasonable tendency to be more interested in pathology than physiology, most work on the problem has concentrated upon neutrophil clearance from the inflamed site. Although neutrophil necrosis and disintegration can occur, examples are usually from sites where uncontrolled inflammation has resulted in tissue damage. A growing body of evidence indicates that intact senescent neutrophils undergoing apoptosis can be removed in a specific and regulated fashion by macrophages and other phagocytes. This appears likely to be an "injury-limiting" disposal mechanism for the extravasated neutrophil. Further dissection of these mechanisms is not only likely to define the fate of the inflammatory neutrophil, but will throw light on the mechanisms by which effete neutrophils are removed from the circulation. Furthermore, new insights into the pathogenesis of persistent inflammation and scarring will be obtained by defining neutrophil clearance mechanisms, as points at which these may break down, hampering resolution, will be identified. Finally, there is the more distant prospect of therapies to hasten neutrophil removal by apoptosis.

7. Acknowledgements

J.S. is a Wellcome Trust Senior Research Fellow in Clinical Science and was formerly a MRC Training Fellow. C.H. was a MRC Senior Clinical Fellow. A large number of colleagues have provided help and advice, but the contributions of Professor Andrew Wyllie, Dr Peter Henson, Dr Laura Meagher, Dr Nancy Hogg and Dr Ian Dransfield deserve special mention.

8. References

Alison, M.R. and Sarraf, C.E. (1992). Apoptosis: a gene-directed programme of cell death. J. Roy. Coll. Phys. Lond. 26, 25–35.

Arai, K.-I., Lee, L., Miyama, A., Miyatake, S., Arai, N. and Yokota, T. (1990). Cytokines: coordinators of immune and inflammatory conditions. Annu. Rev. Biochem. 59, 783–811.

Araki, S., Shimada, Y., Kaji, K. and Hayashi, H. (1990). Apoptosis of endothelial cells induced by fibroblast growth factor deprivation. Biochem. Biophys. Res. Comm. 168, 1194–1199.

Arends, M.J., Morris, R.G. and Wyllie, A.H. (1990). Apoptosis: the role of the endonuclease. Am. J. Path. 136, 593–608.

Asch, A.S., Barnwell, J., Silverstein, R.L. and Nachman, R.L. (1987). Isolation of the thrombospondin membrane receptor. J. Clin. Invest. 79, 1054–1061.

Athens, J.W., Mauer, A.M., Ashenbrucker, H., Cartwright, G.E. and Wintrobe, M.M. (1959). Leukokinetic studies I. A method for labelling leukocytes with di-isopropylfluorophosphate (DFP-32). Blood 14, 303–310.

Athens, J.W., Mauer, A.M., Ashenbrucker, H., Cartwright, G.E. and Wintrobe, M.M. (1960). Leukokinetic studies II. A method for labelling granulocytes in vitro with radioactive di-isopropylfluorophosphate. J. Clin. Invest. 39, 1481–1492.

Athens, J.W., Mauer, A.M., Ashenbrucker, H., Cartwright, G.E. and Wintrobe, M.M. (1961a). Leukokinetic studies III. The distribution of granulocytes in the blood of normal subjects. J. Clin. Invest. 40, 159–167.

Athens, J.W., Raab, O.P., Raab, S.O., Mauer, A.M., Ashenbrucker, H., Cartwright, G.E. and Wintrobe, M.M. (1961b). Leukokinetic studies IV. The total blood, circulating and marginal granulocytes pools and the granulocyte turnover rate in normal subjects. J. Clin. Invest. 40, 989–997.

Ballard, K.J. and Holt, S.J. (1968). Cytological and cytochemical studies on cell death and digestion in the fetal rat foot: the role of macrophages and hydrolytic enzymes. J. Cell Sci. 3, 245–257.

Barres, B.A., Hart, I.K., Coles, H.S.R., Burne, J.F., Voyvodic, J.T., Richardson, W.D. and Raff, M.C. (1992). Cell death and control of cell survival in the oligodendrocyte lineage. Cell 70, 31–46.

Benhamou, L.E., Cazenave, P.A. and Sarthou, P. (1990). Anti-immunoglobulins induce death by apoptosis in WEHI-231 B lymphoma cells. Eur. J. Immunol. 20, 1405–1409.

Bissonnette, R.P., Echeverri, F., Mahoubi, A. and Green, D.R. (1992). Apoptotic cell death induced by c-myc is inhibited by bcl-2. Nature 359, 552–554.

Brewer, D.B. (1964). Electron-microscope phagocytosis of neutrophil polymorphonuclear leukocytes by macrophages. J. Patrol. 88, 307–310.

Buttyan, R., Olsson, C.A., Pintar, J., Chang, C., Bandyk, M., Ng, P.Y. and Sawezuk, I.S. (1989). Induction of the TRPM-2 gene in cells undergoing programmed cell death. Mol. Cell Biol. 9, 3473–3481.

Cagan, R.L. and Ready, D.F. (1989). The emergence of order in the *Drosophila* pupal retina. Dev. Biol. 136, 346–362.

Campbell, E.J. and Campbell, M.A. (1988). Cellular proteolysis by neutrophils in the presence of proteinase inhibitors: effects of substrate opsonization. J. Cell Biol. 106, 667–675.

Chapes, S.K. and Haskill, S. (1983). Evidence for granulocyte-mediated macrophage activation after *C. parvum* immunization. Cell. Immunol. 75, 367–377.

Clark, R.J., Jones, H.A., Rhodes, G.G. and Haslett, C. (1989). Non-invasive assessment in self-limited pulmonary inflammation by external scintigraphy of [111]Indium-labelled neutrophil influx and by measurement of the local metabolic response with positron emission tomography. Am. Rev. Respir. Dis. 139, A58.

Cohen, J.J. (1991). Programmed cell death in the immune system. Adv. Immunol. 50, 55–85.

Cohen, J.J. and Duke, R.C. (1984). Glucocorticoid activation of a calcium dependent endonuclease in thymic nuclei leads to cell death. J. Immunol. 132, 38–42.

Colditz, I.G. and Movat, H.Z. (1984). Kinetics of neutrophil accumulation in acute inflammatory lesions induced by chemotoxins and chemotoxinogens. J. Immunol. 133, 2169–2178.

Dancey, J.T., Deubelbeiss, K.A., Harker, L.A. and Finch, C.A. (1976). Neutrophil kinetics in man. J. Clin. Invest. 58, 706–711.

Dinarello, C.A. (1989). Interleukin-1 and its biologically related cytokines. Adv. Immunol. 44, 153–185.

Dini, L., Autori, F., Lentini, A., Olivierio, S. and Piacentini, M. (1992). The clearance of apoptotic cells in the liver is mediated by the asialoglycoprotein receptor. FEBS Lett. 296, 174–178.

Doherty, D.E., Henson, P.M. and Clark, R.A.F. (1990). Fibronectin fragments containing the RGDS cell binding domain mediate monocyte migration into the rabbit lung. J. Clin. Invest. 86, 1065–1074.

Donald, K.J., Edwards R.L. and McEvoy, J.D.S. (1976). An ultrastructural study of the pathogenesis of tissue injury in limited Wegener's granulomatosis. Pathology 8, 161–169.

Downey, G.P. and Worthen, G.S. (1988). Neutrophil retention in model capillaries. Deformability, geometry and hydrodynamic forces. J. Appl. Physiol. 65, 1861–1871.

Duke, R.C. and Cohen, J.J. (1986). IL-2 addiction: withdrawal of growth factor activates a suicide program in dependent T cells. Lymphokine Res. 5, 289–294.

Duvall, E., Wyllie, A.H. and Morris, R.G. (1985). Macrophage recognition of cells undergoing programmed cell death. Immunology 56, 351–358.

Duvall, E. and Wyllie, A.H. (1986). Death and the cell. Immunol. Today 7, 115–119.

Evan, G.I., Wyllie, A.H., Gilbert, G.S., Littlewood, T.D., Land, H., Brooks, M., Waters, C.M., Penn, L.Z. and Hancock, D.C. (1992). Induction of apoptosis in fibroblasts by c-myc protein. Cell 69, 119–128.

Fadok, V.A., Voelker, D.R., Campbell, P.A., Cohen, J.J., Bratton, D.L. and Henson, P.M. (1992a). Exposure of phosphatidylserine on the surface of apoptotic lymphocytes triggers specific recognition and removal by macrophages. J. Immunol. 148, 2207–2216.

Fadok, V., Savill, J.S., Haslett, C., Bratton, D.L., Doherty, D.E., Campbell, P.A. and Henson, P.M. (1992b). Different populations of macrophages use either the vitronectin receptor or the phosphatidylserine receptor to recognize and remove apoptotic cells. J. Immunol. 149, 4029–4035.

Fanidi, A., Harrington, E.A. and Evan, G.I. (1992). Cooperative interaction between c-myc and bcl-2 proto-oncogenes. Nature 359, 554–556.

Ferguson, D.J.P. and Anderson, T.J. (1981). Ultrastructural observations on cell death by apoptosis in the "resting" human breast. Virchows Arch. 393, 193–203.

Ferguson, M.W.J. (1988). Palate development. Development (Suppl.) 103, 41–60.

Fliedner, T.M., Cronkite, E.P. and Robertson J.S. (1964). Granulocytopoiesis I. Senescence and random loss of neutrophilic granulocytes in human beings. Blood 24, 402–414.

Frazier, W.A. (1987). Thrombospondin: a modular adhesive glycoprotein of platelets and nucleated cells. J. Cell. Biol. 105, 625–632.

Gammon, R. (1982). Leucocytoclastic vasculitis. Clin. Rheum. Dis. 8, 397–413.

Gartner, T.K., Williams, D.C., Minion, F.C. and Phillips, D.R. (1978). Thrombin-induced platelet aggregation is mediated by a platelet plasma membrane-bound pectin. Science 200, 1281–1283.

Grigg, J., Savill J., Sarraf, C., Haslett, C. and Silverman, M. (1991). Neutrophil apoptosis and clearance from neonatal lungs. Lancet 338, 720–722.

Hall, S.E., Savill, J.S. and Haslett, C. (1990). Fibroblast recognition of aged neutrophils is mediated by the RGD adhesion signal and is modulated by charged particles. Clin. Sci. 78 (Suppl. 22), 17p.

Harris, J.E. and Ford, C.E. (1964). Cellular traffic of the thymus: experiments with chromosome markers. Evidence that the thymus plays an instructional part. Nature 201, 884–886.

Haslett, C. (1992). Resolution of acute inflammation and the role of apoptosis in the tissue fate of granulocytes. Clin. Sci. 83, 639–648.

Haslett, C. and Henson, P.M. (1988). In "The Molecular and Cellular Biology of Wound Repair" (eds R.A.F. Clark and P.M. Henson) pp. 185–211. Plenum Publishing Corp., New York.

Haslett, C., Guthrie, L.A., Kopaniak, M.M., Johnston, R.B. and Henson, P.M. (1985). Modulation of multiple neutrophil functions by preparative methods or trace concentrations of bacterial lipopolysaccharide. Am. J. Pathol. 119, 101–110.

Haslett, C., Worthen, G.S., Giclas, P.C., Morrison, D.C., Henson, J.E. and Henson, P.M. (1987). The pulmonary vascular sequestration of neutrophils in endotoxaemia is initiated by an effect of endotoxin on the neutrophil in the rabbit. Am. Rev. Respir. Dis. 136. 9–18.

Haslett, C., Shen, A.S., Fieldsen, D.C., Allen, D., Henson, P.M. and Cherniak, R.M. (1989a). [111]Indium-labelled neutrophil influx into the lungs of bleomycin-treated rabbits assessed non-invasively by external scintigraphy. Am. Rev. Respir. Dis. 140, 756–763.

Haslett, C., Jose, P.J., Giclas, P.C., Williams, T.J. and Henson, P.M. (1989b). Cessation of neutrophil influx in C5a-induced acute experimental arthritis is associated with loss of chemoattractant activity from joint spaces. J. Immunol. 142, 3510–3517.

Henson, P.M. and Johnston, R.B. (1987). Tissue injury in inflammation. Oxidants, proteinases and cationic proteins. J. Clin. Invest. 79, 669–674.

Henson, P.M., Henson, J.E., Fittschen, C., Kimani, G., Bratton, D.L. and Riches, D.W.H. (1988). In "Inflammation: Basic Principles and Clinical Correlates" (eds J.I. Gallin, I.M. Goldstein and R. Snyderman) pp. 363–390. Raven Press, New York.

Hockenberry, D., Nunez, G., Milliman, C., Schreiber, R.D. and Korsmeyer, S.J. (1990). Bcl-2 is an inner mitochondrial membrane protein that blocks programmed cell death. Nature 348, 384–387.

Hogg, J.C. (1987). Neutrophil kinetics and lung injury. Physiol. Rev. 67, 1249–1295.

Hunt, T.K., Banda, M.J. and Silver, I.A. (1985). Cell interactions in post-traumatic fibrosis. Ciba Found. Symp. 114, 127–149.

Hurley, J.V. (1983). In "Acute Inflammation" (ed. J.V. Hurley) pp. 109–117. Churchill Livingstone, London.

Hynes, R.O. (1987). Integrins: a family of cell surface receptors. Cell 48, 549–554.

Hynes, R.O. (1992). Integrins: versatility, modulation, and signalling in cell adhesion. Cell 69, 121–125.

Ignotz, R.A., Heino, J. and Massague, J. (1989). Regulation of cell adhesion receptors by transforming growth factor-β Regulation of vitronectin receptor and LFA-1. J. Biol. Chem. 264, 383–392.

Itoh, N., Yonehara, S., Ishii, A., Yonehara, M., Mizushima, S.-I., Sameshima, M., Hase, A., Seto, Y. and Nagata, S. (1991). The polypeptide encoded by the cDNA for human cell surface antigen Fas can mediate apoptosis. Cell 66, 233–243.

Jacobson, M.D., Burne, J.F., King, M.P., Miyashita, T., Reed, J.C. and Raff, M.C. (1993). Bcl-2 blocks apoptosis in cells lacking mitochondrial DNA. Nature 362, 365–369.

Jaffe, E.A., Leung, L.L.K., Nachman, R.L., Levin, R.I. and Mosher, D.F. (1982). Thrombospondin is the endogenous pectin of human platelets. Nature 295, 246–248.

Janoff, A. (1985). Elastase in tissue injury. Annu. Rev. Med. 36, 207–241.

Janoff, A. and Zweifach, B.W. (1964). Production of inflammatory changes in the microcirculation by cationic proteins. J. Exp. Med. 120, 747–755.

Johnson, R.J., Couser, W.G., Chi, E.Y., Adler, S. and Klebanoff, S.J. (1987). New mechanism for glomerular injury: myeloperoxidase in hydrogen peroxide-halide system. J. Clin. Invest. 79, 1379–1392.

Kadri, A., Moinuddin, M. and De Leeuw (1975). Phagocytosis of blood cells by splenic macrophages in thrombotic thrombocytopaenic purpura. Ann. Intern. Med. 82, 799–802.

Kar, S., Ren, Y., Savill, J.S. and Haslett, C. (1993). Inhibition of macrophage phagocytosis in vitro of aged neutrophils increases release of neutrophil contents. Clin. Sci. in press.

Kay, M.M.B. (1975). Mechanism of removal of senescent cells by human macrophages in situ. Proc. Natl Acad. Sci. USA 72, 3521–3525.

Kerr, J.F.R., Wyllie, A.H. and Currie, A.R. (1972). Apoptosis: a basic biological phenomenon with wide-ranging implications in tissue kinetics. Br. J. Cancer 26, 239–257.

Klebanoff, S.J. (1988). In "Inflammation: Basic Principles and Clinical Correlates" (eds J.I. Gallin, I.M. Goldstein and R. Snyderman) pp. 391–423. Raven Press, New York.

Koury, M.J. and Bondurant, M.C. (1990). Erythropoietin retards DNA breakdown and prevents programmed death in erythroid progenitor cells. Science 246, 378–380.

Krissansen, G.W., Elliott, M.J., Lucas, C.M., Stomski, F.C., Berndt, M.C., Cheresh, D.F., Lopez, A.F. and Burns, G.F. (1990). Identification of a novel integrin β subunit expressed on cultured monocytes (macrophages). J. Biol. Chem. 265, 823–830.

Kyprianou, N., English, H.F. and Isaacs, J.T. (1990). Programmed cell death during regression of PC-82 human prostate cancer following androgen ablation. Cancer Res. 50, 3748–3751.

Lawler, J. (1986). The structural and functional properties of thrombospondin. Blood 67, 1197–1209.

Lawler, J.W., Slater, H.S. and Coligan, J.E. (1978). Isolation and characterization of a high molecular weight glycoprotein from human blood platelets. J. Biol. Chem. 253, 8609–8616.

Lee, A., Young, S.K., Henson P.M. and Haslett, C. (1989). Modulation of neutrophil programmed cell death by inflammatory mediators. FASEB J. 3: A1344.

Liu, Y.J., Joshua, D.E., Williams, G.T., Smith, C.A., Gordon, J. and MacLennan, I.C.M. (1989). Mechanism of antigen-driven selection in germinal centres. Nature 342, 929–931.

MacDonald, H.R. and Lees, R.K. (1990). Programmed death of autoreactive thymocytes. Nature 343, 642–644.

MacNee, W. and Selby, C. (1990). Neutrophil kinetics in the lungs. Clin. Sci. 79, 97–107.

Malech, H.D. and Gallin, J.I. (1988). Neutrophils in human diseases. N. Engl. J. Med. 317, 687–694.

Mangan, D.F., Welch, G.R. and Wahl, S.M. (1991). Lipopolysaccharide, tumour necrosis factor-α and IL-1β prevent programmed cell death (apoptosis) in human peripheral blood monocytes. J. Immunol. 146, 1541–1545.

Massague, J. (1990). The transforming growth factor-β family. Annu. Rev. Cell Biol. 6, 597–621.

McConkey, D.J., Nicotera, P., Hartzell, P., Bellomo, G., Wyllie A.H. and Orrenius, S. (1989). Glucocorticoids activate a suicide process in thymocytes through an elevation of cytosolic Ca^{2+} concentration. Arch. Biochem. Biophys. 269, 365–370.

McCullough, J., Weblen, B.J., Peterson, P.K. and Quie, P.G. (1978). Effects of temperature on granulocyte preservation. Blood 52, 301–305.

Meagher, L.C., Savill, J.S., Baker A., Fuller R. and Haslett, C. (1992). Phagocytosis of apoptotic neutrophils does not induce macrophage release of thromboxane B_2. J. Leukocyte Biol. 52, 269–273.

Menken, V. (1956). Biology of inflammation: chemical mediators and cellular injury. Science 123, 527–534.

Metchnikoff, E. (1893). Lectures on the comparative pathology of inflammation (translated from the French by F.A. Starling and E.H. Starling) Kegan, Paul, Trench and Trubner, London.

Morris, R.G., Hargreaves A.D., Duvall, E. and Wyllie, A.H. (1984). Hormone induced cell death 2. Surface changes in thymocytes undergoing apoptosis. Am. J. Path. 115, 426–436.

Nachman, R.L. and Leung, L.L.K. (1982). Complex formation of platelet glycoproteins IIb and IIIa with fibrinogen. J. Clin. Invest. 69, 263–269.

Nemazee, D.A. and Buerki, K. (1989). Clonal deletion of B lymphocytes in a transgenic mouse bearing anti-MHC class I antibody genes. Nature 337, 562–565.

Newman, S.L., Henson, J.E. and Henson, P.M. (1982). Phagocytosis of senescent neutrophils by human monocyte-derived macrophages and rabbit inflammatory macrophages. J. Exp. Med. 156, 430–442.

Nichols, B.A. and Bainton, D. (1975). In "Mononuclear Phagocytes in Immunity, Infection and Pathology" (ed. R. van Furth) p. 39. Blackwell, London.

Nunez, G., London. L., Hockenberry, D., Alexander, M., McKearn, J.P. and Korsmeyer, S.J. (1990). De-regulated Bcl-2 gene obstruction selectively prolongs survival of growth factor-deprived haemopoietic cell lines. J. Immunol. 144, 3602–3604.

Oberhammer, F.A., Pavelka, M., Sharma, S., Tiefenbacher, R., Purchio, A.F., Bursch, W. and Schulte-Herman, R. (1992). Induction of apoptosis in cultured hepatocytes and in regressing liver by transforming growth factor-β_1. Proc. Natl Acad. Sci. USA 89, 5408–5412.

Oquendo, P., Hundt, E., Lawler, J. and Seed, B. (1989). CD36 directly mediates cytoadherence of *Plasmodium falciparum*-parasitized erythrocytes. Cell 58, 95–101.

Parmely, R.T., Christ, W.M., Ragab, A.H., Boxer, L.A., Malluh, A. and Findley, H. (1981). Phagocytosis of neutrophils by marrow macrophages in childhood benign neutropaenia. J. Pediatr. 98, 207–211.

Pekin, T., Malinin, T.I. and Zwaifler, R. (1967). Unusual synovial fluid findings in Reiter's syndrome. Ann. Intern. Med. 66, 677–684.

Peters, A.M., Saverymuttu, S.H., Keshavarian, A., Bell, R.N. and Lavender, J.P. (1985). Splenic pooling of granulocytes. Clin. Sci. 68, 283–289.

Pietsch, M.C., Polzar, B., Stephan, H., Crompton, T., MacDonald, H.R., Mannherz, H.G. and Tschopp, J. (1993). Characterization of the endogenous deoxyribonuclease involved in nuclear DNA degradation during apoptosis (programmed cell death). EMBO J. 12, 371–377.

Pytela, R., Pierschbacher, M.D. and Ruoslahti, E. (1985). A 125/115 kDa cell surface receptor specific for vitronectin interacts with the arginine-glycine-aspartic acid adhesion sequence derived from fibronectin. Proc. Natl Acad. Sci. USA 82, 5766–5770.

Raff, M.C. (1992). Social controls on cell survival and cell death. Nature 356, 397–400.

Ranadive, N.S. and Cochrane, C.G. (1970). Basic proteins in rat neutrophils that increase vascular permeability. Clin. Exp. Immunol. 6, 905–909.

Ren, Y. and Savill, J.S. (1993). Increased macrophage secretion of thrombospondin is a mechanism by which cytokines potentiate phagocytosis of neutrophils undergoing apoptosis. (Submitted).

Ross, R. (1989). Platelet-derived growth factor. Lancet 1, 1179–1182.

Sanui, H., Yoshida, S.-I., Nomoto, K., Ohhara R. and Adachi, Y. (1982). Peritoneal macrophages which phagocytose autologous polymorphonuclear leucocytes in guinea pigs. I. Induction by irritants and micro-organisms and inhibition by colchicine. Br. J. Exp. Path. 63, 278–285.

Saverymuttu, S.H., Peters, A.M., Danpure, H.J., Reavy, H.J., Osman, S. and Lavender, J.P. (1983). Lung transit of ^{111}Indium-labelled granulocytes: relationship to labelling techniques. Scand. J. Haematol. 30, 151–160.

Savill, J. (1992). Macrophage recognition of senescent neutrophils. Clin. Sci. 83, 649–655.

Savill, J.S., Wyllie, A.H., Henson, J.E., Walport, M.J., Henson, P.M. and Haslett, C. (1989a). Macrophage phagocytosis of aging neutrophils in inflammation. Programmed cell death in the neutrophil leads to recognition by macrophages. J. Clin. Invest. 83, 865–875.

Savill, J.S., Henson, P.M. and Haslett, C. (1989b). Phagocytosis of aged human neutrophils by macrophages is mediated by a novel "charge sensitive" recognition mechanism. J. Clin. Invest. 84, 1518–1527.

Savill, J., Dransfield, I., Hogg, N. and Haslett, C. (1990). Vitronectin receptor mediated phagocytosis of cells undergoing apoptosis. Nature 343, 170–173.

Savill, J., Smith, J., Sarraf, C., Ren, Y., Abbott, F. and Rees, A. (1992a). Glomerular mesangial cells and inflammatory macrophages ingest neutrophils undergoing apoptosis. Kidney Int. 42, 924–936.

Savill, J., Hogg, N., Ren, Y. and Haslett, C. (1992b). Thrombospondin cooperates with CD36 and the vitronectin receptor in macrophage recognition of neutrophils undergoing apoptosis. J. Clin. Invest. 90, 1513–1522.

Savill, J., Fadok, V.A., Henson, P.M. and Haslett, C. (1993). Phagocyte recognition of cells undergoing apoptosis. Immunol. Today (in press).

Schubert, D., Kimura, H., LaCorbiere M., Vaughan, J., Karr, D. and Fischer, W.H. (1990). Activin is a neural cell survival molecule. Nature 344, 686–870.

Schwartz, R.S., Tanaka, Y., Fidler, I.J., Tsun-Yee Chui, D., Lubin, B. and Schroit, A.J. (1985). Increased adherence of sickled and phosphatidylserine-enriched human erythrocytes to cultured human peripheral blood monocytes. J. Clin. Invest. 75, 1965–1972.

Sendtner, M., Kreuzberg, G.W. and Thoenen, H. (1990). Ciliary neurotrophic factor prevents the degeneration of motor neurons after axotomy. Nature 345, 440–442.

Shi, L., Kraut, R.P., Aebersold, R. and Greenberg, A.H. (1992). A natural killer cell protein that induces DNA fragmentation and apoptosis. J. Exp. Med. 175, 553–566.

Shi, Y., Glynn, J.M., Guilbert, L.J., Cotter, T.G., Bissonnette, R.P. and Green, D.R. (1992). Role for c-myc in activation-induced cell death in T cell hybridomas. Science 257, 212–215.

Smith, C.A., Williams, G.T., Kinston, R., Jenkinson, E.J. and Owen, J.J.T. (1989). Antibodies to the CD3/T-cell receptor complex induce death by apoptosis in immature T-cells in thymic cultures. Nature 337, 181–184.

Silverstein, R.L., Leung, L.L.K. and Nachman, R.L. (1986). Thrombospondin: a versatile multifunctional glycoprotein. Arteriosclerosis 6, 245–253.

Spitznagel, J.K. (1990). Antibiotic proteins of neutrophils. J. Clin. Invest. 86, 1851–1854.

Sporn, M.B., Roberts, A.B., Wakefield, L.M. and de Crombrugge, B. (1987). Some recent advances in the chemistry and biology of transforming growth factor-β. J. Cell. Biol. 105, 1039–1041.

Spriggs, R.S., Boddington, M.M. and Mowat, A.G. (1978). Joint fluid cytology in Reiter's syndrome. Ann. Rheum. Dis. 37, 557–560.

Stern, M., Meagher, L.C., Savill, J.S. and Haslett, C. (1992). Apoptosis in human eosinophils. Programmed cell death in the eosinophil leads to phagocytosis by macrophages and is modulated by IL-5. J. Immunol. 148, 3543–3549.

Trauth, B.C., Klas, C., Peters, A.M.J., Matzuku, S., Moller, P., Falk, W., Debatin, K.-M. and Krammer, P.H. (1989). Monoclonal antibody-mediated tumour regression by induction of apoptosis. Science 245, 301–305.

Tusurata, J.K., Wong, K., Fritz, I.B. and Griswold M.D. (1990). Structural analysis of sulfated glycoprotein-2 from aminoacid sequence. Relationship to clusterin and serum protein 40,40. Biochem. J. 268, 571–574.

Undritz, E. (1973). In "Sandoz Atlas of Haematology" (ed. E. Undritz) Sections 137, 412, and 416. Sandoz Ltd., Basel.

Vartio, T., Seppa, H. and Vaheri, A. (1981). Susceptibility of soluble and matrix fibronectin to degradation by tissue proteinases, mast cell chymase and cathepsin G. J. Biol. Chem. 256, 471–477.

Vaux, D.L., Cory, S. and Adams, J.M. (1988). Bcl-2 gene promotes haemopoietic cell survival and cooperates with c-myc to immortalise pre-B cells. Nature 335, 440–442.

Vlassara, H., Brownlee, M. and Cerami, A. (1986). Novel macrophage receptor for glucose-modified proteins is distinct from previously described scavenger receptors. J. Exp. Med. 164, 1301–1309.

Vlassara, H., Valinsky, J., Brownlee, M., Cerami, C., Nishimoto, S. and Cerami, A. (1987). Advanced glycosylation end-products on erythrocyte cell surface induce receptor-mediated phagocytosis by macrophages. J. Exp. Med. 166, 539–549.

Vedder, N.B., Winn, R.K., Rice, C.L., Chi, E.Y., Arfors, K.-E. and Harlan, J.M. (1990). Inhibition of leukocyte adherence by anti-CD18 monoclonal antibody attenuates reperfusion injury in the rabbit ear. Proc. Natl Acad. Sci. USA 87, 2643–2648.

Walker, N.I., Bennett, R.E. and Kerr, J.F.R. (1989). Cell death by apoptosis during involution of the lactating breast in mice and rats. Am. J. Anat. 185, 19–24.

Weiss, S.J. (1989). Tissue destruction by neutrophils. N. Engl. J. Med. 320, 365–375.

Weiss, S.J., Curnette, J.T. and Regani, S. (1986). Neutrophil-mediated solubilization of the subendothelial matrix: oxidative and non-oxidative mechanisms of proteolysis used by normal and chronic granulomatous disease phagocytes. J. Immunol. 136, 636–642.

Whyte, M.K.B., Meagher, L.C., MacDermot, J. and Haslett, C. (1993a). Impairment of function in aging neutrophils is associated with apoptosis. J. Immunol. 150, 5124–5134.

Whyte, M.K.B., Hardwick, S.J., Meagher, L.C., Savill, J.S. and Haslett, C. (1993b). Transient elevations of cytosolic calcium retard neutrophil apoptosis in vitro. J. Clin. Invest. 92, 446–455.

Williams, G.T., Smith, C.A., Spooncer, E., Dexter, T.M. and Taylor, D.R. (1990). Haemopoietic colony stimulating factors promote cell survival by suppressing apoptosis. Nature 343, 76–78.

Worthen, G.S., Schwab, B., Elson, E.L. and Downey, G.P. (1989). Mechanical properties of stimulated neutrophils: cell stiffening induces retention in capillaries. Science 245, 183–186.

Wyllie, A.H. (1980). Glucocorticoid-induced thymocyte apoptosis is associated with endogenous endonuclease activation. Nature 284, 555–556.

Wyllie, A.H., Kerr, J.F.R. and Currie, A.R. (1980). Cell death: the significance of apoptosis. Int. Rev. Cytol. 68, 251–306.

Wyllie, A.H., Morris, R.G., Smith, A.L. and Dunlop. D. (1986). Chromatin cleavage in apoptosis; association with condensed chromatin morphology and dependence on macromolecular synthesis. J. Pathol. 142, 67–77.

Glossary

Note: This glossary is up to date for the current volume only and will be supplemented with each subsequent volume.

α_1-**ACT** α_1-Antichymotrypsin
α**1-AT** α_1-Antiprotease inhibitor *also known as* α_1-antitrypsin
α_1-**PI** α_1-Proteinase inhibitor
A Absorbance
Å Angstrom
AA Arachidonic acid
aa Amino acids
AAb Autoantibody
Ab Antibody
Ab1 Idiotype antibody
Ab2 Anti-idiotype antibody
Ab2α Anti-idiotype antibody which binds outside the antigen binding region
Ab2β Anti-idiotype antibody which binds to the antigen binding region
Ab3 Anti-anti-idiotype antibody
Abcc Antibody dependent cytotoxic activity
ABA-L-GAT Arsanilic acid conjugated with the synthetic polypeptide L-GAT
AC Adenylate cyclase
ACAT Acyl-co-enzyme-A acyltransferase
ACAID Anterior chamber-associated immune deviation
ACE Angiotensin-converting enzyme
ACh Acetylcholine
ACTH Adrenocorticotrophin hormone
ADCC Antibody-dependent cell-mediated cytotoxicity
Ado Adenosine
ADP Adenosine diphosphate
AECA Antibodies to endothelial cells
AES Anti-eosinophil serum
Ag Antigen
AGE Advanced glycosylation end-product
AGEPC 1-*O*-alkyl–2-acetyl-*sn*-glyceryl–3-phosphocholine; *also known as* PAF
AH Acetylhydrolase
AI Angiotensin I
AII Angiotensin II
AID Autoimmune disease
AIDS Acquired immune deficiency syndrome

A/J A Jackson inbred mouse strain
ALP Anti-leukoprotease
cAMP cyclic adenosine monophosphate (adenosine 3', 5'-phosphate)
AM Alveolar macrophage
AML Acute myelogenous leukaemia
AMP Adenosine monophosphate
ANAb Anti-nuclear antibodies
ANCA Anti-neutrophil cytoplasmic autoantibodies
cANCA Cytoplasmic ANCA
pANCA Perinuclear ANCA
AND Anaphylactic degranulation
ANF Atrial natriuretic factor
ANP Atrial natriuretic peptide
Anti-I–A Antibody against class II MHC molecule encoded by I–A locus
Anti-I–E Antibody against class II MHC molecule encoded by I–E locus
anti-Ig Antibody against an immunoglobulin
anti-RTE Anti-tubular epithelium
AP-1 Activator protein–1
APA B-azaprostanoic acid
APAS Antiplatelet antiserum
APC Antigen-presenting cell
APD Action potential duration
ApO-B Apolipoprotein B
APRL Anti-hypertensive polar renal lipid *also known as* PAF
APUD Amine precursor uptake and decarboxylation
AR-CGD Autosomal recessive form of chronic granulomatous disease
ARDS Adult respiratory distress syndrome
AS Ankylosing spondylitis
4-ASA 4-aminosalicylic acid
5-ASA 5-aminosalicylic acid
ASA Acetylsalicylic acid (aspirin)
ATHERO-ELAM A monocyte adhesion molecule
ATL Adult T cell leukaemia
ATP Adenosine triphosphate
ATPγs Adenosine 3' thiotriphosphate
AUC Area under curve

AVP Arginine vasopressin

β_2 **(CD18)** A leucocyte integrin
β_2**M** β_2-Microglobulin
β-**TG** β-Thromboglobulin
B Bursa-derived
BAL Bronchoalveolar lavage
B$_1$receptor Bradykinin receptor subtype
B$_2$receptor Bradykinin receptor subtype
BAF Basophil-activating factor
BAL Bronchoalveolar lavage
BALF Bronchoalveolar lavage fluid
BALT Bronchus-associated lymphoid tissue
B cell Bone marrow-derived lymphocyte
BCF Basophil chemotactic factor
B-CFC Basophil colony-forming cell
BCG Bacillus Calmette-Guérin
bFGF Basic fibroblast growth factor
BG Birbeck granules
BHR Bronchial hyperresponsiveness
Bl-CFC Blast colony-forming cells
b.i.d. *Bis in die* (twice a day)
Bk Bradykinin
BM Bone marrow
BMCMC Bone marrow cultured mast cell
BMMC Bone marrow mast cell
BOC-FMLP Butoxycarbonyl-FMLP
bp Base pair
BPB Para-bromophenacyl bromide
BPI Bacterial permeability-increasing protein
BSA Bovine serum albumin

C1 The first component of complement
C1 inhibitor A serine protease inhibitor which inactivates C1r/C1s
C1q Complement fragment 1q (anaphylatoxin)
C1qR Receptor for C1w; facilitates attachment of immune complexes to mononuclear leucocytes and endothelium
C2 The second component of complement

C3 The third component of complement

iC3 Inactivated C3

C3a Complement fragment 3a (anaphylatoxin)

C3a$_{72-77}$ A synthetic carboxyterminal peptide C3a analogue

C3aR Receptor for anaphylatoxins, C3a, C4a, C5a

C3b Complement fragment 3b (anaphylatoxin)

C3bi Inactivated form of C3b fragment of complement

C4 The fourth component of complement

iC4 Inactivated C4

C4b Complement fragment 4b (anaphylatoxin)

C4BP C4 binding protein; plasma protein which acts as co-factor to factor I inactivate C3 convertase

C5 The fifth component of complement

C5a Complement fragment 5a (anaphylatoxin)

C5aR Receptor for anaphylatoxins C3a, C4a and C5a

C5b Complement fragment 5b (anaphylatoxin)

C6 The sixth component of complement

C7 The seventh component of complement

C8 The eighth component of complement

C9 The ninth component of complement

C$_\epsilon$2 Heavy chain of immunoglobulin E: domain 2

C$_\epsilon$3 Heavy chain of immunoglobulin E: domain 3

C$_\epsilon$4 Heavy chain of immunoglobulin E: domain 4

Ca *The chemical symbol for* calcium

[Ca^{2+}]$_i$ Intracellular free calcium concentration

CAH Chronic active hepatitis

CALLA Common lymphoblastic leukaemia antigen

CALT Conjunctival associated lymphoid tissue

cAMP cyclic adenosine monophosphate (adenosine 3′, 5′-phosphate)

CAM Cell adhesion molecule

CAP57 Cationic protein from neutrophils

CatG Cathepsin G

CB Cytochalasin B

CBH Cutaneous basophil hypersensitivity

CBP Cromolyn-binding protein

CCK Cholecystokinin

CCR Creatinine clearance rate

CD Cluster of differentiation (a system of nomenclature for surface molecules on cells of the immune system); cluster determinant

CD1 Cluster of differentiation 1 *also known as* MHC class I-like surface glycoprotein

CD1a Isoform a *also known as* non-classical MHC class I-like surface antigen

CD1c Isoform c *also known as* non-classical MHC class I-like surface antigen

CD2 Defines T cells involved in antigen non-specific cell activation

CD3 *Also known as* T cell receptor-associated surface glycoprotein on T cells

CD4 Defines MHC class II-restricted T cell subsets

CD5 *Also known as* Lyt 1 in mouse

CD7 Cluster of differentiation 7

CD8 Defines MHC class I-restricted T cell subset

CD10 *Known to be* common acute leukaemia antigen

CD11a *Known to be* an α chain of LFA–1 (leucocyte function antigen–1) present on several types of leucocyte and which mediates adhesion

CD11b *Known to be* an α chain of CR3 (complement receptor type 3) present on several types of leucocyte and which mediates adhesion

CD11c *Known to be* a complement receptor 4 α chain.

CD14 *Known to be* a lipid-anchored glycoprotein

CD15 *Known to be* Lewis X, fucosyl-N-acetyllactosamine

CD16 *Known to be* IgGFc receptor III low affinity *also known as* IgGFcRIII

CD16–1, CD16–2 Isoforms of CD16

CD18 *Known to be* the common β chain of the CD11 family of molecules

CD20 *Known to be* a pan B cell

CD29 *Known to be* Very late antigen beta chain

CD31 *Known to be* on platelets, monocytes, macrophages, granulocytes, B-cells and endothelial cells; *also known as* PECAM

CD32 IgFc receptor II *also known as* IgFcRII

CD33$^+$ *Known to be* a monocyte and stem cell marker

CD34$^-$ *Known to be* a stem cell marker

CD36 *Known to be* a thrombospondin receptor

CD41 *Known to be* a platelet glycoprotein

CD44 *Known to be* a leucocyte adhesion molecule

CD45 *Known to be* a pan leucocyte marker

CD45RO *Known to be* the isoform of leukosialin present on memory T cells

CD46 *Known to be* a membrane cofactor protein

CD49 Cluster of differentiation 49

CD49a-f *Known to be* very late antigen α 1-α 6 chains

CD49d *Known to be* very late antigen α 4 chain

CD51 *Known to be* vitronectin receptor α chain

CD54 *Known to be* Intercellular adhesion molecule–1 *also known as* ICAM–1

CD59 *Known to be* a low molecular weight HRf present to many haematopoetic and non-haematopoetic cells

CD62 *Known to be present on* activated platelets and endothelial cells; *also known as* P-selectin

CD64 *Known to be* IgGFc receptor I high affinity *also known as* IgGFcRI

CD65 *Known to be* fucoganglioside

CDC Complement-dependent cytotoxicity

cDNA Complementary DNA

CDP Choline diphosphate

CDR Complementary-determining region

CD$_{xx}$ Common determinant *xx*

CEA Carcinoembryonic antigen

CETAF Corneal epithelial T cell activating factor

CF Cystic fibrosis

Cf Cationized ferritin

CFA Complete Freund's adjuvant

CFC Colony-forming cell

CFU Colony-forming unit

CFU-S Colony-forming unit, spleen

CGD Chronic granulomatous disease

cGMP cyclic guanosine monophosphate (guanosine 3′, 5′-phosphate)

CGRP Calcitonin gene-related peptide

CH2 Hinge region of human immunoglobulin

CHO Chinese hamster ovary

CI Chemical ionization

CIBD Chronic inflammatory bowel disease

CK Creatine phosphokinase

CKMB The myocardial-specific isoenzyme of creatine phosphokinase

Cl *The chemical symbol for* chloride

CL Chemiluminescent

CLA Cutaneous lymphocyte antigen

CL18/6 Anti-ICAM–1 monoclonal antibody

CLC Charcot-Leyden crystal

CMC Critical micellar concentration
CMI Cell mediated immunity
CML Chronic myeloid leukaemia
CMV Cytomegalovirus
CNS Central nervous system
CO Cyclooxygenase
CoA Coenzyme A
CoA-IT Coenzyme A – independent transacylase
Con A Concanavalin A
COPD Chronic obstructive pulmonary disease
COS Fibroblast-like kidney cell line established from simian cells
CoVF Cobra venom
CP Creatine phosphate
CPJ Cartilage/pannus junction
Cr *The chemical symbol* for chromium
CR Complement receptor
CR1 Complement receptor type 1
CR2 Complement receptor type 2
CR3 Complement receptor type 3
CR3-α Complement receptor type 3-α
CR4 Complement receptor type 4
CRF Corticotrophin-releasing factor
CRH Corticotrophin-releasing hormone
CRI Cross-reactive idiotype
CRP C-reactive protein
CSA Cyclosporin A
CSF Colony-stimulating factor
CSS Churg-Strauss syndrome
CT Computed tomography
CTAP-III Connective tissue-activating peptide
CTD Connective tissue diseases
C terminus Carboxy terminus of peptide
CThp Cytotoxic T lymphocyte precursors
CTL Cytotoxic T lymphocyte
CTMC Connective tissue mast cell
ct.min^{-1} Counts per minute

Da Dalton (the unit of relative molecular mass)
DAF Decay-accelerating factor
DAG Diacylglycerol
DAO Diamine oxidase
D-Arg D-Arginine
DArg-[Hyp³, DPhe⁷]-BK A bradykinin B$_2$ receptor antagonist. Peptide derivative of bradykinin
DArg-[Hyp³, Thi⁵, DTic⁷, Tic⁸]-BK A bradykinin B$_2$ receptor antagonist. Peptide derivative of bradykinin
DC Dendritic cell
DCF Oxidized DCFH
DCFH 2', 7'-dichlorofluorescin
DEC Diethylcarbamazine
desArg⁹-BK Carboxypeptidase N product of bradykinin

desArg¹⁰KD Carboxypeptidase N product of kallidin
DFMO α-Difluoromethyl ornithine
DFP Diisopropyl fluorophosphate
DGLA Dihomo-γ-linolenic acid
DH Delayed hypersensitivity
DHR Delayed hypersensitivity reaction
DIC Disseminated intravascular coagulation
DL-CFU Dendritic cell/Langerhans cell colony forming
DLE Discoid lupus erythematosus
DMARD Disease-modifying anti-rheumatic drug
DMF N,N-dimethylformamide
DMSO Dimethyl sulfoxide
DNA Deoxyribonucleic acid
D-NAME D-Nitroarginine methyl ester
DNase Deoxyribonuclease
DNCB Dinitrochlorobenzene
DNP Dinitrophenol
Dpt4 *Dermatophagoides pteronyssinus* allergen 4
DGW2 An HLA phenotype
DR3 An HLA phenotype
DR7 An HLA phenotype
DREG–2 Murine IgG$_1$ monoclonal antibody against L-selectin
DREG-56 (Antigen) L-selectin
DREG-200 Monoclonal antibody against L-selectin
ds Double-stranded
DSCG Disodium cromoglycate
DST Donor-specific transfusion
DTH Delayed-type hypersensitivity
DTPA Diethylenetriamine pentaacetate
DTT Dithiothreitol
dv/dt Rate of change of voltage within time

ε Molar absorption coefficient
EA Egg albumin
EAE Experimental autoimmune encephalomyelitis
EAF Eosinophil-activating factor
EAR Early phase asthmatic reaction
EAT Experimental autoimmune thyroiditis
EBV Epstein-Barr virus
EC Electron capture
ECD Electron capture detector
ECE Endothelin-converting enzyme
E-CEF Eosinophil cytotoxicity enhancing factor
ECF-A Eosinophil chemotactic factor of anaphylaxis
ECG Electrocardiogram
ECGF Endothelial cell growth factor
ECGS Endothelial cell growth supplement
E. coli *Escherichia coli*
ECP Eosinophil cationic protein

ED$_{35}$ Effective dose producing 35% maximum response
ED$_{50}$ Effective dose producing 50% maximum response
EDF Eosinophil differentiation factor
EDN Eosinophil-derived neurotoxin
EDRF Endothelium-derived relaxant factor
EDTA Ethylenediamine tetraacetic acid *also known* as etidronic acid
EE Eosinophilic eosinophils
EEG Electroencephalogram
EET Epoxyeicosatrienoic acid
EFA Essential fatty acid
EFS Electrical field stimulation
EG1 Monoclonal antibody specific for the cleaved form of eosinophil cationic peptide
EGF Epidermal growth factor
EGTA Ethylene glycol-bis(β-aminoethyl ether) N,N,N',N'-tetraacetic acid
EI Electron impact
eIF–2 Subunit of protein synthesis initiation factor
ELAM Endothelial leucocyte adhesion molecule
ELF Respiratory epithelium lung fluid
ELISA Enzyme-linked immunosorbent assay
EMS Eosinophilia-myalgia syndrome
ENS Enteric nervous system
EO Eosinophil
Eo-CFC Eosinophil colony-forming cell
EOR Early onset reaction
EPA Eicosapentaenoic acid
EpDIF Epithelial-derived inhibitory factor
EpDRF Epithelium-derived relaxant factor
EPO Eosinophil peroxidase
EPOR Erythropoietin receptor
EPR Effector cell protease
EPX Eosinophil protein X
ER Endoplasmic reticulum
ESP Eosinophil stimulation promoter
ESR Erythrocyte sedimentation rate
ET Endothelin
ET–1 Endothelin–1
ETYA Eicosatetraynoic acid

FA Fatty acid
FAB Fast-electron bombardment
Fab Antigen binding fragment
F(ab')2 Fragment of an immunoglobulin produced pepsin treatment
factor B Serine protease in the C3 converting enzyme of the alternative pathway
factor D Serine protease which cleaves factor B
factor H Plasma protein which acts as a co-factor to factor I

factor I Hydrolyses C3 converting enzymes with the help of factor H

FAD Flavine adenine dinucleotide

FBR Fluorescence photobleaching recovery

Fc Crystallizable fraction of immunoglobulin molecule

Fcγ Receptor for Fc portion of IgG

FcγRI Ig Fc receptor I *also known as* CD64

FcγRII Ig Fc receptor II *also known as* CD32

FcγRIII Ig Fc receptor III *also known as* CD16

FcεRI High affinity receptor for IgE

FcεRII Low affinity receptor for IgE

FcR Receptor for Fc region of antibody

FCS Foetal calf (bovine) serum

FEV₁ Forced expiratory volume in 1 second

FGF Fibroblast growth factor

FID Flame ionization detector

FITC Fluorescein isothiocyanate

FKBP FK506-binding protein

FLAP 5-lipoxygenase-activating protein

FMLP *N*-Formyl-methionyl-leucyl-phenylalanine

FNLP Formyl-norleucyl-leucyl-phenylalanine

FPR Formyl peptide receptor

FSG Focal sequential glomerulosclerosis

FSH Follicle stimulating hormone

FTS Facteur thymic serique

5-FU 5-fluorouracil

G Granulocyte

Ga G-protein

G6PD Glucose 6-phosphate dehydrogenase

GABA γ-aminobutyric acid

GAG Glycosaminoglycan

GALT Gut-associated lymphoid tissue

GAP GTPase-activating protein

GBM Glomerular basement membrane

GC Guanylate cyclase

GC-MS Gas chromatography mass spectroscopy

G-CSF Granulocyte colony-stimulating factor

Ge Glycoprotein exocytosis

GM-CSF Granulocyte colony-stimulating factor

GDP Guanosine 5'-diphosphate

GEC Glomerular epithelial cell

GF–1 An insulin-like growth factor

GFR Glomerular filtration rate

GH Growth hormone

GH-RF Growth hormone-releasing factor

Gi Family of pertussis toxin sensitive G-proteins

GI Gastrointestinal

GIP Granulocyte inhibitory protein

GlyCam–1 Glycosylation-dependent cell adhesion molecule–1

GMC Gastric mast cell

GM-CFC Granulocyte-macrophage colony-forming cell

GM-CSF Granulocyte-macrophage colony-stimulating factor

GMP Guanosine monophosphate (guanosine 5'-phosphate)

GMP–140 Granule-associated membrane protein–140

Go Family of pertussis toxin sensitive G-proteins

GP Glycoprotein

gp45–70 Membrane co-factor protein

gp90^{MEL} 90 kD glycoprotein recognized by monoclonal antibody MEL-14; *also known as* L-selectin

GPIIb-IIIa Glycoprotein IIb-IIIa *known to be* a platelet membrane antigen

GppCH₂P Guanyl-methylene diphosphanate *also known* as a stable GTP analogue

GppNHp Guanylyl-imidiodiphosphate also known as a stable GTP analogue

GRGDSP Glycine-arginine-glycine-aspartic acid serine-proline

Gro Growth-related oncogene

GRP Gastrin-related peptide

Gs Stimulatory G protein

GSH Glutathione (reduced)

GSSG Glutathione (oxidized)

GTP Guanosine triphosphate

GTP-γ-S Guanarine 5'*O*-(3-thiotriphosphate)

GTPase Guanidine triphosphatase

GVHD Graft-versus-host-disease

GVHR Graft-versus-host-reaction

H Histamine

H₁ Histamine receptor type 1

H₂ Histamine receptor type 2

H₃ Histamine receptor type 3

H₂O₂ *The chemical symbol* for hydrogen peroxide

Hag Haemagglutinin

Hag-1 Cleaved haemagglutinin subunit-1

Hag-2 Cleaved haemagglutinin subunit-2

H & E Haematoxylin and eosin

hIL Human interleukin

Hb Haemoglobin

HBBS Hank's balanced salt solution

HDC Histidine decarboxylase

HDL High-density lipoprotein

HEL Hen egg white lysozyme

HEPE Hydroxyeicosapentanoic acid

HEPES *N*-2-Hydroxylethylpiperazine-*N'*-ethane sulphonic acid

HES Hypereosinophilic syndrome

HETE 5,8,9,11 and 15 Hydroxyeicosatetraenoic acid

5(S)HETE A stereo isomer of 5-HETE

HETrE Hydroxyeicosatrienoic acid

HEV High endothelial venule

HFN Human fibronectin

HGF Hepatocyte growth factor

HHT 12-Hydroxy–5, 8, 10-heptadecatrienoic acid

HHTrE 12(S)-Hydroxy–5, 8, 10-heptadecatrienoic acid

HIV Human immunodeficiency virus

HL60 Human promyelocytic leukaemia cell line

HLA Human leucocyte antigen

HLA-DR2 Human histocompatability antigen class II

HMG CoA Hydroxylmethylglutaryl coenzyme A

HMW High molecular weight

HMT Histidine methyltransferase

HMVEC Human microvascular endothelial cell

HNC Human neutrophil collagenase (MMP–8)

HNE Human neutrophil elastase

HNG Human neutrophil gelatinase (MMP–9)

HODE Hydroxyoctadecanoic acid

HPETE, 5-HPETE & 15-HPETE 5 and 15-Hydroperoxyeicosatetraenoic acid

HPETrE Hydroperoxytrienoic acid

HPODE Hydroperoxyoctadecanoic acid

HPLC High-performance liquid chromatography

HRA Histamine-releasing activity

HRAN Neutrophil-derived histamine-releasing activity

HRf Homologous-restriction factor

HRF Histamine-releasing factor

HRP Horseradish peroxidase

HSA Human serum albumin

HSP Heat-shock protein

HS-PG Heparan sulphate proteoglycan

HSV Herpes simplex virus

HSV–1 Herpes simplex virus 1

³HTdR Tritiated thymidine

5-HT 5-Hydroxytryptamine *also known as* Serotonin

HUVEC Human umbilical vein endothelial cell

[Hyp³]-BK Hydroxproline derivative of bradykinin

[Hyp⁴]-KD Hydroxproline derivative of kallidin

I_{sc} Short-circuit current
Ia Immune reaction-associated antigen
Ia+ Murine class II major histocompatibility complex antigen
IB4 Anti-CD18 monoclonal antibody
IBD Inflammatory bowel disease
IBMX Isobutylmethylxanthine
IBS Inflammatory bowel syndrome
IC_{50} Concentration producing 50% inhibition
ICAM Intercellular adhesion molecules
ICAM-1 Intercellular adhesion molecule-1
ICAM-2 Intercellular adhesion molecule-2
ICAM-3 Intercellular adhesion molecule-3
ICE IL-1β-converting enzyme
i.d. Intradermal
IDC Interdigitating cell
IDD Insulin-dependent (type 1) diabetes
IEL Intraepithelial leucocyte
IELym Intraepithelial lymphocytes
IFA Incomplete Freund's adjuvant
IFN Interferon
IFNα Interferon α
IFNβ Interferon β
IFNγ Interferon γ
Ig Immunoglobulin
IgA Immunoglobulin A
IgE Immunoglobulin E
IgG Immunoglobulin G
IgG1 Immunoglobulin G class 1
IgG$_{2a}$ Immunoglobulin G class 2a
IgM Immunoglobulin M
IGF-1 Insulin-like growth factor
IgSF Immunoglobulin superfamily
IGSS Immuno-gold silver stain
IHC Immunohistochemistry
IHES Idiopathic hypereosinophilic syndrome
IκB NFκB inhibitor protein
IL Interleukin
IL-1 Interleukin-1
IL-1α Interleukin-1α
IL-1-β Interleukin-1β
IL-1R Interleukin-1 receptor
IL-1Ra Interleukin-1 receptor antagonist
IL-2 Interleukin 2
IL-2R Interleukin-2 receptor
IL-2Rβ Interleukin-2 receptor β
IL-3 Interleukin-3
IL-3R Interleukin-3 receptor
IL-4 Interleukin-4
IL-4R Interleukin-4 receptor
IL-5 Interleukin-5
IL-5R Interleukin-5-receptor
IL-6 Interleukin-6
IL-6R Interleukin-6 receptor
IL-8 Interleukin-8
ILR Interleukin receptor

IMF Integrin modulating factor
IMMC Intestinal mucosal mast cell
INCAM Inducible cell adhesion molecule
INCAM110 Inducible cell adhesion molecule 110
i.p. Intraperitoneally
IP$_3$ Inositol triphosphate
IP$_4$ Inositol tetrakisphosphate
IPF Idiopathic pulmonary fibrosis
IPO Intestinal peroxidase
IpOCOCq Isopropylidene OCOCq
I/R Ischaemia-reperfusion
IRAP IL-1 receptor antagonist protein
IRF-1 Interferon regulatory factor 1
ISCOM Immune-stimulating complexes
ISGF3 Interferon-stimulated gene Factor 3
ISGF3α α subunit of ISGF3
ISGFγ γ subunit of ISGF3
IT Immunotherapy
ITP Idiopathic thrombocytopenic purpura
i.v. Intravenous

K *The chemical symbol for* potassium
K$_a$ Association constant
kb Kilobase
20KDHRF A homologous restriction factor; binds to C8
65KDHRF A homologous restriction factor, also known as C8 binding protein; interferes with cell membrane pore-formation by C5b-C8 complex
Kcat Catalytic constant; a measure of the catalytic potential of an enzyme
K$_d$ Equilibrium dissociation constant
kD Kilodalton
K$_D$ Dissociation constant
KD Kallidin
Ki Antagonist binding affinity
Ki67 Nuclear membrane antigen
KLH Keyhole limpet haemocyanin
KOS KOS strain of herpes simplex virus

λ_{max} Wavelength of maximum absorbance
LAD Leucocyte adhesion deficiency
LAK Lymphocyte-activated killer (cell)
LAM Leucocyte adhesion molecule
LAM-1 Leucocyte adhesion molecule-1
LAR Late-phase asthmatic reaction
L-Arg L-Arginine
LBP LPS binding protein
LC Langerhans cell
LCF Lymphocyte chemoattractant factor
LCR Locus control region

LDH Lactate dehydrogenase
LDL Low-density lipoprotein
LDV Laser Doppler velocimetry
LECAM Lectin adhesion molecule
LECAM-1 Lectin adhesion molecule-1
Le^x(Lewis X) Leucocyte ligand for selectin
LFA Leucocyte function-associated antigen
LFA-1 Leucocyte function-associated antigen-1; a member of the β-2 integrin family of cell adhesion molecules
LG β-Lactoglobulin
LGL Large granular lymphocyte
LH Luteinizing hormone
LHRH Luteinizing hormone-releasing hormone
LI Labelling index
LIS Lateral intercellular spaces
LMP Low molecular mass polypeptide
LMW Low molecular weight
5-LO 5-Lipoxygenase
12-LO 12-Lipoxygenase
15-LO 15-Lipoxygenase
LP(a) Lipoprotein a
LPS Lipopolysaccharide
L-selectin A cell adhesion molecule expressed on leucocytes that recognizes a carbohydrate ligand
LT Leukotriene
LTA$_4$ Leukotriene A$_4$
LTB$_4$ Leukotriene B$_4$
LTC$_4$ Leukotriene C$_4$
LTD$_4$ Leukotriene D$_4$
LTE$_4$ Leukotriene E$_4$
L$_y$-1$^+$ (Cell line)
LX Lipoxin
LXA$_4$ Lipoxin A$_4$
LXB$_4$ Lipoxin B$_4$
LXC$_4$ Lipoxin C$_4$
LXD$_4$ Lipoxin D$_4$
LXE$_4$ Lipoxin E$_4$
zLYCK Carboxybenzyl-Leu-Tyr-CH$_2$Cl

α2-M α_2-Macroglobulin
M Monocyte
M3 Receptor Muscarinic receptor subtype 3
M-540 Merocyanine-540
mAb Monoclonal antibody
mAb IB4 Monoclonal antibody IB4
mAb PB1.3 Monoclonal antibody PB1.3
mAb R 3.1 Monoclonal antibody R 3.1
mAb R 3.3 Monoclonal antibody R 3.3
mAb 6.5 Monoclonal antibody 6.5
mAb 60.3 Monoclonal antibody 60.3
MAC Membrane attack molecule

Mac Macrophage (also abbreviated to MΦ)

Mac–1 Macrophage–1 antigen; a member of the β-2 integrin family of cell adhesion molecules (also abbreviated to MΦ1)

MAF Macrophage-activating factor

MAO Monoamine oxidase

MAP Monophasic action potential

MAPTAM An intracellular Ca^{2+} chelator

MARCKS Myristolated, alanine-rich C kinase substrate; specific protein kinase C substrate

MBP Major basic protein

MBSA Methylated bovine serum albumin

MC Mesangial cells

M cell Microfold or membranous cell of Peyer's patch epithelium

MCP Membrane co-factor protein

M-CSF Macrophage colony-stimulating factor

MC$_T$ Tryptase-containing mast cell

MC$_{TC}$ Tryptase- and chymase-containing mast cell

MDA Malondialdehyde

MDGF Macrophage-derived growth factor

MDP Muramyl dipeptide

MEA Mast cell growth-enhancing activity

MEL Metabolic equivalent level

MEL-14 antigen Monoclonal antibody that recognizes murine-L-selectin

MEM Minimal essential medium

MG Myasthenia gravis

MGSA Melanoma-growth-stimulatory activity

MHC Major histocompatibility complex

MI Myocardial ischaemia

MIF Migration inhibition factor

mIL Mouse interleukin

MI/R Myocardial ischaemia/reperfusion

MIRL Membrane inhibitor of reactive lysis

mix-CFC Colony-forming cell mix

Mk Megakaryocyte

MLC Mixed lymphocyte culture

MLymR Mixed lymphocyte reaction

MLR Mixed leucocyte reaction

MMC Mucosal mast cell

MMCP Mouse mast cell protease

MMP Matrix metalloproteinase

MMP1 Matrix metalloproteinase 1

MNA 6-Methoxy–2-napthylacetic acid

MNC Mononuclear cells

MΦ Macrophage (also abbreviated to Mac)

MPO Myeloperoxidase

MRI Magnetic resonance imaging

mRNA Messenger ribonucleic acid

MS Mass spectrometry

MSS Methylprednisoline sodium succinate

MT Malignant tumour

MW Molecular weight

Na *The chemical symbol for* sodium

NA Noradrenaline *also known as* norepinephrine

NAAb Natural autoantibody

NAb Natural antibody

NADH Reduced nicotinamide adenine dinucleotide

NADP Nicotinamide adenine diphosphate

NADPH Reduced nicotinamide adenine dinucleotide phosphate

L-NAME L-Nitroarginine methyl ester

NANC Non-adrenergic, non-cholinergic

NAP Neutrophil-activating peptide

NAP–1 Neutrophil-activating peptide–1

NAP–2 Neutrophil-activating peptide–2

NBT Nitro-blue tetrazolium

NC1 Non-collagen 1

N-CAM Neural cell adhesion molecule

NCEH Neutral cholesteryl ester hydrolase

NCF Neutrophil chemotactic factor

NDGA Nordihydroguaretic acid

NDP Nucleoside diphosphate

Neca 5'-(*N*-ethyl carboxamido)-adenosine

NED Nedocromil sodium

NEP Neutral endopeptidase (EC 3.4.24.11)

NF-AT Nuclear factor of activated T lymphocytes

NF-χB Nuclear factor-χB

NGF Nerve growth factor

NGPS Normal guinea-pig serum

NIH 3T3 (fibroblasts) National Institute of Health 3T3-Swiss albino mouse fibroblast

NIMA Non-inherited maternal antigens

Nk Neurokinin

NK Natural killer

Nk–1 Neurokinin receptor subtype

Nk–2 Neurokinin receptor subtype

Nk–3 Neurokinin receptor subtype

NkA Neurokinin A

NkB Neurokinin B

L-NMMA L-Nitromonomethyl arginine

NMR Nuclear magnetic resonance

NO *The chemical symbol for* nitric oxide

L-NOARG L-nitroarginine

NPK Neuropeptide K

NPY Neuropeptide Y

NRS Normal rabbit serum

NSAID Non-steroidal anti-inflammatory drug

NSE Nerve-specific enolase

NT Neurotensin

N terminus Amino terminus of peptide

O$_2^-$ Oxygen free radical

OA Osteoarthritis

OAG Oleoyl acetyl glycerol

OD Optical density

ODC Ornithine decarboxylase

ODS Octadecylsilyl

·OH *The chemical symbol for* hydroxyl radical

OT Oxytocin

OVA Ovalbumin

ox-LDL Oxidized low-density lipoprotein

Ψa Apical membrane potential

P Probability

P Phosphate

PAFR Platelet activating factor receptor

P$_a$O$_2$ Arterial oxygen pressure

P$_i$ Inorganic phosphate

p150,95 A member of the β-2-integrin family of cell adhesion molecules; *also known* as CD11c

PA Phosphatidic acid

pA$_2$ Negative logarithm of the antagonist dissociation constant

PADGEM Platelet activation-dependent granule external membrane

PAF Platelet-activating factor *also known as* APRL

PAGE Polyacrylamide gel electrophoresis

PAI Plasminogen activator inhibitor

PAM Pulmonary alveolar macrophages

PAS Periodic acid–Schiff reagent

PBA Polyclonal B cell activators

PBC Primary biliary cirrhosis

PBL Peripheral blood lymphocytes

PBMC Peripheral blood mononuclear cells

PBS Phosphate-buffered saline

PC Phosphatidylcholine

PCA Passive cutaneous anaphylaxis

pCDM8 Eukaryotic expression vector

PCNA Proliferating cell nuclear antigen

PCR Polymerase chain reaction

p.d. Potential difference

PDBu 4*a*-phorbol 12, 13-dibutyrate

PDE Phosphodiesterase

PDGF Platelet-derived growth factor

PDGFR Platelet-derived growth factor receptor

PE Phosphatidylethanolamine
PECAM–1 Platelet endothelial cell adhesion molecule–1; *also known as* CD31
PEG Polyethylene glycol
PET Positron emission tomography
PEt Phosphatidylethanol
PF4 Platelet factor 4
PG Prostaglandin
PGAS Polyglandular autoimmune syndrome
PGF Prostaglandin F
PGI$_2$ Prostaglandin I$_2$ *also known as* prostacyclin
PGD$_2$ Prostaglandin D$_2$
PGE$_1$ Prostaglandin E$_1$
PGE$_2$ Prostaglandin E$_2$
PGF$_{2\alpha}$ Prostaglandin F2α
PGF$_2$ Prostaglandin F$_2$
PGG$_2$ Prostaglandin G$_2$
PGH Prostaglandin H
P$_a$O$_2$ Arterial oxygen pressure
PGH$_2$ Prostaglandin H$_2$
PGI$_2$ Prostaglandin I$_2$
PGP Protein gene-related peptide
Ph^1 Philadelphia (chromosome)
PHA Phytohaemagglutinin
PHD PHD[8(1-hydroxy–3-oxo-propyl)–9, 12-dihydroxy-5, 10 heptadecadienic acid]
PHI Peptide histidine isoleucine
PHM Peptide histidine methionine
P$_i$ Inorganic phosphate
PI Phosphatidylinositol
PI–3,4-P2 Phosphatidylinositol 3, 4-biphosphate
PI–3,4,5-P3 Phosphatidylinositol 3, 4, 5-trisphosphate
PI–3-kinase Phosphatidylinositol–3-kinase
PI–4-kinase Phosphatidylinositol–4-kinase
PI–3-P Phosphatidylinositol–3-phosphate
PI–4-P Phosphatidylinositol–4-phosphate
PI–4, 5-P2 Phosphatidylinositol 4, 5-biphosphate
PIP Phosphatidylinositol monophosphate
PIP$_2$ Phosphatidylinositol biphosphate
PK Protein kinase
PKA Protein kinase A
PKC Protein kinase C
PL Phospholipase
PLA Phospholipase A
PLA$_2$ Phospholipase A$_2$
PLAP Putative phospholipase activity protein
PLC Phospholipase C
PLD Phospholipase D
PLP Proteolipid protein
PLT Primed lymphocyte typing
PMA Phorbol myristate acetate

PMC Peritoneal mast cell
PMD Piecemeal degranulation
PML Polymorphonuclear leucocyte
PMN Polymorphonuclear neutrophil
PMSF Phenylmethylsulphonyl fluoride
PNU Protein nitrogen unit
p.o. *Per os* (by mouth)
PPD Purified protein derivative
PPME A ligand for L-selectin *also known as* polyphosphomannan ester
PRA Percentage reactive activity
PRD Positive regulatory domain
PRD-II Positive regulatory domain II
PR3 Proteinase–3
proET–1 Proendothelin–1
PRL Prolactin
PRP Platelet-rich plasma
PS Phosphatidylserine
PT Pertussis toxin
PTA$_2$ Pinane thromboxane A$_2$
PTCA Percutaneous transluminal coronary angioplasty
PTCR Percutaneous transluminal coronary recanalization
Pte-H$_4$ Tetrahydropteridine
PtX Pertussis toxin
PUFA Polyunsaturated fatty acid
PUMP–1 Punctuated metalloproteinase
PWM Pokeweed mitogen
PYY Peptide YY

Qa Genetic locus encoding a non-classical class I MHC molecule
q.i.d. Quater *in die* (four times a day)
QRS Segment of electrocardiogram

·R Free radical
R15.7 Anti-CD18 monoclonal antibody
RA Rheumatoid arthritis
RANTES A member of the IL8 supergene family (*R*egulated on *a*ctivation, *n*ormal *T* *e*xpressed and *s*ecreted)
RAST Radioallergosorbent test
RBC Red blood cell
RBF Renal blood flow
RBL Rat basophilic leukaemia
RE RE strain of herpes simplex virus type 1
REA Reactive arthritis
REM Relative electrophoretic mobility
RER Rough endoplasmic reticulum
RF Rheumatoid factor
RF$_L$-6 Rat foetal lung–6
RFLP Restriction fragment length polymorphism
RGD Arginine-glycine-asparagine
rh- Recombinant human – (prefix usually referring to peptides)

RIA Radioimmunoassay
RMCP Rat mast cell protease
RMCPII Rat mast cell protease II
RNA Ribonucleic acid
RNase Ribonuclease
RNHCl *N*-Chloramine
RNL Regional lymph nodes
ROM Reactive oxygen metabolite
ROS Reactive oxygen species
R-PIA *R*-(1-methyl–1-phenyltheyl)-adenosine
RPMI 1640 Roswell Park Memorial Institute 1640 medium
RS Reiter's syndrome
RSV Rous sarcoma virus
RTE Rabbit tubular epithelium
RTE-a-5 Rat tubular epithelium antigen a–5
r-tPA Recombinant tissue-type plasminogen activator
RW Ragweed

S Svedberg (unit of sedimentation density)
SALT Skin-associated lymphoid tissue
SAZ Sulphasalazine
SC Secretory component
SCF Stem cell factor
SCFA Short-chain fatty acid
SCG Sodium cromoglycate
SCID Severe combined immunodeficiency sydrome
sCR1 Soluble type–1 complement receptors
SCW Streptococcal cell wall
SD Standard deviation
SDS Sodium dodecyl sulphate
SDS-PAGE Sodium dodecyl sulphate-polyacrylamide gel electrophoresis
SEM Standard error of the mean
SGAW Specific airway conductance
SHR Spontaneously hypertensive rat
SIRS Soluble immune response suppressor
SK Streptokinase
Sl Murine Steel mutation
SLE Systemic lupus erythematosus
SLe^x Sialyl Lewis X antigen
SLO Streptolysin-O
SLPI Secretory leucocyte protease inhibitor
SM Sphingomyelin
SNAP *S*-Nitroso-*N*-acetylpenicillamine
SNP Sodium nitroprusside
SOD Superoxide dismutase
SOM Somatostatin *also known* as somatotrophin release-inhibiting factor
SOZ Serum-opsonized zymosan
SP Sulphapyridine
S Protein vitronectin
SR Systemic reaction

SRBC Sheep red blood cells
SRS Slow-reacting substance
SRS-A Slow-reacting substance of anaphylaxis
Sub P Substance P

T Thymus-derived
$t_{1/2}$ Half-life
T84 Human intestinal epithelial cell line
TauNHCl Taurine monochloramine
TBM Tubular basement membrane
TCA Trichloroacetic acid
T cell Thymus-derived lymphocyte
TCP Toxin co-regulated pilus
TCR T cell receptor α/β or γ/δ heterodimeric forms
TDI Toluene diisocyanate
TDID$_{50}$ Tissue culture infectious dose – 50%
TEC Tubular epithelial cell
TF Tissue factor
Tg Thyroglobulin
TGF Transforming growth factor
TGFα Transforming growth factor α
TGFβ Transforming growth factor β
TGFβ$_1$ Transforming growth factor β_1
T$_H$ T helper cell
T$_H$H T Helper o
T$_H$p T helper precursor
T$_H$0, T$_H$1, T$_H$2 Subsets of helper T cells
THP-1 Human monocytic leukaemia
Thy 1+ Murine T cell antigen
t.i.d. *Ter in die* (three times a day)
TIL Tumour-infiltrating lymphocytes

TIMP Tissue inhibitors of metalloproteinase
TIMP-1 Tissue inhibitor of metalloproteinases-1
TIMP-2 Tissue inhibitor of metalloproteinases-2
Tla Thymus leukaemia antigen
TLC Thin-layer chromatography
TLCK Tosyl-lysyl-CH$_2$Cl
TLP Tumour-like proliferation
Tm T memory
TNF Tumour necrosis factor
TNF-α Tumour necrosis factor-α
tPA Tissue-type plasminogen activator
TPA 12-O-tetradeconylphorbol–13-acetate
TPCK Tosyl-phenyl-CH$_2$Cl
TPK Tyrosine protein kinases
TPP Transpulmonary pressure
Tris Tris(hydroxymethyl)aminomethane
TSH Thyroid-stimulating hormone
TSP Thrombospondin
TTX Tetrodotoxin
TX Thromboxane
TXA$_2$ Thromboxane A$_2$
TXB$_2$ Thromboxane B$_2$
Tyk$_2$ Tyrosine kinase

U937 (cells) Histiocytic lymphoma, human
UC Ulcerative colitis
UDP Uridine diphosphate
UPA Urokinase-type plasminogen activator
UTP Uridine triphosphate
UV Ultraviolet

VC Veiled cells
VCAM Vascular cell adhesion molecule
VCAM-1 Vascular cell adhesion molecule-1
VF Ventricular fibrillation
VIP Vasoactive intestinal peptide
VLA Very late activation antigen (β 1 integrins)
VLA-1 Very late activation antigen-1
VLA-2 Very late activation antigen-2
VLA-3 Very late activation antigen-3
VLA-4 Very late activation antigen-4
VLA-5 very late activation antigen-5
VLA-6 Very late activation antigen-6
VLDL Very low-density lipoprotein
*V*max Maximal velocity
*V*min Minimal velocity
vp Viral protein
VP Vasopressin
VPB Ventricular premature beat
VT Ventricular tachycardia

W Murine dominant white spotting mutation
WBC White blood cell
WGA Wheat germ agglutinin

XO Xanthine oxidase
Y1/82A A monoclonal antibody detecting a cytoplasmic antigen in human macrophages

ZA Zonulae adherens
ZAS Zymosan-activated serum
ZO Zonulae occludentes

Key to Illustrations

 Helper
lymphocyte

 Suppressor
lymphocyte

 Killer
lymphocyte

 Plasma cell

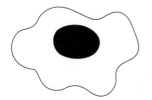 Bacterial or
Tumour cell

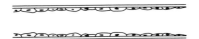 Blood vessel
lumen

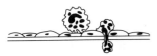 Eosinophil
passing through
vessel wall

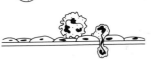 Neutrophil
passing through
vessel wall

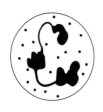 Resting neutrophil

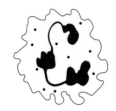 Activated neutrophil

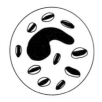 Resting eosinophil

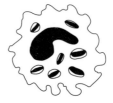 Activated eosinophil

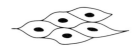 Smooth muscle

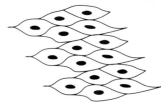 Smooth muscle thickening

 Smooth muscle contraction

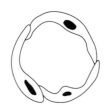 Normal blood vessel

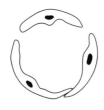 Endothelial cell permeability

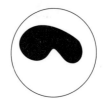 Resting macrophage

 Activated macrophage

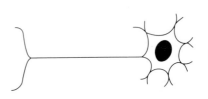 Nerve

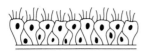 Intact epithelium

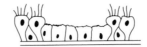 Damaged epithelium

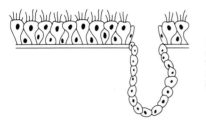 Intact epithelium with submucosal gland

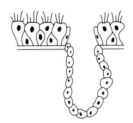 Normal submucosal gland

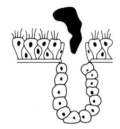 Hypersecreting submucosal gland

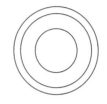 Normal airway

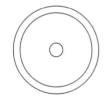 Oedema

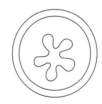 Bronchospasm

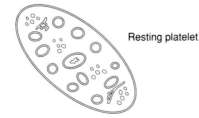 Resting platelet

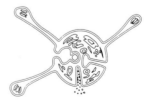 Activated platelet

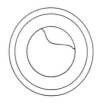 Airway hypersecreting mucus

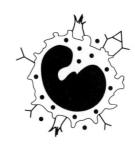

Resting
basophil

Activated
basophil

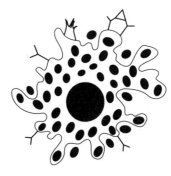

Resting
mast cell

Activated
mast cell

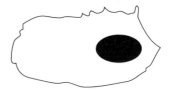

Resting
chondrocyte

Activated
chondrocyte

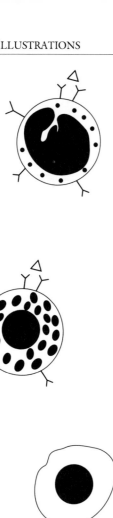

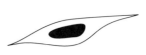

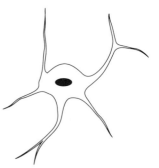

Fibroblast

Cartilage

Dendritic cell/
Langerhans cell

Arteriole

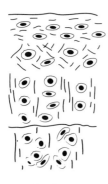

Venule

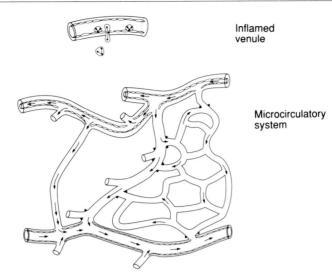

Inflamed
venule

Microcirculatory
system

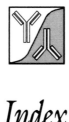

Index